Assessment and Treatment of Substance Use Disorders

Assessment and Treatment of Substance Use Disorders

Edited by Esther Brock

AMERICAN
MEDICAL PUBLISHERS
www.americanmedicalpublishers.com

American Medical Publishers,
41 Flatbush Avenue,
1st Floor, New York,
NY 11217, USA

Visit us on the World Wide Web at:
www.americanmedicalpublishers.com

ISBN: 978-1-63927-089-7

Cataloging-in-Publication Data

Assessment and treatment of substance use disorders / edited by Esther Brock.
p. cm.
Includes bibliographical references and index.
ISBN 978-1-63927-089-7
1. Substance abuse. 2. Substance abuse--Diagnosis. 3. Substance abuse--Treatment. I. Brock, Esther.
RC564 .A77 2022
616.86--dc23

Table of Contents

Preface

Substance use disorder refers to the condition of using one or more substances which cause impairment or distress. It is also known as drug use disorder. These substances include alcohol, caffeine, cannabis, hallucinogens, such as inhalants, opioids, sedatives, hypnotics, stimulants, tobacco, etc. Some of the mental, behavioral and physical symptoms of the disorder are loss of control, strain in life, tremors, sweating, etc. The treatment and management of this type of disorder cane be done through three major ways - detoxification, drug rehabilitation therapy and medication assisted treatment. The topics covered in this extensive book deal with the core subjects of substance use disorders. This book brings forth some of the unexplored concepts related to the assessment and treatment of substance use disorders. Coherent flow of topics, student-friendly language and extensive use of examples make this book an invaluable source of knowledge.

This book has been the outcome of endless efforts put in by authors and researchers on various issues and topics within the field. The book is a comprehensive collection of significant researches that are addressed in a variety of chapters. It will surely enhance the knowledge of the field among readers across the globe.

It gives us an immense pleasure to thank our researchers and authors for their efforts to submit their piece of writing before the deadlines. Finally in the end, I would like to thank my family and colleagues who have been a great source of inspiration and support.

Editor

1

Cigarette Smoke Exposure during Pregnancy Alters Fetomaternal Cell Trafficking Leading to Retention of Microchimeric Cells in the Maternal Lung

Anja Vogelgesang[1,2], Cristina Scapin[1,5], Caroline Barone[1], Elaine Tam[4,6], Anna Blumental Perry[3,6], Christiane E. L. Dammann[1,4]*

1 Division of Newborn Medicine, Department of Pediatrics, Floating Hospital for Children at Tufts Medical Center, Boston, Massachusetts, United States of America, **2** Hanover Medical School, Hanover, Germany, **3** Department of Surgery, Tufts Medical Center, Boston, Massachusetts, United States of America, **4** Sackler School of Graduate Biomedical Sciences, Tufts University School of Medicine, Boston, Massachusetts, United States of America, **5** Genetic and Cellular Biology Division, Dibit. San Raffaele Scientific Institute, Milan, Italy, **6** Department of Biomedical Sciences, Mercer School of Medicine and Department of Laboratory Oncology Research, Anderson Cancer Institute, Memorial University Medical Center, Savannah, Georgia, United States of America

Abstract

Cigarette smoke exposure causes chronic oxidative lung damage. During pregnancy, fetal microchimeric cells traffic to the mother. Their numbers are increased at the site of acute injury. We hypothesized that milder chronic diffuse smoke injury would attract fetal cells to maternal lungs. We used a green-fluorescent-protein (GFP) mouse model to study the effects of cigarette smoke exposure on fetomaternal cell trafficking. Wild-type female mice were exposed to cigarette smoke for about 4 weeks and bred with homozygote GFP males. Cigarette smoke exposure continued until lungs were harvested and analyzed. Exposure to cigarette smoke led to macrophage accumulation in the maternal lung and significantly lower fetal weights. Cigarette smoke exposure influenced fetomaternal cell trafficking. It was associated with retention of GFP-positive fetal cells in the maternal lung and a significant reduction of fetal cells in maternal livers at gestational day 18, when fetomaternal cell trafficking peaks in the mouse model. Cells quickly clear postpartum, leaving only a few, difficult to detect, persisting microchimeric cells behind. In our study, we confirmed the postpartum clearance of cells in the maternal lungs, with no significant difference in both groups. We conclude that in the mouse model, cigarette smoke exposure during pregnancy leads to a retention of fetal microchimeric cells in the maternal lung, the site of injury. Further studies will be needed to elucidate the effect of cigarette smoke exposure on the phenotypic characteristics and function of these fetal microchimeric cells, and confirm its course in cigarette smoke exposure in humans.

Editor: Colette Kanellopoulos-Langevin, Xavier Bichat Medical School, INSERM-CNRS - Université Paris Diderot, France

Funding: Supported by grants from the National Heart, Lung, and Blood Institute (HL-085648)(CD), ATS and FAMRI research awards (ABP), Konrad-Adenauer-Foundation scholarship (AV), and R25 HL007785 (Building Diversity in Biomedical Sciences Program) (ET). The funders had no role in study design, data collection and analysis, decision to publish, or preparation of the manuscript.

Competing Interests: The authors have declared that no competing interests exist.

* E-mail: cdammann@tuftsmedicalcenter.org

These authors contributed equally to this work.

Introduction

Each year, more than 443,000 Americans die of tobacco-related illnesses such as chronic obstructive pulmonary disease (COPD) and lung cancer [1]. These illnesses cause more deaths in women than breast cancer does. Smoking during pregnancy is still a widespread problem. About 14% of women in the United States state that they are smoking during pregnancy [2]. Cigarette smoke (CS) exposure causes oxidative damage to lung tissue and an impairment of the capacity of alveolar macrophages to clear bacteria and apoptotic cells [3], contributing to chronic lung injury in smoking mothers. CS exposure during pregnancy is associated with preterm delivery, low birth weight, and an increased morbidity in the newborn [4]. Animal studies have shown that fetal nicotine exposure may affect the development of the lungs and multiple other organs, and cause long-lasting effects on body adiposity and endocrine function [5].

During pregnancy, fetal cells enter the maternal circulation and are detected as microchimeric cells [6]. Some of these cells persist through one's life [7], but their distribution, impact on maternal health, and preferred organ of residence is not clearly understood. Their presence might be acutely beneficial for the repair of damaged tissue due to their potential stem cell-like properties, but they might also contribute to the development of autoimmune diseases and cancer in women after a certain number of years [8]. In the mouse models, it has been shown that fetal chimeric cells are found in the maternal circulation peaking towards the end of pregnancy. Most of these microchimeric cells are cleared around postpartum day (PD)5–6. The highest number of these cells has been found in the maternal lungs, their likely port of entry [9]. The chimeric cells represent a mixed population of cells, some with stem cell-like properties, and some with more differentiated characteristics [10]. It has been shown that fetal chimeric cells are attracted to the site of severe acute injury [11] and that overall cell trafficking is promoted during loss of pregnancy [12]. The intensity of microchimeric cell trafficking is influenced by the genetic background [13], but both the intensity and the distribution of microchimeric cells in milder chronic, more diffuse injury settings is unclear.

We hypothesized that chronic CS exposure during pregnancy affects trafficking, attraction, and distribution of fetal chimeric cells. Here we present the effects of a mild chronic diffuse lung injury on fetomaternal cell trafficking using a green-fluorescent-protein (GFP) mouse model.

Materials and Methods

Mice and cigarette smoke experiments

All animal use was approved by the Institutional Animal Care and Use Committee of Tufts University and Tufts Medical Center (Assurance number: A3775-01). Female wild-type (wt) C57BL/6 mice were obtained from Jackson Laboratories (Bar Harbor, ME, USA); male homozygous C57BL/6-Tg (CAG-EGFP) C14-Y01-FM131Osb Mice were from Riken BioResource Center (Ibaraki, Japan). Eight-week-old female mice were exposed to CS (1R5F research cigarettes, Tobacco and Health Research Institute, University of Kentucky, Lexington, KY, USA) using a standard smoking machine, as previously published [14]. Intake was slowly increased to an exposure of four cigarettes per day for five days per week for approximately 15–46 days (33 days in average) prior to successful mating. CS-exposed wt mice were mated with homozygous GFP-positive C57BL/6 males to generate GFP-heterozygous fetuses. CS exposure was continued until mice were sacrificed (Figure 1). Non smoke-exposed control animals were mated similarly and used as controls. Pregnant mice as well as non-pregnant control mice (smokers and non-smokers) were anesthetized with ketamine (10 mg/ml) on gestational day (GD)18 of pregnancy or postpartum (postnatal day (PD)4–6, or 6 month after pregnancy). Lungs were perfused free of blood from the right ventricle with 10 mL ice-cold phosphate buffered saline. The trachea was exposed and the left lung was ligated, cut off, frozen on dry ice, and stored at −80°C for DNA isolation. The remaining right lung was either injected intra-tracheally with 2 ml of dispase (undiluted liquid; BD, Bedford, MA, USA, cat no: 354235) and 1% low-melt agarose (Bio-Rad, Hercules, CA, USA, cat no: 161–3111) for fluorescent activated cell sorting (FACS) analysis or inflated with 10% neutral buffered formalin at a constant pressure of 25 cm H_2O for 10 minutes. After inflation, the trachea was ligated and the inflated lungs were removed, fixed in formalin for 24 hours, parted in lobes, and transferred into phosphate buffered saline for later paraffin embedding and cutting. Livers were frozen at -80°C for DNA analysis.

Mac3 immunohistochemistry staining

To identify alveolar macrophages, lung sections were stained with macrophage specific Mac3. Sections were melted and washed with xylene and ethanol. Antigen retrieval was performed in a steamer with Target Retrieval Solution (Dako, Carpinteria, CA, USA, cat no: S1699) for 30 minutes. Slides were blocked with Peroxidase Blocking Reagent (Dako, cat no: S2001) and 5% goat serum, followed by incubation in Avidin/Biotin Block (Vector, Burlingame, CA, USA, cat no: SP-2001) for 15 minutes each. Staining with Mac3 antibody (rat anti-mouse Mac3 antibody; BD Pharmingen, San Diego, CA, USA, cat no: 550292) was performed overnight at 4°C. After staining with the biotin-conjugated goat anti-rat IgG (Vector, cat-no: BA-4000) for 2 hours at 4°C, an additional peroxidase blocking was performed with 3% H_2O_2 in MeOH for 10 minutes, which was followed by incubation with ABC reagent (Vector, cat no: PK-6100) for 30 minutes. Sections were incubated in diaminobenzidine solution (DAB Peroxidase Substrate Kit, 3,3′- diaminobenzidine; Vector, cat no: SK-4100) until desired stain intensity developed. They were then rinsed in tap water, counterstained with hematoxylin (Mayer's Hematoxylin; Rowley Biochemical, Danvers, MA, USA, cat no: L-756-1A), rinsed, dehydrated in ascending series of ethanol, and finally mounted in Cytoseal (Cytoseal-60; Fisher Scientific, Ottawa, ON, USA, cat no: 23-244-257). Macrophages were counted and numbers normalized per mm lung tissue using lung morphometry as described in Shapiro et al [15]. Airspace was quantified by average Chord Length measurements obtained using a previously published, automated image processing algorithm, and Scion image processing software (National Institutes of Health). The software program automatically created a binary black and white image by separating original images into tissue and airspace after large airways, blood vessels, and other nonalveolar structures were manually removed from the images. Pre-drawn horizontal and vertical grids of one pixel width were laid over the individual image. Lines ending on or intercepting with alveolar tissue were counted by analyzing the number of pixels in every object. The image only included lines of one pixel width so that this measurement served as a length. According to methods adapted from Dunhill, this number was used to calculate the average Chord Length [16]. The amount of macrophages was normalized to millimeter of alveolar wall using the following formula:

$$I = 0.3925/CL \cdot 10^3$$

CL: Chord Length (mean value given by Excel during morphometry)

I: Amount of macrophages per mm lung tissue

(10^3 because CL is in µm and I is in mm).

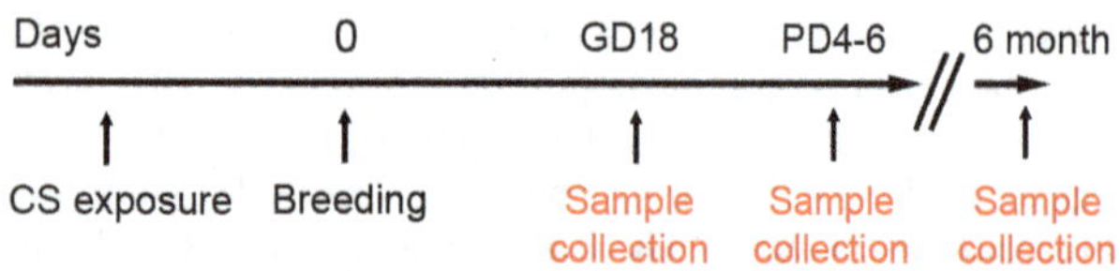

Figure 1. Cigarette smoke exposure model. Cigarette smoke exposure model: After approximately 4 weeks of CS exposure, wild-type female mice were bred with GFP-homozygous males to generate GFP heterozygous fetuses. Pregnant and non-pregnant control females continued to smoke and were sacrificed at gestational day (GD)18, at postpartum day (PD)4–6 and after 6 month. Maternal lungs and livers (GD 18 only) were analyzed for the presence of inflammation and GFP-positive cells.

GFP immunohistochemistry staining

Immunostaining with GFP antibodies was performed in frozen lung sections. The primary antibody has successfully been used for GFP detection before [17]. The procedure and reagents were similar to the immunostaining of macrophages with the following exceptions: After fixation of frozen sections in pre-cooled acetone, antigen retrieval was performed for 10 minutes. The primary antibody (rabbit anti-GFP IgG; Invitrogen, Grand Island, NY, USA, cat no: A11122) was incubated for 1 hour at 37°C, followed by staining with the biotinylated goat anti-rabbit antibody for 30 minutes at 37°C. During incubation with diaminobenzidine, the desired diaminobenzidine intensity was checked under the microscope using the lung section of a GFP-positive animal.

GFP immunofluorescence

After fixation in pre-cooled acetone, nuclear staining was performed with Hoechst (Bisbenzamide; Sigma-Aldrich, St. Louis, MO, USA, cat no: B2883) for 30 seconds and slides were mounted. Cryostat sections of mice at GD18 and non-pregnant controls were evaluated for GFP-positive cells with a confocal laser scanning microscope (TCS SP2, Leica).

Flow cytometry of GFP-labeled cells

To evaluate the number of fetal cells entering the maternal lungs during pregnancy, the number of GFP-positive cells was analyzed in maternal lung tissue. Right lungs were removed, minced, and incubated in dispase/collagenase (final concentration: 2 mg/ml; Roche Applied Sciences, Indianapolis, IN, USA, cat no: 10269638001) in PBS for 45 minutes at 37°C. 0.025 mg/ml DNase (Sigma-Aldrich, St. Louis, MO, USA, cat no: D4527) was added for 4 minutes on ice and digested tissue was filtered through 100 μm and 40 μm filters. Cells were resuspended in 3% paraformaldehyde, fixed for 20 minutes at 4°C, and analyzed in 10% fetal bovine serum in phosphate buffered saline by FACS using a Cytomation MoFlo (Beckman Coulter, Indianapolis, IN, USA). Data of the whole cell suspension were collected and analyzed for GFP-fluorescence based on FL1 (Argon laser for excitation at 488 nm). Data were analyzed with Cytomation Summit software (Cytomation, Fort Collins, CO, USA). Gating was performed according to the controls. Lungs of virgin wild-type female C57BL/6 mice were used as negative controls and lungs of non-exposed GFP-positive pups (GD18) were used as GFP-positive controls. Data were presented as total number of GFP-positive cells per right lung.

Quantitative real-time PCR (qPCR)

Genomic DNA was extracted using the Qiagen DNeasy Blood and Tissue kit (Qiagen, Valencia, CA, USA, cat-no: 69504) following the manufacturer's instructions. DNA elution was performed twice using 100 μl H20 followed by 100 μl AE buffer. The DNA yield was quantified with a spectrometer and DNA stored at 4°C until further analysis. 600 ng DNA was loaded per well for GFP and 100 ng for Apolipoprotein B (ApoB) analysis in a total volume of 50 μl, as previously published [18]. Pan et al have shown that in a titration curve using GFP-concentrations of 100% to 0.001% in a total of 1000 ng DNA the Threshold Cycle Number (Ct) for ApoB remained constant, while the Ct for GFP showed an appropriate decrease in the concentration of GFP. When loading serial dilutions (from 1:1 to 1:100,000) of GFP-positive DNA with one GFP copy per cell, the Delta of the Threshold Cycle Number (DCt) remained constant, which indicates that the PCR efficiency for GFP and ApoB is similar. These authors finally used 1000 ng of DNA for all further experiments compared, while we have, similar to Fujiki *et al*, used 600 ng [9]. Each sample was loaded in triplicates. PCR-Primers and FAM labeled probes were designed and synthesized by Applied Biosystems (Carlsbad, CA, USA). The following primers and probe sequences were used for GFP: Forward primer: 5′ - TGCTGCTGCCCGACAA-3′, reverse primer: 5′ - TGTGATCGCGCTTCTCGTT-3′, Taqman probe: 5′ - FAM-CCACTACCTGAGCACCC-3′ [11]. Apolipoprotein B (ApoB) was used as an internal control to measure the total content of DNA. Forward primer: 5′-CGTGGGCTCCAGCATTCTA-3′, reverse primer: 5′-TCACCAGTCATTTCTGCCTTTG-3′, Taqman probe: 5′-FAM-CCTTGAGCAGTGCCCGAC-CATTC-TAMRA-3′ [19]. Real-Time qPCR analysis was performed using the Applied Biosystems, 7900 HT FAST Real-Time PCR system and SDS2.2.2 software for analysis. Thermal profile: First cycle: 2 minutes at 50°C, 10 minutes at 95°C, 40 cycles: 15 seconds at 95°C, and 1 minute at 60°C. Each threshold cycle number was determined as the first cycle at which a threshold value in fluorescence signal was reached. Single difference in threshold cycle (DCt) values were calculated for GFP by subtracting the Ct of ApoB from the cycle of GFP. Each sample was loaded as triplicates so that averages of Ct values were used. DDCt values of CS-exposed samples were determined by subtracting the mean of the DCt of the controls of that specific PCR run from the mean of the CS-exposed sample's DCt. The DDCt value expresses the difference of the content of GFP in CS-exposed samples compared to controls. A negative value indicates a smaller DCt, which means that the threshold of the GFP fluorescent signal is reached in an earlier cycle assuming a constant ApoB signal. To better understand if the increased number of GFP positive cells found in maternal lungs were a result of an overall increase in trafficking of microchimeric cells or a redistribution of trafficking fetal cells towards the injured maternal lung, we also performed additional qPCR of maternal livers at GD18. DNA of liver tissue was isolated and processed similarly to lung samples.

Statistics

For the statistical analysis, unpaired two-tailed or one-tailed t-tests were used where appropriate. All data were presented as mean ± standard error of the mean (SEM) unless otherwise stated.

Results

Validation of CS exposure model in pregnant mice

A) CS exposure results in inflammation of and an increased number of macrophages in maternal lungs. It has been shown that inhalation of CS leads to cell injury, cell death, and inflammation with recruitment of neutrophils, macrophages, and T cells. Inhalation of CS also results in impaired activity of inflammatory cells, leading to slow, progressive lung destruction [14]. In mouse models of CS exposure, macrophage accumulation can be detected as early as 4 weeks. We evaluated macrophage recruitment in parasagittal lung sections obtained from smoker and control animals about 6 weeks after starting the CS exposure, using immunohistochemistry staining for Mac3, an antigen expressed in macrophages (Figure 2A). The number of Mac3-positive cells was calculated per mm of the alveolar wall using a published morphometric analysis[14]. CS exposure resulted in a significant increase in the number of macrophages in the lungs independent of pregnancy (Figure 2B). Mean number of macrophages per mm of alveolar wall was 15±1.09 in non-pregnant smokers (n = 3) and 16±0.16 in pregnant smokers (n = 2). In lungs of non CS-exposed mice, the mean number of macrophages was 9±0.29 in non-pregnant (n = 4) and 10±0.74 in pregnant (n = 3) mice. The increase of macrophages in smokers compared to non-smokers was statistically significant for both groups non-pregnant and pregnant (non-pregnant smokers versus non-pregnant non-smokers: p = 0.0284, pregnant smokers versus pregnant non-smokers: p = 0.0187). Again, there were no further differences in the macrophage numbers between pregnant and non-pregnant smokers (non-pregnant versus pregnant non-smokers: p = 0.1994, non-pregnant versus pregnant smokers: p = 0.3866) indicating that the duration of CS exposure or of the presence of fetal microchimeric cells was too short to see a significant impact on macrophage numbers. In summary, our results confirm that our CS exposure injury model produced an inflammation in lungs of smokers.

B) CS exposure leads to lower weight in newborn mice. CS exposure is known to affect weight of humans and

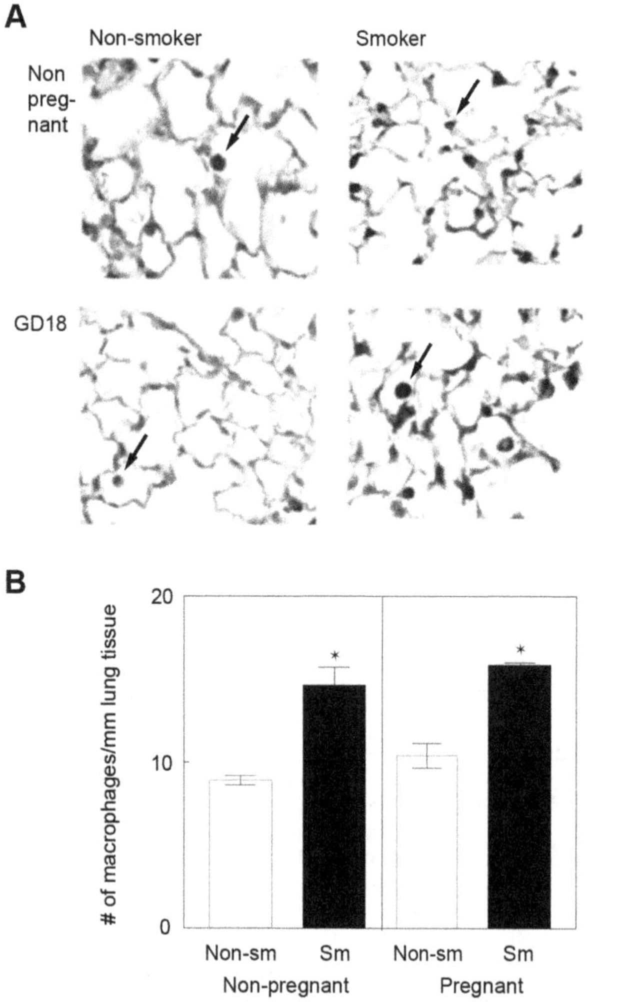

Figure 2. CS exposure increases macrophages in maternal lungs. (A): Immunohistochemical staining in non-pregnant (upper panel) non-smoking (left) and smoking females (right) and in gestational day (GD) 18 pregnant (lower panel) non-smoking (left) and smoking (right) females. Original magnification is 200×. Arrows point to alveolar macrophages. (B): For quantification, macrophages were counted and normalized per mm lung tissue. CS-exposed samples were compared to non-exposed controls (*$p<0.05$, mean ± SEM, n = 2–4).

mice [20,21,22]. In our model, a short 3-week CS exposure prior to breeding resulted in a modest 2.6% decrease in weight of smoking mice (18.53±0.22 g, n = 31) compared to non-smoking mice (19.01±0.25 g, n = 19, p = 0.1497). The absence of a statistical significance might be explained by the short duration of CS exposure, leading only to a trend in weight decrease (Figure 3A). Importantly, intrauterine CS exposure led to a significantly lower weight in newborns (1.16 g±0.01 g, n = 49) when compared to the non-exposed littermates (1.29 g±0.01 g, n = 81, p<0.0001) (Figure 3B). Furthermore, we observed that the rate of pregnancies after overnight mating was decreased in CS-exposed mice (17.39%, n = 46) compared to non-exposed controls (23.81%, n = 42). A high number of CS-exposed offspring died (17 out of 63), while none of the non CS-exposed offspring died (total of 106). There was no difference in the number of pups per litter between the CS-exposed litter (mean 7.87, n = 15) and control litter (mean 7.88, n = 24).

CS exposure during pregnancy leads to a retention of trafficking fetal cells in the maternal lungs at GD18

In order to compare the pulmonary retention of fetal cells in non-smoking mothers to smoking mothers, we analyzed the maternal lungs at gestational day (GD)18, when the number of fetal cells in maternal organs is known to be highest [9]. At GD18, fetal chimeric cells were detected in maternal lungs of smokers and non-smokers by immunohistochemical staining, as well as by fluorescence analyses using a confocal microscope (Figure 4A). The fetal GFP-positive cells were easily distinguishable from autofluorescent macrophages in slides of CS-exposed lungs, due to their uninterrupted bright fluorescence in contrast to the irregular fluorescence in the granules of macrophages. The very low number of fetal cells per test field made quantification via this method impossible. We therefore performed FACS analysis in the right side of the maternal lung. A total of 8 to 18 million cells (mean number 12 million cells) were obtained by digesting the right lung into a single cell suspension, which was used for analysis. Quantitative analysis by FACS showed that the number of fetal cells at GD18 was increased in CS-exposed lungs (834±112, n = 5) compared to non-exposed control lungs (633±68, n = 4, p = 0.1756) (Figure 4B). This difference did not reach statistical significance. The actual number of GFP positive cells, identified by FACS, might be slightly underestimated due to their preferred presence on the outskirts of the gate for GFP positivity. Populations of GFP positive cells were seen at the outskirt of the gate, making it difficult to define a clear cut-off between positive and negative cells (Figure 4C). This is a known phenomenon previously reported by others [9]. Since FACS and qPCR analysis are the most common sensitive methods to detect microchimeric cells [23,24], we confirmed our FACS results with qPCR analyses. qPCR revealed a statistically significant increase in GFP-positive DNA and therefore a negative DDCt value of −1.41±0.71 (n = 7) in CS-exposed maternal lungs when compared to non-exposed lungs (n = 7, p = 0.0469) (Figure 4D). We therefore concluded that CS exposure results in an increased retention of fetal cells in the maternal lungs.

CS exposure leads to lower numbers of fetal cells in maternal livers at GD18

Intrauterine blood flow directs fetal cells to enter the maternal circulation through the maternal pulmonary arteries, leading to a presumed higher frequency of fetal cells in the maternal lung [9]. Fetal cells travelling to the mother pass through the lungs before reaching other organs [9,25]. CS injures the lung and increases the retention of microchimeric cells. In order to verify if this phenomenon is due to an increased trafficking or redistribution of microchimeric cells, we analyzed the maternal liver for the number of chimeric cells. We used the more quantitative approach with qPCR analyses. CS exposure led to a significant decrease of GFP-positive DNA (DDCt = 2.17±0.40, n = 6) in the maternal liver at GD18 compared to livers from non CS-exposed control mice (n = 3, p = 0.0028) (Figure 4D). Therefore, we concluded that CS exposure alters the distribution of fetal cells, with a decrease of fetal cells in the maternal liver and their retention in the maternal lungs, which is the site of injury and inflammation.

CS exposure does not change the postpartum clearance of fetal cells from maternal lungs

To analyze the effect of CS exposure on the clearance rate of fetal cells from the maternal lungs, we studied the presence of fetal cells at postpartum days (PD) 4–6. It is known that most microchimeric cells are cleared at this time point making them

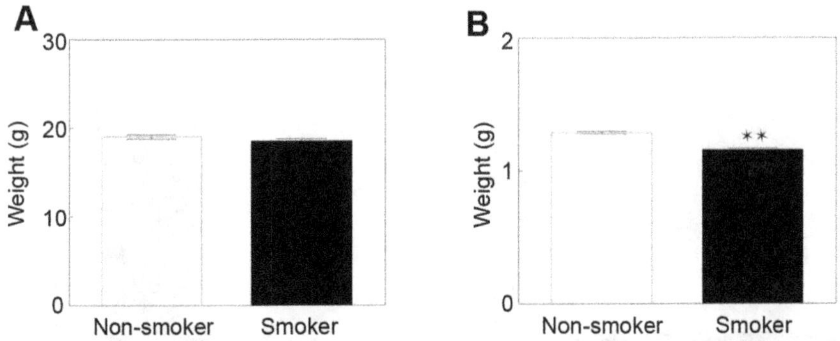

Figure 3. CS exposure decreases weights in the offspring. (A): CS exposure did not reduce weight of adult virgin mice (mean ± SEM, n = 19–31). (B): CS exposure significantly reduced weights of offspring at birth (**p<0.0001, mean ± SEM, n = 49–81).

almost non-detectable [9]. FACS analysis was performed on 5 million to 26 million cells (mean number 12 million cells). CS did not significantly change the clearance of fetal cells, although there may be a trend towards a faster clearance in lungs of smokers (4.5±1.23, n = 6) compared to non-smokers (6.83±2.02, n = 6, p = 0.3535) (Figure 5A). These FACS results were again confirmed by qPCR analyses. The trend towards faster clearance in CS-exposed lungs (DDCt = 0.79±0.59, n = 5, p = 0.2548), when compared to non CS-exposed control lungs (n = 10) was confirmed by qPCR (Figure 5B); however, neither result reached statistical significance. This might be due to the overall low number of fetal cells at PD4-6 in syngeneic strains (1–10 cells in smokers and 4–15 cells for non-smokers). Indeed, it has been shown that fetal cell trafficking is higher and fetal cells persist longer in mice of allogeneic crossing [26]. In allogeneic crossings of C57BL/6 with transgenic mixed genetic background mice, we found about 90,000 cells on PD6 in the maternal lungs of non-smokers, while less than half that number existed in the CS-exposed lungs (own unpublished data).

In humans, fetal cells have been found in the lungs even 27 years after pregnancy [7]. Therefore, we tested whether GFP-positive cells can be detected long after pregnancy in lungs of mice exposed to CS. Lungs of mice exposed to CS starting one month before pregnancy and ending 6 months after were harvested and analyzed for the presence of GFP-positive cells by FACS analysis, compared to their non-smoking pregnant controls. 8 to 11 million cells (mean number 10 million cells) were counted by MoFlo software as described in Material and Methods. We were unable to detect any GFP-positive cells (n = 4) independent of exposure to CS. We concluded that there is no preferential significant long-term retention of fetal cells in the lungs of syngeneic crossbred mice.

Discussion

Fetomaternal cell trafficking has been demonstrated in healthy mice [9] and human pregnancies [7]. In mice, it has been demonstrated that trafficking and distribution of fetal cells can be influenced by acute localized injury, attracting fetal cells to the site of injury [11,27]. It is not known if injury leads to an overall increase in cell trafficking or altered retention of chimeric fetal cells in the injured maternal organs. Very limited information is available on the effects of chronic, relatively mild diffuse injury on fetomaternal cell trafficking. In this study, we used maternal CS exposure, a mild, slowly-progressing diffuse inflammatory injury to the lung, to study its effect on fetomaternal trafficking. First, we validated our CS exposure animal model and confirmed that CS exposure induced lung inflammation as previously seen [3]. The presence of almost double the amount of macrophages in the lungs of smokers compared to non-smokers is indicative of both inflammatory and possible reparative responses triggered by CS exposure. There was no difference in cell number between non-pregnant and pregnant smokers, indicating that pregnancy-induced changes including the presence of microcimeric cells do not affect this inflammatory response after short-term CS exposure. The role of macrophages in CS-induced damage is a focus of vigorous investigation, as these cells secrete numerous proteases that eventually add to CS-induced tissue destruction later in the course of injury. It is assumed that macrophages, which are recruited as M1-phenotypes pro-inflammatory cells in CS, are causing reprogramming of alveolar macrophages into partially M2-polarized macrophages with tissue remodeling properties [28]. But this develops much later in the course of exposure and we here focused our analysis on the days of the known peaks of intrauterine cell trafficking at GD18 and its quick postpartum clearance [9].

Secondly, we confirmed effects of CS exposure on the intrauterine environment, finding lower weights in the offspring of smoking mothers, also reported by others [29]. In addition to the lower weights, we observed a higher incidence of stillbirth in CS-exposed pregnancies. An association between maternal smoking during pregnancy and stillbirth has been shown before in human pregnancies [4].

CS exposure was associated with an increase in the number of fetal cells in the maternal lungs and a significant decrease of cells in the maternal livers at the known peak of naturally occurring microchimerism at GD18. It has been suggested that in mouse models of acute injuries, injury most likely attracts microchimeric cells by altered tissue attraction of exciting cells. Acute cardiac injury leads to selective retention of fetal cells to the maternal heart [30]. This was also shown in a brain injury model, where the overall number of fetal cells was not significantly increased, but cells were attracted to the site of injury [11]. The injury caused by CS develops slowly, is diffuse, and will lead to anatomic lung injury after years of exposure. We here present new insights on this mild chronic diffuse injury model being able to result in retention of microchimeric fetal cells at the site of injury. This is an important discovery, because mild chronic injuries are more common in life than focal acute injuries. The mild chronic injury we induced led only to a small but significant increase in the number of fetal cells in the maternal lung. This is in alignment with studies in humans [31] and mice [32,33] indicating that the presence of chimerism relates to the extent and degree of injury. Additionally, CS-exposed fetuses are significantly smaller than non-exposed controls, and smaller litter weight is known to result in a smaller

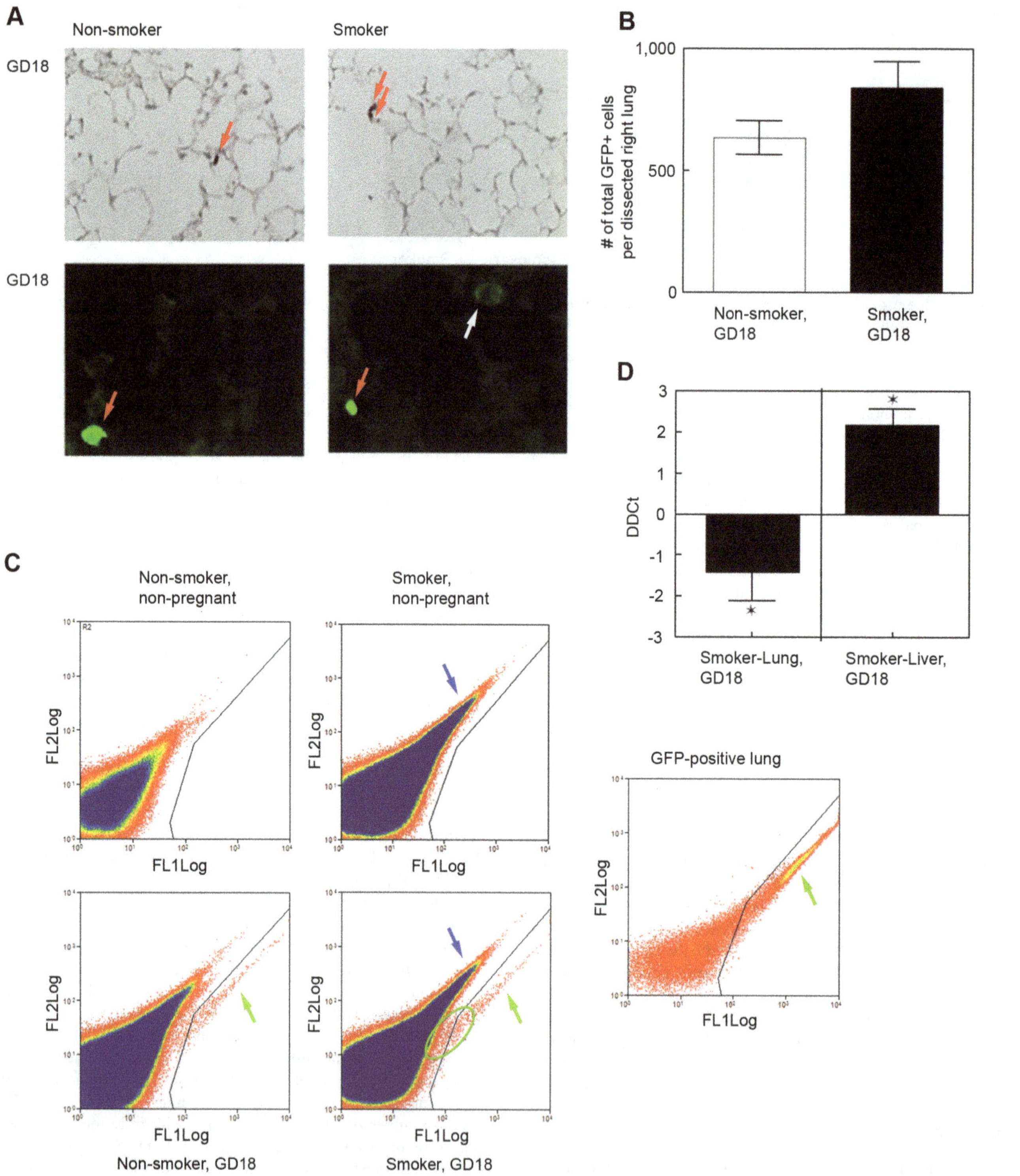

Figure 4. Analysis of fetomaternal trafficking on GD18. (A): Fetal GFP-positive cells were detectable by immunohistochemistry (IHC) (upper panel) and immunofluorescence (IF) (lower panel) at GD18 of pregnancy. For IHC sections primary rabbit anti-GFP IgG was used (magnification is 200×). IF pictures were taken with a confocal microscope. CS-exposed macrophages are known to acquire autofluorescence (white arrow), but they were clearly distinguishable from GFP-positive cells (red arrows). (B–D): GFP-positive cells were quantified by FACS analysis (B, C) and by qPCR analysis (D). (B): Quantification of GFP-positive cells in lungs of pregnant non-smokers and smokers by FACS. Bars represent mean ± SEM of total number of GFP-positive cells included in the gate per dissected right lung (mean ± SEM, n = 4–5). (C): Samples from non-pregnant mice were used as negative (upper graphs), and lungs of GFP-positive pups as positive controls for gating (graph in third column, green arrow points to GFP-positive cells). Samples of CS-exposed mice showed autofluorescent cells (right upper and lower graph, blue arrow), which were easily distinguishable from GFP-positive cells (green arrow). The area included in the ellipse contains potential GFP-positive cells outside of the GFP-positive gate. Those cells were not included in the calculation of the number of GFP-positive cells by FACS shown in B. (D): Quantification of GFP content in maternal lung (left) and liver (right) on GD18 of pregnancy by qPCR. Means of DCt values of non-exposed controls were compared to CS-exposed samples. Results are shown as DDCt values. (lung: *$p<0.05$ one-sided, mean ± SEM, n = 7) (liver: *$p<0.05$, mean ± SEM, n = 3–6).

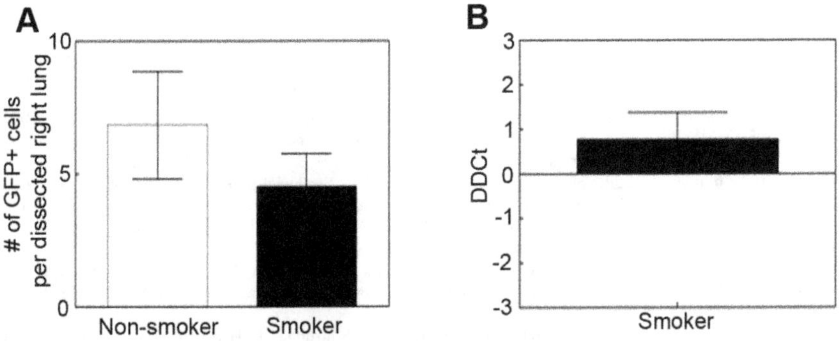

Figure 5. Analysis of postpartum clearance of fetal cells from the maternal lungs. Postpartum clearance of fetal cells is independent of CS measured at PD4–6 by FACS (A) and qPCR analyses (B). Samples were processed and analyzed similarly to GD18 (mean ± SEM, n = 6 (A), n = 5–10 (B)).

number of trafficking fetal cells [9,10]. Another reason for our small increase in the number of microchimeric cells detected in the maternal lung after CS exposure is the fact that some of these fetal cells might be damaged by CS exposure and might undergo apoptosis following removal by macrophages.

The clinical impact of retention of these fetal cells on an injured organ is not clear. Knowing that fetal microcimeric cells have potential stem cell like properties [34], one could assume that fetal cells can contribute to the repair processes. Indeed, in some cases the fetal progenitors cells have acquired tissue-specific characteristics after entering the maternal organism during pregnancy [34], emphasizing this assumption of their contribution in repair processes. At present, it is not clear if these cells are able to proliferate [35], differentiate [35,36,37], or fuse with organ-specific cells [37,38]. Recent publications have reported that fetal cells seem to differentiate into various cell types [34,39]. In human breast cancer, fetal cells were found in 9 out of 10 samples, whereas no cells where found in non-diseased control samples [40]. Similarly in human papillary thyroid cancer, 11 fetal cells per 1 million maternal cells were found in the diseased tissue, while only 2 cells per million were detected in non-affected tissue [41]. In autoimmune thyroiditis, human fetal cells were not only found in the diseased tissue [42], but also increased in the peripheral blood [43]. Despite the clear evidence of an increase of fetal microchimerism in affected tissue, the question of its function in the disease processes and its influence on maternal health is as yet unresolved.

Our finding of the short duration in the maternal lung after pregnancy, suggests that CS exposure might have negative adverse effects on survival, regeneration capacity, migratory ability, and the cytokines profiles of these chimeric cells, which has been reported before [3,44,45]. The trend towards a faster postpartum clearance of fetal cells from the smoker lungs supports this idea and may reflect a more rapid senescence of these cells in the setting of continuous CS exposure, as has been described for other stem cells in oxidative stress injury [46]. We did not detect fetal cells in the lungs of smokers 6 month after pregnancy. It may be that only a few fetal cells are retained in the lungs of smoking mothers and they are not detectable using our methods. We did not examine possible anti-GFP alloresponse that might be triggered by the mobilization of macrophages and the known T cell immunogenicity of GFP, resulting in a clearance of these GFP cells.

The impact of CS on health is well known. The impact of the retention of fetal cells in the maternal lung and the observation of fewer cells in the maternal liver are very intriguing findings, but its impact is not clear. It can be explained by a few non-exclusive possibilities. First, CS exposure could cause retention of fetal cells at the site of injury as an inconsequential response to tissue damage, decreasing the pool of trafficking cells to other organs. Second, CS exposure may result in altered capacity for movement and retention of damaged fetal cells, keeping them in the lungs, the port of entry. A third possibility is that CS-injured alveolar macrophages cannot remove them. Fourth, CS exposure may affect the ability of fetal cells to migrate efficiently to other organs. Indeed, it has been demonstrated that CS exposure affects the Rho and Rac GTPase balance, which is crucial for efficient cell movements [3,47]. And fifth, fetal chimeric cells might have originated from the placenta [30,48]. Considering the effects of maternal CS exposure on placental blood flow and the trophoblasts itself in humans [4], it could be most likely that these fetal cells entering the maternal organism are already affected in their biology, specifically their potential for movement.

A weakness of our study is that we have not been able to study the biology and function of these microchimeric cells or the effects of a longer duration of CS exposure on trafficking. However, to our knowledge, this study is the first to analyze CS exposure in combination with analysis of fetomaternal trafficking. Our research focused on the maternal lung tissue; CS might influence trafficking to other organs. Since the highest median number of chimeric cells have been found in the lungs, liver, and spleen [9], and these numbers are already at the border of detection by FACS and qPCR analyses, analysis of other organs seems almost impossible and even more challenging. In summary we here demonstrate that CS exposure during pregnancy alters fetomaternal trafficking, leading to retention of fetal cells in the maternal lung and a concomitant decrease in the maternal liver. It can be assumed that this model of a chronic, very common lung injury is comparable to other chronic mild injuries in pregnancy, like inflammation due to chorioamnionitis.

Acknowledgments

We would like to thank Diana Bianchi and Kirby Johnson for providing homozygous GFP-positive males and for their help with qPCR analyses. We are grateful to Allen Parmalee for assistance with FACS and Carine Tarazi for proofreading the manuscript. In addition we would like to thank Frauke-Gesche Gerdts for her help smoking the animals and Cristina Scapin for all her technical support and involvement with the allogeneic cross breeding.

Author Contributions

Conceived and designed the experiments: ABP CD CS. Performed the experiments: AC CS CB ET. Analyzed the data: AV CS CB ET. Contributed reagents/materials/analysis tools: ABP CD. Wrote the paper: AV ABP CD.

References

1. CDC (2010) CDC grand rounds: current opportunities in tobacco control. MMWR Morb Mortal Wkly Rep 59: 487–492.
2. Tong VT, Jones JR, Dietz PM, D'Angelo D, Bombard JM (2005) Trends in smoking before, during, and after pregnancy - pregnancy risk assessment monitoring system (PRAMS), United States, 31 sites, 2000–2005. MMWR Morb Mortal Wkly Rep 58: 1–29.
3. Minematsu N, Blumental-Perry A, Shapiro SD (2010) Cigarette smoke inhibits engulfment of apoptotic cells by macrophages through inhibition of actin rearrangement. Am J Respir Cell Mol Biol 44: 474–482.
4. Rogers JM (2009) Tobacco and pregnancy. Reprod Toxicol 28: 152–160.
5. Oliveira E, Moura EG, Santos-Silva AP, Fagundes ATS, Rios AS, et al. (2009) Short- and long-term effects of maternal nicotine exposure during lactation on body adiposity, lipid profile, and thyroid function of rat offspring. J Endocrinol 202: 397–405.
6. Gammill HS, Nelson JL (2010) Naturally acquired microchimerism. Int J Dev Biol 54: 531–543.
7. Bianchi DW, Zickwolf GK, Weil GJ, Sylvester S, DeMaria MA (1996) Male fetal progenitor cells persist in maternal blood for as long as 27 years postpartum. PNAS 93: 705–708.
8. Nelson JL, Furst DE, Maloney S, Gooley T, Evans PC, et al. (1998) Microchimerism and HLA-compatible relationships of pregnancy in scleroderma. Lancet 351: 559–562.
9. Fujiki Y, Johnson KL, Tighiouart H, Peter I, Bianchi DW (2008) Fetomaternal trafficking in the mouse increases as delivery approaches and is highest in the maternal lung. Biol Reprod 79: 841–848.
10. Fujiki Y, Johnson KL, Peter I, Tighiouart H, Bianchi DW (2009) Fetal cells in the pregnant mouse are diverse and express a variety of progenitor and differentiated cell markers. Biol Reprod 81: 26–32.
11. Tan X-W, Liao H, Sun L, Okabe M, Xiao Z-C, et al. (2005) Fetal microchimerism in the maternal mouse brain: A novel population of fetal progenitor or stem cells able to cross the blood–brain barrier? Stem Cells 23: 1443–1452.
12. Johnson KL, Tao K, Stroh H, Kallenbach LR, Peter I, et al. (2010) Increased fetal cell trafficking in murine lung following complete pregnancy loss from exposure to lipopolysaccharide. Fertil Steril 93: 1718–1721.
13. Kallenbach LR, Bianchi DW, Peter I, Stroh H, Johnson KL (2011) Maternal background strain influences fetal–maternal trafficking more than maternal immune competence in mice. J Reprod Immunol 90: 188–194.
14. Hautamaki RD, Kobayashi DK, Senior RM, Shapiro SD (1997) Requirement for macrophage elastase for cigarette smoke–induced emphysema in mice. Science 277: 2002–2004.
15. Shapiro SD, Goldstein NM, Houghton AM, Kobayashi DK, Kelley D, et al. (2003) Neutrophil elastase contributes to cigarette smoke-induced emphysema in mice. Am J Pathol 163: 2329–2335.
16. Dunhill MS (1962) Quantitative methods in the study of pulmonary pathology. Thorax 17: 320–328.
17. Swenson ES, Price JG, Brazelton T, Krause DS (2007) Limitations of green fluorescent protein as a cell lineage marker. Stem Cells 25: 2593–2600.
18. Pan D (2002) Biodistribution and toxicity studies of VSVG-pseudotyped lentiviral vector after intravenous administration in mice with the observation of in vivo transduction of bone marrow. Mol Ther 6: 19–29.
19. Khosrotehrani K (2004) Fetal cell-free DNA circulates in the plasma of pregnant mice: relevance for animal models of fetomaternal trafficking. Hum Reprod 19: 2460–2464.
20. Albanes D, Jones DY, Micozzi MS, Mattson ME (1987) Associations between smoking and body weight in the US population- analysis of NHANES. Am J Public Health 77: 439–444.
21. Chen H, Vlahos R, Bozinovski S, Jones J, Anderson GP, et al. (2005) Effect of short-term cigarette smoke exposure on body weight, appetite and brain neuropeptide Y in mice. Neuropsychopharmacology 30: 713–719.
22. Chen H, Hansen MJ, Jones JE, Vlahos R, Anderson GP, et al. (2008) Long-term cigarette smoke exposure increases uncoupling protein expression but reduces energy intake. Brain Res 1228: 81–88.
23. Gammill HS, Adams Waldorf KM, Aydelotte TM, Lucas J, Leisenring WM, et al. (2011) Pregnancy, microchimerism, and the maternal grandmother. PLoS ONE 6: e24101.
24. Drabbels JJM, van de Keur C, Kemps BM, Mulder A, Scherjon SA, et al. (2011) HLA-targeted flow cytometric sorting of blood cells allows separation of pure and viable microchimeric cell populations. Blood 118: 149–155.
25. Rosner M, Hengstschläger M (2013) Amniotic fluid stem cells and fetal cell microchimerism. Trends Mol Med 19: 271–272.
26. Vernochet C, Caucheteux SM, Kanellopoulos-Langevin C (2007) Bi-directional cell trafficking between mother and fetus in mouse placenta. Placenta 28: 639–649.
27. Nguyen Huu S, Oster M, Uzan S, Chareyre F, Aractingi S, et al. (2007) Maternal neoangiogenesis during pregnancy partly derives from fetal endothelial progenitor cells. Proc Natl Acad Sci U S A 104: 1871–1876.
28. Shaykhiev R, Krause A, Salit J, Strulovici-Barel Y, Harvey BG, et al. (2009) Smoking-dependent reprogramming of alveolar macrophage polarization: implication for pathogenesis of chronic obstructive pulmonary disease. J Immunol 183: 2867–2883.
29. Esposito ER, Horn KH, Greene RM, Pisano MM (2008) An animal model of cigarette smoke-induced in utero growth retardation. Toxicology 246(2–3): 193–202.
30. Kara RJ, Bolli P, Karakikes I, Matsunaga I, Tripodi J, et al. (2012) Fetal cells traffic to injured maternal myocardium and undergo cardiac differentiation. Circ Res 110: 82–93.
31. Kleeberger W, Versmold A, Rothämel T, Glöckner S, Bredt M, et al. (2003) Increased chimerism of bronchial and alveolar epithelium in human lung allografts undergoing chronic injury. Am J Pathol 162: 1487–1494.
32. Khosrotehrani K, Reyes RR, Johnson KL, Freeman RB, Salomon RN, et al. (2006) Fetal cells participate over time in the response to specific types of murine maternal hepatic injury. Hum Reprod 22: 654–661.
33. Nassar D, Droitcourt C, Mathieu-d'Argent E, Kim MJ, Khosrotehrani K, et al. (2012) Fetal progenitor cells naturally transferred through pregnancy participate in inflammation and angiogenesis during wound healing. FASEB J 26: 149–157.
34. Khosrotehrani K, Leduc Ml, Bachy Vr, Nguyen Huu S, Oster Ml, et al. (2008) Pregnancy allows the transfer and differentiation of fetal lymphoid progenitors into functional T and B cells in mothers. J Immunol 180: 889–897.
35. Watt FM (2000) Out of eden: stem cells and their niches. Science 287: 1427–1430.
36. Zengin E, Chalajour F, Gehling UM, Ito WD, Treede H, et al. (2006) Vascular wall resident progenitor cells: a source for postnatal vasculogenesis. Development 133: 1543–1551.
37. Spees JL, Whitney MJ, Sullivan DE, Lasky JA, Laboy M, et al. (2007) Bone marrow progenitor cells contribute to repair and remodeling of the lung and heart in a rat model of progressive pulmonary hypertension. FASEB J 22: 1226–1236.
38. Herzog EL, Van Arnam J, Hu B, Zhang J, Chen Q, et al. (2007) Lung-specific nuclear reprogramming is accompanied by heterokaryon formation and Y chromosome loss following bone marrow transplantation and secondary inflammation. FASEB J 21: 2592–2601.
39. Carraro G, Perin L, Sedrakyan S, Giuliani S, Tiozzo C, et al. (2008) Human amniotic fluid stem cells can integrate and differentiate into epithelial lung lineages. Stem Cells 26: 2902–2911.
40. Dubernard G, Aractingi S, Oster M, Rouzier R, Mathieu M-C, et al. (2008) Breast cancer stroma frequently recruits fetal derived cells during pregnancy. Breast Cancer Res 10: R14.
41. Cirello V, Recalcati MP, Muzza M, Rossi S, Perrino M, et al. (2008) Fetal cell microchimerism in papillary thyroid cancer: a possible role in tumor damage and tissue repair. Cancer Res 68: 8482–8488.
42. Klintschar M (2006) Fetal microchimerism in hashimoto's thyroiditis: a quantitative approach. Eur J Endocrinol 154: 237–241.
43. Lepez T, Vandewoestyne M, Hussain S, Van Nieuwerburgh F, Poppe K, et al. (2011) Fetal microchimeric cells in blood of women with an autoimmune thyroid disease. PLoS ONE 6: e29646.
44. Asano H, Horinouchi T, Mai Y, Sawada O, Fujii S, et al. (2012) Nicotine- and tar-free cigarette smoke induces cell damage through reactive oxygen species newly generated by PKC-dependent activation of NADPH oxidase. J Pharmacol Sci 118: 275–287.
45. Weiss DJ, Bertoncello I, Borok Z, Kim C, Panoskaltsis-Mortari A, et al. (2011) Stem cells and cell therapies in lung biology and lung diseases. Proc Am Thorac Soc 8: 223–272.
46. Shao L, Li H, Pazhanisamy SK, Meng A, Wang Y, et al. (2011) Reactive oxygen species and hematopoietic stem cell senescence. Int J Hematol 94: 24–32.
47. Richens TR, Linderman DJ, Horstmann SA, Lambert C, Xiao YQ, et al. (2009) Cigarette smoke impairs clearance of apoptotic cells through oxidant-dependent activation of RhoA. Am J Respir Crit Care Med 179: 1011–1021.
48. Pritchard S, Wick HC, Slonim DK, Johnson KL, Bianchi DW (2012) Comprehensive analysis of genes expressed by rare microchimeric fetal cells in the maternal mouse lung. Biol Reprod 87.

2

Water-Pipe Smoking and Albuminuria: New Dog with Old Tricks

Iqra Ishtiaque[1], Kashif Shafique[2,3]*, Zia Ul-Haq[3,4], Abdul Rauf Shaikh[5], Naveed Ali Khan[6], Abdul Rauf Memon[7], Saira Saeed Mirza[8], Afra Ishtiaque[9]

1 University Medical and Dental College, Faisalabad, Pakistan, **2** School of Public Health, Dow University of Health Sciences, Karachi, Pakistan, **3** Institute of Health and Wellbeing, Public Health, University of Glasgow, Glasgow, United Kingdom, **4** Institute of Public Health and Social Sciences, Khyber Medical University, Peshawar, KPK, Pakistan, **5** Department of Community Medicine, Dow University of Health Sciences, Karachi, Pakistan, **6** Department of Surgery, Dow University of Health Sciences, Karachi, Pakistan, **7** Department of Medicine, Dow University of Health Sciences, Karachi, Pakistan, **8** Department of Epidemiology, University of Rotterdam, Rotterdam, The Netherlands, **9** King Edward Medical University, Lahore, Pakistan

Abstract

Water-pipe (WP) smoking is on rise worldwide for the past few years, particularly among younger individuals. Growing evidence indicates that WP smoking is as harmful as cigarette smoking. To date, most of the research has focused on acute health effects of WP smoking, and evidence remains limited when it comes to chronic health effects in relation to long-term WP smoking. Therefore, the aim of this study was to examine the association between WP smoking and albuminuria in apparently healthy individuals. This analysis was conducted on data of a population-based cross-sectional study—the Urban Rural Chronic Diseases Study (URCDS). The study sample was recruited from three sites in Pakistan. Trained nurses carried out individual interviews and obtained the information on demographics, lifestyle factors, and past and current medical history. Measurements of complete blood count, lipid profile, fasting glucose level, and 24-hour albuminuria were also made by using blood and urine samples. Albumin excretion was classified into three categories using standard cut-offs: normal excretion, high-normal excretion and microalbuminuria. Multiple logistic regression models were used to examine the relationship between WP smoking and albuminuria. The final analysis included data from 1,626 health individuals, of which 829 (51.0%) were males and 797 (49.0%) females. Of 1,626 individuals, 267 (16.4%) were current WP smokers and 1,359 (83.6%) were non-WP smokers. WP smoking was significantly associated with high-normal albuminuria (OR = 2.33, 95% CI 1.68-3.22, p-value <0.001) and microalbuminuria (OR = 1.75, 95% CI 1.18-2.58, p-value 0.005) after adjustment for age, sex, BMI, social class, hypertension, and diabetes mellitus. WP smoking was significantly associated with high-normal albuminuria and microalbuminuria when analysis was stratified on hypertension and diabetes mellitus categories. WP smoking has a strong association with albuminuria in apparently healthy individuals. More research is warranted to evaluate the temporality of this association between WP smoking and albuminuria.

Editor: Natalie Walker, The National Institute for Health Innovation, New Zealand

Funding: These authors have no support or funding to report.

Competing Interests: The authors have declared that no competing interests exist.

* E-mail: k.shafique@duhs.edu.pk

Introduction

Water-pipe (WP) also named as shisha, narghile, hookah and arghile is an ancient device which has had a re-birth in recent years [1,2]. A perforated aluminium foil is used in a typical WP which splits the burning charcoal from tobacco. This charcoal and tobacco is connected to a water bowl through a pipe. The air is drawn through the mouthpiece of a hose when a smoker inhale it and this results in burning of both charcoal and tobacco, while the smoke bubbles through the water in this inhaling process [1,2]. There is a misconception that the course of smoke over the water makes it "filtered" and its potential harmful effects on human health are reduced if not completely removed by this so-called "filtering" process [3,4]. There are many similarities between traditional and modern WPs in terms of its configuration as well as the contents used in these devices. Perhaps the only difference between the old and modern WPs is that the charcoal and tobacco is more refined in the later while they were in raw form in the old WPs.

WP smoking trend has dramatically increased in recent years especially among younger individuals [2,5]. Some variations in prevalence of WP smoking are also reported in different regions of the world such as: Arab Americans (12%-15%), Arabic Gulf region (9%-16%), Estonia (21%), and Lebanon (25%) [2,5]. The highest prevalence was reported among University students of Syria (25.5%) [6] and it also remained fairly high (24.5%) among younger individuals (18-24 years of age) in the United States (US) [7]. Pakistan has also seen a rise in WP smoking in last few years with approximately 33% of student being current smokers and nearly half of the University students have tried it once. [8].

In recent years, harmful effects of WP smoking have been reported with particular attention to respiratory and cardiovascular effects [9], although the evidence is limited to acute harmful properties of WP smoking on cardio-respiratory health [9,10]. A recent population-based study suggested that WP smokers had double risk of having metabolic syndrome compared to non-users with more pronounced effects among women [11]. The harmful effects of WP smoking are mainly attributed to toxicants in the smoke which are similar toxicants as in the cigarettes [1,12]. Interestingly, some even suggested that the CO content in WP smoke is three to ten times higher than in cigarette smoke [1,13,14]. Furthermore, WP smokers showed significantly higher blood nicotine levels than cigarette smokers [15].

Urinary albumin excretion is a very sensitive marker of renal injury and its role has also been identified in risk of cardiovascular diseases among healthy as well as diabetic individuals [16,17]. Cigarette smoking has been previously linked with albuminuria and abnormal renal function in humans [18]. Moreover, smoking less than and greater than 20 cigarettes per day shown increased risk of microalbuminuria (Relative risk 1.92, 95% CI 1.54-2.39) and (Relative risk 2.15, 95% CI 1.52-3.03) respectively, among healthy as well as diabetic individuals [19,20].

Given that growing evidence now indicates that WP smoking is as harmful as cigarette smoking, its impact on other aspects of health need to be investigated. To date, most of the research has focused on acute health effects of WP smoking, and the scientific evidence on chronic conditions (cardiovascular and renal) and its association with long-term WP smoking remains scarce. If the toxicants in WP smoke are fairly similar to those of cigarette smoke, there may be a relationship between WP smoking and abnormal renal functions as cigarette smoking has well known adverse effects on kidneys. Therefore, the aim of this analysis was to determine the association between WP smoking and albuminuria in seemingly healthy individuals.

Methods

Cohort selection and study participants

This study was conducted using the data of the Urban Rural Chronic Diseases Study (URCDS) - a cross-sectional study conducted in urban and rural settings of Pakistan to examine the development and prognosis of chronic diseases. The details of this study design and characteristics of the study sample have been explained elsewhere [11]. In brief, the study sample was drawn from the northeast of Punjab province in Faisalabad city (an urban centre) and a village (a rural centre) nearly 35 kilometres away from the centre of the city. Faisalabad is third biggest city of Pakistan with a population of approximately six million when this cross-sectional survey was conducted. Three hospitals (two urban and a rural) were involved in data collection process i.e. Afra General Hospital, Haider Medicare Hospital and New Lahore Hospital.

To increase the participation rate of community in this baseline survey, potential participants were contacted using a variety of different approaches. Participants were requested to participate in this study by personalised letters using the regional voter list as a sampling frame which have individuals older than 18 years but we only sampled from those who were 30 years or above at the time of sampling. Simple random sampling was carried out through Stata software using voter list as sampling frame. Furthermore, announcements in community gatherings, study information dissemination through local key informants, political leaders and religious heads. Healthy adults of age 30 to 75 years living in the vicinity of above mentioned hospitals were eligible to participate in the study. Three clinics were especially set-up in hospitals and all participants who visited during the period of 1st January 2006 to 31st June 2009 were included in this study. Both males and females, employed or un-employed as well as retired from their jobs were eligible to be included in the study. Individuals accompanying patients for their routine health check-ups were also approached and included in the study, if consented.

All eligible individuals were interviewed by a trained staff nurse, followed by a physical examination by a medical specialist at specially set-up clinic. The interview included demographic detail (age, sex, occupation, income, area of residence), lifestyle habits (including cigarette smoking, water-pipe smoking and physical activity) and general health questions. Social class was used as a measure of socio-economic status and every individual was classified to a category based on their occupation. The classification included "Upper class"- including professional individuals holding a management level post in either private or government setup, "middleclass" was assigned to non-manual employees who were skilled office workers and "lower-class" was labelled to manual labour (unskilled workers or farmers). Women were either classified the social class of their husbands or parents depending on their marital status. Following the initial interview, physical examination for measurements of weight, height, waist circumference and blood pressure were taken. Blood samples were obtained by trained nurses for the measurements of lipid profile and glucose level. A subgroup of individuals was also investigated for C-reactive protein and albuminuria. Trained nurses provided oral as well as written information to participants about the method to collect 24-hour urine samples. Participants were also requested to delay the urine collection if they have fever, urinary tract infection or menstruation. They were also informed cease the heavy exercise at least for 24 hours of urine collection. Participants were requested to keep the urine cold (at 4°C) before the visit to clinic but not more than two days. Measurements of urine volume and albumin were obtained in respective laboratories attached to hospitals.

Albuminuria definitions

We used the standard definition to define microalbuminuria i.e. an albumin excretion of 30 to 300 mg/24 hours. As some evidence also suggests that the risk of cardiovascular and renal diseases may rise even at a lower cut-off point than what is considered as pathologic, we also created a group of individuals who had albumin excretion between 15 to 30 mg/24 hours and classified them as high-normal albuminuria as in previously reported studies.

Ethics statement

This study was reviewed and approved by the Ethical Review Committee at the, Afra General Hospital, Faisalabad. This study was also carried out in accordance with the Declaration of Helsinki guidelines. The approvals were also obtained from all three hospitals – Afra General Hospital, Haider Medicare Hospital and New Lahore Hospital. Study participants provided written informed consent prior to their participation in the study.

Sample size estimation

The sample size for this study was estimated to detect a 2% difference in prevalence of albuminuria (assuming 20% prevalence of albuminuria among WP smokers) between groups. The significance level was at 0.05 and power of the study at 80% using two sided comparisons. Both X^2 using the Yates' continuity correction and Fisher Exact Test were used to compute the sample size. A total of 1535 individuals were required to be included in the study to conduct this survey with an allocation ratio of 1.

Data analysis

We used STATA software version 11 (StataCorp, College Station, TX, USA) for data analysis. The study sample was categorized into two groups such as "WP smokers" and "non-WP smokers". Current water-pipe smokers were defined as those who regularly smoked WP at least once in a week in the previous year. Non-WP smoker group included those who were never WP smokers as well as who quit smoking (ex-WP smokers). Those who quitted WP smoking at least twelve months before the beginning of this study were defined as Ex-smokers those who quitted less than a year's time were considered as smokers. Age was categorised into 10 year age bands except the highest age group which was a 15 years age band due to smaller number of individuals in that group.

For the estimation of raised blood pressure and glucose level, new variables were created using the IDF specific criteria. Hypertension was defined as systolic blood pressure of at least 140 mm Hg, diastolic blood pressure of at least 90 mm Hg, or history of use of antihypertensive drugs. Diabetes mellitus was defined as a fasting plasma glucose level of >126 mg/dL, a random plasma glucose level of >180 mg/dL or greater, or the use of antidiabetic medication. Therefore, wherever hypertension or diabetes mellitus is mentioned in this manuscript, it reflects increased level or previously known condition, or both.

Independent sample t-test was used to compare continuous variables between two groups while chi-square test was used for comparison between categorical variables. We used multiple logistic regressions to examine the association between WP smoking and high-normal albuminuria as well as microalbuminuria. Separate multivariable logistic regression models were ran to explore the association between WP smoking and high albuminuria and microalbuminuria after adjusting for age, sex, BMI, social class, hypertension and diabetes mellitus. A stratified analysis was also carried out to estimate the effect of WP smoking on albuminuria based on hypertension and diabetes mellitus categories.

A total of 2700 individuals were included in this study however there were some information missing i.e. blood pressure data (n = 75), self-reported diabetes mellitus and blood glucose (n = 47), height and weight (n = 24), social class and triglycerides level(n = 79), Those who had missing information for any of these were excluded from the final analysis. Furthermore, those who were cigarette smokers (n = 128) or combine users of cigarette and WP (n = 443) were also excluded from the present analysis. The data on albumin excretion was also not available for 406 individuals, so they were also excluded from this analysis.

Results

Data from 1,626 healthy individuals were used for final analysis which included 829 (51.0%) males and 797 (49.0%) females. Of 1,626 individuals, 267 (16.4%) were current WP smokers and 1,359 (83.6%) were non-WP smokers. Number of ex-WP smokers was fairly small (n = 13), we performed a sub-analysis by excluding these ex-WP smokers but overall association between WP and albuminuria remained unchanged so they were included in the non-WP smoking category. There was no significant difference in duration of WP smoking among three groups of albumin excretion (p-value 0.20), while the overall mean duration of WP smoking was 14.9±10.8 years. Out of the total 1,626, 1011 (62.3%) had albumin excretion within normal range, 340 (20.9%) had high-normal albumin excretion and 273 (16.8%) had microalbuminuria. No statistically significant differences of age at baseline examination, sex, BMI and social class were observed between three groups of albumin excretion. Furthermore diabetics, hypertensives and current WP smokers were significantly more likely to have microalbuminuria compared with non-diabetics, normotensives and non-WP smokers, respectively. Table 1, shows the demographic and lifestyle characteristics of study sample.

Water-pipe smoking and high-normal albuminuria

The frequency of high-normal albuminuria was significantly higher among WP smokers compared with non-WP smokers. Univariable analysis showed that WP smokers were 2.4 times higher risk to have high-normal albuminuria compared with non-WP smokers (OR = 2.40, 95% CI .75-3.28, p-value <0.001). Furthermore on univariable analysis, individuals who were, older (p-value <0.001), females (p-value 0.002), obese (p-value 0.001), had diabetes mellitus (p-value 0.001) and hypertension (p-value 0.002) were significantly more likely to have high-normal albuminuria compared with youngers, males, desirable weight individuals, non-diabetics and normotensives respectively (table 2). Conversely, manual workers were 30% less likely to have high-normal albuminuria compared with professionals (OR = 0.61, 95% CI 0.43-0.87, p-value 0.001). On multivariable analysis, WP smoking was significantly associated with high-normal albuminuria (OR = 2.33, 95% CI 1.68-3.22, p-value <0.001) after adjustment for age, sex, BMI, social class, hypertension and diabetes mellitus (table 2).

Water-pipe smoking and microalbuminuria

The frequency of microalbuminuria was significantly higher among WP smokers compared to non-WP smokers (p-value 0.001). Univariable analysis showed that WP smokers were 2.3 times more likely to have high microalbuminuria compared with non-WP smokers (OR = 2.27, 95% CI 1.62-3.19, p-value <0.001). Furthermore on univariable analysis, older individuals (p-value <0.001), females (p-value 0.002), obese individuals (p-value 0.001), individuals with diabetes mellitus (p-value 0.001) and individuals with hypertension (p-value 0.002) were significantly more likely to have high microalbuminuria compared to younger, male, desirable weight, non-diabetics and normotensive individuals respectively (table 3). Conversely, manual workers were 64% less likely to have high-normal albuminuria compared with professionals (OR = 0.36, 95% CI 0.25-0.53, p-value 0.001). On multivariable analysis, WP smoking was significantly associated with high microalbuminuria (OR = 1.75, 95% CI 1.18-2.58, p-value 0.005) after adjustment for age, sex, BMI, social class, hypertension and diabetes mellitus (table 3).

Water-pipe smoking and albuminuria in relation to hypertension and diabetes mellitus

A stratified analysis based on hypertension and diabetes mellitus status of individuals was also carried out to understand the relationship between WP smoking and albuminuria. WP smokers were two times more likely to have high-normal albuminuria compared with non-WP smokers regardless of hypertension status. However, WP smokers who had diabetes mellitus were 3.5 times more likely to have high-normal albuminuria compared to non-WP smokers; a slightly higher odds ratio compared to non-diabetics (figure 1A). The effect of WP smoking on microalbuminuria among diabetic and hypertensive individuals was higher when these effects were compared to non-diabetic and normotensive individuals (figure 1B).

Discussion

This is the first population-based study providing some insights in to the effect of WP smoking on renal function of apparently healthy population. This study indicates a harmful relationship between WP smoking and albuminuria. The observed positive association between WP smoking and albuminuria was independent of age at baseline, sex, BMI, social class, hypertension and diabetes mellitus. The association between WP smoking and

Table 1. Baseline characteristics of study participants by albumin excretion.

	Albumin excretion			P-value*
	Normal	High-normal	Microalbuminuria	
	<15 mg/L	15-30 mg/L	>30-300 mg/L	
	(n = 1011)	(n = 340)	(n = 274)	
	n (%)	n (%)	n (%)	
Age at screening (continuous)	47.97±11.9	53.33±13.0	57.18±12.2	<0.001
Age at screening (years)				
30-39	295 (76.2)	61 (15.8)	31 (8.0)	<0.001
40-49	307 (71.9)	75 (17.6)	45 (10.5)	
50-59	196 (57.1)	80 (23.3)	67 (19.6)	
60-75	213 (45.6)	124 (26.6)	130 (27.8)	
Sex				
Male	569 (68.7)	159 (19.2)	100 (12.1)	<0.001
Female	442 (55.4)	181 (22.8)	173 (21.8)	
Social class				
Professional	129 (50.6)	63 (24.7)	63 (24.7)	<0.001
Non-manual workers	384 (60.6)	128 (20.2)	122 (19.2)	
Manual workers	498 (67.7)	149 (20.3)	88 (12.0)	
Body mass index (continuous)	25.6±3.9	26.6±3.9	28.0±4.6	<0.001
Body mass index (kg/m^2)				
Desirable < 23	258 (72.7)	62 (17.4)	35 (9.9)	<0.001
Overweight >23-27.5	500 (66.5)	155 (20.6)	97 (12.9)	
Obese > 27.5	253 (48.9)	123 (23.8)	141 (27.3)	
Blood pressure				
Normotensive	855 (69.6)	236 (19.2)	137 (11.2)	<0.001
Hypertensive	156 (39.4)	104 (26.3)	136 (34.3)	
Diabetes mellitus				
No	886 (66.7)	266 (20.0)	176 (13.3)	<0.001
Yes	125 (42.2)	74 (25.0)	97 (32.8)	
Waterpipe smoking				
Non smokers	891 (65.7)	25 (18.9)	209 (15.4)	<0.001
Current smokers	120 (44.9)	83 (31.1)	64 (24.0)	

P-value was calculated using the chi-squared test.

albuminuria changed a little when analysis was stratified on presence or absence of hypertension and diabetes mellitus.

Many previous studies have investigated the adverse influence of cigarette smoking on renal function but there is no previous evidence of detrimental effects of WP smoking on renal function. It is well established that the urinary albumin level is a sensitive marker of glomerular injury [19] and the fact that the cigarette smoking is associated with albuminuria indicates a direct or indirect relationship of cigarette smoking in initiation and progression of kidney damage [21]. The finding of this study that WP smoking is related to declining renal function is biologically plausible. Given that the WP smoke contains similar toxicants as cigarettes, kidney damage may have been a result of WP smoking through similar mechanisms as suggested for cigarette smoking. Several mechanisms have been proposed through which cigarette smoking can lead to renal injury.

The increase in glomerular filtration rate (GFR) caused by cigarette smoking may have some role in initiation and development of renal injury and chronic renal diseases [22,23]. The increase in GFR due to cigarette smoking may possibly be a response to nicotine content of smoke which leads to increased excretion of sodium, chloride and urine flow [24,25]. This observation also indicates that the release of catecholamine from adrenal medulla may have been responsible for nicotine action on the kidney. Another possible mechanism by which nicotine can alter GFR is the altered cervical parasympathetic tone may cause increase in vasopressin release which ultimately leads to increase in GFR [26,27]. There is also a possibility that the increase in GFR may be a response to increased blood pressure secondary to smoking nicotine products. Other renal functions such as altered proximal tubular function, increased excretion of N-acetyl-ß3-glucoasmindase and impairment of organic cation transport are also a consequence of cigarette smoking, which are particularly related with the amount of tobacco smoked over time. [28].

The findings of this study could be a result of some biases inherent in epidemiological studies. There is a chance of some

Table 2. Relationship between water-pipe smoking and high-normal albumin excretion.

	Univariable analysis			Multivariable analysis$		
	Odds Ratio (95% CI)		p value	Odds Ratio (95% CI)		p value
Waterpipe smoking						
Non smokers		1			1	
Current smokers	2.40	(1.75, 3.28)	<0.001	2.33	(1.68, 3.22)	<0.001
Age at screening (years)						
30-39		1			1	
40-49	1.18	(0.81, 1.72)	0.38	1.09	(0.75, 1.60)	0.65
50-59	1.97	(1.35, 2.88)	<0.001	1.66	(1.12, 2.47)	0.01
60-75	2.82	(1.98, 4.01)	<0.001	2.08	(1.40, 3.09)	<0.001
Sex						
Male		1			1	
Female	1.47	(1.45, 1.88)	0.002	1.53	(1.18, 1.98)	<0.001
Social class						
Professional		1			1	
Non-manual workers	0.68	(0.48, 0.98)	0.04	0.96	(0.61, 1.50)	0.84
Manual workers	0.61	(0.43, 0.87)	0.006	1.00	(0.60, 1.65)	0.23
Body mass index (kg/m^2)						
Desirable < 23		1			1	
Overweight >23-27.5	1.29	(0.93, 1.80)	0.13	0.90	(0.64, 1.29)	0.57
Obese > 27.5	2.02	(1.42, 2.87)	<0.001	1.28	(0.82, 2.02)	0.28
Blood pressure *						
Normotensive		1			1	
Hypertensive	2.42	(1.81, 3.21)	<0.001	1.65	(1.19, 2.28)	0.002
Diabetes mellitus *						
No		1			1	
Yes	1.97	(1.43, 2.71)	<0.001	1.19	(0.83, 1.71)	0.34

$All estimates were adjusted for age at screening, sex, BMI, social class blood pressure and diabetes mellitus. * indicate increased level of specific measure or a previously diagnosed condition.

selection bias which could be due to exclusion of those individuals who used to smoke both cigarettes and WP. The main reason for excluding these individuals was the inability to understand the true effect of WP smoke on albuminuria because of simultaneous cigarette smoking. Moreover, significant differences were observed in age at baseline examination, sex, BMI, social class, hypertension and diabetes mellitus of three study arms i.e. normal albumin excretion, high-normal albumin excretion and microalbuminuria. Differential distribution of these factors may have confounded the observed association between WP smoking and albuminuria, however, multivariable adjustment did not alter the findings of this study. Furthermore, stratified analyses were also carried out based on all these baseline factors but the relationship between WP smoking and albuminuria remained consistent (data not shown).

Diabetes mellitus and hypertension are independently associated with albuminuria so the stratified analyses were also carried out based on these variables. The overall associations between WP smoking and high-normal albuminuria were similar both in hypertension and diabetes mellitus categories. However, there was some evidence of differential effect of WP smoking on microalbuminuria with more pronounced effect among hypertensive and diabetic individuals. This may be combined effect of WP smoking with these morbidities to cause renal damage; a further study on healthy population without any morbidity may explain the true effect of WP smoking on microalbuminuria. Another important concern can be the exposure to second-hand smoke due to WPs, which may have influenced the findings of this study because WPs are usually smoked in social meetings with a few people around. Some participants of this study classified as non-WP smokers in this study may actually have been exposed to second-hand smoke through polluted air and may have developed impairment in their renal profile. This misclassification is not likely to change the overall outcome of this study because, if some of the non-WP smoker were actually exposed to second-hand smoke, the harmful effect of WP in this study may have been attenuated and underestimated while the actual effect of WP may even be greater than the one reported here.

This was the first population-based study with large sample size, which assessed the relationship between WP smoking and albuminuria. Generally, the adverse health effects of WP smoking are not very well understood yet and most of the health conditions are unexamined in association with WP smoking. Furthermore, the quality of evidence is fairly low which has been suggested by a reviews [29]. There are some limitations of this study as well which need to be accounted when drawing any conclusions from present analysis. Firstly, the study sample was drawn from one region of Pakistan which mainly represents only one ethnic group (which is approximately 60% of national population) living in this country

Table 3. Relationship between water-pipe smoking and microalbuminuria.

	Univariable analysis			Multivariable analysis$		
	Odds Ratio (95% CI)		p value	Odds Ratio (95% CI)		p value
Water-pipe smoking						
Non smokers		1			1	
Current smokers	2.27	(1.62, 3.19)	<0.001	1.75	(1.18, 2.58)	0.005
Age at screening (years)						
30-39		1			1	
40-49	1.39	(0.86, 2.26)	0.18	1.07	(0.64, 1.77)	0.8
50-59	3.25	(2.05, 5.17)	<0.001	1.86	(1.12, 3.08)	0.02
60-75	5.81	(3.78, 8.92)	<0.001	2.64	(1.63, 4.30)	<0.001
Sex						
Male		1			1	
Female	2.23	(1.69, 2.93)	<0.001	2.22	(1.63, 3.01)	<0.001
Social class						
Professional		1			1	
Non-manual workers	0.65	(0.45, 0.94)	0.02	1.09	(0.69, 1.73)	0.36
Manual workers	0.36	(0.25, 0.53)	<0.001	0.93	(0.54, 1.60)	0.78
Body mass index (kg/m²)						
Desirable < 23		1			1	
Overweight >23-27.5	1.43	(0.94, 2.16)	0.09	0.75	(0.48, 1.18)	0.22
Obese > 27.5	4.11	(2.73, 6.18)	<0.001	1.75	(1.04, 2.95)	0.34
Blood pressure*						
Normotensive		1			1	
Hypertensive	5.44	(4.06, 7.29)	<0.001	2.91	(2.07, 4.09)	<0.001
Diabetes mellitus*						
No		1			1	
Yes	3.91	(2.86, 5.33)	<0.001	1.63	(1.22, 2.35)	0.01

$All estimates were adjusted for age at screening, sex, BMI, social class blood pressure and diabetes mellitus. * indicate increased level of specific measure or a previously diagnosed condition.

so the findings of the present study may not be generalizable to other regions and ethnicities living in Pakistan. Secondly, selection of study sample was based on different types of invitations to increase the participation rate which may have led to some selection bias. However, our previous analysis has showed that the distribution of many risk factors i.e. obesity, hypertension and diabetes mellitus, is comparable with published studies from this region [11] so any effect is unlikely due to differential distribution of background risk factors in the study sample. Lastly, in this part of the country, traditional WPs are commonly used and these were mainly smoked by the study participants. There can be some argument that the raw charcoal and raw tobacco may not be similar in terms of smoke toxicants produced by the modern fashionable WPs. However, some evidence suggests that flavouring of tobacco and charcoal did not cut down the potential adverse effects of WPs [30–32].

Public health implications

WP smoking has markedly increased globally in recent years. Given the injurious effects of WP smoking on renal function observed in this study, WP smoking may significantly increase the burden of renal diseases in future, however, confirmation of a causal relationship between WP smoking and renal damage is required before initiating wider public health actions. Further prospective studies including younger individuals and using different varieties of tobacco in WPs may be useful in understanding the relationship of WP smoking in development of renal and other chronic diseases. Health education and awareness programs specific to target groups are the only interventions which are critical to eliminate the false beliefs of WP harmlessness. Although, the target groups for such interventions can be broad but particular attention to younger age individuals will be important to reduce the future burden of diseases associated with WP smoking.

Conclusion

This study observed a significant independent positive relationship between WP smoking and albuminuria among middle and old aged individuals. Future research using prospective cohort and including younger age individuals would be useful to understand the mechanism and temporal association between WP smoking and albuminuria.

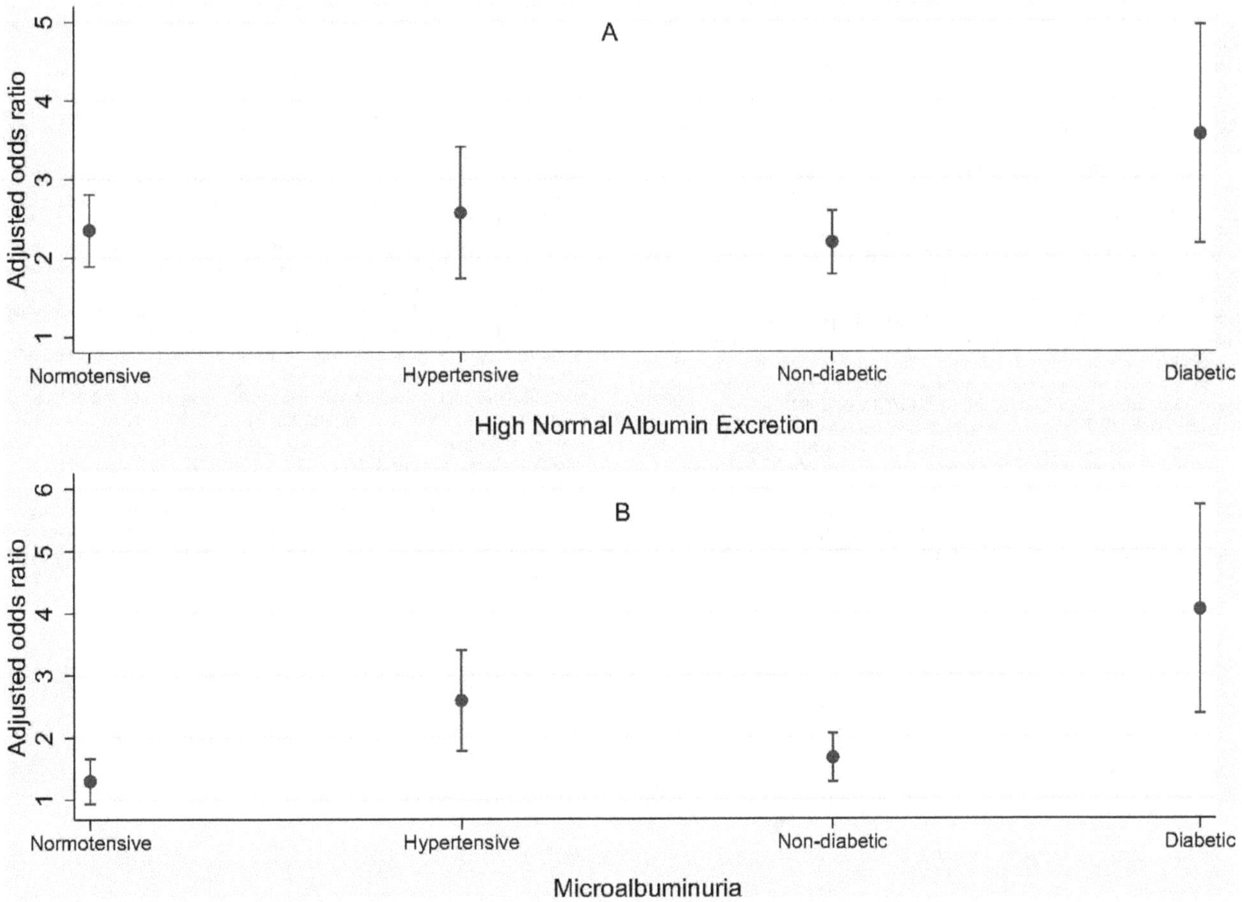

Figure 1. Association between and water-pipe smoking and albuminuria based on hypertension and diabetes mellitus categories. All estimates were adjusted for age, sex, BMI and social class.

Acknowledgments

Authors are grateful to Dr. Itfaque, Dr. Rubina Itfaque and Mr. Muhammad Asif for their role in data collection and compilation.

Author Contributions

Conceived and designed the experiments: KS AI ZUH. Performed the experiments: II AI. Analyzed the data: SSM ZUH. Wrote the paper: II KS NAK ARS ARM.

References

1. Eissenberg T, Shihadeh A (2009) Waterpipe tobacco and cigarette smoking: direct comparison of toxicant exposure. Am J Prev Med 37: 518-523. doi: 10.1016/j.amepre.2009.07.014.
2. Maziak W (2011) The global epidemic of waterpipe smoking. Addict Behav 36: 1-5. doi: 10.1016/j.addbeh.2010.08.030.
3. Maziak W, Eissenberg T, Rastam S, Hammal F, Asfar T, et al. (2004) Beliefs and attitudes related to narghile (waterpipe) smoking among university students in Syria. Ann Epidemiol 14: 646-654. doi:10.1016/j.annepidem.2003.11.003.
4. Roskin J, Aveyard P (2009) Canadian and English students' beliefs about waterpipe smoking: a qualitative study. BMC Public Health 9: 10. doi: 10.1186/1471-2458-9-10.
5. Akl EA, Gunukula SK, Aleem S, Obeid R, Jaoude PA, et al. (2011) The prevalence of waterpipe tobacco smoking among the general and specific populations: a systematic review. BMC Public Health 11: 244. doi: 10.1186/1471-2458-11-244.
6. Maziak W, Hammal F, Rastam S, Asfar T, Eissenberg T, et al. (2004) Characteristics of cigarette smoking and quitting among university students in Syria. Prev Med 39: 330-336. doi: 10.1016/j.ypmed.2004.01.024.
7. Smith JR, Edland SD, Novotny TE, Hofstetter CR, White MM, et al. (2011) Increasing hookah use in California. Am J Public Health 101: 1876-1879. doi: 10.2105/AJPH.2011.300196.
8. Jawaid A, Zafar AM, Rehman TU, Nazir MR, Ghafoor ZA, et al. (2008) Knowledge, attitudes and practice of university students regarding waterpipe smoking in Pakistan. Int J Tuberc Lung Dis 12: 1077-1084.
9. Shaikh RB, Vijayaraghavan N, Sulaiman AS, Kazi S, Mohammed Shafi MS (2008) The acute effects of Waterpipe smoking on the cardiovascular and respiratory systems. J Prev Med Hyg 49: 101-107.
10. Khabour OF, Alzoubi KH, Bani-Ahmad M, Dodin A, Eissenberg T, et al. (2012) Acute exposure to waterpipe tobacco smoke induces changes in the oxidative and inflammatory markers in mouse lung. Inhal Toxicol 24: 667-675. doi: 10.3109/08958378.2012.710918.
11. Shafique K, Mirza SS, Mughal MK, Arain ZI, Khan NA, et al. (2012) Water-pipe smoking and metabolic syndrome: a population-based study. PLoS One 7: e39734. doi: 10.1371/journal.pone.0039734.
12. Neergaard J, Singh P, Job J, Montgomery S (2007) Waterpipe smoking and nicotine exposure: a review of the current evidence. Nicotine Tob Res 9: 987-994. doi: 10.1080/14622200701591591.
13. Daher N, Saleh R, Jaroudi E, Sheheitli H, Badr T, et al. (2010) Comparison of carcinogen, carbon monoxide, and ultrafine particle emissions from narghile waterpipe and cigarette smoking: Sidestream smoke measurements and assessment of second-hand smoke emission factors. Atmos Environ 44: 8-14. doi: 10.1016/j.atmosenv.2009.10.004.
14. Jacob P III, Abu Raddaha AH, Dempsey D, Havel C, Peng M, et al. (2011) Nicotine, carbon monoxide, and carcinogen exposure after a single use of a water pipe. Cancer Epidemiol Biomarkers Prev 20: 2345-2353. doi: 10.1158/1055-9965.EPI-11-0545.
15. Shafagoj YA, Mohammed FI, Hadidi KA (2002) Hubble-bubble (water pipe) smoking: levels of nicotine and cotinine in plasma, saliva and urine. Int J Clin Pharmacol Ther 40: 249-255.

16. Svensson MK, Cederholm J, Eliasson B, Zethelius B, Gudbjornsdottir S (2013) Albuminuria and renal function as predictors of cardiovascular events and mortality in a general population of patients with type 2 diabetes: A nationwide observational study from the Swedish National Diabetes Register. Diab Vasc Dis Res 10: 520-529. doi: 10.1177/1479164113500798.
17. Doggen K, Nobels F, Scheen AJ, Van Crombrugge P, Van Casteren V, et al. (2013) Cardiovascular risk factors and complications associated with albuminuria and impaired renal function in insulin-treated diabetes. J Diabetes Complications 27: 370-375. doi: 10.1016/j.jdiacomp.2013.02.008.
18. Orth SR, Ritz E (2002) The renal risks of smoking: an update. Curr Opin Nephrol Hypertens 11: 483-488.
19. Orth SR (2002) Smoking and the kidney. J Am Soc Nephrol 13: 1663-1672.
20. Pinto-Sietsma SJ, Mulder J, Janssen WMT, Hillege HL, de Zeeuw D, et al. (2000) Smoking is related to albuminuria and abnormal renal function in nondiabetic persons. Ann Intern Med 133: 585-591.
21. Orth SR, Hallan SI (2008) Smoking: a risk factor for progression of chronic kidney disease and for cardiovascular morbidity and mortality in renal patients--absence of evidence or evidence of absence? Clin J Am Soc Nephrol 3: 226-236. Smoking is related to albuminuria and abnormal renal function in nondiabetic persons. Ann Intern Med 133: 585-59110.2215/CJN.03740907.
22. Hostetter TH (1995) Progression of renal disease and renal hypertrophy. Annu Rev Physiol 57: 263-278. doi: 10.1146/annurev.ph.57.030195.001403.
23. Neuringer JR, Brenner BM (1993) Hemodynamic theory of progressive renal disease: a 10-year update in brief review. Am J Kidney Dis 22: 98-104.
24. Cooper RG (2008) Renal function in male Sprague-Dawley rats concurrently exposed to long-term nicotine (3-{1-methyl-2-pyrrolidinyl}pyridine) and methylated spirits (methyl alcohol). Ren Fail 30: 107-114. doi: 10.1080/08860220701742179.
25. Tamaoki L, Oshiro-Monreal FM, Helou CM (2009) Effects of nicotine exposure on renal function of normal and hypercholesterolemic rats. Am J Nephrol 30: 377-382 doi:10.1159/000235622.
26. Andersson K, Siegel R, Fuxe K, Eneroth P (1983) Intravenous injections of nicotine induce very rapid and discrete reductions of hypothalamic catecholamine levels associated with increases of ACTH, vasopressin and prolactin secretion. Acta Physiol Scand 118: 35-40. doi: 10.1111/j.1748-1716.1983.tb07237.x.
27. Lightman S, Langdon N, Todd K, Forsling M (1982) Naloxone increases the nicotine-stimulated rise of vasopressin secretion in man. Clin Endocrinol (Oxf) 16: 353-358.
28. Wong LT, Smyth DD, Sitar DS (1992) Interference with renal organic cation transport by (-)- and (+)-nicotine at concentrations documented in plasma of habitual tobacco smokers. J Pharmacol Exp Ther 261: 21-25.
29. Warnakulasuriya S (2011) Waterpipe smoking, oral cancer and other oral health effects. Evid Based Dent 12: 44-45. doi: 10.1038/sj.ebd.6400790.
30. Al Ali R, Rastam S, Ibrahim I, Bazzi A, Fayad S, et al. (2013) A comparative study of systemic carcinogen exposure in waterpipe smokers, cigarette smokers and non-smokers. Tob Control. doi: 10.1136/tobaccocontrol-2013-051206.
31. Cobb CO, Shihadeh A, Weaver MF, Eissenberg T (2011) Waterpipe tobacco smoking and cigarette smoking: a direct comparison of toxicant exposure and subjective effects. Nicotine Tob Res 13: 78-87. doi: 10.1093/ntr/ntq212.
32. Daher N, Saleh R, Jaroudi E, Sheheitli H, Badr T, et al. (2010) Comparison of carcinogen, carbon monoxide, and ultrafine particle emissions from narghile waterpipe and cigarette smoking: Sidestream smoke measurements and assessment of second-hand smoke emission factors. Atmos Environ (1994) 44: 8-14. doi: 10.1016/j.atmosenv.2009.10.004.

3

Influenza Virus-Induced Lung Inflammation Was Modulated by Cigarette Smoke Exposure in Mice

Yan Han[1], Man To Ling[1], Huawei Mao[1], Jian Zheng[1], Ming Liu[2], Kwok Tai Lam[1], Yuan Liu[1], Wenwei Tu[1]*, Yu-Lung Lau[1]*

1 Department of Paediatrics and Adolescent Medicine, Li Ka Shing Faculty of Medicine, University of Hong Kong, Hong Kong Special Administrative Region, People's Republic of China, 2 State Key Laboratory of Respiratory Diseases, Guangzhou Institute of Respiratory Diseases, First Affiliated Hospital, Guangzhou Medical College, Guangzhou, People's Republic of China

Abstract

Although smokers have increased susceptibility and severity of seasonal influenza virus infection, there is no report about the risk of 2009 pandemic H1N1 (pdmH1N1) or avian H9N2 (H9N2/G1) virus infection in smokers. In our study, we used mouse model to investigate the effect of cigarette smoke on pdmH1N1 or H9N2 virus infection. Mice were exposed to cigarette smoke for 21 days and then infected with pdmH1N1 or H9N2 virus. Control mice were exposed to air in parallel. We found that cigarette smoke exposure alone significantly upregulated the lung inflammation. Such prior cigarette smoke exposure significantly reduced the disease severity of subsequent pdmH1N1 or H9N2 virus infection. For pdmH1N1 infection, cigarette smoke exposed mice had significantly lower mortality than the control mice, possibly due to the significantly decreased production of inflammatory cytokines and chemokines. Similarly, after H9N2 infection, cigarette smoke exposed mice displayed significantly less weight loss, which might be attributed to lower cytokines and chemokines production, less macrophages, neutrophils, $CD4^+$ and $CD8^+$ T cells infiltration and reduced lung damage compared to the control mice. To further investigate the underlying mechanism, we used nicotine to mimic the effect of cigarette smoke both *in vitro* and *in vivo*. Pre-treating the primary human macrophages with nicotine for 72 h significantly decreased their expression of cytokines and chemokines after pdmH1N1 or H9N2 infection. The mice subcutaneously and continuously treated with nicotine displayed significantly less weight loss and lower inflammatory response than the control mice upon pdmH1N1 or H9N2 infection. Moreover, α7 nicotinic acetylcholine receptor knockout mice had more body weight loss than wild-type mice after cigarette smoke exposure and H9N2 infection. Our study provided the first evidence that the pathogenicity of both pdmH1N1 and H9N2 viruses was alleviated in cigarette smoke exposed mice, which might partially be attributed to the immunosuppressive effect of nicotine.

Editor: Dominik Hartl, University of Tübingen, Germany

Funding: This work was supported by the Area of Excellence program on Influenza, the University Grants Committee of the Hong Kong SAR, China (AoE/M-12/06); General Research Fund, Research Grants Council of Hong Kong; a Commission Grant from the Research Fund for the Control of Infectious Diseases (RFCID) of the Health, Welfare and Food Bureau of the Hong Kong SAR Government (2009-2014, Lab-11); Edward Sai-Kim Hotung Paediatric Education and Research Fund. The funders had no role in study design, data collection and analysis, decision to publish, or preparation of the manuscript.

Competing Interests: The authors have declared that no competing interests exist.

* E-mail: lauylung@hku.hk (Y. Lau); wwtu@hku.hk (WT)

Introduction

Influenza A viruses cause regular outbreaks worldwide with significant morbidity and mortality in humans and animals [1,2]. In 2009, a new swine-origin pandemic H1N1 (pdmH1N1) rapidly spread throughout the world [3]. By 2012, 284,500 deaths were associated with pdmH1N1, majority of which occurred in people younger than 65 years and most of them occurred in Africa and Southeast Asia [4]. H9N2 avian influenza A virus (H9N2/G1) has caused recurrent human infections in Asia since 1998 [5]. Until 2003, 8 cases of H9N2 infection have been reported in China, all with mild influenza-like symptoms and recovered [6,7]. The new pandemic outbreak of pdmH1N1 and continuous sporadic reports of human infection with H9N2 highlight the ever-existing threat of influenza A virus infection on public health [1,7,8].

Cigarette smoke has been considered the main risk factor for morbidity and mortality related to cardiovascular disease, cancer, and chronic obstructive pulmonary disease [9,10]. Although the adverse effect of cigarette smoke on human health is well documented, there is evidence showing that cigarette smoke might decrease the incidence of some inflammatory and neurodegenerative diseases, including ulcerative colitis, endometriosis, pigeon breeders' disease, sarcoidosis and Parkinson's disease [11]. Mainstream cigarette smoke produces almost 5,000 chemicals, among which, nicotine is mainly responsible for initiation and maintenance of tobacco dependence [12,13]. Nicotine has immune-suppressive effect by binding to α7 nicotinic acetylcholine receptor (α7 nAChR) and hence activating cholinergic anti-inflammatory pathway [14].

Current epidemiological investigations showed that smokers are at increased risk of influenza virus infection compared with non-smokers [15–19], which might be due to the immunosuppressive effect of cigarette smoke. It was reported that such immunologic abnormalities in smokers could be resolved within 6 weeks after cigarette smoke cessation [9]. However, all these studies were on the seasonal influenza (A/H3N2, A/H1N1 and Type B) viruses.

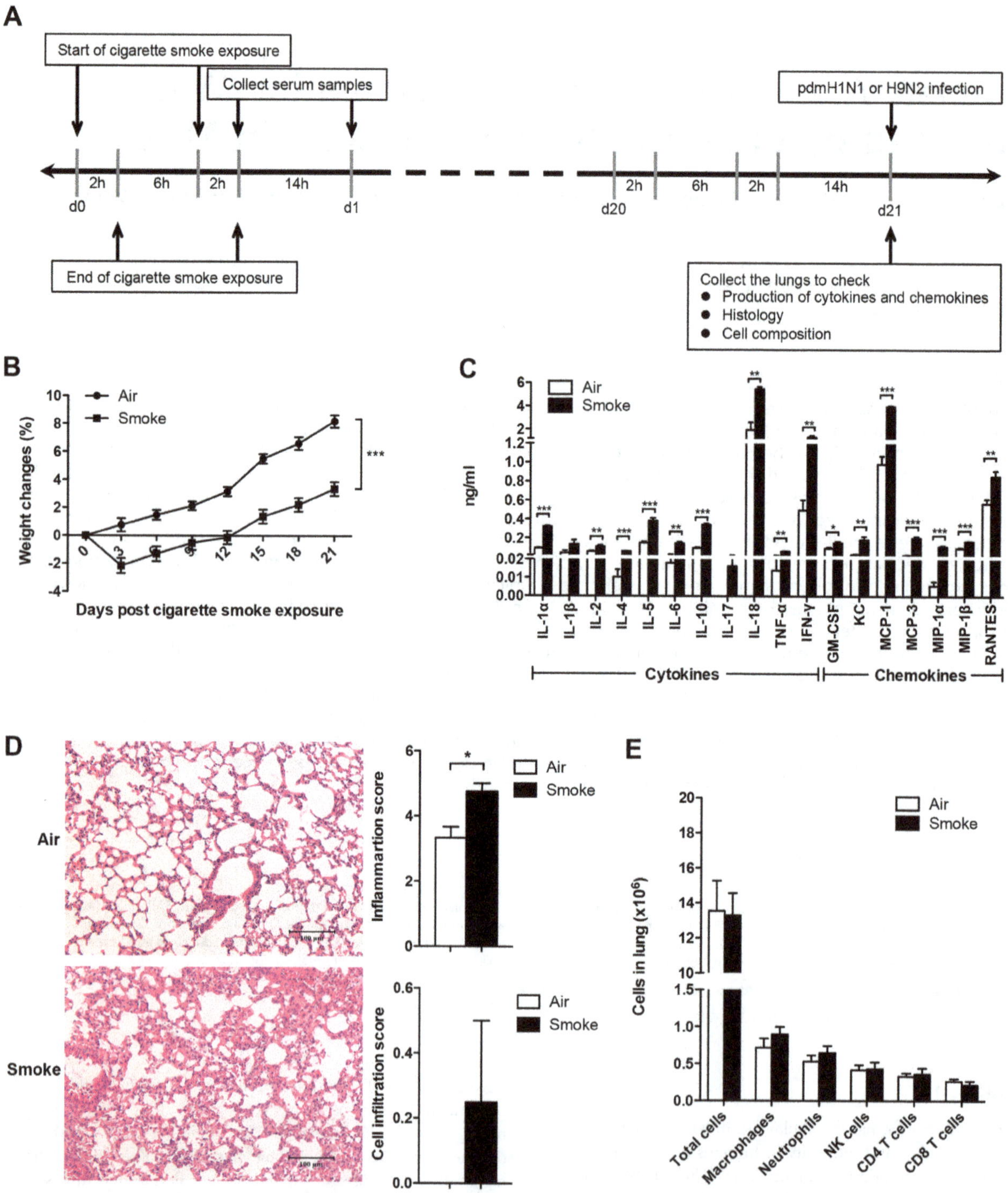

Figure 1. Cigarette smoke exposure alone up-regulated the inflammation of mice. A) Study design for cigarette smoke exposure model. The mice were exposed to 4% (vol/vol, smoke/air) cigarette smoke for 2 hours per episode, 2 episodes per day for 21 days and then infected with pdmH1N1 or H9N2 virus. B) Body weight changes of the mice exposed to room air or cigarette smoke for 21 days. There were 50 mice per group. Data are representative of three independent experiments. C) Production of cytokines and chemokines in lung homogenates on day 21 of air or cigarette smoke exposed mice (fourteen hours after the last cigarette smoke exposure). Data are representative of three independent experiments. D) Histopathological analysis of pulmonary tissues collected on day 21 of air or cigarette smoke exposure (fourteen hours after the last cigarette smoke exposure). Results are representative pictures (200X) of hematoxylin and eosin stained pulmonary tissues. Scale bar: 100 μm. Inflammation score and cell infiltration score were evaluated by a board-certified pathologist. E) Absolute number of lung cells on day 21 of air or cigarette smoke exposure (fourteen hours after the last cigarette smoke exposure). Macrophages ($CD11b^+$, $F4/80^+$), neutrophils ($CD11b^+$, $Ly\text{-}6G^+$), NK cells ($CD3^-$, $NK1.1^+$), $CD4^+$ T cells ($CD3^+$, $CD4^+$) and $CD8^+$ T cells ($CD3^+$, $CD8a^+$). There were 4 mice per group (C, D, and E). Results represent mean ± SEM. $^*p<0.05$; $^{**}p<0.01$; $^{***}p<0.001$.

Until now, there is no report related to the susceptibility and severity of pdmH1N1 or avian H9N2 influenza virus infection in smokers. As pdmH1N1 and H9N2 can infect mice [20] and mice are widely used to examine the influenza pathology [21], we chose a mouse model to investigate the risk of pdmH1N1 and H9N2 infection in cigarette smoke exposed mice. We hypothesized that the disease severity of pdmH1N1 and H9N2 infection would be exacerbated by cigarette smoke exposure, and we also used nicotine to mimic the effect of cigarette smoke.

Materials and Methods

Ethics Statement

Written consent for the use of buffy coat for research purposes was obtained from the donors by the Hong Kong Red Cross Blood Transfusion Services at the time of blood donation. The use of buffy coat for this experiment was approved by the Institutional Review Board of the University of Hong Kong/Hospital Authority Hong Kong West Cluster (IRB reference number: UW 07–390).

All manipulations on animal work in this manuscript were performed in compliance with "Code of Practice for Care and Use of Animals for Experimental Purposes (2004)" and approved by the Committee on the Use of Live Animals in Teaching and Research (CULATR), the University of Hong Kong (reference number: 2631-12 and 2819-12).

Influenza virus preparation and titration

Influenza virus A/California/04/2009 (pdmH1N1) was grown in embryonated chicken eggs. Influenza virus A/Quail/Hong Kong/G1/97 (H9N2) was propagated in Madin-Darby canine kidney (MDCK) cells with modified Eagle's medium (Invitrogen, Grand Island, NY, USA) containing 2 mg/L N-Tosyl-L-Phenylalanine Chloromethyl Ketone-treated trypsin (Sigma, St. Louis, MO, USA). MDCK cell line was purchased from ATCC (American Type Culture Collection, Manassas, VA, USA) and routinely maintained in our lab. Viruses were purified by ultracentrifugation as described previously [20,22]. The virus titer was determined by titration in MDCK cells, with daily observation of cytopathogenic effect, and confirmed by hemagglutination assay. The tissue culture infective dose affecting 50% of the cultures ($TCID_{50}$)/ml was calculated by the Reed-Muench formula.

Smoking mouse model and virus infection

Female C57B6/N mice of 6–8 weeks were obtained from Laboratory Animal Unit, the University of Hong Kong; α7 nAChR knockout mice and wild-type mice were purchased from the Jackson Laboratory. The mice were exposed to 4% (vol/vol, smoke/air) cigarette smoke for 2 hours per episode, 2 episodes per day with commercially available cigarette (Camel; filters, Japan Tobacco INC) for 21 days (Fig. 1A) using the modified ventilated cigarette smoke exposure chambers as described [23,24]. Control mice were exposed only to fresh air (0%, vol/vol, smoke/air) in another ventilated chamber with the same procedure. Fourteen hours after the last cigarette smoke exposure, the mice were anesthetized and inoculated intranasally with 30 μl of 5×10^3 $TCID_{50}$ pdmH1N1, or 10^5 $TCID_{50}$ H9N2 virus. Simultaneously, control mice were treated with PBS in the same way. The well-being of animals was monitored three times daily after cigarette smoke exposure and influenza virus infection. The criteria that we used to monitor the well-being of the mice including appearance, food and water intake, clinical signs (temperature, cardiac and respiratory rates) and behavior (natural or provoked). The mice were humanely euthanized when they showed any one of the following termination criteria: body weight loss ≥30%, body temperature ±2°C, cardiac/respiratory rate ±50%, and sign of severe pneumonia (very weak and pre-comatose). All animal care and experimental protocols were conducted in accordance with the CULATR guidelines of the University of Hong Kong.

These results demonstrated that the peak mortality in the control mice on day 5 post-pdmH1N1 infection might partially be attributed to the hyper-cytokine response. This mortality was significantly reduced by cigarette smoke exposure, which might be due to the significantly decreased production of inflammatory cytokines, as well as reduced pulmonary tissues pathology. The immunosuppressive effect of cigarette smoke exposure was independent of virus replication.

Quantitation of cotinine

The half-life of nicotine is very short and will be metabolized into different metabolites. The average eradication half-life of nicotine in mouse plasma is approximately 6–7 minutes and cotinine is the major stable metabolite of nicotine [25]. Then serum level of cotinine instead of nicotine was measured using commercially available kit (Neogen, KY, USA) following the manufacturer's instructions. All measurements were performed in duplicate.

Preparation of mouse lung homogenates

The mouse lungs were harvested at the specific time points and homogenized using a tissue homogenizer (Omni International, Kennesaw, GA, USA) as previously described [20,26]. The homogenates were centrifuged at 1500 *g* for 10 minutes at 4°C. The supernatants were collected and separated into aliquots. Virus titer was determined immediately and the remaining supernatants were stored at −70°C for cytokines and chemokines detection.

Cytokines and chemokines determination

Expression levels of interleukin (IL) 1α, IL-1β, IL-2, IL-4, IL-5, IL-6, IL-8, IL-10, IL-17, IL-18, tumor necrosis factor (TNF) α, interferon (IFN) γ, granulocyte-macrophage colony-stimulating factor (GM-CSF), keratinocyte chemoattractant (KC), monocyte chemotactic protein (MCP) 1, MCP-3, macrophage inflammatory proteins (MIP) 1α, MIP-1β, monokine induced by interferon gamma (MIG), regulated and normal T-cell expressed and secreted (RANTES) in the lung homogenates or cell supernatants were quantitatively determined by flow cytometry based immunoassay (eBioscience, San Diego, CA, USA) according to the manufacturer's protocol [20]. The samples were acquired on a LSRII (BD, San Diego, CA, USA) and the amount (ng/ml) was calculated by FlowCytomix™ Pro 3.0 software (eBioscience).

Pulmonary histopathology

The lung tissues were fixed in 10% formalin, embedded in paraffin, cut and stained with hematoxylin and eosin to analyze inflammation-associated lung damage. Histopathologic inflammation score of lung tissues was evaluated by a board-certified pathologist blinded to experimental design. Lung inflammatory changes were graded using a semi-quantitative scoring system based on the following parameters: peri-bronchiolar and bronchial infiltrates, bronchiolar and bronchial luminal exudates, perivascular infiltrates, parenchymal pneumonia, and edema, as previously described [20,27]. Each parameter was graded on a scale of 0–4 with 0, absent; 1, slight; 2, mild; 3, moderate; and 4, severe. The total lung inflammation score was expressed as the sum of the scores for each parameter. The degree of cell infiltration was

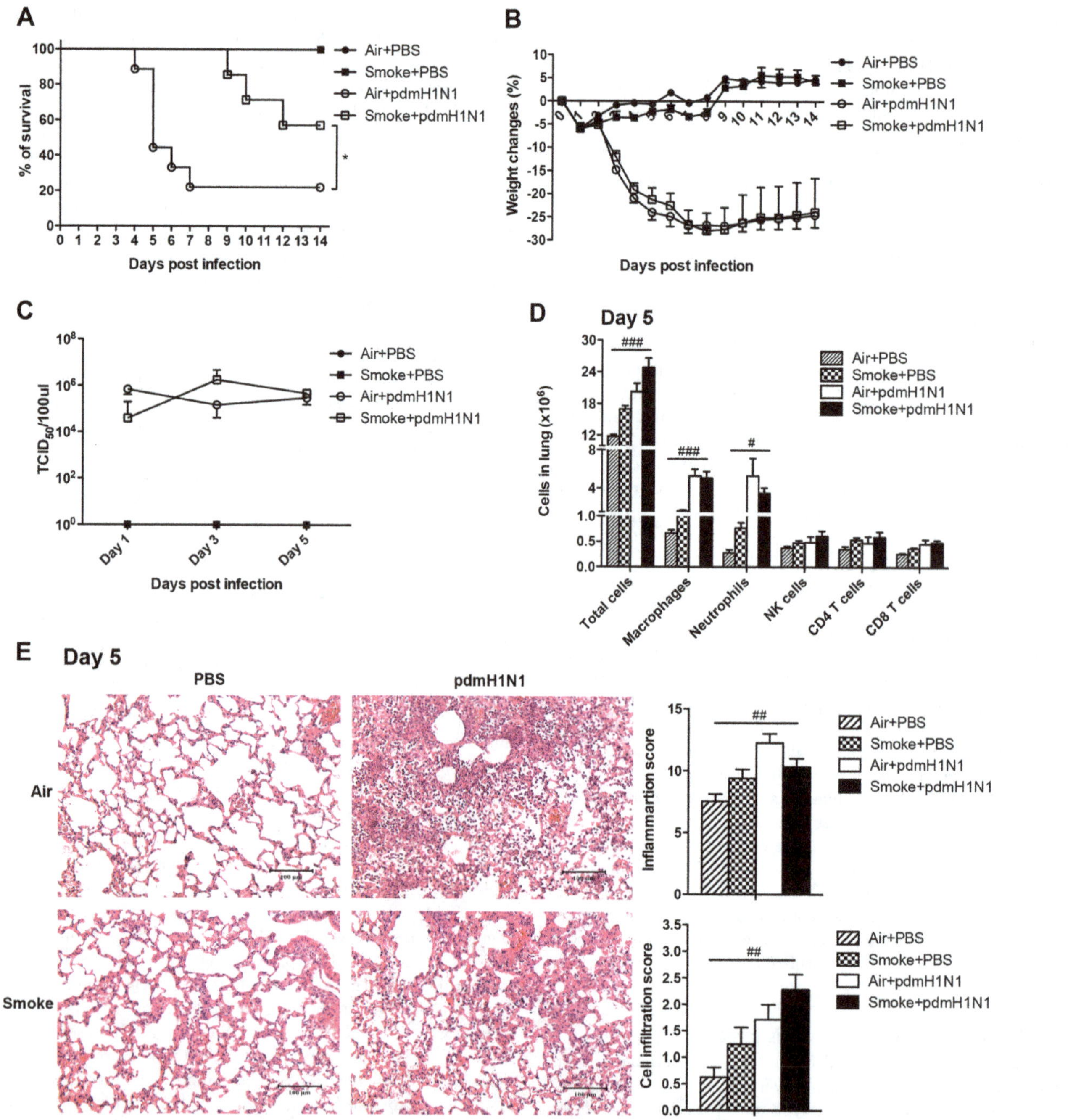

Figure 2. Cigarette smoke exposure decreased the severity of pdmH1N1 infection in mice. The mice were exposed to room air or cigarette smoke for 21 days and then infected with pdmH1N1 virus. A) Survival curve of mice infected with pdmH1N1 virus. There were 6-9 mice per group. Data are representative of three independent experiments. B) Body weight changes of mice infected with pdmH1N1 virus. There were 6–9 mice per group. Data are representative of three independent experiments. C) Lung virus titers of pdmH1N1 infected mice. There were 4–10 mice per group. Data are representative of two independent experiments. D) Absolute number of lung cells on day 5 of pdmH1N1 infection. Macrophages ($CD11b^+$, $F4/80^+$), neutrophils ($CD11b^+$, $Ly\text{-}6G^+$), NK cells ($CD3^-$, $NK1.1^+$), $CD4^+$ T cells ($CD3^+$, $CD4^+$) and $CD8^+$ T cells ($CD3^+$, $CD8a^+$). There were 4–5 mice per group. E) Histopathological analysis of pulmonary tissues collected on day 5 of pdmH1N1 infection. Results are representative pictures (200X) of hematoxylin and eosin stained pulmonary tissues. Scale bar: 100 μm. Inflammation score and cell infiltration score were evaluated by a board-certified pathologist. There were 4–8 mice per group. Data are representative of two independent experiments. Results represent mean ± SEM. *$p<0.05$ was determined by Log-rank (Mantel-Cox) test; $^{\#}p<0.05$, $^{\#\#}p<0.01$; $^{\#\#\#}p<0.001$ were tested by ANOVA of four groups.

independently scored of 0–3 with 0, no cells; 1, few cells; 2, moderate influx of cells; and 3, extensive influx of cells [20,26].

To summarize, after H9N2 virus infection, cigarette smoke exposed mice had less weight loss, possibly due to less cytokines production, lower cellular infiltration and less lung damage compared to the control mice.

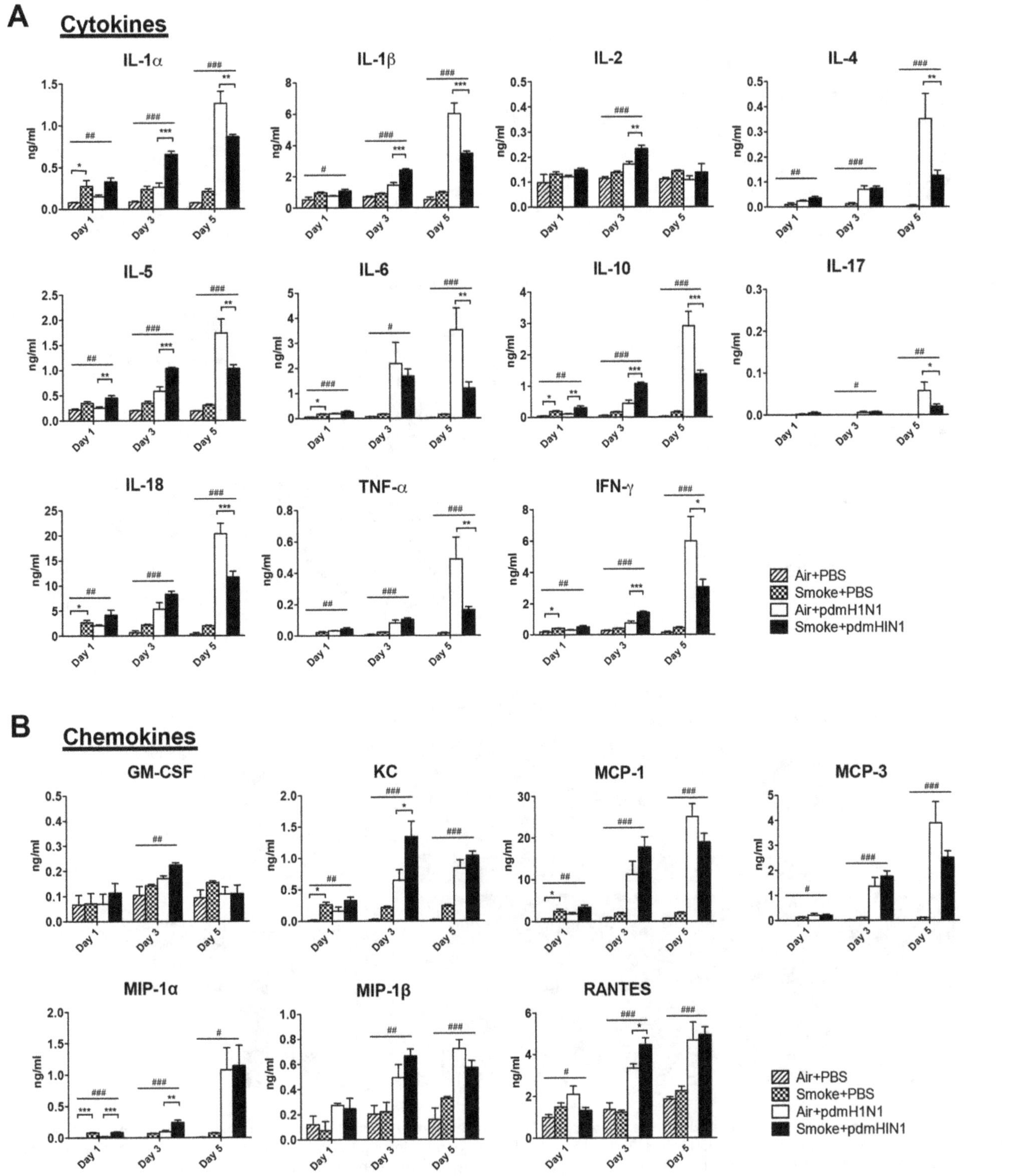

Figure 3. Cigarette smoke exposure suppressed the production of cytokines at later time point of pdmH1N1 infection. The mice were exposed to room air or cigarette smoke for 21 days and then infected with pdmH1N1 virus. The lungs were collected on day 1, 3 and 5 after pdmH1N1 infection. A) The production of cytokines. B) The production of chemokines. Results represent mean ± SEM of 4–10 mice per group. Data are representative of two independent experiments. $^{\#}p<0.05$, $^{\#\#}p<0.01$; $^{\#\#\#}p<0.001$ were tested by ANOVA of four groups; $^{*}p<0.05$; $^{**}p<0.01$; $^{***}p<0.001$ were determined by Tukey post hoc test.

Lung cells isolation and flow cytometric analysis

The mouse lungs were cut into small pieces and incubated in Iscove's Modified Dulbecco's Medium (Invitrogen) containing 1mg/ml collagenase D (Roche, Mannheim, Germany) and 20 U/ml DNase I (Roche) at 37°C with shaking for 1–2 hours. After treating with Ammonium-Chloride-Potassium lysing buffer and

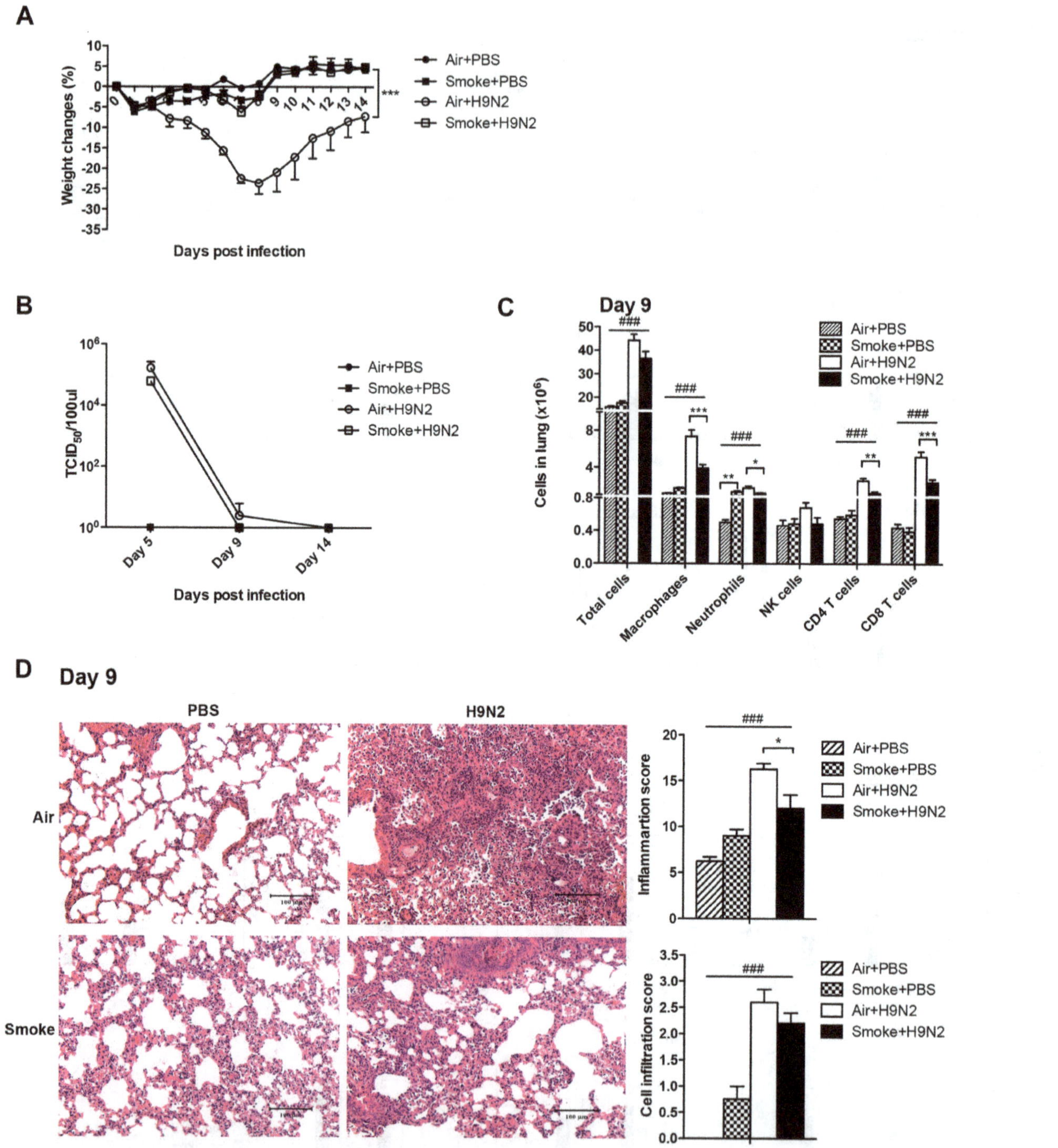

Figure 4. Cigarette smoke exposure reduced the severity of H9N2 infection in mice. The mice were exposed to room air or cigarette smoke for 21 days and then infected with H9N2 virus. A) Body weight changes of mice infected with H9N2 virus. There were 6–7 mice per group. Data are representative of three independent experiments. ***$p<0.001$ was compared between Air+H9N2 and Smoke+H9N2 and was examined by multiple regression analysis adjusted for time. B) Lung virus titers of H9N2 infected mice. There were 4–7 mice per group. C) Absolute number of lung cells on day 9 of H9N2 infection. Macrophages ($CD11b^+$, $F4/80^+$), neutrophils ($CD11b^+$, $Ly\text{-}6G^+$), NK cells ($CD3^-$, $NK1.1^+$), $CD4^+$ T cells ($CD3^+$, $CD4^+$) and $CD8^+$ T cells ($CD3^+$, $CD8a^+$). There were 4–5 mice per group. D) Histopathological analysis of pulmonary tissues collected on day 9 of H9N2 infection. Results are representative pictures (200X) of hematoxylin and eosin stained pulmonary tissues. Scale bar: 100 μm. Inflammation score and cell infiltration score were evaluated by a board-certified pathologist. There were 4 mice per group. Results represent mean ± SEM. ###$p<0.001$ was tested by ANOVA of four groups; *$p<0.05$; **$p<0.01$; ***$p<0.001$ were determined by Tukey post hoc test (C and D).

filtering by a 70 μm nylon mesh, 1×10^6 cells were stained with a combination of monoclonal antibodies (mAbs) of PE-Cy5-anti-CD11b (M1/70, eBioscience), eFluor 450-anti-F4/80 (BM8, eBioscience), and Alexa Fluor 700-anti-Ly-6G (RB6-8C5, eBioscience); or a combination of mAbs of eFluor 450-anti-CD3 (17A2, eBioscience), FITC-anti-NK1.1 (PK136, BioLegend, San

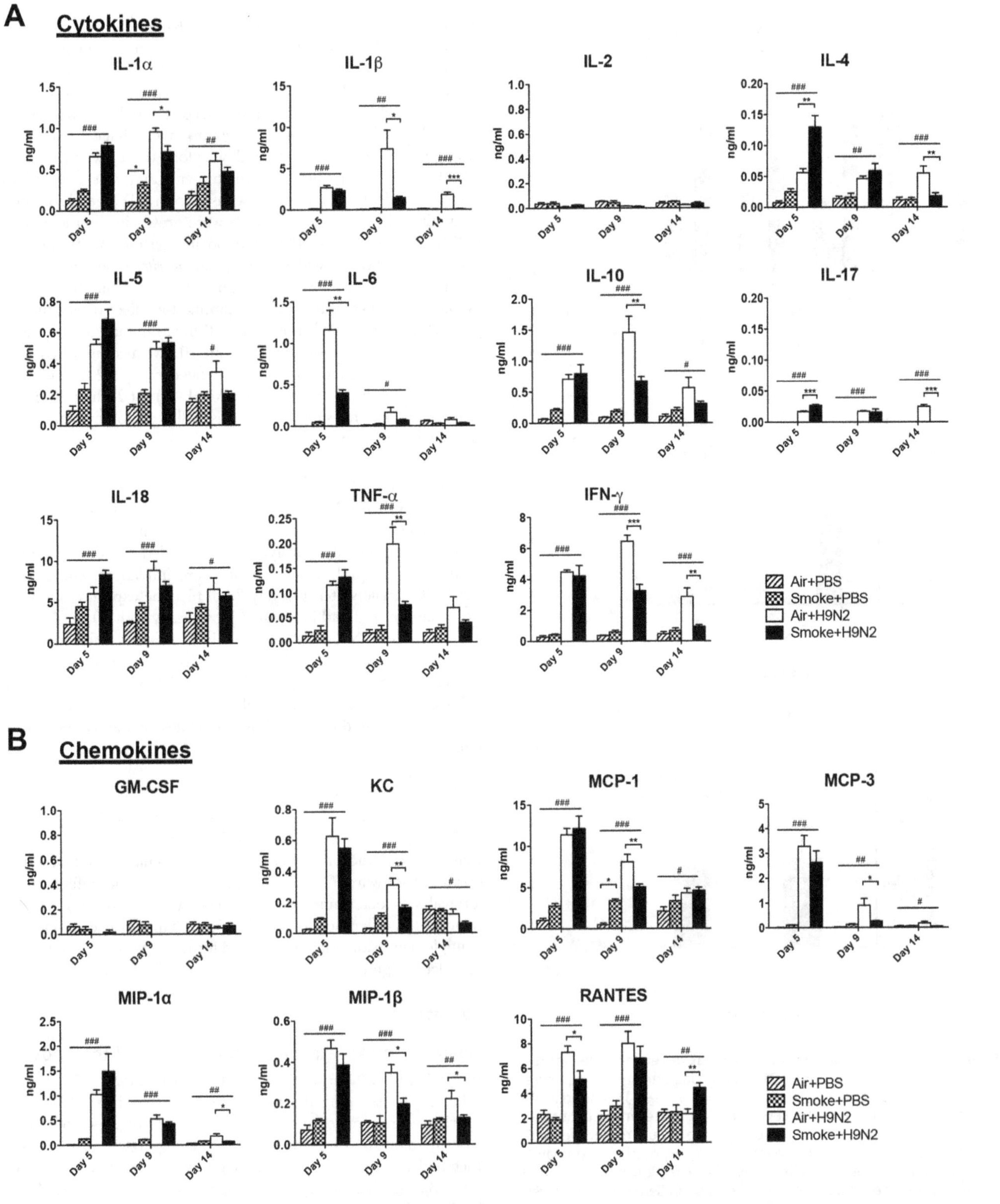

Figure 5. Cigarette smoke exposure suppressed the production of cytokines and chemokines of H9N2 infected mice. The mice were exposed to room air or cigarette smoke for 21 days and then infected with H9N2 virus. The lungs were collected on day 5, 9 and 14 after H9N2 infection. A) The production of cytokines. B) The production of chemokines. Results represent mean ± SEM of 4–7 mice per group. $^{\#}p<0.05$, $^{\#\#}p<0.01$; $^{\#\#\#}p<0.001$ were tested by ANOVA of four groups; $^{*}p<0.05$; $^{**}p<0.01$; $^{***}p<0.001$ were determined by Tukey post hoc test.

Diego, CA, USA), PE-anti-CD4 (RM4-5, BD), and APC-anti-CD8a (53-6.7, BD); or their relevant isotype-specific antibodies as described previously [26,28]. Before running samples, counting beads were added into the stained cells (Molecular Probes, Carlsbad, CA, USA). All samples were acquired on LSR II and analyzed by FlowJo software (TreeStar, Ashland, OR, USA).

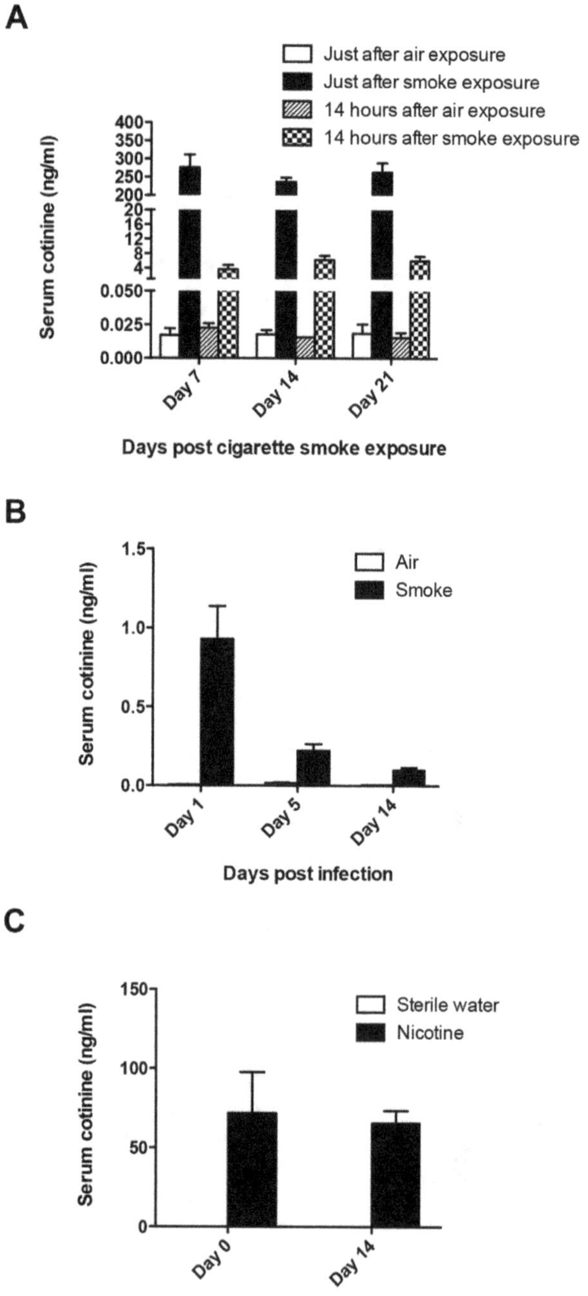

Figure 6. Mouse serum cotinine levels at different time points. A) Serum cotinine levels during 21 days of cigarette smoke exposure. The serum samples were collected on day 7, day 14 and day 21 (immediately or 14 hours after cessation of cigarette smoke exposure). (n = 2 and n = 4 for air and smoke exposure group respectively). B) Serum cotinine levels of air or cigarette smoke exposed mice on day 1, day 5 and day 14 after pdmH1N1/H9N2 virus infection. (n = 2 and n = 4 for air and smoke exposure group respectively). C) Serum cotinine levels of sterile water or nicotine treated mice on day 0 and day 14 after pdmH1N1/H9N2 virus infection. (n = 4 for both sterile water and nicotine treatment groups). Results represent mean ± SEM.

Nicotine treatment and virus infection of the cells.

Peripheral blood mononuclear cells (PBMC) were isolated from buffy coat of healthy donors (from Hong Kong Red Cross) by Lymphoprep™ (Fresenius Kabi Norge AS) gradient centrifugation. The research protocol was approved by the Institutional Review Board of the University of Hong Kong/Hospital Authority Hong Kong West Cluster. Primary human macrophages were generated from PBMC as described [29]. Briefly, the monocytes were cultured in RPMI 1640 medium (Invitrogen) supplemented with 5% autologous serum and were seeded into the 24-well plates, cultured for 14 days to differentiate into macrophages. The purity of monocytes was examined by flow cytometry (LSRII) with anti-CD14 monoclonal antibody (Invitrogen), and was consistently over 90%. A549 cell line was purchased from ATCC and routinely maintained in our lab. A549 cells were grown in the medium of RPMI 1640 contains 10% fetal bovine serum. A549 cells are cancer cells and are widely used as an *in vitro* model for type II pulmonary epithelial cells [30]. Thus primary human macrophages and A549 cells were used to examine the effect of nicotine on pdmH1N1 or H9N2 virus infection. Primary human macrophages and A549 cells were pre-treated with 10 μM nicotine (Sigma) or PBS for 72 h with the medium changed every 12 h; and then infected with pdmH1N1 or H9N2 (MOI = 2). At 24 h or 48 h post virus infection, the supernatant was collected for cytokines and chemokines measurement.

Nicotine *in vivo* study

Female C57B6/N mice of 6–8 weeks were anesthetized and implanted with Alzet (Cupertino, CA, USA) micro-osmotic pumps (model 1004) subcutaneously, which provided nicotine at rate of 24 mg/kg/day [31]. Control mice were implanted with pumps filled with sterile water. On day 22 of nicotine exposure, the mice were anesthetized and inoculated intranasally with 30 μl of 5×10^3 $TCID_{50}$ pdmH1N1, or 10^5 $TCID_{50}$ H9N2 viruses. After infection, the mice were weighed and monitored every day. The pumps kept deliver nicotine after pdmH1N1 or H9N2 virus infection. All animal care and experimental protocols were conducted in accordance with the CULATR guidelines of the University of Hong Kong.

Statistical analysis

Data are expressed as mean ± SEM. Statistical analysis was performed by unpaired two-tailed Student's *t test* or one-way analysis of variance (ANOVA) followed by Tukey post hoc test in Prism 5.0 software (GraphPad). The p value of the difference for survival was determined by Log-rank (Mantel-Cox) test. The p value of the difference for body weight change was examined by multiple regression analysis adjusted for time. A p value <0.05 was considered significant.

Results

Cigarette smoke exposure alone decreased the body weight gain and elevated lung inflammation

Before investigating the impact of influenza virus infection in cigarette smoke exposed mice, the influence of cigarette smoke exposure alone on mice was determined. Cigarette smoke exposed mice had significantly less body weight gain than the control mice (Fig. 1B). Significantly higher production of IL-1α, IL-2, IL-4, IL-5, IL-6, IL-10, IL-18, TNF-α, IFN-γ, GM-CSF, KC, MCP-1, MCP-3, MIP-1α, MIP-1β and RANTES were shown in cigarette smoke exposed mice than that in control mice (Fig. 1C). Cigarette smoke exposed mice had increased lung damage than control mice, with thickening of intra-alveolar septa and hemorrhages. Moreover, cigarette smoke exposure significantly increased the inflammation score and mildly enhanced the cell infiltration score (Fig. 1D). For the lung cell composition, there were no differences for the number of total cells, macrophages, neutrophils, NK cells,

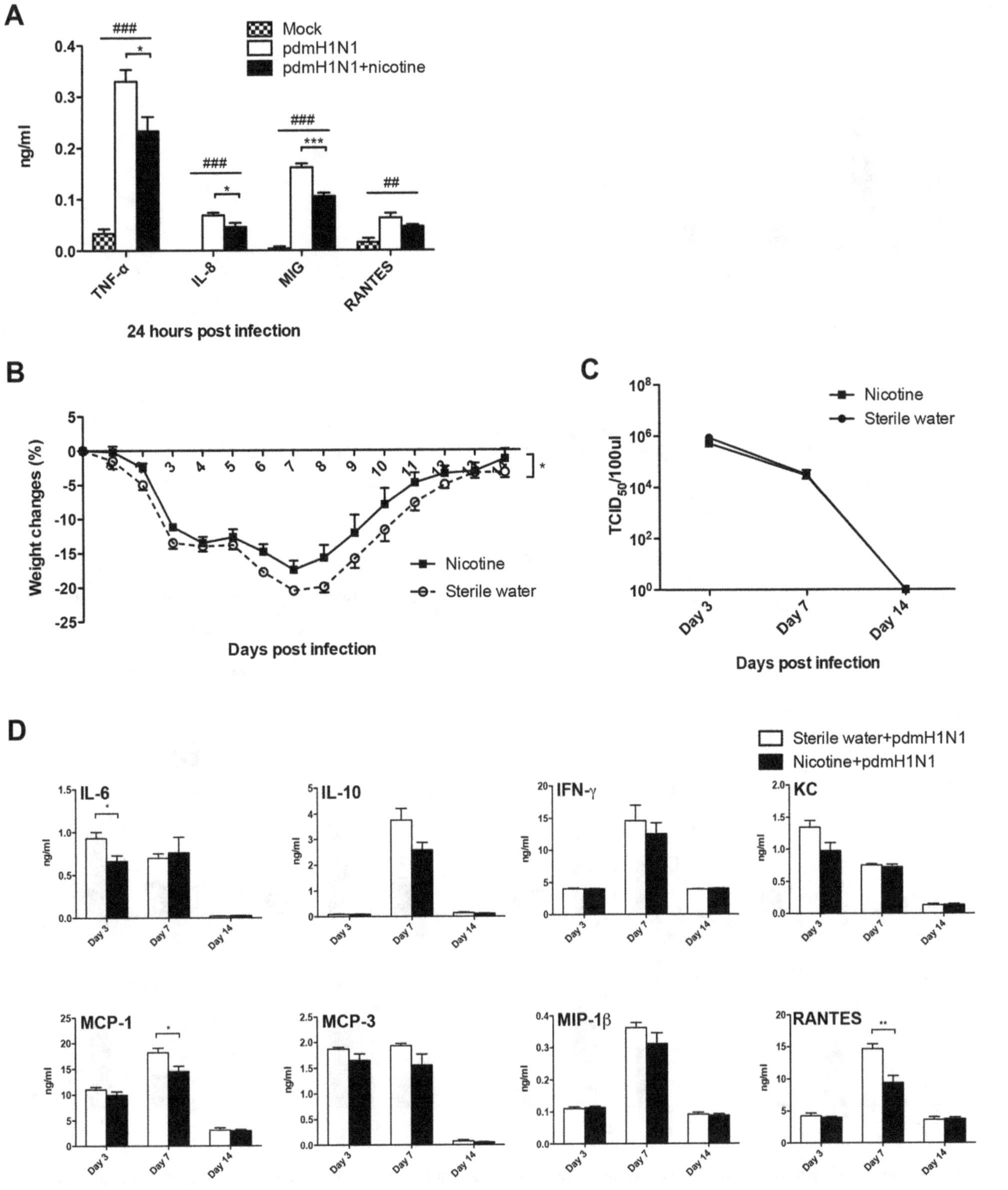

Figure 7. Nicotine suppressed the inflammatory response induced by pdmH1N1 infection *in vitro* and *in vivo*. A) Nicotine inhibited the pdmH1N1-induced production of cytokines and chemokines in primary human macrophages. Primary human macrophages were pre-treated with 10 μM nicotine for 72 h, and then infected with pdmH1N1 virus. Data represent 4–5 independent experiments. ##$p<0.01$ and ###$p<0.001$ were tested by ANOVA of three groups; *$p<0.05$ and ***$p<0.001$ were determined by Tukey post hoc test. B) Body weight changes of nicotine treated mice after pdmH1N1 virus infection. The mice were pre-treated with nicotine subcutaneously for 21 days and then infected by pdmH1N1 virus. There were 5 mice per group. Data are representative of two independent experiments. *$p<0.05$ was examined by multiple regression analysis adjusted for time. C) Lung virus titers of nicotine treated mice at indicated time points after pdmH1N1 infection. There were 4 mice per group. D) Production of cytokines and chemokines in the lung homogenates from nicotine treated mice after pdmH1N1 virus infection. There were 4–5 mice per group. *$p<0.05$ and **$p<0.01$ were performed by unpaired two-tailed Student's *t test*. Results represent mean ± SEM.

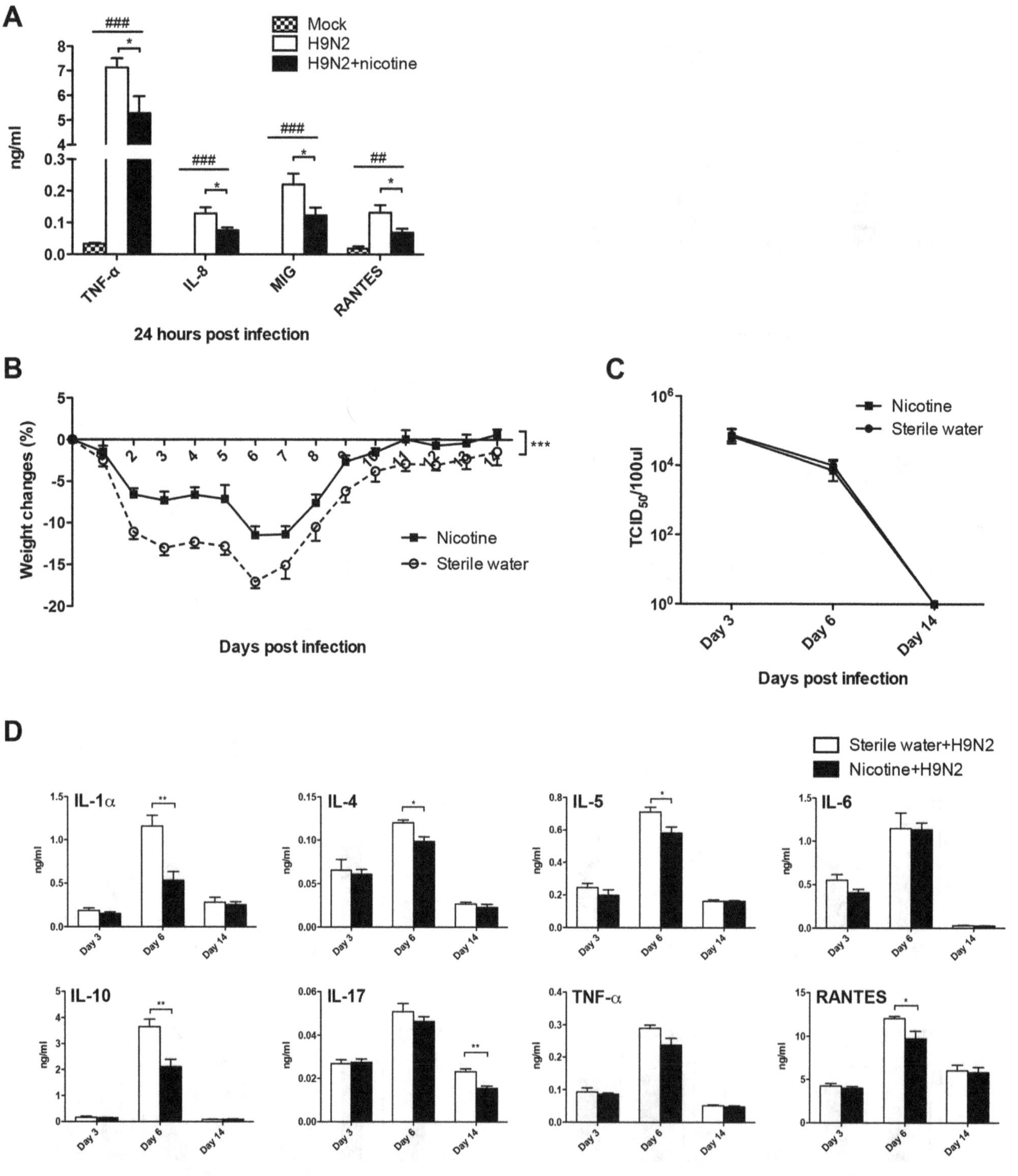

Figure 8. Nicotine inhibited the inflammatory response induced by H9N2 infection *in vitro* and *in vivo*. A) Nicotine suppressed the H9N2-induced production of cytokines and chemokines in primary human macrophages. Primary human macrophages were pre-treated with 10 μM nicotine for 72 h, and then infected with H9N2 virus. Data represent 4–5 independent experiments. $^{\#\#}p<0.01$ and $^{\#\#\#}p<0.001$ were tested by ANOVA of three groups; $^{*}p<0.05$ was determined by Tukey post hoc test. B) Body weight changes of nicotine treated mice after H9N2 virus infection. The mice were pre-treated with nicotine subcutaneously for 21 days and then infected by H9N2 virus. There were 5 mice per group. Data are representative of two independent experiments. $^{***}p<0.001$ was examined by multiple regression analysis adjusted for time. C) Lung virus titers of nicotine treated mice at indicated time points after H9N2 infection. There were 4 mice per group. D) Production of cytokines and chemokines in the lung homogenates from nicotine treated mice after H9N2 virus infection. There were 4–5 mice per group. $^{*}p<0.05$ and $^{**}p<0.01$ were performed by unpaired two-tailed Student's *t test*. Results represent mean ± SEM.

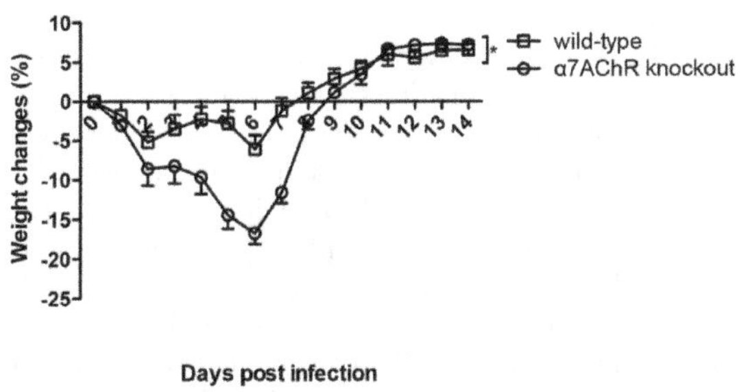

Figure 9. Cigarette smoke exposure resulted in increased body weight loss in α7 nAChR knockout mice as compared to wild-type mice after H9N2 virus infection. Wild-type and α7 nAChR knockout mice were exposed to cigarette smoke for 21 days and then infected with H9N2 virus. The body weight changes were monitored for 14 days. Results represent mean ± SEM. N = 4 and n = 6 for α7 nAChR knockout and wild-type mice respectively. $^{*}p<0.05$ was determined by multiple regression analysis adjusted for time.

$CD4^+$ T cells and $CD8^+$ T cells between cigarette smoke exposed mice and control mice (Fig. 1E).

Collectively, cigarette smoke exposure could induce less body weight gain, which might be attributed to up-regulated production of inflammatory cytokines, and increased lung damage compared with the control mice. However, cigarette smoke exposure could not change the lung cell composition.

Mortality rate of pdmH1N1 infection was decreased by prior cigarette smoke exposure

In order to investigate the role of upregulated inflammation caused by the prior cigarette smoke exposure on the subsequent influenza A virus infection, the mice were infected with pdmH1N1 virus after 21 days of cigarette smoke exposure. Cigarette smoke exposure significantly decreased the mice mortality (Fig. 2A) but had no effect on body weight changes (Fig. 2B) compared to air exposure after pdmH1N1 infection. Because the mice began to die on day 4, early time points of day 1, 3, and 5 after pdmH1N1 infection were selected for the following measurements. There was no difference for lung virus titer at all time points between air and cigarette smoke exposed mice upon pdmH1N1 infection (Fig. 2C). After pdmH1N1 virus infection, cigarette smoke exposed mice had significantly higher production of IL-1α, IL-1β, IL-2, IFN-γ, KC, RANTES on day 3; IL-5, IL-10 and MIP-1α both on day 1 and day 3 in the lungs than the control mice. However on day 5, the phenomenon was reversed, cigarette smoke exposed mice produced significantly lower cytokines than the control mice, including IL-1α, IL-1β, IL-4, IL-5, IL-6, IL-10, IL-17, IL-18, TNF-α and IFN-γ (Fig. 3). For lung cell composition, cigarette smoke exposure could not affect the number of total cells, macrophages, neutrophils, NK cells, $CD4^+$ T cells and $CD8^+$ T cells in the lung on day 5 after pdmH1N1 infection (Fig. 2D). Less lung damage was observed in cigarette smoke exposed mice on day 5 after pdmH1N1 infection than the control mice; however, the difference was not statistically significant (Fig. 2E).

Severity of H9N2 infection was reduced by prior cigarette smoke exposure

To further investigate whether the immunosuppressive effect of cigarette smoke exposure was independent of influenza subtypes, we tested avian H9N2 virus. Cigarette smoke exposed mice showed significantly lower body weight loss than the control mice (Fig. 4A). There was no death from H9N2 infection; the mice were sacrificed on day 5, 9 and 14 post-infection and the mouse lungs were collected for the following measurements. There was no difference for virus titer at all time points between air and cigarette smoke exposed mice after H9N2 infection (Fig. 4B). For inflammatory response, cigarette smoke exposed mice had significantly lower production of IL-1α, IL-1β, IL-10, TNF-α, IFN-γ, KC, MCP-1, MCP-3 and MIP-1β on day 9, IL-6 and RANTES on day 5 after H9N2 infection compared with the control mice (Fig. 5). Cigarette smoke exposed mice displayed significantly less number of macrophages, neutrophils, $CD4^+$ T cells and $CD8^+$ T cells than the control mice on day 9 after H9N2 infection (Fig. 4C). Moreover, significantly less lung damage was observed in cigarette smoke exposed mice than in control mice on day 9 after H9N2 infection (Fig. 4D).

PdmH1N1-induced inflammatory response and disease severity were suppressed by nicotine *in vitro* and *in vivo* respectively

The above data demonstrated that the severity of pdmH1N1 or H9N2 infection was alleviated by cigarette smoke exposure via decreasing the inflammatory response. The underlying mechanisms were further investigated. Nicotine is one of the major components in cigarette smoke but its half-life is short. The serum concentration of cotinine, a major metabolite of nicotine, was about 250 ng/ml, which was comparable to the serum cotinine levels in cigarette smokers [32], immediately after cessation of cigarette smoke exposure, and decreased to around 4 ng/ml at 14 hour after cessation of cigarette smoke exposure (Fig. 6A). Moreover, the mean serum cotinine concentration was 0.93 ng/ml, 0.22 ng/ml and 0.10 ng/ml on day 1, day 5 and day 14 post pdmH1N1 or H9N2 virus infection respectively (Fig. 6B). This data demonstrated that the effect of nicotine might be on-going during the 14 days of pdmH1N1 or H9N2 virus infection. Then we hypothesized that it is nicotine in cigarette smoke that might be responsible for the immunosuppressive effect.

We firstly used *in vitro* method to test our hypothesis. In primary human macrophages, pdmH1N1-induced production of TNF-α, IL-8 and MIG was significantly inhibited by nicotine (Fig. 7A). In the human lung alveolar epithelial cell line A549, nicotine could decrease the production of MCP-1 at 24 h, IL-8 at 48 h post-pdmH1N1 infection respectively (Fig. S1A). For the *in vivo* study, we chose the dose of 24 mg/kg/day because the serum cotinine concentration was maintained at around 70 ng/ml both on day 0 and day 14 after pdmH1N1 or H9N2 virus infection (Fig. 6C), which was within the range of serum cotinine concentration of the cigarette smoke exposure group (Fig. 6A). Our data demonstrated that there was no death in both sterile water and nicotine delivery groups after pdmH1N1 infection. However, nicotine treated mice had significantly less body weight loss after pdmH1N1 infection compared to control mice (Fig. 7B). There was no difference for lung virus titer at indicated time points between nicotine treated and control mice after pdmH1N1 infection (Fig. 7C). For the inflammatory response, nicotine treated mice had significantly less production of IL-6 on day 3, MCP-1 and RANTES on day 7 after pdmH1N1 infection compared with control mice (Fig. 7D). In summary, the inflammatory response and disease severity induced by pdmH1N1 virus could be suppressed by nicotine.

H9N2-induced inflammatory response and disease severity were inhibited by nicotine *in vitro* and *in vivo* respectively

We further investigated whether the immunosuppressive effect of nicotine was independent of influenza subtypes and then tested

H9N2 virus. H9N2 induced expression of TNF-α, IL-8, MIG and RANTES was significantly suppressed by nicotine in primary human macrophages (Fig. 8A). Nicotine could also suppress the expression of IL-8 at 24 h post-H9N2 infection in A549 cells (Fig. S1B). There was no mortality in both sterile water and nicotine delivery groups after H9N2 infection. However, nicotine treated mice had significantly less body weight loss after H9N2 infection compared to control mice (Fig. 8B). There was no difference for lung virus titer at indicated time points between nicotine treated and control mice after H9N2 infection (Fig. 8C). For the inflammatory response, nicotine could suppress the secretion of IL-1α, IL-4, IL-5, IL-10 and RANTES on day 6 and IL-17 on day 14 significantly after H9N2 infection compared with control mice (Fig. 8D). Taken together, nicotine had immunosuppressive effect on H9N2 infection.

Cigarette smoke exposure resulted in increased body weight loss in α7 nAChR knockout mice as compared to wild-type mice after H9N2 virus infection

Nicotine exerts its immunosuppressive effect by binding to α7 nAChR and hence activating cholinergic anti-inflammatory pathway [14]. In order to further test the hypothesis that it is nicotine in cigarette smoke that might be responsible for the immunosuppressive effect, we used α7 nAChR knockout mice and wild-type mice to perform the mechanistic study. Wild-type and α7 nAChR knockout mice were exposed to cigarette smoke for 21 days and then infected with H9N2 virus at fourteen hours after the last cigarette smoke exposure. Our data demonstrated that cigarette smoke exposure resulted in significantly increased body weight loss in α7 nAChR knockout mice than in wild-type mice after H9N2 virus infection (Fig. 9).

Discussion

The present study demonstrated that cigarette smoke exposure alone up-regulated the mouse lung inflammation. The pathogenicity caused by pdmH1N1 or H9N2 virus infection was alleviated by such prior cigarette smoke exposure. The beneficial effect was due to the immunosuppressive effect of cigarette smoke exposure that down-regulated the influenza virus induced hyper-inflammatory response. Indeed, the immunosuppressive effect of cigarette smoke has been previously reported, including macrophages extracted from smokers or smoke exposed mice have reduced inflammation in response to LPS or poly I:C stimulation [33,34]. Furthermore, this study demonstrated that the immunosuppressive effect of cigarette smoke was partially attributed to nicotine.

Our findings of the beneficial effect of cigarette smoke exposure in pdmH1N1 and H9N2 virus infected mice are contrary to the current epidemiological evidence that showed the mortality and hospitalization rates were increased in smokers who had seasonal influenza infection [15,16,19]. This discrepancy could be explained by both viral and host determinants. Both 2009 pdmH1N1 and H9N2 viruses, that crossed species from swine and bird to human respectively, are more virulent than seasonal influenza virus [35,36]. Therefore, epidemiological data regarding the impact of cigarette smoke on seasonal influenza virus infection might not be applicable to pdmH1N1 and H9N2 virus directly. There is an urgent need to conduct epidemiological investigations to fully understand the impact of smoking on the severity of pdmH1N1 or H9N2 virus infection.

The interaction of cigarette smoke exposure and influenza virus infection in mouse model is complex. Due to the differences in the composition of cigarette smoke, the method and duration of smoke exposure, the dose and subtypes of the influenza A virus, the results of different animal studies might be contradictory. Gualano *et al.*, using BALB/C mice exposed to smoke with 9 Winfield Red cigarettes per day for 4 days, and infected with H3N1 virus, found that smoke exposure prior to influenza virus infection led to more lung inflammation, higher viral burden and greater body weight loss [37]. Another study, using C57BL/6 mice exposed to 1R3 cigarettes smoke for 3–5 months and infected with low dose or high dose H1N1-A/FM/1/47, demonstrated that cigarette smoke attenuated the inflammatory response to low dose virus infection, while high dose infection resulted in higher inflammation and significant morbidity [38]. Our study, using C57BL/6 mice, ventilated cigarette smoke exposure system, 21 days of cigarette smoke exposure and pdmH1N1 or H9N2 virus, demonstrated that prior cigarette smoke exposure decreased the severity of influenza virus infection by attenuating the hyper-inflammatory response.

Inflammation is a double-edged sword; adequate inflammation is necessary for the development of immune response, clearance of pathogens and recovery from tissue injuries, while excessive inflammatory response would be life threatening. PdmH1N1 and H9N2 influenza viruses could produce excessive inflammatory cytokines compared with seasonal influenza virus [35,36], which might contribute to the more severe disease. In support with these observation, here, we also found that, comparing with cigarette smoke exposed mice, control mice had hyper-inflammatory response with higher production of several cytokines, including IL-1α, IL-1β, IL-6, IL-10, TNF-α and IFN-γ on day 5 of pdmH1N1 and day 9 of H9N2 infection, coinciding with the mice having peak mortality and body weight loss respectively. Other studies also demonstrated the deleterious role of dysregulation of cytokines. Enhanced secretion of IL-1α and IL-1β could lead to acute pulmonary inflammatory pathology upon influenza A virus infection in mouse model [39]. Elevated IL-6 levels are associated with disease severity triggered by pdmH1N1 infection in mice [40]. Anti-TNF-α agents could decrease lung inflammation and prolong survival of A/PR/8 infected mice; reduce weight loss and illness severity in mice upon influenza A X31 infection [41]. The expression of IFN-γ is significantly increased in pdmH1N1 infected patients [42]. The deleterious role of hyper-production of IL-10 is supported by IL-10 deficiency mice having enhanced survival upon high-dose influenza virus infection [43]. In our study, cigarette smoke exposure significantly suppressed the production of these inflammatory cytokines after pdmH1N1 and H9N2 infection, leading to the decreased inflammatory response in the lung. The suppressed inflammation can explain the lower mortality after pdmH1N1 infection; less body weight loss, lung injury and immune cells infiltration after H9N2 infection in cigarette smoke exposed mice.

The cell types infiltrating into the lung were mostly neutrophils and macrophages at early time points, with lymphocytes predominant at later time points of infection in our study (data not shown). The hyper-expression of chemokines, such as KC, MCP-1, MCP-3 and MIP-1β in control mice might coordinate the increased recruitment of neutrophils and macrophages on day 9 post-H9N2 infection. Moreover, the increased production of RANTES on day 5, which is chemotactic for T cells, might contribute to higher infiltration of $CD4^+$ and $CD8^+$ T cells in the control mice at day 9 after H9N2 infection. IL-6, except for its role in resolution of innate immunity, is also an important cytokine to regulate the shift from innate immune response to adaptive immune response and enhance the proliferation of T cells and influenza-specific T memory cells [44,45]. Therefore, the significantly higher production of IL-6 on day 5 might contribute to the significantly higher recruitment of $CD4^+$ and $CD8^+$ T cells in the control mice at day 9 after H9N2 infection. The excessive number of macrophages, neutrophils, $CD4^+$ and $CD8^+$ T cells might lead to deleterious lung immunopathology. By releasing the oxygen radicals and proteolytic enzymes, such as neutrophil elastase and matrix metalloproteinases-8 (MMP-8), MMP-9 and MMP-12, neutrophils and macrophages could cause lung damage [46]. The recruitment of macrophages in the lung could also contribute to the alveolar epithelial cell destruction and apoptosis [47]. More $CD4^+$ T cells could induce more inflammatory cytokines, such as IL-6, IL-10 and IFN-γ, leading to more inflammatory response. Furthermore, $CD4^+$ T cells could directly lead to severe immunopathology and tissue damage via a cytokine-independent manner in influenza infection [48]. $CD8^+$ CTLs could exacerbate influenza viral pathology and induce mortality at high viral dose infection [49]. Our data of significantly increased immune cells number in the lung of control mice upon H9N2 infection corroborated this observation. Cigarette smoke exposure significantly improved this deleterious effect.

In our study, cigarette smoke had no effect on viral burden, which is consistent with other investigations [50]. Some studies however showed increased virus titer in cigarette smoke exposed mice [37] and in smokers [51,52]. Interestingly, Robbins *et al.* found that cigarette smoke exposure enhanced the viral burden in low dose influenza A virus infection, but had no effect in high dose influenza infection [38]. Taken together, these data indicate that the immunosuppressive effect of cigarette smoke on influenza A virus infection is independent of viral burden.

The immunosuppressive effect of nicotine has been previously reported, including ameliorating inflammatory diseases, such as ulcerative colitis [53,54] and cutaneous inflammation [55]. Transcutaneous nicotine administration could attenuate the LPS-induced systemic inflammatory response in human subjects [56]. Our *in vitro* and *in vivo* experiments confirmed such immunosuppressive effect of nicotine. Other studies also demonstrated that H1N1-A/PR/8/34-induced morbidity and mortality were decreased by nicotine treatment in mice [57,58]. However, they found that nicotine promoted influenza infection with increased lung virus titer, which is contrary to our results that nicotine could not affect lung virus replication. Together with our study, these observations suggest that the immunosuppressive effect of nicotine might be independent of virus replication.

For safety consideration, we could not expose the mice to cigarette smoke after pdmH1N1 or H9N2 virus infection. Although the half-life of nicotine is very short, the cotinine could still be detectable on day 14 after pdmH1N1 or H9N2 virus infection. This data demonstrated that the effect of nicotine might be on-going during the 14 days of pdmH1N1 or H9N2 virus infection.

Although we suggested that cigarette smoke exposure decreased the severity of influenza A virus infection, we are not intent to encourage people to smoke. The immunosuppressive effect of cigarette smoke plays a protective role just in our mouse model, when encountering highly virulent influenza virus infection that induces hyper-reaction of inflammatory responses. However, the immunosuppressive effect of cigarette smoke will be deleterious for people suffering from seasonal influenza virus infection [15,16,19], which produces appropriate inflammation that is necessary for the generation of immune responses, elimination of pathogens and recovery from tissue injuries [9,59].

Our study provides the first *in vivo* evidence that cigarette smoke, mediated partially by nicotine, could alleviate the pathogenicity of both pdmH1N1 and H9N2 viruses. Future epidemiological studies of pdmH1N1/H9N2 infection in smokers would be important to clarify the implications of our findings in humans.

Supporting Information

Figure S1 Nicotine suppressed the expression of chemokines after pdmH1N1 and H9N2 infection in A549 cells. A549 cells were pre-treated with 10 μM nicotine for 72 h, and then infected with pdmH1N1 or H9N2 virus. A) Effect of nicotine in pdmH1N1-induced inflammatory response. B) Impact of nicotine on H9N2-induced inflammatory response. Data are mean ± SEM and represent 4 independent experiments. $^{\#}p<0.05$ and $^{\#\#\#}p<0.001$ were tested by ANOVA of three groups; $^{**}p<0.01$ and $^{***}p<0.001$ were determined by Tukey post hoc test.

Acknowledgments

We thank Dr. Judith Choi Wo Mak in the Department of Medicine in the University of Hong Kong and Prof. Chi Hin Cho in the School of Biomedical Sciences in the Chinese University of Hong Kong for establishing the ventilated cigarette smoke exposure system. We also thank University Postgraduate Studentship and University Postgraduate Fellowship in The University of Hong Kong.

Author Contributions

Conceived and designed the experiments: YH HM WT Y. Lau. Performed the experiments: YH MTL JZ KTL Y. Liu. Analyzed the data: YH HM ML WT Y. Lau. Contributed reagents/materials/analysis tools: YH. Wrote the paper: YH. Reviewed and critically revised the manuscript: WT Y. Lau.

References

1. Itoh Y, Shinya K, Kiso M, Watanabe T, Sakoda Y, et al. (2009) In vitro and in vivo characterization of new swine-origin H1N1 influenza viruses. Nature 460: 1021–1025.
2. Kuiken T, Riteau B, Fouchier RA, Rimmelzwaan GF (2012) Pathogenesis of influenza virus infections: the good, the bad and the ugly. Curr Opin Virol 2: 276–286.
3. WHO (2009) Acute Respiratory Infections (Update September 2009).
4. Dawood FS, Iuliano AD, Reed C, Meltzer MI, Shay DK, et al. (2012) Estimated global mortality associated with the first 12 months of 2009 pandemic influenza A H1N1 virus circulation: a modelling study. Lancet Infect Dis 12: 687–695.
5. Butt KM, Smith GJ, Chen H, Zhang LJ, Leung YH, et al. (2005) Human infection with an avian H9N2 influenza A virus in Hong Kong in 2003. J Clin Microbiol 43: 5760–5767.
6. WHO (1999) 1999- Influenza A(H9N2) in Hong Kong Special Administrative Region (SAR) and China – Update.
7. WHO (2003) Influenza A(H9N2) in Hong Kong Special Administrative Region of China (SAR).
8. Khoufache K, Berri F, Nacken W, Vogel AB, Delenne M, et al. (2013) PAR1 contributes to influenza A virus pathogenicity in mice. J Clin Invest 123: 206–214.
9. Arcavi L, Benowitz NL (2004) Cigarette smoking and infection. Arch Intern Med 164: 2206–2216.
10. Goncalves RB, Coletta RD, Silverio KG, Benevides L, Casati MZ, et al. (2011) Impact of smoking on inflammation: overview of molecular mechanisms. Inflamm Res 60: 409–424.
11. Sopori M (2002) Effects of cigarette smoke on the immune system. Nat Rev Immunol 2: 372–377.
12. Gardi C, Valacchi G (2012) Cigarette smoke and ozone effect on murine inflammatory responses. Ann N Y Acad Sci 1259: 104–111.
13. Jackson KJ, Walters CL, Miles MF, Martin BR, Damaj MI (2009) Characterization of pharmacological and behavioral differences to nicotine in C57Bl/6 and DBA/2 mice. Neuropharmacology 57: 347–355.
14. Andersson U, Tracey KJ (2012) Reflex principles of immunological homeostasis. Annu Rev Immunol 30: 313–335.
15. Rogot E, Murray JL (1980) Smoking and causes of death among U.S. veterans: 16 years of observation. Public Health Rep 95: 213–222.

16. Kark JD, Lebiush M (1981) Smoking and epidemic influenza-like illness in female military recruits: a brief survey. Am J Public Health 71: 530–532.
17. Kark JD, Lebiush M, Rannon L (1982) Cigarette smoking as a risk factor for epidemic a(h1n1) influenza in young men. N Engl J Med 307: 1042–1046.
18. Hanshaoworakul W, Simmerman JM, Narueponjirakul U, Sanasuttipun W, Shinde V, et al. (2009) Severe human influenza infections in Thailand: oseltamivir treatment and risk factors for fatal outcome. PLoS One 4: e6051.
19. Wilson KM, Pier JC, Wesgate SC, Cohen JM, Blumkin AK (2013) Secondhand tobacco smoke exposure and severity of influenza in hospitalized children. J Pediatr 162: 16–21.
20. Ling MT, Tu W, Han Y, Mao H, Chong WP, et al. (2012) Mannose-binding lectin contributes to deleterious inflammatory response in pandemic H1N1 and avian H9N2 infection. J Infect Dis 205: 44–53.
21. Doherty PC, Turner SJ, Webby RG, Thomas PG (2006) Influenza and the challenge for immunology. Nat Immunol 7: 449–455.
22. Tu W, Mao H, Zheng J, Liu Y, Chiu SS, et al. (2010) Cytotoxic T lymphocytes established by seasonal human influenza cross-react against 2009 pandemic H1N1 influenza virus. J Virol 84: 6527–6535.
23. Chan KH, Ho SP, Yeung SC, So WH, Cho CH, et al. (2009) Chinese green tea ameliorates lung injury in cigarette smoke-exposed rats. Respir Med 103: 1746–1754.
24. Wong HP, Li ZJ, Shin VY, Tai EK, Wu WK, et al. (2009) Effects of cigarette smoking and restraint stress on human colon tumor growth in mice. Digestion 80: 209–214.
25. Matta SG, Balfour DJ, Benowitz NL, Boyd RT, Buccafusco JJ, et al. (2007) Guidelines on nicotine dose selection for in vivo research. Psychopharmacology (Berl) 190: 269–319.
26. Tu W, Zheng J, Liu Y, Sia SF, Liu M, et al. (2011) The aminobisphosphonate pamidronate controls influenza pathogenesis by expanding a gammadelta T cell population in humanized mice. J Exp Med 208: 1511–1522.
27. Goodman AG, Fornek JL, Medigeshi GR, Perrone LA, Peng X, et al. (2009) P58(IPK): a novel "CIHD" member of the host innate defense response against pathogenic virus infection. PLoS Pathog 5: e1000438.
28. Zheng J, Liu Y, Qin G, Chan PL, Mao H, et al. (2009) Efficient induction and expansion of human alloantigen-specific CD8 regulatory T cells from naive precursors by CD40-activated B cells. J Immunol 183: 3742–3750.
29. Qin G, Liu Y, Zheng J, Ng IH, Xiang Z, et al. (2011) Type 1 responses of human Vgamma9Vdelta2 T cells to influenza A viruses. J Virol 85: 10109–10116.
30. Foster KA, Oster CG, Mayer MM, Avery ML, Audus KL (1998) Characterization of the A549 cell line as a type II pulmonary epithelial cell model for drug metabolism. Exp Cell Res 243: 359–366.
31. Dickson PE, Rogers TD, Lester DB, Miller MM, Matta SG, et al. (2011) Genotype-dependent effects of adolescent nicotine exposure on dopamine functional dynamics in the nucleus accumbens shell in male and female mice: a potential mechanism underlying the gateway effect of nicotine. Psychopharmacology (Berl) 215: 631–642.
32. Hukkanen J, Jacob P 3rd, Benowitz NL (2005) Metabolism and disposition kinetics of nicotine. Pharmacol Rev 57: 79–115.
33. Chen H, Cowan MJ, Hasday JD, Vogel SN, Medvedev AE (2007) Tobacco smoking inhibits expression of proinflammatory cytokines and activation of IL-1R-associated kinase, p38, and NF-kappaB in alveolar macrophages stimulated with TLR2 and TLR4 agonists. J Immunol 179: 6097–6106.
34. Gaschler GJ, Zavitz CC, Bauer CM, Skrtic M, Lindahl M, et al. (2008) Cigarette smoke exposure attenuates cytokine production by mouse alveolar macrophages. Am J Respir Cell Mol Biol 38: 218–226.
35. Kang YM, Song BM, Lee JS, Kim HS, Seo SH (2011) Pandemic H1N1 influenza virus causes a stronger inflammatory response than seasonal H1N1 influenza virus in ferrets. Arch Virol 156: 759–767.
36. Zhou J, Law HK, Cheung CY, Ng IH, Peiris JS, et al. (2006) Differential expression of chemokines and their receptors in adult and neonatal macrophages infected with human or avian influenza viruses. J Infect Dis 194: 61–70.
37. Gualano RC, Hansen MJ, Vlahos R, Jones JE, Park-Jones RA, et al. (2008) Cigarette smoke worsens lung inflammation and impairs resolution of influenza infection in mice. Respir Res 9: 53.
38. Robbins CS, Bauer CM, Vujicic N, Gaschler GJ, Lichty BD, et al. (2006) Cigarette smoke impacts immune inflammatory responses to influenza in mice. Am J Respir Crit Care Med 174: 1342–1351.
39. Schmitz N, Kurrer M, Bachmann MF, Kopf M (2005) Interleukin-1 is responsible for acute lung immunopathology but increases survival of respiratory influenza virus infection. J Virol 79: 6441–6448.
40. Paquette SG, Banner D, Zhao Z, Fang Y, Huang SS, et al. (2012) Interleukin-6 is a potential biomarker for severe pandemic H1N1 influenza A infection. PLoS One 7: e38214.
41. Darwish I, Mubareka S, Liles WC (2011) Immunomodulatory therapy for severe influenza. Expert Rev Anti Infect Ther 9: 807–822.
42. Liu Y, Chen H, Sun Y, Chen F (2012) Antiviral role of Toll-like receptors and cytokines against the new 2009 H1N1 virus infection. Mol Biol Rep 39: 1163–1172.
43. McKinstry KK, Strutt TM, Buck A, Curtis JD, Dibble JP, et al. (2009) IL-10 deficiency unleashes an influenza-specific Th17 response and enhances survival against high-dose challenge. J Immunol 182: 7353–7363.
44. Jones SA (2005) Directing transition from innate to acquired immunity: defining a role for IL-6. J Immunol 175: 3463–3468.
45. Longhi MP, Wright K, Lauder SN, Nowell MA, Jones GW, et al. (2008) Interleukin-6 is crucial for recall of influenza-specific memory CD4 T cells. PLoS Pathog 4: e1000006.
46. Brusselle GG, Joos GF, Bracke KR (2011) New insights into the immunology of chronic obstructive pulmonary disease. Lancet 378: 1015–1026.
47. Herold S, Steinmueller M, von Wulffen W, Cakarova L, Pinto R, et al. (2008) Lung epithelial apoptosis in influenza virus pneumonia: the role of macrophage-expressed TNF-related apoptosis-inducing ligand. J Exp Med 205: 3065–3077.
48. Damjanovic D, Small CL, Jeyananthan M, McCormick S, Xing Z (2012) Immunopathology in influenza virus infection: uncoupling the friend from foe. Clin Immunol 144: 57–69.
49. Moskophidis D, Kioussis D (1998) Contribution of virus-specific CD8+ cytotoxic T cells to virus clearance or pathologic manifestations of influenza virus infection in a T cell receptor transgenic mouse model. J Exp Med 188: 223–232.
50. Bauer CM, Zavitz CC, Botelho FM, Lambert KN, Brown EG, et al. (2010) Treating viral exacerbations of chronic obstructive pulmonary disease: insights from a mouse model of cigarette smoke and H1N1 influenza infection. PLoS One 5: e13251.
51. Jaspers I, Horvath KM, Zhang W, Brighton LE, Carson JL, et al. (2010) Reduced expression of IRF7 in nasal epithelial cells from smokers after infection with influenza. Am J Respir Cell Mol Biol 43: 368–375.
52. Noah TL, Zhou H, Monaco J, Horvath K, Herbst M, et al. (2011) Tobacco smoke exposure and altered nasal responses to live attenuated influenza virus. Environ Health Perspect 119: 78–83.
53. Lunney PC, Leong RW (2012) Review article: Ulcerative colitis, smoking and nicotine therapy. Aliment Pharmacol Ther 36: 997–1008.
54. Guslandi M (1999) Nicotine treatment for ulcerative colitis. Br J Clin Pharmacol 48: 481–484.
55. Misery L (2004) Nicotine effects on skin: are they positive or negative? Exp Dermatol 13: 665–670.
56. Wittebole X, Hahm S, Coyle SM, Kumar A, Calvano SE, et al. (2007) Nicotine exposure alters in vivo human responses to endotoxin. Clin Exp Immunol 147: 28–34.
57. Razani-Boroujerdi S, Singh SP, Knall C, Hahn FF, Pena-Philippides JC, et al. (2004) Chronic nicotine inhibits inflammation and promotes influenza infection. Cell Immunol 230: 1–9.
58. Sopori ML, Kozak W, Savage SM, Geng Y, Soszynski D, et al. (1998) Effect of nicotine on the immune system: possible regulation of immune responses by central and peripheral mechanisms. Psychoneuroendocrinology 23: 189–204.
59. Huttunen R, Heikkinen T, Syrjanen J (2011) Smoking and the outcome of infection. J Intern Med 269: 258–269.

4

Abnormal White Matter Integrity in the Corpus Callosum among Smokers: Tract-Based Spatial Statistics

Wakako Umene-Nakano[1]*, Reiji Yoshimura[1], Shingo Kakeda[2], Keita Watanabe[2], Kenji Hayashi[1], Joji Nishimura[2], Hidehiko Takahashi[3], Junji Moriya[2], Satoru Ide[2], Issei Ueda[2], Hikaru Hori[1], Atsuko Ikenouchi-Sugita[1], Asuka Katsuki[1], Kiyokazu Atake[1], Osamu Abe[4], Yukunori Korogi[2], Jun Nakamura[1]

1 Department of Psychiatry, University of Occupational and Environmental Health, Kitakyushu, Japan, **2** Department of Radiology, University of Occupational and Environmental Health, Kitakyushu, Japan, **3** Department of Psychiatry, Kyoto University Graduate School of Medicine, Kyoto, Japan, **4** Department of Radiology, School of Medicine, Nihon University, Tokyo, Japan

Abstract

In the present study, we aimed to investigate the difference in white matter between smokers and nonsmokers. In addition, we examined relationships between white matter integrity and nicotine dependence parameters in smoking subjects. Nineteen male smokers were enrolled in this study. Eighteen age-matched non-smokers with no current or past psychiatric history were included as controls. Diffusion tensor imaging scans were performed, and the analysis was conducted using a tract-based special statistics approach. Compared with nonsmokers, smokers exhibited a significant decrease in fractional anisotropy (FA) throughout the whole corpus callosum. There were no significant differences in radial diffusivity or axial diffusivity between the two groups. There was a significant negative correlation between FA in the whole corpus callosum and the amount of tobacco use (cigarettes/day; $R = -0.580$, $p = 0.023$). These results suggest that the corpus callosum may be one of the key areas influenced by chronic smoking.

Editor: Gianluigi Forloni, "Mario Negri" Institute for Pharmacological Research, Italy

Funding: Professor Jun Nakamura has received grant support from Dainippon Sumitomo Pharma Co. Ltd. and Otsuka Pharmaceutical Co. Ltd in 2012. The funders had no role in study design, data collection and analysis, decision to publish, or preparation of the manuscript.

Competing Interests: The authors have the following interests: This study was supported by Dainippon Sumitomo Pharma Co. Ltd. and Otsuka Pharmaceutical Co. Ltd. There are no patents, products in development or marketed products to declare. This does not alter the authors' adherence to all the PLOS ONE policies on sharing data and materials, as detailed online in the guide for authors.

* E-mail: wakako-u @med.uoeh-u.ac.jp

Introduction

The most prevalent substance dependence issue worldwide is tobacco smoking. Smoking leads to serious public health problems and preventable early deaths [1]. In neuroimaging researches, smoking has been associated with large-scale structural brain alterations [2,3,4]. Particularly, recent voxel-based morphometry (VBM) study, smoking was associated with reductions in cerebral grey matter in the prefrontal, anterior cingulate, parietal, and temporal cortices and the cerebellum [3] [4]. There was an inverse relationship between cortical volume or cortical thickness and exposure to smoking [3] [5]. Furthermore, lower gray matter density in the prefrontal cortex and higher density in the insula have also been observed in smokers [6]. In short, the results of previous studied were consistent.

Diffusion tensor imaging (DTI) is sensitive to water diffusion characteristics and has been developed as a tool for investigating the local properties of brain white matter [7]. There are three diffusion metrics derived from DTI data: fractional anisotropy (FA), which reflects the directionality of water diffusion and the coherence of white matter fiber tracts; axial diffusivity (AD), which measures the magnitude of diffusivity along the principle diffusion direction; and radial diffusivity (RD), which reflects the magnitude of diffusivity perpendicular to the principle diffusion direction [8] [9]. Furthermore, the mean diffusivity (MD) was also calculated from DTI data. In a previous study, higher FA was measured in the corpus callosum of smokers compared with age-matched nonsmokers [10]. Jacobsen et al. [11] examined FA among adolescent smokers and nonsmokers with and without prenatal exposure to maternal smoking. In this study, both prenatal exposure and adolescent exposure to tobacco smoke was associated with increased FA in the anterior cortical white matter. Adolescent smoking was also associated with increased FA in regions of the internal capsule that contain auditory thalamocortical and corticofugal fibers. Thus, the effect of smoking on FA was inconsistent, and the regions affected were various.

The novel voxel-wise approach of tract-based spatial statistics (TBSS) was recently introduced [12], restricting the evaluation of diffusion parameters to a white matter skeleton common to all subjects. Voxel-based DTI analysis is not a mainstream of SPM (Statistical Parametric Mapping; Institute of Neurology, London, UK) and not officially supported. Therefore, there has not been a consensus about the method to spatially normalize FA images and the size of the smoothing kernel. To overcome these problems TBSS has been proposed [12].

To date, only two studies existed investigated white matter in smokers using TBSS. First, Zhang et al. [13] investigated FA using TBSS analysis methods in smokers with schizophrenia and healthy age-matched control subjects. The authors reported lower FA in the prefrontal white matter of a subsample of highly nicotine-dependent smokers and a negative correlation between FA and nicotine dependence, as measured by the Fagerström score. Second, Lin et al. [14] also reported that compared with nonsmokers, heavy smokers had lower FA in the left anterior corpus callosum. The results of two former studies were controversial, and the influence of smoking on white matter still remains unclear.

The objectives of the current study were 1) to investigate differences between smokers and nonsmokers in white matter, and 2) to examine relationships between white matter integrity and nicotine dependence parameters in the smokers.

Methods

Participants

Twenty smokers met the DSM-IV criteria for nicotine dependence; the score on the Tobacco Dependence Screener Scale (TDS) was used to diagnose nicotine dependence [15] The exclusion criteria included a current or past history of any comorbid neurological disorder, significant medical conditions, abnormal results on laboratory screening tests, or addiction to alcohol or other substances (with the exception of nicotine). We also performed the Mini International Neuropsychiatric Interview (MINI) [16] to rule out past or present history of comorbid psychiatric disorders. Finally, nineteen males were enrolled of this study. As part of the initial clinical evaluation, all smokers were asked to complete baseline questionnaires that assessed detailed demographic information and smoking-related clinical variables. The expiratory carbon monoxide (CO) levels of the smokers were measured using the Smokerlyzer system (Bedfont Scientific Ltd., Rochester, UK). Nicotine dependence levels were assessed with the Fagerström Test for Nicotine Dependence (FTND) [17]. Twenty age-matched nonsmokers with no current or past psychiatric history were included as controls. Finally, eighteen males were enrolled of this study. Alcohol use levels were assessed with the Alcohol Use Disorders Identification Test (AUDIT) [18] [19]. This study was approved by the Ethics Committee of the University of Occupational and Environmental Health. All the participants gave written informed consent to participate in the study.

Diffusion Tensor Images: Magnetic Resonance Imaging Scanning Protocol

All MR examinations were performed with a 3T MR system (Signa EXCITE 3T; GE Healthcare, Milwaukee, WI) with an 8-channel brain-phased array coil. The brain volume data were obtained with a three-dimensional fast spoiled gradient recalled acquisition with steady state (3D-FSPGR), which was acquired with parameters of 10/4.1/700 (repetition time msec/echo time msec/inversion time msec), a flip angle of 10 degree, a 24-cm field of view, and 1.2-mm-thick sections with $0.47 \times 0.47 \times 1.2$ mm resolution. Diffusion tensor images were acquired using a single-shot, spin-echo echo-planar sequence with the following parameters: TR/TE = 12000/83.3 msec, 4-mm slice thickness, no gap, 26-cm field of view; number of excitation = 1, and a spatial resolution of $1.02 \times 1.02 \times 4$ mm. Diffusion gradients (b value of 1,000 sec/mm^2) were always applied on each axis simultaneously around the 180-degree pulse. The diffusion properties were measured along 25 noncollinear directions. The structural distortion of diffusion-weighted MR images was corrected based on each T2-weighted planar image (b = 0 sec/mm^2) [20].

Volume Imaging Processing

All images were corrected for image distortion caused by gradient nonlinearity using "GradWarp" [21] and for intensity inhomogeneity using "N3" [22]. Image processing for VBM, a fully automatic technique for the computational analysis of differences in regional brain volume throughout the entire brain, was conducted using SPM8. The 3D-FSPGR images in native space were spatially normalized, segmented into grey matter (GM), white matter (WM), and cerebrospinal fluid images, and intensity-modulated using the Diffeomorphic Anatomical Registration Through Exponential Lie Algebra (DARTEL) toolbox on SPM8 [23]. Age was treated as confounding covariates. The DARTEL was proposed by Ashburner as an alternative method of normalization in the SPM package [24]. In an intensity modulation step, the voxel values of the segmented images were multiplied by the measure of warped and unwarped structures derived from the nonlinear step of the spatial normalization. This step converted the relative regional GM and WM density into absolute volume, expressed as the amount of per-unit volume of brain tissue before spatial normalization. The resulting modulated GM and WM images were smoothed with an 8-mm Gaussian kernel. An analysis of covariance model was used to examine group differences in GM and WM, with age as a covariate. These analyses yielded statistical parametric maps {SPM (t)} based on a voxel-level height threshold of $p<0.001$. Topological false discovery rate (FDR) correction was applied. The significance level was set at FDR-corrected $p<0.05$.

DTI Image Processing using TBSS

FA maps were computed for all subjects from the diffusion-tensor images after eddy current correction and automatic brain extraction using the FMRIB Diffusion Toolbox, which is part of the Functional MR Imaging of the Brain Software Library (FMRIB) Software Library [25]. The data were corrected for spatial distortion caused by gradient nonlinearity using grad_unwarp [21]. A voxel-wise statistical analysis of the DTI data was performed using TBSS [12] and implemented in the FMRIB Software Library 4.1.6 (University of Oxford, Oxford, UK) [25]. The FA, AD, RD and MD images were created by fitting a tensor model to the raw diffusion data. Brain extraction was performed using the Brain Extraction Tool 2.1 [26]. The FA data for all the subjects were aligned into a common space via nonlinear registration [27]. Next, a mean FA image was created and thinned to create a mean FA skeleton representing the centers of all tracts common to the group. This skeleton had a threshold of FA>0.20. Each subject's aligned FA data were then projected onto this skeleton, and the resulting data were fed into a voxel-wise cross-subject statistical analysis. Subsequently, other relevant DTI output images (AD, RD, MD) were projected onto the mean FA skeleton to compare other diffusivity values between groups in the same spatial location.

Diffusion tensor metrics were compared between groups with unpaired t test adjusted for the subject's age using TBSS analysis. The significance threshold for between-group differences was set at $p<0.05$; this was corrected for multiple comparisons across voxels using the threshold-free cluster-enhancement option. The number of permutations was set to 20,000 in all voxel-wise analyses.

DTI Imaging Process Tract-Specific Analysis

FA maps were computed using dTV II and VOLUMEONE1.72, developed by Masutani et al. [28] (University of Tokyo; diffusion tensor visualizer available at http://www.volume-one.org/). Diffusion tensors were computed, and fiber tracts were created by interpolation along the z-axis to obtain data (voxel size 2.0×2.0×3.0 mm^3). Color coded maps were created using 26 sets of images (25 sets with b = 1,000 s/mm^2, 0 set with b = 0 s/mm^2). Fiber tracts were based on a fiber assignment that was made using the continuous tracking approach [29] to obtain a three-dimensional tract reconstruction. The fiber tracts were initiated by placing a seed area in the anatomical regions through which the particular fibers were expected to course [26]. Tract measurements of the corpus callosum were performed by one of the authors (K.W.), who was blind to the status of each subject. The seed ROI was placed manually, including the entirety of the corpus callosum, on a reconstructed midsagittal image with a non-diffusion-weighted image (b = 0 s/mm^2). Tractographic images of the corpus callosum were generated with threshold values of line-tracking termination FA>0.18. Voxelization along the corpus callosum was then performed. To reduce the partial volume effect of the peripheral portion of the tract and to eliminate small incidental artifactual lines, we used a shape-processing technique based on mathematical morphology [28]. In this shape-processing technique, we dilated the voxels once and eroded them twice. The FA values in coregistered voxels were calculated.

Statistical Analysis

All statistical analyses were conducted using SAS Version 9.3 (SAS Institute, Cary, North Carolina, USA). The Mann-Whitney U test and the chi-squared test were used to compare the variables between the smokers and nonsmokers. Pearson's correlation coefficient was used to examine the relationship between FA levels and smoking-related clinical variables. The level of significance was set at $p<0.05$.

Results

Subject Demographics

Table 1 shows the backgrounds of the smokers (N = 19) and the nonsmokers (N = 18). All were males and there was no significant difference in the distributions of age (Smokers: 40.5±8.6, Nonsmokers: 40.5±8.6) Detailed information about smoking-related clinical variables and the AUDIT scores was not available for three subjects (N = 16). The mean AUDIT score for the smokers was significantly higher compared to that of the nonsmokers (smokers: 9.1±6.3, nonsmokers: 4.9±4.4; $p = 0.022$).

Total Volumes

There was no significant difference in the global brain volume (total gray matter and total white matter) between the smokers and the nonsmokers (Table 1). The regional volumetric analysis showed no significant group difference in any regions.

TBSS and Tract-Specific Analysis Results

Compared with the nonsmokers, the smokers exhibited a significant decrease in FA throughout the corpus callosum (Figure 1). There were no significant differences in AD or RD. In addition, there was a significant negative correlation between FA throughout the whole corpus callosum and the amount of tobacco use (cigarettes/day) covariant age ($R = -0.580$, $p = 0.023$; Figure 2), but there were no significant correlations between the amount of tobacco use and AD, RD or MD ($p = 0.522$, $p = 0.678$, $p = 0.850$). No significant correlations were observed between FA and the duration of tobacco use, the Brinkman index, the TDS scores, the FTND scores, CO levels, or the mean AUDIT scores.

Discussion

The current study provides novel evidence of decreased FA throughout the whole corpus callosum in smokers. Based on this result, we evaluated the relationship between FA levels of corpus callosum and smoking-related clinical variables using tract-specific analysis. This analysis has the advantage of detecting abnormalities in specific white matter tracts, whereas TBSS can influence the outcome by multiple comparisons [30]. We found a significant inverse correlation between FA levels and the amount of tobacco consumptions. No significant differences regarding AD, RD or MD in any region of brain were observed. Our finding is concordant with the results of Lin et al. [14], which observed decreased FA in the left anterior corpus callosum, but not concordant with a significantly decreased AD and a significantly increased RD. It is generally believed that AD mainly reflects axonal integrity [31] and RD is more related to the integrity and thickness of the myelin sheaths covering the axons [32]. Animal

Table 1. Background of smokers and non-smokers.

	Smokers (N = 19)*	Non-Smokers (N = 18)	P
Age (years)	40.5±8.6 (27–54)	36.4±8.0 (30–61)	0.094
AUDIT	9.1±6.3	4.9±4.4	0.022
Age of first use (years)	19.6±1.4		
Duration of use (years)	19.8±8.5		
Amount of use (cigarettes/day)	18.8±7.4		
Brinkman index (daily number of cigarettes × year)	394.1±271.0		
Scores of TDS	6.9±1.7		
Scores of FTND	3.7±1.5		
CO levels (ppm)	16.4±12.8		
Total gray matter volume	718.5±52.9	738.5±52.1	0.186
Total white matter volume	541.2±46.8	545.2±39.5	0.750

Abbreviation. AUDIT: Alcohol Use Disorders Identification Test; TDS: Tobacco Dependence Screener Scale; FTND: Fagerström Test for Nicotine Dependence; CO; carbon monoxide.

*Detailed information about the smoking-related clinical variables and the AUDIT scores of three subjects (N = 16) were not available. The mean AUDIT scores of the smokers (N = 16) was significantly higher than that of the nonsmokers (N = 18; smokers: 9.1±6.3; nonsmokers: 4.9±4.4; p = 0.022).

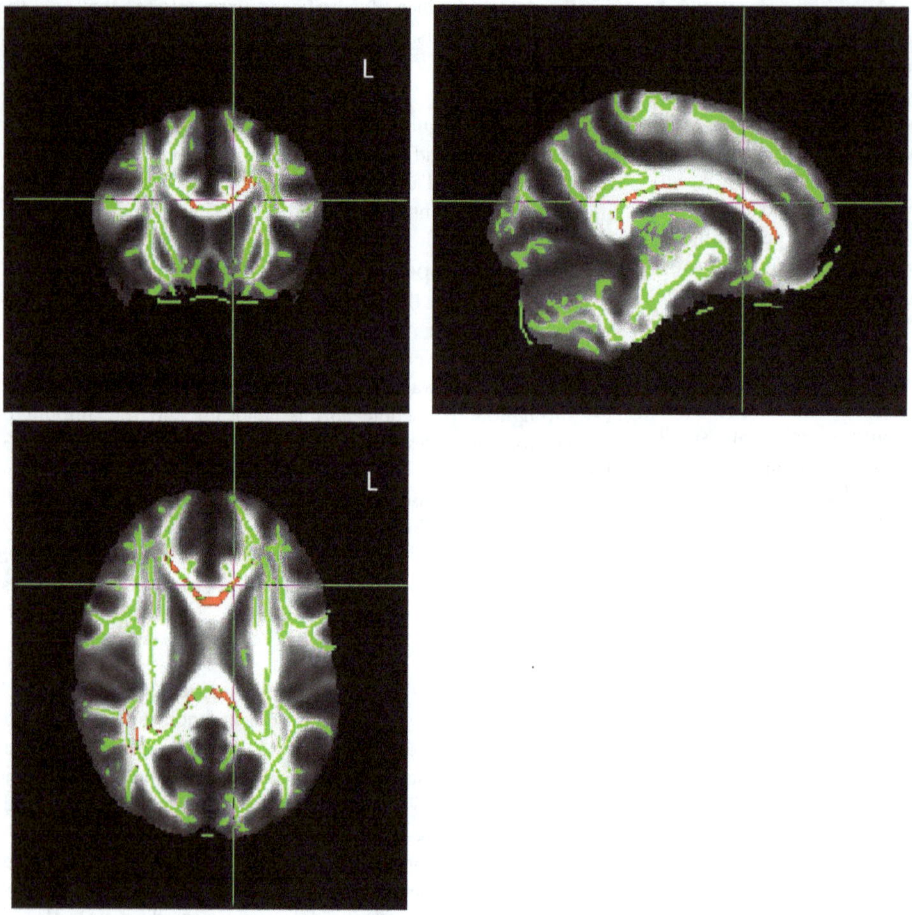

Figure 1. TBSS and tract-specific analysis results. The red voxels represent the areas where the fractional anisotropy (FA) levels of smokers were significantly reduced with respect to those of nonsmokers. Compared with nonsmokers, the smokers exhibited a significant decrease in FA throughout the whole corpus callosum.

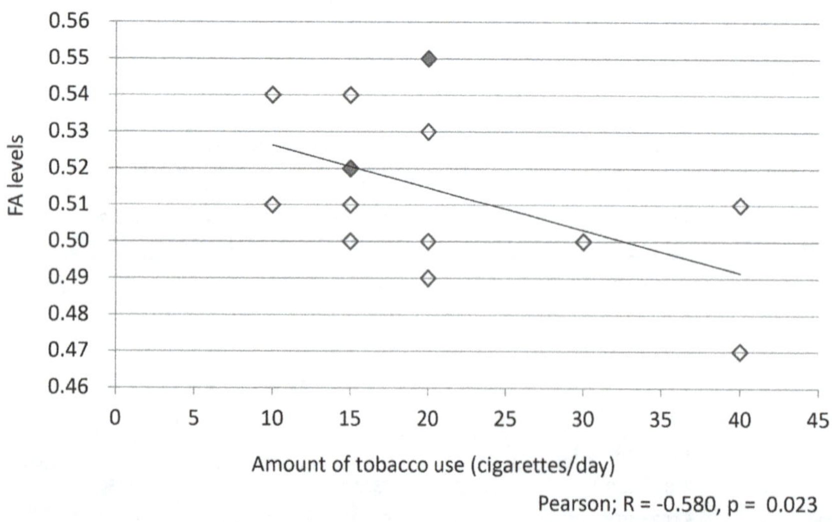

Figure 2. The correlation between FA levels throughout the whole corpus callosum and the amount of tobacco use (N = 16). There was a significant negative correlation between FA levels throughout the whole corpus callosum and the amount of tobacco use covariant age (cigarettes/day; R = − 0.580, p = 0.023). The number of spots was decreased from 16 to 13 because three spots represented the same data (three represented the FA level = 0.52 and N = 15, and two represented the FA level = 0.55 and N = 20; these spots are shown in gray spots).

DTI studies have demonstrated that decreased AD with the degeneration, and increased RD with demyelination [32,33]. And the decreased FA in corpus callosum of smokers is likely the manifestation of axonal damage and disrupted myelin integrity in the region. Our subjects were lower FTND score rather than Lin et al. [14], which suggests our samples were not heavy smokers. In other words, not much amount of smoking might influence only in FA.

Zhang et al. [13] also reported lower-than-normal FA in a section of the left prefrontal white matter in a subsample of highly dependent smokers, and no smoking-related differences in other white matter areas. This inconsistency may arise from the comorbidity of psychiatry disorder in a part of our samples both smokers and healthy controls.

The corpus callosum connects the brain hemispheres and facilitates communication between left- and right-side brain structures; it is the largest white matter fiber tract connecting the neocortex of the two hemispheres [34]. The anterior parts of the corpus callosum connect the frontal cortices, while the body and the splenium connect the parietal, temporal, and occipital homotopic regions [35]. Compromised fiber connectivity within the corpus callosum has been previously reported in subjects with substance addictions [36]. Decreased FA in the genu, body and splenium of the corpus callosum has been associated with alcohol-dependent subjects [37]. Significant reductions in FA in the genu and rostral body [38] and in the body and splenium of the corpus callosum [39] have been reported in cocaine-dependent subjects. Methamphetamine abusers showed reduced white matter integrity in the genu [40] and the rostral body [41] of the corpus callosum. There was a significant reduction in FA in the genu and the isthmus of the corpus callosum in opiate-dependent subjects [42]. Qiu et al. [43] recently reported that heroin-dependent individuals had significantly lower FA throughout the brain, including the genu and the isthmus of the corpus callosum, compared with controls. Taken together, these findings suggest that substance abuse may be associated with reduced FA levels that reflect less microstructural integrity. In contrast, Paul et al. [10] reported that smokers exhibited higher levels of FA in the corpus callosum than nonsmokers did. The authors hypothesized that either nicotine-induced cytotoxic cell swelling secondary to nicotine-induced osmotic imbalances or vasogenic swelling characterized by plasma fluid leaking into the parenchymal interstitial space might lead to alterations in the white matter. According to Hudkins et al. [44], FA may rise during the early years of smoking and subsequently decline with continued smoking in later years. Negative correlations between the age at which the subjects began smoking and FA have been observed [41]. Our finding in the present study is in accordance with that of Hudkins et al. [41]. In short, it is plausible that nicotine bidirectionally influences FA in the corpus callosum based on smoking duration or/and smoking amount. The subjects of Lin et al. [14] were also older ages. The reason of discrepancy about location of corpus callosum between whole corpus callosum in this study and anterior corpus callosum in Lin et al. [14] study might be differences sample characteristics (our subject was only male), level of cigarette smoking (our subject was lower FTND score) and alcohol consumption.

There were several limitations to our study. First, the sample size was small and this might lead absence of finding a change in the frontal cortex in the RD and AD Second, we did not evaluate healthy controls using any structured interviewed. Therefore, we might not completely exclude comorbidity psychiatric disorders among both samples. Third, the results may have been influenced by alcohol intake, given the higher AUDIT scores among the smokers (Table 1) and we could not evaluate comparing two groups covariant with scores of AUDIT. The level of score of AUDIT among smokers did not correspond to alcoholism, and there was not a significant correlation between FA level and mean AUDIT scores. Taking together, it is not ruled out that cigarette smoking increases alcohol consumptions, which might influence the results. Forth, we did not measure plasma levels of nicotine and cotinine, a metabolite of nicotine. We are currently undergoing the new study taking account of above problems.

In conclusion, we found that FA in smokers was significantly decreased compared with that of nonsmokers. Moreover, an inverse correlation between the amount of cigarette smoking and FA throughout the whole corpus callosum, which may shed light on the vulnerability of the region after long-term exposure in nicotine.

Author Contributions

Conceived and designed the experiments: WU-N RY SK HT. Performed the experiments: WU-N SK KH HH AI-S AK KA J. Nishimura. Analyzed the data: WU-N SK KW. Contributed reagents/materials/analysis tools: WU-N RY SK KW KH JM SI IU. Wrote the paper: WU-N RY SK KW HT OA YK J. Nakamura.

References

1. Benowitz NL (2008) Clinical pharmacology of nicotine: implications for understanding, preventing, and treating tobacco addiction. Clin Pharmacol Ther 83: 531–541.
2. Azizian A, Monterosso J, O'Neill J, London ED (2009) Magnetic resonance imaging studies of cigarette smoking. Handb Exp Pharmacol: 113–143.
3. Brody AL, Mandelkern MA, Jarvik ME, Lee GS, Smith EC, et al. (2004) Differences between smokers and nonsmokers in regional gray matter volumes and densities. Biol Psychiatry 55: 77–84.
4. Gallinat J, Meisenzahl E, Jacobsen LK, Kalus P, Bierbrauer J, et al. (2006) Smoking and structural brain deficits: a volumetric MR investigation. Eur J Neurosci 24: 1744–1750.
5. Kuhn S, Schubert F, Gallinat J (2010) Reduced thickness of medial orbitofrontal cortex in smokers. Biol Psychiatry 68: 1061–1065.
6. Zhang X, Salmeron BJ, Ross TJ, Geng X, Yang Y, et al. (2011) Factors underlying prefrontal and insula structural alterations in smokers. Neuroimage 54: 42–48.
7. Le Bihan D (2003) Looking into the functional architecture of the brain with diffusion MRI. Nat Rev Neurosci 4: 469–480.
8. Basser PJ, Pierpaoli C (1996) Microstructural and physiological features of tissues elucidated by quantitative-diffusion-tensor MRI. J Magn Reson B 111: 209–219.
9. Song SK, Sun SW, Ramsbottom MJ, Chang C, Russell J, et al. (2002) Dysmyelination revealed through MRI as increased radial (but unchanged axial) diffusion of water. Neuroimage 17: 1429–1436.
10. Paul RH, Grieve SM, Niaura R, David SP, Laidlaw DH, et al. (2008) Chronic cigarette smoking and the microstructural integrity of white matter in healthy adults: a diffusion tensor imaging study. Nicotine Tob Res 10: 137–147.
11. Jacobsen LK, Picciotto MR, Heath CJ, Frost SJ, Tsou KA, et al. (2007) Prenatal and adolescent exposure to tobacco smoke modulates the development of white matter microstructure. J Neurosci 27: 13491–13498.
12. Smith SM, Jenkinson M, Johansen-Berg H, Rueckert D, Nichols TE, et al. (2006) Tract-based spatial statistics: voxelwise analysis of multi-subject diffusion data. Neuroimage 31: 1487–1505.
13. Zhang X, Stein EA, Hong LE (2010) Smoking and schizophrenia independently and additively reduce white matter integrity between striatum and frontal cortex. Biol Psychiatry 68: 674–677.
14. Lin F, Wu G, Zhu L, Lei H (2012) Heavy smokers show abnormal microstructural integrity in the anterior corpus callosum: a diffusion tensor imaging study with tract-based spatial statistics. Drug Alcohol Depend 129: 82–87.
15. Kawakami N, Takatsuka N, Inaba S, Shimizu H (1999) Development of a screening questionnaire for tobacco/nicotine dependence according to ICD-10, DSM-III-R, and DSM-IV. Addict Behav 24: 155–166.
16. Sheehan DV, Lecrubier Y, Sheehan KH, Amorim P, Janavs J, et al. (1998) The Mini-International Neuropsychiatric Interview (M.I.N.I.): the development and validation of a structured diagnostic psychiatric interview for DSM-IV and ICD-10. J Clin Psychiatry 59 Suppl 20: 22–33;quiz 34–57.

17. Heatherton TF, Kozlowski LT, Frecker RC, Fagerstrom KO (1991) The Fagerstrom Test for Nicotine Dependence: a revision of the Fagerstrom Tolerance Questionnaire. Br J Addict 86: 1119–1127.
18. Reinert DF, Allen JP (2007) The alcohol use disorders identification test: an update of research findings. Alcohol Clin Exp Res 31: 185–199.
19. Hiro H, Shima S (1996) Availability of the Alcohol Use Disorders Identification Test (AUDIT) for a complete health examination in Japan. Nihon Arukoru Yakubutsu Igakkai Zasshi 31: 437–450.
20. Haselgrove JC, Moore JR (1996) Correction for distortion of echo-planar images used to calculate the apparent diffusion coefficient. Magn Reson Med 36: 960–964.
21. Jovicich J, Czanner S, Greve D, Haley E, van der Kouwe A, et al. (2006) Reliability in multi-site structural MRI studies: effects of gradient non-linearity correction on phantom and human data. Neuroimage 30: 436–443.
22. Sled JG, Zijdenbos AP, Evans AC (1998) A nonparametric method for automatic correction of intensity nonuniformity in MRI data. IEEE Trans Med Imaging 17: 87–97.
23. Ashburner J (2009) Computational anatomy with the SPM software. Magn Reson Imaging 27: 1163–1174.
24. Ashburner J (2007) A fast diffeomorphic image registration algorithm. Neuroimage 38: 95–113.
25. Smith SM, Jenkinson M, Woolrich MW, Beckmann CF, Behrens TE, et al. (2004) Advances in functional and structural MR image analysis and implementation as FSL. Neuroimage 23 Suppl 1: S208–219.
26. Smith SM (2002) Fast robust automated brain extraction. Hum Brain Mapp 17: 143–155.
27. Rueckert D, Sonoda LI, Hayes C, Hill DL, Leach MO, et al. (1999) Nonrigid registration using free-form deformations: application to breast MR images. IEEE Trans Med Imaging 18: 712–721.
28. Masutani Y, Aoki S, Abe O, Hayashi N, Otomo K (2003) MR diffusion tensor imaging: recent advance and new techniques for diffusion tensor visualization. Eur J Radiol 46: 53–66.
29. Mori S. Wakana S, Van Zijl PCM (2004) *MRI Atlas* of Human White Matter. Elisevier, Amsterdam.
30. Kamagata K, Motoi Y, Tomiyama H, Abe O, Ito K, et al (2013). Relationship between cognitive impairment and white-matter alteration in Parkinson's disease with dementia: tract-based spatial statistics and tract-specific analysis. Eur Radiol 23: 1946–1955.
31. Sun SW, Liang HF, Trinkaus K, Cross AH, Armstrong RC, et al. (2006) Noninvasive detection of cuprizone induced axonal damage and demyelination in the mouse corpus callosum. Magn Reson Med 55: 302–308.
32. Song SK, Yoshino J, Le TQ, Lin SJ, Sun SW, et al. (2005) Demyelination increases radial diffusivity in corpus callosum of mouse brain. Neuroimage 26: 132–140.
33. Wu Q, Butzkueven H, Gresle M, Kirchhoff F, Friedhuber A, et al. (2007) MR diffusion changes correlate with ultra-structurally defined axonal degeneration in murine optic nerve. Neuroimage 37: 1138–1147.
34. de Lacoste MC, Kirkpatrick JB, Ross ED (1985) Topography of the human corpus callosum. J Neuropathol Exp Neurol 44: 578–591.
35. Abe O, Masutani Y, Aoki S, Yamasue H, Yamada H, et al. (2004) Topography of the human corpus callosum using diffusion tensor tractography. J Comput Assist Tomogr 28: 533–539.
36. Arnone D, Abou-Saleh MT, Barrick TR (2006) Diffusion tensor imaging of the corpus callosum in addiction. Neuropsychobiology 54: 107–113.
37. De Bellis MD, Van Voorhees E, Hooper SR, Gibler N, Nelson L, et al. (2008) Diffusion tensor measures of the corpus callosum in adolescents with adolescent onset alcohol use disorders. Alcohol Clin Exp Res 32: 395–404.
38. Moeller FG, Hasan KM, Steinberg JL, Kramer LA, Dougherty DM, et al. (2005) Reduced anterior corpus callosum white matter integrity is related to increased impulsivity and reduced discriminability in cocaine-dependent subjects: diffusion tensor imaging. Neuropsychopharmacology 30: 610–617.
39. Lim KO, Wozniak JR, Mueller BA, Franc DT, Specker SM, et al. (2008) Brain macrostructural and microstructural abnormalities in cocaine dependence. Drug Alcohol Depend 92: 164–172.
40. Salo R, Nordahl TE, Buonocore MH, Natsuaki Y, Waters C, et al. (2009) Cognitive control and white matter callosal microstructure in methamphetamine-dependent subjects: a diffusion tensor imaging study. Biol Psychiatry 65: 122–128.
41. Moeller FG, Steinberg JL, Lane SD, Buzby M, Swann AC, et al. (2007) Diffusion tensor imaging in MDMA users and controls: association with decision making. Am J Drug Alcohol Abuse 33: 777–789.
42. Bora E, Yucel M, Fornito A, Pantelis C, Harrison BJ, et al. (2012) White matter microstructure in opiate addiction. Addict Biol 17: 141–148.
43. Qiu Y, Jiang G, Su H, Lv X, Zhang X, et al. (2013) Progressive white matter microstructure damage in male chronic heroin dependent individuals: a DTI and TBSS study. PLoS One 8: e63212.
44. Hudkins M, O'Neill J, Tobias MC, Bartzokis G, London ED (2012) Cigarette smoking and white matter microstructure. Psychopharmacology (Berl) 221: 285–295.

5

Prevalence and Correlates of Cigarette Smoking among Chinese Schizophrenia Inpatients Receiving Antipsychotic Mono-Therapy

Yan-Min Xu[1,2], Hong-Hui Chen[3,4]*, Fu Li[3], Fang Deng[3], Xiao-Bo Liu[3], Hai-Chen Yang[2], Li-Guo Qi[2], Jin-Hong Guo[2], Tie-Bang Liu[2]*

1 Department of Psychology, Normal College of Shenzhen University, Shenzhen, China, **2** Shenzhen Institute of Mental Health, Shenzhen Kangning Hospital, Shenzhen Mental Health Center, Shenzhen, China, **3** Affiliated Mental Health Center, Tongji Medical College of Huazhong University of Science and Technology, Wuhan, China, **4** Health and Family Planning Commission of Wuhan Municipality, Wuhan, China

Abstract

Objective: To investigate the prevalence rate of cigarette smoking and its socio-demographic and clinical correlates in Chinese schizophrenia inpatients receiving antipsychotic mono-therapy.

Methods: This study was a cross-sectional, two-site, hospital-based survey. Four hundred and twenty-nine schizophrenia patients (male/female: 66.9% vs. 33.1%) were consecutively recruited from psychosis inpatient wards of two large specialty psychiatric hospitals in mainland China. Patients were assessed using a cigarette smoking questionnaire, the Positive and Negative Symptom Scale, the Simpson Angus Scale, the Barnes Akathisia Rating Scale, and the Abnormal Involuntary Movement Scale. Socio-demographic and other clinical data were also collected. We calculated the prevalence of current smoking in our sample as well as its indirectly standardized prevalence ratio (ISPR) using data from the 2010 Global Adult Tobacco Survey in China.

Results: The prevalence rate of current smoking was 40.6% in our sample, and 57.5% in males and 6.3% in females. The ISPRs of all patients, men and women were 1.11(95%CI: 0.95~1.29), 1.07(95%CI = 0.91~1.24) and 4.64(95%CI = 2.12~8.82), respectively. The overall and male-specific prevalence of current smoking did not differ significantly between patients and the general population. In multiple logistic regression analysis, male sex, older age, poor marital status, alcohol use, use of first-generation antipsychotics, longer duration of illness, more frequent hospitalizations, and more severe negative symptoms were independently associated with current smoking.

Conclusion: Male Chinese inpatients with schizophrenia who received a mono-therapy of antipsychotics were not more likely to smoke than the general population. Cigarette smoking is more common in schizophrenia patients with more severe illness.

Editor: Jerson Laks, Federal University of Rio de Janeiro, Brazil

Funding: This work was supported by grant from Wuhan Planning Project of Science and Technology (grant number: 200860923434) (HH Chen, PI). The funders had no role in study design, data collection and analysis, decision to publish, or preparation of the manuscript.

Competing Interests: The authors have declared that no competing interests exist.

* E-mail: Dr.Chen_Honghui@hotmail.com (H-HC); liutbsz@gmail.com (T-BL)

Introduction

It has been recognized for many years that there is a much higher prevalence of smoking in schizophrenia patients than in the general population or patients with other mental disorders [1–3]. A meta-analysis based on worldwide studies has revealed that, the pooled smoking prevalence rates in Western schizophrenia patients were 76% for males, 50% for females, and 67% for both genders, respectively [3]. Furthermore, schizophrenia patients are not only more likely to smoke, but also smoke more heavily, have longer smoking duration, and have lower rate of smoking cessation than individuals without schizophrenia [4]. Consequently, high rate of smoking may contribute to reduction in life expectancy and excess morbidity and mortality among people with schizophrenia [5–8]. In addition, cigarette smoking also has been demonstrated to be associated with more frequent hospital readmissions, increased financial burden, and higher rate of attempted suicide [9–12].

Although cultural context contribute to cigarette smoking [13], the majority of the studies on smoking in schizophrenia patients come from Western countries, whereas few reports have come from Asian countries, especially regarding Chinese patients with schizophrenia. In recent years, a limited number of prevalence studies focusing on smoking of schizophrenia patients have been carried out in mainland China [14–20]. Compared with most figures reported in Western literature, the smoking prevalence rates of Chinese schizophrenia patients were relatively lower in men (median = 49%, mean = 48.7%) [15,17,21], and considerably lower in women (mean = 4.1%) [14,19]. Although these Chinese studies varied with regard to sampling methods (i.e., consecutive vs. convenience sampling), samples (i.e., inpatient vs. outpatient), and definitions of current smoking (i.e., currently smoke daily vs. currently smoke every day or on some days), the notable discrepancies in the smoking rates between Chinese and Western patients may still indicate the smoking characteristics of schizophrenia patients have ethnic and/or socio-cultural differences. Thus, the findings of Western studies on smoking might not generalize to Chinese patients.

The underlying causal mechanisms of high frequency of smoking in schizophrenia patients are unclear, especially whether smoking is a risk indicator for the development of the illness, a marker of a more severe illness, or an attempt at self-medication [1,4,18]. Several studies viewed smoking as an environment risk factor that causes schizophrenia [22,23]. In a historical–prospective cohort study, Weiser et al. followed 14,248 male adolescents for 4–16 years, and found a statistically significant association between the number of cigarettes smoked before the onset of illness and risk of developing later schizophrenia in smoking adolescents, with heavier smoking being associated with an almost two-fold increase in risk of schizophrenia [24]. A replication study regarding the relationship between smoking initiation and schizophrenia in Chinese population also found that daily smoking was significantly associated with vulnerability to schizophrenia [25]. On the contrary, another longitudinal study over a 27-year follow-up period revealed that smoking was associated with lower risk of subsequently developing schizophrenia and suggested that smoking might be an independent protective factor for schizophrenia [26]. In China, a study by Ma X et al. showed similar findings, in which, the authors found that smoking may delay full symptoms onset of schizophrenia by reducing some cognitive impairment in the illness and thus smoking might be a protective factor [18]. Hence, the evidence for the association between smoking and vulnerability to schizophrenia is inconclusive.

Previous studies on the clinical features of smoking schizophrenia patients also yielded inconsistent findings. Some found that smoking was significantly correlated with younger age, earlier age at onset (AAO) of illness, increased number of hospitalizations, elevated risk of suicide, higher doses of antipsychotic agents, more antipsychotic drug induced side-effects, and more severe psychotic symptoms [2,9,12,18,27–30]. Thus schizophrenia smokers may be more serious cases, supporting the viewpoint of smoking as a marker of more severe illness process. However, the self-medication hypothesis argues that individuals with schizophrenia smoke to alleviate negative symptoms and side effects of antipsychotic medication [31]. Several studies found schizophrenia patients who were current smokers had significantly fewer negative symptoms [15,17,32] and less extrapyramidal side effects (EPS) [15,17,33] than non-smoking patients, supporting the self-medication theory [34]. Unfortunately, any one of these theories mentioned above, could not be used to explain all the clinical findings of existing studies, as there were still many exceptions. For example, studies found that there were no statistically significant differences between schizophrenia smokers and non-smokers with regard to the severity of negative symptoms [14,16,19], dystonia and dyskinesia [35,36]. In general, research regarding the clinical characteristics of smoking individuals with schizophrenia has produced mixed results, which may be primarily due to limitations of study design. Many studies had insufficient sample sizes, used convenient samples, lacked standardized assessment tools, failed to fully address confounding (i.e., antipsychotic medication use), restricted study sample to be patients of one hospital, and, in most cases, recruited chronic rather than acute schizophrenia samples, thus only capturing data of part of the schizophrenia population.

Schizophrenia and related psychotic syndromes can be understood as disorders of adaptation to social context[37]. There is substantial evidence that schizophrenia represents the extreme of a psychosis continuum rather than a discrete illness entity, environmental factors such as taking psychoactive drugs during adolescence and young adulthood, have critical roles in the transition process from less severe levels of psychotic disorder phenotypes to schizophrenia [37–39]. Twin and adoption studies suggest that inherited genes make a person vulnerable to schizophrenia and then environmental factors act on this vulnerability to trigger the disorder [37,40]. Therefore, investigating the smoking pattern of schizophrenia smokers in the context of Chinese society, especially age at regular smoking onset and heavy smoking, and the association between psychotic symptoms and smoking, might increase our understanding of the underlying mechanisms of schizophrenia. Moreover, understanding the prevalence of smoking and its clinical correlates in schizophrenia patients is important and helpful for mental health professionals to develop effective strategies to reduce its harmful consequences. Given the inconclusive findings and limitations of current studies, this study aimed to investigate the prevalence of cigarette smoking and its socio-demographic and clinical correlates in a consecutive sample of schizophrenia inpatients using a single antipsychotic agent in Wuhan and Shenzhen, China.

Methods

Ethics Statement

The study protocol was approved by the Ethic Committees of Wuhan Mental Health Center and Shenzhen Kangning Hospital. Before respondents were interviewed, written consent was obtained from all of the subjects and their guardians, and declarations of anonymity and confidentiality had been made. Verbal consent also obtained from each included inpatient's responsible physician. For the compensation of time spent in participating in this study, each respondent had been given a gift prior to the interview.

Settings and subjects

This cross-sectional, two-site, hospital-based survey was conducted between January 2011 and June 2013. Subjects were recruited by consecutively screening patients with schizophrenia who attended the psychosis inpatient wards of Wuhan Mental Health Center and Shenzhen Kangning Hospital in Wuhan and Shenzhen, two of the largest cities in China. These two cities, one located in south-central area and the other located in southeastern coastal area of China, are typical examples of the metropolitan regions of mainland China, in terms of their financial conditions and levels of health care service. Both hospitals are the largest specialty psychiatric hospitals of local areas, with 610 and 450 hospital beds, respectively. They are responsible for mental health services of the residents of Wuhan and Shenzhen, and thus have a catchments area of approximately 10,020,000 and 10,547,400, respectively.

Patients who satisfied the following inclusion criteria were invited to participate in the study: 1) age 18–60 years; 2) men and women with a DSM-IV diagnosis of schizophrenia; 3) inpatients of psychosis wards; 4) had been treated with a stable dose of oral antipsychotic mono-therapy for at least four weeks before entry into the study, irrespective of the presence or absence of combination use of other non-antipsychotic drugs. Subjects with severe medical conditions, obvious intellectual disorders, active non-nicotine substance dependence, and organic psychosis, and who were prescribed two or more classes of antipsychotic agents, were excluded from this study. Although our subjects were inpatients, they were allowed to smoke regularly every day, except the time for sleep and taking drugs. Patients could easily buy cigarettes of most cigarette brands at reasonable prices in their psychiatric wards.

Instruments and assessment

The cross-sectional data of patients' demographic and clinical characteristics and prescriptions of antipsychotic drugs were recorded using a standardized protocol and data collection procedure. Data on patients' socio-demographic variables and clinical characteristics were collected through a questionnaire designed for this study. AAO refers to age at the first psychotic symptom reported by the patients themselves or informants [41]. Alcohol user was defined as a person who drank at least one alcoholic beverage per month in the past year [42]. Case records of included subjects were additionally reviewed for the following clinical variables: number of hospitalizations, length of illness, family history of psychiatric disorders, and types and doses of current antipsychotic drugs. Unclear or inaccurate answers were confirmed again with patients themselves and/or their guardians. Discrepancies were solved by consensus between patients and their guardians or responsible psychiatrists. Because of different types of neuroleptics used, daily doses were converted into chlorpromazine equivalents (CPZ-eqs) for statistical analysis [43,44].

We also administered a standardized cigarette smoking questionnaire to record smoking habit of each subject, including the average number of cigarettes smoked per day. Items of smoking questionnaire were adapted from the instruments of 2008 US National Health Interview Survey (hereafter refer to "NHIS definition" of smoking) [45]. It comprised of two questions. The first question, asked of all respondents, is "have you smoked at least 100 cigarettes in your entire life?" Respondents answering "yes" are classified as ever smokers, and those who answer "no" are classified as never smokers and excluded from subsequent cigarette use questions. Ever smokers are then asked a second question: "do you now smoke cigarettes every day, some days or not at all?" Respondents who answer "every day" or "some days" are classified as current smokers and those who answer "not at all" are categorized into former smokers. Heavy smokers were defined as those smoking at least 20 cigarettes daily [46].

Psychopathology of schizophrenia in the 4-week period preceding the interview was measured using the Chinese version of Positive and Negative Symptom Scale (PANSS) with subscales for positive symptoms (PANSS-P), negative symptoms (PANSS-N), and general psychopathological symptoms (PANSS-G) [47]. Drug-related extrapyramidal side effects (EPS) were assessed using Simpson Angus Scale (SAS) [48], Barnes Akathisia Rating Scale (BARS) [49], and Abnormal Involuntary Movement Scale (AIMS) [50]. The diagnostic threshold scores for the presence of pseudoparkinsonism and akathisia were ≥7 in SAS [51] and ≥2 in BARS global clinical assessment item [49], respectively. A score of 3 or more on any of the first 7 AIMS items, or a score of 2 or more on any two of the first 7 AIMS items, was taken to be indicative of dyskinesia [52]. The Chinese versions of these assessment instruments have been shown to be reliable and valid for measuring the psychotic symptoms and drug-related EPS of Chinese schizophrenia patients [53–56], the internal consistency of all the rating instruments (three subscales of PANSS, SAS, BARS, and AIMS) was good in this study (Cronbach α coefficients ranged between 0.74 and 0.93).

Two raters, an experienced psychiatrist and a clinical psychologist, were responsible for all of the assessments. Prior to the study, both raters underwent a training course on the use of PANSS, SAS, BARS, and AIMS. Before the beginning of this study, an inter-rater correlation coefficients ranging from 0.81 to 0.93 was obtained in 11 voluntary schizophrenia patients between the two raters for all assessment scales.

Once participants agreed to participate in this study, they were told that the main goal of this study was to help clinicians understand the relationship between schizophrenia and smoking, and the results might be helpful for the management and rehabilitation of schizophrenia. Hence, supplying real information about the smoking behaviors was of vitally importance for this study. Our raters were also required to be patient to help respondents recall their smoking details during the course of interview. The completeness of all interview and physical examination records was checked daily by the survey team leader. Errors, omissions and other flaws were solved during the fieldwork period of this survey.

Statistical analysis

For the analysis, we used the SPSS software for Windows, version 15.0 (SPSS Ltd.). According to the smoking status diagnosed by NHIS definition, prevalence rates for ever, current and former cigarette smoking were calculated. Because the number of former smoker in our sample was very small ($N = 3$), the following univariate and multivariate analyses only focused on current and never smokers. In univariate analysis, the comparison between current smokers and never smokers with respect to socio-demographic and clinical characteristics was performed by independent sample t-test, Mann-Whitney U test, and chi-square test as appropriate. Multivariate logistic regression was used to identify factors associated with current smoking. Associations between current smoking and all potential predictors were assessed in univariate analyses, followed by multivariate analyses of the selected subsets. A variable was selected if it was statistically significant at the nominal two-sided 0.05 level in univariate analysis. We quantified associations of predictors and current smoking by calculating odds ratios (ORs) with 95% confidence intervals (CIs) for each variable.

To clarify whether schizophrenia inpatients have higher current smoking rate than Chinese general population, we introduced the latest smoking data from the 2010 Global Adult Tobacco Survey in China (2010 GATS China) [57–59] as the comparison reference. The 2010 GATS China was a nationally representative household survey of non-institutional men and women aged 15 and older, and was conducted between December 2009 and March 2010. The survey was completed with high response rate (96.0%) and high qualities by strict quality control measures, and successfully collected 13,354 Chinese adults' tobacco use data. Since our study sample and the external standard population, 2010 GATS China sample, were not comparable in terms of age and gender structures, we compared the smoking rates between schizophrenia and the general population by calculating the Indirectly Standardized Prevalence Ratios (ISPRs) [60,61]. Specifically, this indirect standardization approach applied the stratum specific smoking rates (i.e., age and gender specific rates) of 2010 GATS China population to the number of individuals in the corresponding stratum in our sample. An expected number of smokers was generated for each stratum, and the total expected was used in the denominator. The numerator was the total number of observed smokers in our schizophrenia sample. ISPR was the ratio of the observed number of smokers in our study sample over the expected number of smokers in the general population. Its 95%CI was estimated through formulas proposed by Rothman and Boice [62].

Results

Characteristics of subjects

Out of 976 schizophrenia inpatients who were screened during the study period, 617 were on antipsychotic mono-therapy treatment and fulfilled the inclusion criteria. Among them, 56 refused, 93 did not complete assessment, and 39 were ineligible for other reasons, leaving 429 (69.5%) patients completed the interview and physical examination. The mean age at the time of this survey was 33.1 years (standard deviation [SD] = 10.2, range = 18~60), and 66.9% of the subjects were male. The numbers of patients using promethazine, perphenazine, chlorpromazine, sulpiride, paliperidone, clozapine, risperidone, quetiapine, olanzapine, amisulpride, and aripiprazole were 2, 19, 76, 5, 1, 117, 95, 24, 53, 2, and 35, respectively. Therefore, for the antipsychotics used, the second-generation antipsychotic (SGA) mono-therapy was used more often compared to the first-generation antipsychotic (FGA) (77.4% vs. 22.6%) mono-therapy. Other socio-demographic and clinical characteristics of the schizophrenia inpatients are displayed in the first three columns of Table 1.

Smoking patterns of schizophrenia inpatients

Of the 429 patients, 177 (41.3%) were identified as ever smokers, 3 as former smokers (0.7%) and 174 as current smokers (40.6%); 57.5% of male (N = 165) and 6.3% of female patients (N = 9) were current smokers. Among the current smokers, the mean number of cigarettes consumed per day was 16.1 (SD = 9.0, range = 2–40), while 15.2% of them smoked ≤ 9 cigarettes daily, 43.5% of them smoked 10–19 cigarettes, and 41.4% smoked ≥ 20 cigarettes (heavy smoking). For current smokers, the mean age at regular smoking onset was 20.6 (SD = 4.6) years, and the mean AAO for schizophrenia was 24.9 (SD = 7.4) years, with 75.8% starting regular smoking before the onset of schizophrenia. The age of regular smoking start in patients was significantly earlier than their age of illness onset (paired-samples t test, t = 13.38, P<0.001).

The ISPRs of all patients, male and female patients were 1.11(95%CI: 0.95~1.29), 1.07 (95%CI: 0.91~1.24) and 4.64(95%CI: 2.12~8.82), respectively (Table 2). These results mean that only female patients had a statistically higher prevalence of current smoking than the general population, whereas all patients and female patients did not. Compared with smokers of the general population, current smokers with schizophrenia had significantly lower percentage of heavy smokers (41.4% vs. 51.9%, Z = 2.77, P = 0.023). There was no statistically

Table 1. Socio-demographic and clinical characteristics of inpatients with schizophrenia, split by smoking status.

	All subjects (N = 429)		Current smokers (N = 174)		Never smokers (N = 252)		Statistics	
Variables	n	%	n	%	n	%	$\chi2$	P
Study site (Wuhan)	306	71.3	119	68.4	187	74.2	1.71	0.19
Male	287	66.9	165	94.8	119	47.2	105	<0.001
Without medical insurance	232	54.1	98	56.3	133	52.8	0.52	0.47
Marital status							16.74	<0.001
Married/re-married/co-habiting	146	34	43	24.7	101	40.1		
Never-married	227	52.9	97	55.7	129	51.2		
Divorced/widowed/separated	56	13.1	34	19.5	22	8.7		
Being unemployed	178	41.5	73	42	104	41.3	0.02	0.89
Alcohol use	121	28.2	82	47.1	37	14.7	53.8	<0.001
Family history of psychiatric disease	92	21.4	37	21.3	53	21	0.003	0.95
Taking FGAs	97	22.6	60	34.5	37	14.7	22.9	<0.001
Pseudoparkinsonism	60	14	6	3.4	54	27.5	60.3	<0.001
Akathisia	94	21.9	21	12.1	73	29	17.1	<0.001
Dyskinesia	85	19.8	31	17.8	54	21.4	0.84	0.36
	Mean	SD	Mean	SD	Mean	SD	t/Z	P
Age (years)	33.1	10.2	35.5	9.7	31.3	10.2	4.19	<0.001
Education level (years)	11.2	3.4	11.1	2.8	11.4	3.8	1.01	0.32
Age at onset (years)	24.9	7.4	25.7	7.8	24.2	7.1	2.11	0.035
Length of illness (years)	7.6	8.7	8.9	8.4	6.7	8.9	3.44	0.001*
Duration of antipsychotic treatment	6.2	7.9	7.7	8.2	5.1	7.6	4.46	<0.001*
Number of hospitalizations	3.3	3.7	4.4	4.7	2.6	2.5	5.48	<0.001*
Neuroleptic dose (CPZ eqs, mg/day)	372.6	318.7	390.8	312.3	353.5	333.1	0.67	0.45*
PANSS total score	56.7	21.4	61.5	24	52	17.1	4.77	<0.001
PANSS-P subscore	16.2	6.8	17.3	7.4	15.1	5.8	3.43	<0.001
PANSS-N subscore	13.2	6.1	14.2	6.6	12.2	5.3	3.46	<0.001
PANSS-G subscore	27.3	12.8	30	14	24.7	10.8	4.4	<0.001

Note: FGA, first-generation antipsychotics. CPZ eqs, chlorpromazine equivalents; PANSS, positive and negative symptom scale; *Mann-Whitney U test.

significant difference in age of initiation of regular smoking between current smoking patients and the general population (mean age at smoking initiation in 2010 GATS China =21.2 years, one-sample t test, t=1.72, P=0.087).

Correlates of current smoking

The socio-demographic and clinical characteristics of current and never smokers are shown in the fourth to seventh columns of Table 1. Univariate analysis (the last two columns of Table 1) showed that current smokers were more likely to be male, be in poor marital status (never married, divorced, widowed, or separated), use alcohol, take FGAs, have less pseudoparkinsonism, have less akathisia, be older, have later AAO, have longer duration of illness, receive long-term antipsychotic treatment, be hospitalized more frequently, be scored higher in PANSS, PANSS-P, PANSS-N, and PANSS-G scales. Multivariate logistic regression analysis (Table 3) considering all variables statistically significant in the univariate analysis (with a Backward: Wald $\chi 2$ selection method) revealed that male sex, older age, poor marital status, alcohol use, use of FGAs, longer duration of illness, more frequent hospitalizations, and more severe negative symptoms remained independently associated with smoking after adjustment for all other variables.

Discussion

This study demonstrated that the prevalence of current smoking was 40.6% and the ISPR was 1.11 in Chinese schizophrenia inpatients currently receiving a mono-therapy of antipsychotics. However, both the overall and male-specific prevalence rates of current smoking did not differ significantly between patients and the general population. Only female Chinese inpatients with schizophrenia seem to have higher smoking risk than the general population, but the absolute difference (equals to 3.9%) between the two prevalence rates is really too small. Considering the finding that the female-specific prevalence (6.3%) was too low, and the comparable prevalence between the whole sample and the general population, it is difficult to conclude that Chinese inpatients with schizophrenia are more likely to smoke than the general population. This study further demonstrated that current smokers of patients had significantly lower rate of heavy smoking than those of the general population, indicating that Chinese schizophrenia smokers are not heavy cigarette smokers. Although we found the majority of smokers (75.8%) started regular smoking before the disease onset, the mean age of starting to smoke (20.6 years) was similar to that of the general population; these phenomena might not support the viewpoint that schizophrenia patients start regular smoking in greater numbers during adolescence than the normal population in Western countries [63]. Furthermore, the similar overall prevalence of smoking between our patient sample and the general population may indicate that smoking in Chinese schizophrenia patients is an ingrained habit. In Chinese culture, smoking is a deeply rooted tradition, as most of the Chinese people have already been accustomed to offering others cigarettes or smoking cigarettes provided by others as a gesture of hospitality and friendship[64]. The studied psychiatric hospitals also supplied relatively free environments to let their patients smoke. There is a possibility that Chinese schizophrenia patients and the general population had comparable prevalence of smoking before hospitalization. Under the circumstances, individuals with schizophrenia would still keep their smoking habit even after their admission in the hospital, therefore, no statistically significant difference in the overall prevalence of current smoking was found between the two groups in this study. Another finding that almost all of the ever smokers were current smokers in our study sample seems consistent with such hypothesis.

In addition to showing the differences in smoking characteristics between individuals with schizophrenia and the general population, our study also found lower current smoking prevalence, including gender-specific and overall prevalence, of schizophrenia inpatients than those reported previously in Western studies [US (males: 91%, females:70%) [65], Canada (both genders: 63%) [66], Germany (males: 70%) [67], Spain (males: 81%, females: 13%) [68], and Ireland (males: 92% females: 82%) [69]]. These low prevalence rates in our study are somewhat consistent with the

Table 2. Indirectly standardized prevalence ratios of current smoking in schizophrenia inpatients, calculating using the results of 2010 Global Adult Survey in China as the standard populations.

Sample	Parameter for indirect standardization	Age group (years) 16~24	25~34	35~44	45~54	55~60	Total	Indirectly standardized prevalence ratio (95% CI)
Males	No. of subjects	59	105	67	48	8	287	1.07(0.91, 1.24)
	Prevalence of current smoking in patients (%)	33.9	64.8	58.2	70.8	50	57.5	
	Age-specific prevalence of current smoking in general population (%)	33.6	53.0	63.7	66.3	58.9	—	
	No. of observed current smokers	20	68	39	34	4	165	
	No. of expected current smokers	19.8	55.7	42.7	31.8	4.7	154.7	
Females	No. of subjects	49	41	31	20	1	142	4.64(2.12, 8.82)
	Prevalence of current smoking in patients (%)	8.2	2.4	6.5	10	0.0	6.3	
	Age-specific prevalence of current smoking in general population (%)	0.7	0.3	2.4	3.5	2.8	—	
	No. of observed current smokers	4	1	2	2	0	9	
	No. of expected current smokers	0.34	0.12	0.74	0.70	0.03	1.94	

Table 3. Multiple logistic regression for correlates of current smoking.

Variables	Reference category	Beta	Standard error	Wald $\chi 2$	P	OR(95%CI)
Male gender	Female gender	2.90	0.41	51.23	<0.001	18.18(8.20, 40.0)
Age (years)	—*	0.09	0.02	17.42	<0.001	1.09(1.05, 1.14)
Never-married	Married/re-married/co-habiting	1.16	0.35	10.76	0.001	3.18(1.59, 6.34)
Divorced/widowed/separated	Married/re-married/co-habiting	1.43	0.45	9.90	0.002	4.17(1.71, 10.14)
Alcohol use	No alcohol use	1.87	0.31	35.73	<0.001	6.50(3.52, 12.00)
FGAs	SGAs	1.38	0.33	17.52	<0.001	3.98(2.08, 7.58)
Length of illness (years)	—*	0.09	0.02	16.15	<0.001	1.09(1.05, 1.14)
Number of hospitalizations	—*	0.16	0.05	9.92	0.002	1.17(1.06, 1.29)
PANSS-N subscore	—*	0.06	0.03	4.54	0.013	1.06(1.01, 1.12)

Note: *continuous variable.

findings of previously published Chinese schizophrenia inpatient studies (males: 42.2%~52.0%, females: 4.5%~6.3%) [14,18,20]. The discrepancies in the smoking rates between Chinese and Western studies could be due to the exclusion of patients with alcohol/heroin dependence (smoking rate in such patients is expected to be high) [70], and the potential selection bias that only patients using a single antipsychotic agent was included in this study. Moreover, in most literature from western countries, the smoking rate of female schizophrenia patients is very close to that of males[3], but in Chinese schizophrenia patients, women's smoking prevalence is obviously lower than men's. The high ratio of male-to-female smoking prevalence rates is in line with that of the normal population in 2010 GATS China survey[57]. The dramatic gender difference reflects the cultural differences between China and western countries. In general, China is still a male dominated society, and smoking is regarded as the patent and privileges of men. Chinese females who smoke are typically viewed as women with either a wild streak or loose morals. Thus the cultural resistance against women smoking in modern China remains very strong[16], this cultural phenomenon should also be applicable to Chinese patients with schizophrenia, which leads to the low smoking rate in female patients compared with western female patients.

When we study the association between smoking and schizophrenia, as measured by OR, it is noteworthy that the estimated ORs have close relationship with the smoking prevalence rates of the general population, because the conclusions regarding whether patients have higher, lower or comparable risk of smoking, highly depending on the control population used. For example, two studies conducted in Turkey and US reported similar smoking rates in their schizophrenia sample (50% and 51%) [71,72], but the corresponding smoking rates in Turkey and US general population were quite different (43% and 23%), therefore, a non-significant OR of 1.3 for Turkey patients and a statistically significant OR of 3.5 for US patients were obtained [3]. In our study, we not only found a lower prevalence of smoking, but also revealed a comparable smoking prevalence between patients and the general population. Schizophrenia smokers in our sample are less likely to be heavy smokers as Western smokers with schizophrenia [2]. As a result, smoking might not be associated with the vulnerability to schizophrenia in Chinese population. The potential socio-cultural, biological and public anti-smoking policy factors for these differences need to be further explored.

Analyses of correlates of current smoking revealed that, in schizophrenia inpatients, smoking was more prevalent among patients who were male, were older, were in poor marital status, used alcohol, took FGAs, had longer illness duration, had multiple hospitalizations, and had more severe negative symptoms. These findings indicate that the potential etiologies of smoking in schizophrenia are complex and multifactorial. In this study, male sex, older age (below 60 years old), and unmarried status were identified as significantly risk factors for smoking, these findings are in line with previous reports for both the general population [59,73] and schizophrenia patients [16,19,20]. In general, alcohol drinkers usually smoke and vice versa, as both behaviors are strongly influenced by some shared genetic factors [74]. In agreement with the findings of earlier studies [16,17], smoking was significantly associated with alcohol use in our schizophrenia sample. Several studies have shown a higher prevalence of smoking in schizophrenia patients with lower educational attainment [2,19]; however, we did not find such association in our sample, which is consistent with three previous studies [12,16,17]. This discrepancy might be attributable to the differences in sample characteristic. Also, other risk factors could mask or affect the role of education level.

It has been suggested that individuals with schizophrenia use tobacco to gain relief from EPS induced by antipsychotic medication. Cigarette smoking increases the activity of hepatic CYP 1A2 enzymes, thus decreasing the concentration of antipsychotic drugs [28,75]. Therefore, patients on FGAs are more likely to smoke as a result of much EPS from FGA treatment. This study partly replicates earlier findings [15,16,31,33], as its univariate analysis found that a higher likelihood of smoking was associated with less EPS (pseudoparkinsonism and akathisia) and use of FGAs. Smoking could increase clearance of antipsychotics, which in turn makes schizophrenia smokers require higher dosages of antipsychotics than non-smokers, but there was no statistically significant difference in the neuroleptic dosage between smokers and never-smokers in the present study. Moreover, more severe negative symptoms were found to be correlated with current smoking. These findings might suggest the undertreatment of inpatients with schizophrenia. Another reasonable explanation for this phenomenon is that there was a significantly higher proportion of FGA use in smokers, but FGAs are not good at reducing the negative symptoms. Hence, the association between more severe negative symptoms and smoking was found. Although nicotine might alleviate negative symptoms of smokers through stimulating release of dopamine and serotonin in the brain [76], these positive effects might have been weakened by the increased clearance of antipsychotics and undertreatment. Other factor correlated with EPS may mask the role of EPS to smoking, so the statistically significant association between less EPS and smoking disappeared in the multiple logistic regression model. The finding of more severe negative symptoms in smokers when compared to never-smokers is similar to the results of several previous studies [29,30,77].

After adjusting confounders, smoking was still associated with more hospital admissions and longer illness duration; both findings indicated that our smoking cases have a more severe disease course. Previous studies also support these findings [15,17,29,30,77]. Presence of smoking has been reported to be associated with increased risk of hospital readmission and longer duration of hospitalization [78]. The increased severity of illness also may be attributed to high prevalence of alcohol use, as alcohol consumption was founded to be associated with increased risk of hospital admissions in cases with physical disease [79]. There is evidence that severe, treatment resistant schizophrenia is associated with smoking in patients with schizophrenia regardless of gender or alcohol use [80]; this is similar to our finding that smoking was related to more severe illness.

The strength of this study was ensuring the analysis on the association of smoking with types and doses of antipsychotic agents in subjects receiving neuroleptic mono-therapy treatment, by eliminating the masked effect of patients receiving multiple antipsychotic medications. However, this study has several limitations that should be noted. First, our study sample consists of inpatients on antipsychotic mono-therapy only and can't represent all patients with schizophrenia. Therefore, the results may not be applicable to outpatients and inpatients on antipsychotic poly-therapy. In addition, our sample was selected from specialty psychiatric hospitals of two large cities in mainland China. Although the prevalence and correlates identified in our study seem consistent with several findings in previous reports, whether they also apply to other institutions of China is still questionable. So the findings from this study should be generalized with caution. Second, our study was a cross-sectional, observational study in nature, thus the cause-consequence relationships between smoking and risk factors could not be created. Third, the definition of smoking used in the present study is broader, because it defines a current smoker as an ever smoker who currently smokes daily or on some days [81]. On the contrary, most of the previous clinical studies restricted current smokers to be ever smokers who currently smoke daily. Hence, we may overestimate the smoking prevalence of our schizophrenia sample. Fourth, this study used a questionnaire to record the smoking status of schizophrenia patients, which is not as accurate as several laboratory indicators, such as measuring the level of cotinine (a metabolite of nicotine) in the blood samples. Although we had taken some quality control measures to minimum the measurement bias, biases due to memory effect and social desirability response might still be inevitable in the present study. Finally, since the number of identified female smokers was very limited, males accounted for 95% the smokers; on the other hand, the sample size of female patients in our sample is also small. Thus, those identified correlates of smoking may not be applied to female schizophrenia patients and the prevalence estimation of smoking in female patients is unstable. The smoking characteristics of female people with schizophrenia need to be further studied.

Conclusions

In summary, smoking in Chinese male schizophrenia inpatients, who were receiving antipsychotic mono-therapy, is as prevalent as the general population, and the overall prevalence of smoking in Chinese schizophrenia inpatients is lower than most figures reported in Western literature. Smoking had relationship with gender, age, and marital status; Illness severity-related indicators seemed to have close relationship with smoking in this patient population. Smoking may serve as an important clinical marker of severe illness in individuals with schizophrenia. Given the harmful consequences and its association with more severe illness, effective measures to promote smoking cessation in schizophrenia should be implemented in Chinese patients with schizophrenia.

Acknowledgments

The authors thank all the research staff for their team collaboration work and all the patients involved in this study for their cooperation and support.

Author Contributions

Conceived and designed the experiments: HHC TBL. Performed the experiments: YMX FL FD XBL. Analyzed the data: YMX HHC. Contributed reagents/materials/analysis tools: HCY LGQ JHG. Wrote the paper: YMX HHC.

References

1. Sagud M, Mihaljević-Peles A, Mück-Seler D, Pivac N, Vuksan-Cusa B, et al. (2009) Smoking and schizophrenia. Psychiatr Danub 21: 371–375.
2. Dickerson F, Stallings C, Origoni AE, Vaughan C, Khushalani S, et al. (2013) Cigarette smoking among persons with schizophrenia or bipolar disorder in routine clinical settings, 1999–2011. Psychiatr Serv 64: 44–50.
3. de Leon J, Diaz FJ (2005) A meta-analysis of worldwide studies demonstrates an association between schizophrenia and tobacco smoking behaviors. Schizophr Res 76: 135–157.
4. Kelly C, McCreadie R (2000) Cigarette smoking and schizophrenia. Adv Psychiatr Treat 6: 327–331.
5. Hennekens CH, Hennekens AR, Hollar D, Casey DE (2005) Schizophrenia and increased risks of cardiovascular disease. Am Heart J 150: 1115–1121.
6. Brown S, Kim M, Mitchell C, Inskip H (2010) Twenty-five year mortality of a community cohort with schizophrenia. Br J Psychiatry 196: 116–121.
7. Kelly DL, McMahon RP, Wehring HJ, Liu F, Mackowick KM, et al. (2011) Cigarette smoking and mortality risk in people with schizophrenia. Schizophr Bull 37: 832–838.
8. Curkendall SM, Mo J, Glasser DB, Rose Stang M, Jones JK (2004) Cardiovascular disease in patients with schizophrenia in Saskatchewan, Canada. J Clin Psychiatry 65: 715–720.
9. Kobayashi M, Ito H, Okumura Y, Mayahara K, Matsumoto Y, et al. (2010) Hospital readmission in first-time admitted patients with schizophrenia: smoking patients had higher hospital readmission rate than non-smoking patients. Int J Psychiatry Med 40: 247–257.
10. Steinberg M, Williams J, Ziedonis D (2004) Financial implications of cigarette smoking among individuals with schizophrenia. Tob Control 13: 206.
11. Hooman S, Zahra H, Safa M, Hassan FM, Reza MM (2013) Association between cigarette smoking and suicide in psychiatric inpatients. Tob Induc Dis 11: 5.
12. Kao YC, Liu YP, Cheng TH, Chou MK (2011) Cigarette smoking in outpatients with chronic schizophrenia in Taiwan: relationships to socio-demographic and clinical characteristics. Psychiatry Res 190: 193–199.
13. Parry O, Thomson C, Fowkes G (2002) Cultural context, older age and smoking in Scotland: qualitative interviews with older smokers with arterial disease. Health Promot Int 17: 309–316.
14. Zhang X, Chen DC, Xiu MH, Haile CN, He SC, et al. (2013) Cigarette smoking, psychopathology and cognitive function in first-episode drug-naive patients with schizophrenia: a case-control study. Psychol Med 43: 1651–1660.
15. Zhang XY, Liang J, Chen DC, Xiu MH, He J, et al. (2012) Cigarette smoking in male patients with chronic schizophrenia in a Chinese population: prevalence and relationship to clinical phenotypes. PLoS One 7: e30937.
16. Hou YZ, Xiang YT, Yan F, Ungvari GS, Dickerson F, et al. (2011) Cigarette smoking in community-dwelling patients with schizophrenia in China. J Psychiatr Res 45: 1551–1556.
17. Wang CY, Xiang YT, Weng YZ, Bo QJ, Chiu HF, et al. (2010) Cigarette smoking in patients with schizophrenia in China: prospective, multicentre study. Aust N Z J Psychiatry 44: 456–462.
18. Ma X, Li C, Meng H, Du L, Wang Q, et al. (2010) Premorbid tobacco smoking is associated with later age at onset in schizophrenia. Psychiatry Res 178: 461–466.

19. Tang YL, George TP, Mao PX, Cai ZJ, Chen Q (2007) Cigarette smoking in Chinese male inpatients with schizophrenia: a cross-sectional analysis. J Psychiatr Res 41: 43–48.
20. Tang YL, Gillespie CF, Epstein MP, Mao PX, Jiang F, et al. (2007) Gender differences in 542 Chinese inpatients with schizophrenia. Schizophr Res 97: 88–96.
21. Zhang XY, Chen DC, Xiu MH, Yang FD, Haile CN, et al. (2012) Gender differences in never-medicated first-episode schizophrenia and medicated chronic schizophrenia patients. J Clin Psychiatry 73: 1025–1033.
22. Quednow BB, Brinkmeyer J, Mobascher A, Nothnagel M, Musso F, et al. (2012) Schizophrenia risk polymorphisms in the TCF4 gene interact with smoking in the modulation of auditory sensory gating. Proc Natl Acad Sci U S A 109: 6271–6276.
23. Kelly C, McCreadie RG (1999) Smoking habits, current symptoms, and premorbid characteristics of schizophrenic patients in Nithsdale, Scotland. Am J Psychiatry 156: 1751–1757.
24. Weiser M, Reichenberg A, Grotto I, Yasvitzky R, Rabinowitz J, et al. (2004) Higher rates of cigarette smoking in male adolescents before the onset of schizophrenia: a historical-prospective cohort study. Am J Psychiatry 161: 1219–1223.
25. Zhang XY, Li CB, Li M, Zheng YL, Zhang CX, et al. (2010) Smoking initiation and schizophrenia: a replication study in a Chinese Han population. Schizophr Res 119: 110–114.
26. Zammit S, Allebeck P, Dalman C, Lundberg I, Hemmingsson T, et al. (2003) Investigating the association between cigarette smoking and schizophrenia in a cohort study. Am J Psychiatry 160: 2216–2221.
27. Lowe EJ, Ackman ML (2010) Impact of tobacco smoking cessation on stable clozapine or olanzapine treatment. Ann Pharmacother 44: 727–732.
28. Goff DC, Henderson DC, Amico E (1992) Cigarette smoking in schizophrenia: relationship to psychopathology and medication side effects. Am J Psychiatry 149: 1189–1194.
29. Chong SA, Choo HL (1996) Smoking among Chinese patients with schizophrenia. Aust N Z J Psychiatry 30: 350–353.
30. Patkar AA, Gopalakrishnan R, Lundy A, Leone FT, Certa KM, et al. (2002) Relationship between tobacco smoking and positive and negative symptoms in schizophrenia. J Nerv Ment Dis 190: 604–610.
31. Winterer G (2010) Why do patients with schizophrenia smoke? Curr Opin Psychiatry 23: 112–119.
32. Smith RC, Singh A, Infante M, Khandat A, Kloos A (2002) Effects of cigarette smoking and nicotine nasal spray on psychiatric symptoms and cognition in schizophrenia. Neuropsychopharmacology 27: 479–497.
33. Barnes M, Lawford BR, Burton SC, Heslop KR, Noble EP, et al. (2006) Smoking and schizophrenia: is symptom profile related to smoking and which antipsychotic medication is of benefit in reducing cigarette use. Aust N Z J Psychiatry 40: 575–580.
34. Kumari V, Postma P (2005) Nicotine use in schizophrenia: the self medication hypotheses. Neurosci Biobehav Rev 29: 1021–1034.
35. Liao DL, Yang JY, Lee SM, Chen H, Tsai SJ (2002) Smoking in chronic schizophrenic inpatients in taiwan. Neuropsychobiology 45: 172–175.
36. Zhang XY, Yu YQ, Sun S, Zhang X, Li W, et al. (2011) Smoking and tardive dyskinesia in male patients with chronic schizophrenia. Prog Neuropsychopharmacol Biol Psychiatry 35: 1765–1769.
37. van Os J, Kenis G, Rutten BP (2010) The environment and schizophrenia. Nature 468: 203–212.
38. Linscott RJ, van Os J (2013) An updated and conservative systematic review and meta-analysis of epidemiological evidence on psychotic experiences in children and adults: on the pathway from proneness to persistence to dimensional expression across mental disorders. Psychol Med 43: 1133–1149.
39. Johns LC, van Os J (2001) The continuity of psychotic experiences in the general population. Clin Psychol Rev 21: 1125–1141.
40. Mäki P, Veijola J, Jones PB, Murray GK, Koponen H, et al. (2005) Predictors of schizophrenia–a review. Br Med Bull 73–74: 1–15.
41. Rajji TK, Ismail Z, Mulsant BH (2006) Age at onset and cognition in schizophrenia: meta-analysis. Br J Psychiatry 195: 286–293.
42. Xiang YT, Ma X, Lu JY, Cai ZJ, Li SR, et al. (2009) Alcohol-related disorders in Beijing, China: prevalence, socio-demographic correlates, and unmet need for treatment. Alcohol Clin Exp Res 33: 1111–1118.
43. Rey MJ, Schulz P, Costa C, Dick P, Tissot R (1989) Guidelines for the dosage of neuroleptics. I: Chlorpromazine equivalents of orally administered neuroleptics. Int Clin Psychopharmacol 4: 95-104.
44. Woods SW (2003) Chlorpromazine equivalent doses for the newer atypical antipsychotics. J Clin Psychiatry 64: 663–667.
45. Ryan H, Trosclair A, Gfroerer J (2012) Adult current smoking: differences in definitions and prevalence estimates–NHIS and NSDUH, 2008. J Environ Public Health: DOI:10.1155/2012/918368.
46. Qian J, Cai M, Gao J, Tang S, Xu L, et al. (2010) Trends in smoking and quitting in China from 1993 to 2003: National Health Service Survey data. Bulletin of the World Health Organization 88: 769–776.
47. He Y, Zhang M (1997) Use of the Positive and Negative Syndrome Scales (PANSS). Journal of Clinical Psychological Medicine 7: 353–355.
48. Simpson GM, Angus JW (1970) A rating scale for extrapyramidal side effects. Acta Psychiatr Scand Suppl 212: 11–19.
49. Barnes TR (1989) A rating scale for drug-induced akathisia. Br J Psychiatry 154: 672–676.
50. Victoria M, Farrell SP (2002) Schizophrenia, Tardive Dyskinesia, and the Abnormal Involuntary Movement Scale (AIMS). Journal of the American Psychiatric Nurses Association 8: 51–56.
51. Janno S, Holi MM, Tuisku K, Wahlbeck K (2005) Validity of Simpson-Angus Scale (SAS) in a naturalistic schizophrenia population. BMC Neurol 5:5.
52. Tohen M, Chengappa KN, Suppes T, Baker RW, Zarate CA, et al. (2004) Relapse prevention in bipolar I disorder: 18-month comparison of olanzapine plus mood stabiliser v. mood stabiliser alone. Br J Psychiatry 184: 337–345.
53. Si T, Yang J, Shu L, Wang X, Kong Q, et al. (2004) The reliability, validity of PANSS and its implication. Chin Ment Health J 18: 45–47.
54. Fan B (1990) Abnormal Inventory Movement Scale (AIMS). Shanghai Arch Psychiatry 2: 65–66.
55. Xiao Z, Yan W (1990) Tardive Dyskinesia Rating Scale (TDRS). Shanghai Arch Psychiatry 2: 66–67.
56. Zhang M (1998) Handbook of Psychistric Scales. Changsha: Hunan Science and Technology Press.
57. Giovino GA, Mirza SA, Samet JM, Gupta PC, Jarvis MJ, et al. (2012) Tobacco use in 3 billion individuals from 16 countries: an analysis of nationally representative cross-sectional household surveys. Lancet 380: 668–679.
58. China CDC (2010) Global Adult Tobacco Survey (GATS) China 2010 Country Report. Beijing, China: China's Three Gorge Press.
59. Li Q, Hsia J, Yang G (2011) Prevalence of smoking in China in 2010. N Engl J Med 364: 2469–2470.
60. Ulm K (1990) A simple method to calculate the confidence interval of a standardized mortality ratio. American Journal of Epidemiology 131: 373–375.
61. Deddens JA, Petersen MR (2008) Approaches for estimating prevalence ratios. Occup Environ Med 65: 481, 501–506.
62. Rothman KJ, Boice JD (1979) Epidemiologic analysis with a programmable calculator. Washington, DC: Government Printing Office.
63. de Leon J (1996) Smoking and vulnerability for schizophrenia. Schizophr Bull 22: 405–409.
64. Pan Z (2004) Socioeconomic predictors of smoking and smoking frequency in urban China: evidence of smoking as a social function. Health Promot Int 19: 309–315.
65. de Leon J, Diaz FJ, Rogers T, Browne D, Dinsmore L (2002) Initiation of daily smoking and nicotine dependence in schizophrenia and mood disorders. Schizophr Res 56: 47–54.
66. Challis GB (1999) Level of activity and prevalence of smoking in psychiatric patients. Can J Psychiatry 44: 711.
67. Steinert T, Wolfersdorf M, Thoma H, Marpert M (1996) Does long-term hospitalization modify cardiovascular morbidity in schizophrenic patients. Fortschr Neurol Psychiatr 64: 212–220.
68. LLerena A, de la Rubia A, Peñas-Lledó EM, Diaz FJ, de Leon J (2003) Schizophrenia and tobacco smoking in a Spanish psychiatric hospital. Schizophr Res 60: 313–317.
69. Masterson E, O'Shea B (1984) Smoking and malignancy in schizophrenia. Br J Psychiatry 145: 429–432.
70. McCool RM, Paschall Richter K (2003) Why do so many drug users smoke? J Subst Abuse Treat 25: 43–49.
71. Uzun O, Cansever A, Basoğlu C, Ozşahin A A (2003) Smoking and substance abuse in outpatients with schizophrenia: a 2-year follow-up study in Turkey. Drug Alcohol Depend 70: 187–192.
72. Sandyk R, Kay SR (1991) Tobacco addiction as a marker of age at onset of schizophrenia. Int J Neurosci 57: 259–262.
73. Cho HJ, Khang YH, Jun HJ, Kawachi I (2008) Marital status and smoking in Korea: the influence of gender and age. Soc Sci Med 66: 609–619.
74. De Leon J, Rendon D, Baca-Garcia E, Aizpuru F, Gonzalez-Pinto A, et al. (2007) Association between smoking and alcohol use in the general population: stable and unstable odds ratios across two years in two different countries. Alcohol Alcohol 42: 252–257.
75. Leonard S, Mexal S, Freedman R (2007) Smoking, Genetics and Schizophrenia: Evidence for Self Medication. J Dual Diagn 3: 43–59.
76. Levin ED, Rezvani AH (2007) Nicotinic interactions with antipsychotic drugs, models of schizophrenia and impacts on cognitive function. Biochem Pharmacol 74: 1182–1191.
77. Okan E, Aslı E (2012) Cigarette smoking in patients with schizophrenia in Turkey: relationships to psychopathology, socio-demographic and clinical characteristics. Düşünen Adam: The Journal of Psychiatry and Neurological Sciences 25: 321–329.
78. Hvidtfeldt UA, Rasmussen S, Grønbaek M, Becker U, Tolstrup JS (2010) Influence of smoking and alcohol consumption on admissions and duration of hospitalization. Eur J Public Health 20: 376–382.
79. Hart CL, Smith GD (2008) Alcohol consumption and mortality and hospital admissions in men from the Midspan collaborative cohort study. Addiction 103: 1979–1986.
80. Meszaros ZS, Dimmock JA, Ploutz-Snyder RJ, Abdul-Malak Y, Leontieva L, et al. (2011) Predictors of smoking severity in patients with schizophrenia and alcohol use disorders. Am J Addict 20: 462–467.
81. Diaz FJ, James D, Botts S, Maw L, Susce MT, et al. (2009) Tobacco smoking behaviors in bipolar disorder: a comparison of the general population, schizophrenia, and major depression. Bipolar Disord 11: 154–165.

6

Genetic Determinants of Chronic Obstructive Pulmonary Disease in South Indian Male Smokers

Cholendra Arja[1], Rajasekhara Reddy Ravuri[2], Venugopal N. Pulamaghatta[3], Krishna Mohan Surapaneni[4], Premanand Raya[5], Chandrasekhar Adimoolam[3], Kodanda Reddy Kanala[1]*

1 Department Of Anthropology, Division Of Human Genetics, Sri Venkateswara University, Tirupati, Andhra Pradesh, India, **2** Department Of Human Genetics, Punjabi University, Patiala, Punjab, India, **3** Anthropological Survey Of India, Southern Regional Centre, Mysore, Karnataka, India, **4** Department Of Biochemistry, Saveetha Medical College & Hospital, Faculty Of Medicine, Saveetha University, Chennai, Tamil Nadu, India, **5** Premananda Allergy And Chest Hospital, Tirupati, Andhra Pradesh, India

Abstract

The development of chronic obstructive pulmonary disease, upon exposure to tobacco smoke, is the cumulative effect of defects in several genes. With the aim of understanding the genetic structure that is characteristic of our patient population, we selected forty two single nucleotide polymorphisms of twenty genes based on previous studies and genotyped a total of 382 samples, which included 236 patients and 146 controls using Sequenom MassARRAY system. Allele frequencies of rs2276109 (MMP12) and rs1800925 (IL13) differed significantly between patients and controls ($p = 0.013$ and 0.044 respectively). Genotype analysis showed association of rs2276109 (MMP12) under additive and dominant models ($p = 0.017$, $p = 0.012$ respectively), rs1800925 (IL13) under additive model ($p = 0.047$) and under recessive model, rs1695 (GSTP1; $p = 0.034$), rs729631, rs975278, rs7583463 (SERPINE2; $p = 0.024$, 0.024 and 0.012 respectively), rs2568494, rs10851906 (IREB2; $p = 0.026$ and 0.041 respectively) and rs7671167 (FAM13A; $p = 0.029$). The minor alleles of rs1695 (G), rs7671167 (T), rs729631 (G), rs975278 (A) and rs7583463 (A) showed significant negative association whereas those of rs2276109 (G), rs2568494 (A), rs10851906 (G) and rs1800469 (T; TGF-β) showed significant positive association with lung function under different genetic models. Haplotypes carrying A allele of rs2276109, G allele of rs1695 showed negative correlation with lung function. Haplotypes carrying major alleles of rs7671167 (C) of FAM13A and rs729631 (C), rs975278 (G), rs7583463 (C) of SERPINE2 had protective effect on lung function. Haplotypes of IREB2 carrying major alleles of rs2568494 (G), rs2656069 (A), rs10851906 (A), rs965604 (C) and minor alleles of rs1964678 (T), rs12593229 (T) showed negative correlation with lung function. In conclusion, our study replicated the results of most of the previous studies. However, the positive correlation between the minor alleles of rs2568494 (A) and rs10851906 (G) of IREB2 and lung function needs further investigation.

Editor: Balraj Mittal, Sanjay Gandhi Medical Institute, India

Funding: The Indian Council of Medical Research (ICMR; New Delhi) provided the grant for completing this research (IRIS ID: 2009-07590; File no. 54/08/2009/HUM-BMS). The funders had no role in study design, data collection and analysis, decision to publish, or preparation of the manuscript.

Competing Interests: The authors have declared that no competing interests exist.

* E-mail: Kanalakr@yahoo.com

Introduction

The spectrum of Chronic Obstructive Pulmonary Disease (COPD) involves two pathological conditions, chronic bronchitis and emphysema. In India, tobacco smoke and exposure to biomass fuel exhaust (animal dung cakes, wood and crop residues) are the risk factors in males and females respectively [1]. In India an estimated 82.3% of males with COPD are smokers [2]. According to the estimation of World Health Organization (WHO) in 2002, COPD was responsible for over half a million deaths in India, placing the country second in the world in COPD mortality [3].

Alpha 1-antitrypsin deficiency is the only established genetic factor that invariably results in COPD in smokers. However, this is found only in about one percent of cases [4]. Linkage studies and subsequent association studies carried out with positional candidate genes or genes selected based on their presumptive role in pathophysiology have identified numerous genetic markers falling into the classes of antioxidants, proteases, antiproteases and inflammatory mediators [5]. However, the replication of genetic associations across different populations has not always been consistent [6]. While sample size, subject selection criteria and study designs contribute their share, the complex interplay between various molecules that are involved in the maintenance of lung integrity, which makes COPD polygenic, renders consistency across different population settings rather unlikely. Nevertheless, such studies helped us understand the pathogenesis of COPD under the headings of oxidant-antioxidant imbalance theory, the protease-antiprotease imbalance theory and inflammation. This genetic complexity and hence the pathophysiological heterogeneity together with the variability attributed to the disease by the environment, rendered COPD an incurable disease so far.

Identifying a common pathway(s) that links exposure to emphysema is possible only when genes implicated in the pathogenesis of COPD in one population are validated in other populations. To this end we selected forty two SNPs across twenty genes by referring to previous studies on COPD to identify the genetic makeup that is signature of our patient population.

Materials and Methods

Subjects

A total of 386 males (236 patients and 150 controls) were included in the study. All subjects were *bidi* (tobacco wrapped in tendu leaf (*Diospyros melanoxylon*)) smokers and were over 40 years of age with a smoking history >10 pack years. COPD diagnosis and staging was done using GOLD criteria [7]. Spirometry was performed while the patients were in stable condition using SpiroWin Model No. 99 spirometer (Genesis Medical Systems, Hyderabad, Andhra Pradesh, India.). All patients were requested to withhold their COPD medications for six hours (for short acting bronchodilators) or twelve hours (for long acting bronchodilators). Patients were required to have a post FEV_1/FVC ratio <70%. Subjects with a history of lung cancer, bronchial asthma, bronchiectasis, cystic fibrosis and fibrosis of pulmonary tuberculosis were excluded from the study. Patients were requested to stop all the medications they were using for a period of 24 hours prior to the day of testing. Reversibility of air flow obstruction was tested within 10–15 min after administering 0.5% salbutamol nebulizer solution at a dosage of 0.02 ml/kg body-weight diluted to 2 ml with isotonic saline with a compressed air driven nebulizer (Pulmo-Aide 5610, Devilbiss; DeVilbiss Healthcare, Somerset, PA, USA). Patients who showed reversibility ≥12% predicted and ≥200 ml of the absolute value of FEV_1 were excluded from the study.

While patients were available at the clinic, controls matching patients for age, smoking medium and pack years had to be searched for and could be reached only at their work places. Hence a portable spirometer (Vitalograph copd-6; Vitalograph Inc., Lenexa, KS, USA) which gave FEV_6 was used to diagnose controls. Prior to use with controls, the portable spirometer was tested against the standard spirometer at the clinic to assess the validity of the former's readings. Apparently normal individuals, strictly with an FEV_1/FEV_6 ratio >70% were selected as controls. Irrespective of the spirometry values, subjects were excluded from the control group if they reported difficulty in breathing while walking or working at any point of time in their life, have/had exposure to risk factors other than smoking (biomass fuel exhaust, diesel exhaust, grain dust, cotton dust), ceased to smoke at any point of time in their life due to breathing problems or visited any physician due to respiratory problems. A written informed consent was obtained from all the subjects prior to their participation in the study. The study protocol was approved by the Human Ethics Committee of Sri Venkateswara University (No:SVUHEC/ANTH/2010-09).

SNP Selection and Genotyping

Forty two SNPs from twenty genes were selected based on previous studies on COPD (Table S1). Genomic DNA was extracted from about 10 ml of whole peripheral blood using standard phenol-chloroform method. All subjects were genotyped using Sequenom's MassARRAY system (Sequenom Inc., San Diego, California, USA) according to manufacturer's specifications for the iPlex chemistry using 10 ng genomic DNA. Prior to further analysis, the assay performance and genotype calls were qualified by evaluating genotype cluster plots.

Statistical Analyses

Descriptive statistics were calculated using SPSS v16.0 (SPSS Inc., Chicago, IL, USA). Discontinuous variables are presented with percentages. Mean and standard deviation were calculated for clinical characteristics and compared between patients and controls using unpaired Student's *t*-test after adjusting for age, pack years and age - pack years interaction. Genetic analyses were carried out using PLINK software [8]. All the SNPs were checked for deviation from Hardy-Weinberg equilibrium in controls. Allele frequency variations were compared between patients and controls using Pearson's Chi-square test to generate odds ratio with 95% confidence limits. The contribution of each genotype to COPD susceptibility was evaluated using logistic regression under additive, dominant and recessive genetic models after adjusting for age and pack years. A linear regression model was used to study the association of SNPs with two COPD phenotypes (FEV_1 and FEV_1/FVC) under three genetic models with age and pack years as covariates. Haplotypes were generated using a sliding window method and their association was tested against COPD and its phenotypes using regression model after adjusting for age and pack years. The sliding window approach implemented in PLINK sequentially examines smaller sets of SNPs within the region. For example, using a 4-SNP overlapping sliding window, one would first conduct a haplotype analysis of SNPs 1–4, followed by SNPs 2–5, followed by SNPs 3–6, and so on until the last SNP in the region is reached [9,10]. A p value less than 0.05 was considered as significant throughout the analyses. The Benjamini–Hochberg False Discovery Rate method was used to correct for multiple hypothesis testing for allele and genotype association [11], whereas maxT permutation of 10000 steps was used to generate adjusted empirical p value for haplotype association tests [8].

Results

Demographics and clinical characteristics of the study population are presented in table 1. The age of the study population ranged from 40–80 years. Most of the subjects were older than 60 years (69.5% in patients, 55.5% in controls). There were more patients (42.4%) with BMI <18.5 kg/m2 compared to controls (17.9%). The majority of patients and controls were heavy smokers (69.06% and 74.7% respectively). The smoking intensity (calculated as pack years) was greater in control group than in patients (48.24±25.76 vs. 42.96±23.53; $p=0.03$). GOLD COPD staging identified most of the patients in stages III and IV (44.1% and 39.4% respectively).

The SNPs genotyped and genes studied along with results of allelic association are presented in table S1. Four control subjects had insufficient DNA quality and had to be excluded. Hence 146 control samples were genotyped. None of the SNPs deviated significantly from Hardy-Weinberg equilibrium in controls ($p>0.05$). Two SNPs in SERPINA3 (rs1800463 and rs17473), which had minor allele frequency <0.01 were excluded from further analysis. The minor allele frequencies of two SNPs, one in MMP12 (rs2276109) and another in IL13 (rs1800925) differed significantly between patients and controls (OR = 0.476, 95% CI: 0.263–0.863, $p=0.013$ and OR = 1.453, 95% CI: 1.009–2.091, $p=0.044$ respectively). The significance was lost after correcting for multiple testing. Logistic regression analysis after adjustment for age and smoking history under different genetic models revealed association of MMP12 (rs2276109) under additive and dominant models ($p=0.017$, $p=0.012$ respectively), IL13 (rs1800925) under additive model ($p=0.047$) and GSTP1 (rs1695, $p=0.034$), SERPINE2 (rs729631, $p=0.024$; rs975278, $p=0.024$; rs7583463, $p=0.012$), IREB2 (rs2568494, $p=0.026$; rs10851906, $p=0.041$) and FAM13A (rs7671167, $p=0.029$) under recessive model (table S2). None of the SNPs retained significance after correction for multiple testing.

Among the SNPs genotyped, nine SNPs showed significant association with FEV_1, and/or FEV_1/FVC (Table 2). The T allele of FAM13A (rs7671167) showed significant negative association with FEV_1 under additive and recessive models ($p=0.013$ and

Table 1. Demographics and clinical characteristics of the patients and controls.

		COPD (n = 236)	Controls (n = 150)	*t*-value	*p*-value
		Mean (SD)	Mean (SD)		
Age		63.19 (8.79)	61.07 (9.05)	2.272	0.02
Pack years®¥		42.96 (23.53)	48.24 (25.76)	2.01	0.03
BMI‡		19.82 (3.84)	22.01 (3.17)	6.04	0.07
FEV1%‡		36.82 (13.67)	71.68 (11.77)	26.42	0
FEV_1/FVC‡		55.42 (9)	85.98* (7.67)	35.37	0
Occupation (%)	Agriculture	56.8	52.1		
	Labor	13.6	17.8		
	Business	14.8	8.2		
	Employees	14.8	21.9		
GOLD COPD staging (%)	I	0.8			
	II	15.7			
	III	44.1			
	IV	39.4			

® p - value adjusted for age.
‡p-value adjusted for age and pack years.
*FEV_1/FEV_6.
¥Pack years were calculated by multiplying the number of bidis smoked per day with number of years of smoking, and then dividing the product by 24 (number of bidis in a packet) [42].

0.011 respectively) and with FEV_1/FVC under recessive model (p = 0.036). The G allele of GSTP1 (rs1695) showed significant negative association with FEV_1 under additive (p = 0.043) and recessive models (p = 0.001) and with FEV_1/FVC under recessive model (p = 0.023). The association of rs1695 under recessive model with FEV_1 remained significant even after correction for multiple testing (p-FDR = 0.026). The G allele of MMP12 (rs2276109) showed significant positive association with FEV_1 under dominant model (p = 0.050) and with FEV_1/FVC under additive (p = 0.015) and dominant models (p = 0.007). Two SNPs in IREB2 (rs2568494-A and rs10851906-G) showed marginal positive association with only FEV_1 under recessive model (p = 0.052). The T allele of TGF-β showed association with FEV_1/FVC under dominant model (p = 0.028). Three SNPs in SERPINE2 (rs729631-G, rs975278-A, rs7583463-A), showed significant positive association with both the phenotypes under recessive model (FEV_1, p = 0.002; FEV_1/FVC, p = 0.011, 0.011, 0.007 respectively). The p values remained significant after correction for multiple testing only for FEV_1 (p-FDR = 0.026).

Using a sliding window approach we generated haplotypes of 2, 3 and 4 SNPs and analyzed their association with COPD, FEV_1 and FEV_1/FVC. The haplotypes showing nominal significant association are presented in table S3. Haplotypes carrying the G allele of rs2276109 (MMP12) had a significant protective effect against developing COPD. Haplotypes of MMP12 carrying the A allele of both rs652438 and rs2276109 conferred significant risk of developing the disease. The IREB2 haplotypes containing the major alleles of rs2568494, rs2656069, rs10851906, rs965604 and minor alleles of rs1964678 and rs12593229 showed significant negative association with both COPD and lung function

Table 2. Single nucleotide polymorphisms showing association with COPD phenotypes.

GENE	SNP ID	Allele	β- FEV_1	P1*	Model#	P-FDR	β-FEV_1/FVC	P2*	Model#	P-FDR
FAM13A	rs7671167	T	−3.913, −6.773	0.013, 0.011	A, R	0.302, 0.087	−4.436	0.036	R	0.290
GSTP1	rs1695	G	−3.425, −13.25	0.043, 0.001	A, R	0.694, 0.026	−7.184	0.023	R	0.220
MMP12	rs2276109	G	6.557	0.050	D	0.943	6.024, 7.095	0.015, 0.007	A, D	0.371, 0.359
SERPINE2	rs729631	G	−10.89	0.002	R	0.026	−7.195	0.011	R	0.133
SERPINE2	rs975278	A	−10.89	0.002	R	0.026	−7.195	0.011	R	0.133
SERPINE2	rs7583463	A	−9.523	0.002	R	0.026	−6.655	0.007	R	0.133
IREB2	rs2568494	A	9.445	0.052	R	0.275				
IREB2	rs10851906	G	6.524	0.052	R	0.275				
TGF -β	rs1800469	T					3.857	0.028	D	0.4467

P1*: p-value for FEV_1 adjusted for age and pack years. P2*: p-value for FEV_1/FVC adjusted for age and pack years.
P-FDR: p-value corrected for multiple hypothesis testing by Benjamini-Hochberg False Discovery Rate method.
#A: Additive, R: Recessive, D: Dominant.

parameters. The SERPINE2 haplotypes containing major alleles of rs729631, rs975278, rs7583463 and minor allele of rs16865421 had a significantly greater frequency in controls and were positively associated with lung function. The two SNP haplotype of GSTP1 containing the minor allele G of rs1695 was negatively associated with FEV_1. This effect appeared to be profound when in combination with the risk haplotype AA of MMP12. However, G allele of rs1695 did not seem to be sufficient enough to produce the detrimental effect when in combination with the protective haplotype AG of MMP12. The 2, 3 and 4 SNP haplotypes constructed out of SNPs of the genes studied on chromosome 4 (GC, FAM13A, HHIP), showed that the haplotypes carrying the C allele of FAM13A had a protective effect on lung function. There were more controls carrying the haplotype CTCA (rs4588-rs7041-rs7671167-rs1828591) than patients. The frequencies of the two SNP haplotypes of EPHX1 did not differ significantly between patients and controls (data not shown). However, the presence of EPHX1 haplotype carrying minor allele C of rs1051740 and G of rs2234922 was found to have a protective effect ($\beta = 6.44$, $p = 0.037$). None of the haplotypes retained their significance after adjusting for multiple testing.

Discussion

In this study, we aimed at understanding the genetic structure that underlies the risk of developing COPD in our study population. To accomplish this, subjects were screened for single nucleotide polymorphisms of the genes falling into the classes of antioxidants, detoxification, proteases, antiproteases, inflammatory mediators and also those identified recently through GWAS. In agreement with the pathophysiological heterogeneity of the disease associations were found with the genes belonging to different classes.

MMP12 is an elastase which is predominantly produced by the alveolar macrophages. The lung tissues of the patients with advanced emphysema abound in MMP12 protein [12] and mice lacking MMP12 activity are protected against cigarette smoke induced emphysema [13]. The *A* allele of MMP12 SNP rs2276109 (−82 A→G) is associated with higher gene expression [14]. The functional impact of SNP rs652438 (1082A→G) on MMP12 activity is not known. In the present study, the frequency of rs2276109 *G* allele is significantly higher in controls. A significant positive correlation was also found between the rs2276109 G allele and FEV_1 under dominant model ($\beta = 6.557$, $p = 0.050$) and FEV_1/FVC under dominant ($\beta = 7.095$, $p = 0.007$) and additive models ($\beta = 6.024$, $p = 0.015$). Though the frequency of G allele of rs652438 was higher in controls, it did not reach significance level (0.061 in cases vs. 0.075 in controls, OR = 0.803, 95% CI: 0.452–1.427, $p = 0.454$). The deleterious effect of the A alleles of both rs2276109 and rs652438 is evident throughout the haplotype analysis. The frequency of AA haplotype was significantly higher in cases than in controls (0.894 and 0.836 respectively, $p = 0.031$). But the AA haplotype alone was not able to significantly decrease lung function (FEV_1: $\beta = -2.53$, $p = 0.26$; FEV_1/FVC: $\beta = -3.27$, $p = 0.066$ respectively). However 3 and 4 SNP haplotypes in which A allele of either SNP was present showed significant negative association with the lung function. Our result with respect to MMP12 is in agreement with previous studies [15,16].

Studies in murine models showed that over expression of IL13 produces cathepsin and matrix metalloproteinase dependent emphysema, mucus metaplasia and inflammation [17]. The SNP rs1800925 (−1111 C→T) which results in increased production of IL13 [18] showed association with COPD in earlier studies [19,20]. In our study too, the *T* allele of IL-13 showed significant association with the risk of developing COPD (OR = 1.453, 95% CI: 1.009–2.091, $p = 0.044$). In addition to this our genotype tests showed significant association of rs1800925 with COPD under additive genetic model (OR = 1.443, 95% CI: 1.005–2.071, $p = 0.047$).

Studies on animal models showed that decreased TGF- β signaling results in emphysema through alterations in macrophage MMP12 expression [21,22]. The SNP rs1800469 of TGF- β (-509 C→T) is associated with increased expression [23]. Consistent with the physiological role of TGF- β in emphysema, earlier study [24] found association of *C* allele with COPD. In our study the *T* allele frequency was higher in controls, but the difference between patients and controls was not statistically significant (0.350 in cases vs. 0.404 in controls, OR = 0.793, 95% CI: 0.587–1.071, $p = 0.129$). However, in the regression analysis, the *T* allele showed a significant positive correlation with FEV_1/FVC ($\beta = 3.857$, $p = 0.028$) under dominant model.

GSTs are a family of enzymes that catalyze the conjugation of reduced glutathione and subsequent detoxification of wide range of electrophilic substrates. Among the isoenzymes of GST, GSTP1 is the predominant form in human lung [25]. Two polymorphisms in GSTP1 have been investigated in COPD till date; rs1695 (A→G, Ile105Val,) and rs1138272 (C→T, Ala114Val). The replacement of Ile with less bulkier Val increases the catalytic activity of the enzyme towards polycyclic aromatic hydrocarbon diol epoxides [26,27]. But contrary to what could be expected, this increased catalytic activity was found to be associated with several forms of cancer including that of lung [28,29]. Studies in COPD with GSTP1 polymorphisms have shown mixed results. Some studies showed association of 105Ile variant with the disease [30,31] while some showed association with 105Val variant [32,33]. In our study, the SNP rs1695 showed association with COPD under recessive model (OR = 2.756, 95% CI: 1.081–7.026, $p = 0.034$). The rs1695 G allele showed significant negative correlation with FEV_1 under recessive ($\beta = -13.25$, $p = 0.001$) and additive model ($\beta = -3.425$, $p = 0.043$) and with FEV_1/FVC under recessive model ($\beta = -7.184$, $p = 0.023$). Significant negative correlations were also found between rs1695 G- rs1138272 C haplotype and FEV_1 ($\beta = -4.59$, $p = 0.010$). The haplotypes carrying the A allele of rs1695 had significant positive effect on FEV_1 ($\beta = 3.43$, $p = 0.043$).

FAM13A is a tumor suppressor gene. Earlier studies [34,35] showed that the C allele of FAM13A rs7671167 (T→C) has a protective effect on COPD and our study supports the same. The frequency of T allele was greater in patients than in controls, but the difference was not significant (0.492 in cases vs. 0.432 in controls, $p = 0.094$). The SNP rs7671167 showed association with COPD under recessive model (OR = 1.853, 95% CI: 1.066–3.223, $p = 0.029$). The T allele also showed significant negative correlation with lung function (FEV_1: $\beta = -6.773$, $p = 0.011$, recessive model; $\beta = -3.913$, $p = 0.013$, additive model) (FEV_1/FVC: $\beta = -4.436$, $p = 0.036$, recessive model).

SERPINE2 is a member of serine protease inhibitor family and is capable of inhibiting thrombin, urokinase, plasmin and trypsin. Two major studies [36,37], showed association of SERPINE2 polymorphisms with COPD. Another study [38] conducted in Japanese population showed association of rs975278 of SERPINE2 with emphysema under recessive model. In our study SNPs rs729631 (OR = 2.558, 95% CI: 1.131–5.788, $p = 0.024$), rs975278 (OR = 2.558, 95% CI: 1.131–5.788, $p = 0.024$), rs7583463 (OR = 2.407, 95% CI: 1.212–4.781, $p = 0.012$) of SERPINE2 showed significant association with COPD under recessive model. The same SNPs also showed significant negative correlation with FEV_1 and FEV_1/FVC under recessive model.

IREB2 together with IREB1 is involved in the regulation of cellular iron metabolism. Increased levels of IREB2 m-RNA have been reported in the lungs of smokers and COPD patients [39]. The polymorphisms of IREB2 have no known functional impact. Since the presence of excess iron in lung tissues can contribute to oxidative stress, abnormalities in IREB2 functioning or expression are likely to influence the pathology of COPD by augmenting oxidative stress. The minor allele frequency of all the IREB2 SNPs studied, with the exception of rs965604 was higher in controls than in cases. However, the difference was not significant. The SNPs rs2568494 and rs10851906 showed association with COPD under recessive model (OR = 0.336, 95% CI: 0.129–0.876, p = 0.026 and OR = 0.512, 95% CI: 0.270–0.972, p = 0.041 respectively). Further, rs2568494-A and rs10851906-G alleles showed marginal positive correlation with FEV_1 ($\beta = 9.445$, $p = 0.052$ and $\beta = 6.524$, $p = 0.052$ respectively). The protective effect of rs2568494-A allele is contrary to earlier findings [39,40,41]. Further the major alleles rs1964678-C and rs12593229-G were reported to confer risk in a previous study [39] Contrary to this, the haplotypes carrying the minor alleles rs1964678-T and rs12593229-T were associated with the significant risk of developing the disease and showed significant negative correlation with lung function. The associations found with respect to IREB2 in our study cannot be considered conclusive and generalized to the population from which the sample was drawn because of our small sample size. Further, there is also a chance that these associations could be affected by the SNPs of nearby genes with which the IREB2 SNPs are in LD.

Our study has few limitations. Firstly, only male subjects were included in the study. This was due to lack of affected female subjects available under smoking category. Exposure to biomass fuel smoke (wood, cow dung cakes etc) is the predominant risk factor for COPD in females in India. Therefore only smokers were chosen with the assumption that the mechanism by which tobacco smoke, which is a carrier of several Group I and Group II carcinogens, initiates COPD could be different from that of biomass fuel smoke. Second limitation of our study is the sample size. One factor that greatly contributed to this was the strict adherence to *bidi* smokers. Cigarette is expensive than bidi. As most of the interviewed subjects were daily wage labors, the choice of smoking medium depended highly on the person's day to day variable financial status. There were subjects who smoked both bidi and cigarette. Such subjects were excluded to avoid misinterpretation of pack years. Lastly, our patient population is not uniformly distributed across different GOLD stages of COPD. COPD was unknown to all our subjects until diagnosis (in case of patients) or our visit (in case of controls). Patients consulted physician only when they had severe respiratory problems due to disease progression. Therefore, at the time of initial diagnosis, most of the patients were either in GOLD stage III or GOLD stage IV.

Conclusion

Our study managed to reinforce the theories of oxidant-antioxidant imbalance, protease-antiprotease imbalance and inflammation upon which the etiology of COPD has been built. While most of the associations found in this study have been reported elsewhere, the associations found with IREB2 need to be investigated with larger sample sizes.

Author Contributions

Conceived and designed the experiments: KRK PR CSA KMS. Performed the experiments: CA RRR. Analyzed the data: CA RRR VNP. Wrote the paper: AC RRR KRK.

References

1. Jain NK, Thakkar MS, Jain N, Rohan KA, Sharma M (2011) Chronic obstructive pulmonary disease: Does gender really matter? Lung India 28: 258–262.
2. Jindal SK, Aggarwal AN, Gupta D (2001) A review of population studies from India to estimate national burden of chronic obstructive pulmonary disease and its association with smoking. Indian J.Chest Dis. Allied Sci 43: 139–47.
3. Lopez AD, Shibuya K, Rao C, Mathers CD, Hansell AL, et al. (2006) Chronic obstructive pulmonary disease: current burden and future projections. Eur Respir J 27: 397–412.
4. Mahadeva R, Lomas D (1998) Alpha1-antitrypsin deficiency, cirrhosis and emphysema. Thorax 53: 501–505.
5. Wood AM, Stockley RA (2006) The genetics of chronic obstructive pulmonary disease. Respir Res 7: 130.
6. Hersh CP, DeMeo DL, Silverman EK (2008) National Emphysema Treatment Trial State of the Art. Genetics of Emphysema. Proc Am Thorac Soc 5: 486–493.
7. Global Initiative for Chronic Obstructive Lung Disease. Global strategy for the diagnosis, management, and prevention of COPD. Executive summary. National Institutes of Health. 2006. Available: http://www.who.int/respiratory/copd/GOLD_WR_06.pdf. Accessed: 2012 Nov. 22.
8. Purcell S, Neale B, Todd-Brown K, Thomas L, Ferreira MAR (2007) PLINK: A Tool Set for Whole-Genome Association and Population-Based Linkage Analyses. Am J Hum Genet. 81: 559–575.
9. Purcell S, Daly MJ, Sham PC (2007) WHAP: haplotype-based association analysis. Bioinformatics. 23: 255–6.
10. Shili Lin, Hongyu Zhao (2010) Handbook on analyzing human genetic data: computational approaches and software. Heidelberg; New York: Springer.
11. Benjamini Y, Hochberg Y (1995) Controlling the false discovery rate: a practical and powerful approach to multiple testing. J R Statist Soc B 57: 289–300.
12. Caramori G, Di Gregorio C, Carlstedt I, Casolari P, Guzzinati I, et al. (2004) Mucin expression in peripheral airways of patients with chronic obstructive pulmonary disease. Histopathology 45: 477–484.
13. Hautamaki RD, Kobayashi DK, Senior RM, Shapiro SD (1997) Requirement for macrophage elastase for cigarette smoke-induced emphysema in mice. Science 277: 2002–2004.
14. Jormsjo S, Ye S, Moritz J, Walter DH, Dimmeler,S, etal. (2000) Allele-specific regulation of matrix metalloproteinase-12 gene activity is associated with coronary artery luminal dimensions in diabetic patients with manifest coronary artery disease. Circ Res 86: 998–1003.
15. Elkington PT, Cooke GS (2010) MMP12, lung function, and COPD in high-risk populations. N Engl J Med 362: 1241.
16. Haq I, Chappell S, Johnson SR, Lotya J, Daly L, et al. (2010) Association of MMP-2 polymorphisms with severe and very severe COPD: a case control study of MMPs-1, 9 and 12 in a European population. BMC Med Genet 11: 7.
17. Zheng T, Zhu Z, Wang Z, Homer RJ, Ma B, et al. (2000) Inducible targeting of IL-13 to the adult lung causes matrix metalloproteinase- and cathepsin-dependent emphysema. J Clin Invest 106: 1081–93.
18. van der Pouw Kraan TC, van Veen A, Boeije LC, van Tuyl SA, de Groot ER, et al. (1999) An IL-13 promoter polymorphism associated with increased risk of allergic asthma. Genes Immun 1: 61–65.
19. van der Pouw Kraan TCTM, Küçükaycan M, Bakker AM, Baggen JMC, van der Zeehttp://www.nature.com/gene/journal/v3/n7/abs/6363896a.html - aff4 JS, et al. (2002) Chronic obstructive pulmonary disease is associated with the -1055 IL-13 promoter polymorphism. Genes and Immunity 3: 436–439.
20. Sadeghnejad A, Meyers DA, Bottai M, Sterling DA, Bleecker ER, et al. (2007) IL13 promoter polymorphism 1112C/T modulates the adverse effect of tobacco smoking on lung function. Am J Respir Crit Care Med 176: 748–52.
21. Morris DG, Huang X, Kaminski N, Wang Y, Shapiro SD, et al. (2003) Loss of integrin alpha(v)beta6-mediated TGFbeta activation causes Mmp12-dependent emphysema. Nature 422: 169–73.

22. Roberts AB (2003) Medicine: Smoke signals for lung disease. Nature 422: 130–1.
23. Grainger DJ, Heathcote K, Chiano M, Snieder H, Kemp PR, et al. (1999) Genetic control of the circulating concentration of transforming growth factor type beta1. Hum. Mol. Genet 8: 93–97.
24. Celedón JC, Lange C, Raby BA, Litonjua AA, Palmer LJ, et al. (2004) The transforming growth factor-beta1 (TGFB1) gene is associated with chronic obstructive pulmonary disease (COPD). Hum Mol Genet 13: 1649–56.
25. Cantlay AM, Smith CA, Wallace WA, Yap PL, Lamb D, et al. (1994) Heterogeneous expression and polymorphic genotype of glutathione S-transferases in human lung. Thorax 49: 1010–4.
26. Zimniak P, Nanduri B, Pikula S, Bandorowicz-Pikula J, Singhal SS, et al. (1994) Naturally occurring human glutathione S-transferase GSTP1–1 isoforms with isoleucine and valine in position 104 differ in enzymic properties. Eur. J. Biochem 224: 893–899.
27. Sundberg K, Johansson A, Stenberg G, Widersten M, Seidel A, et al. (1998) Differences in the catalytic efficiences of allelic variants of glutathione transferase P1–1 towardscarcinogenic diol epoxides of polycyclic aromatic hydrocarbons.Carcinogenesis, 19: 433–436.
28. Ryberg D, Skaug V, Hewer A, Phillips DH, Harries LW, et al. (1997) Genotypes of glutathione transferase M1 and P1 and their significance for lung DNA adduct levels and cancer risk. Carcinogenesis 18: 1285–9.
29. Harries LW, Stubbins MJ, Forman D, Howard GCW, Wolf CR (1997) Identification of genetic polymorphisms at the glutathione Stransferase Pi locus and association with susceptibility to bladder, testicular and prostate cancer. Carcinogenesis 18: 641–644.
30. Ishii T, Matsuse T, Teramoto S, Matsui H, Miyao M, et al. (1999) Glutathione S-transferase P1 (GSTP1) polymorphism in patients with chronic obstructive pulmonary disease. Thorax 54: 693–6.
31. He JQ, Ruan J, Connett JE, Anthonisen NR, Paré PD, et al. (2002) Antioxidant gene polymorphisms and susceptibility to a rapid decline in lung function in smokers. Am J Respir Crit Care Med 166: 323–8.
32. Vibhuti A, Arif E, Deepak D, Singh B, Qadar Pasha MA (2007) Genetic polymorphisms of GSTP1 and mEPHX correlate with oxidative stress markers and lung function in COPD. Biochem Biophys Res Commun 359: 136–42.
33. He JQ, Connett JE, Anthonisen NR, Paré PD, Sandford AJ. (2004) Glutathione S-transferase variants and their interaction with smoking on lung function. Am J Respir Crit Care Med 170: 388–94.
34. Young RP, Hopkins RJ, Hay BA, Whittington CF, Epton MJ, et al. (2010) FAM13A locus in COPD is independently associated with lung cancer - evidence of a molecular genetic link between COPD and lung cancer. Appl Clin Genet 4: 1–10.
35. Cho MH, Boutaoui N, Klanderman BJ, Sylvia JS, Ziniti JP, et al. Variants in FAM13A are associated with chronic obstructive pulmonary disease. Nat Genet 42: 200–202.
36. Demeo DL, Mariani TJ, Lange C, Srisuma S, Litonjua AA, et al. (2006) The SERPINE2 gene is associated with chronic obstructive pulmonary disease. Am J Hum Genet 78: 253–64.
37. Zhu G, Warren L, Aponte J, Gulsvik A, Bakke P, et al. (2007) The SERPINE2 gene is associated with chronic obstructive pulmonary disease in two large populations. Am J Respir Crit Care Med 176: 167–73.
38. Fujimoto K, Ikeda S, Arai T, Tanaka N, Kumasaka T, et al. (2010) Polymorphism of SERPINE2 gene is associated with pulmonary emphysema in consecutive autopsy cases. BMC Med Genet 11: 159.
39. DeMeo DL, Mariani T, Bhattacharya S, Srisuma S, Lange C, et al. (2009) Integration of genomic and genetic approaches implicates IREB2 as a COPD susceptibility gene.Am J Hum Genet 85: 493–502.
40. Chappell SL, Daly L, Lotya J, Alsaegh A, Guetta-Baranes T, et al. (2011) The role of IREB2 and transforming growth factor beta-1 genetic variants in COPD: a replication case-control study. BMC Med Genet 12: 24.
41. Kim WJ, Wood AM, Barker AF, Brantly ML, Campbell EJ, et al. (2012) Association of IREB2 and CHRNA3 polymorphisms with airflow obstruction in severe alpha-1 antitrypsin deficiency. Respir Res13: 16.
42. Kumar R, Prakash S, Kushwah AS, Vijayan VK (2010) Breath carbon monoxide concentration in cigarette and bidi smokers in India. Indian J Chest Dis Allied Sci 52: 19–24.

7

The Effects of Smoking on Levels of Endothelial Progenitor Cells and Microparticles in the Blood of Healthy Volunteers

Fariborz Mobarrez[1]*, Lukasz Antoniewicz[1], Jenny A. Bosson[2], Jeanette Kuhl[1], David S. Pisetsky[3,4], Magnus Lundbäck[1]

1 Karolinska Institutet, Department of Clinical Sciences, Division of Cardiovascular Medicine, Danderyd Hospital, Stockholm, Sweden, **2** Department of Public Health and Clinical Medicine, Division of Medicine/Respiratory Medicine, Umeå University, Umeå, Sweden, **3** Medical Research Service, Durham VA Hospital, Durham, North Carolina, United States of America, **4** Department of Medicine, Duke University Medical Center, Durham, North Carolina, United States of America

Abstract

Background: Cigarette smoking, both active and passive, is one of the leading causes of morbidity and mortality in cardiovascular disease. To assess the impact of brief smoking on the vasculature, we determined levels of circulating endothelial progenitor cells (EPCs) and circulating microparticles (MPs) following the smoking of one cigarette by young, healthy intermittent smokers.

Materials and Methods: 12 healthy volunteers were randomized to either smoking or not smoking in a crossover fashion. Blood sampling was performed at baseline, 1, 4 and 24 hours following smoking/not smoking. The numbers of EPCs and MPs were determined by flow cytometry. MPs were measured from platelets, leukocytes and endothelial cells. Moreover, MPs were also labelled with anti-HMGB1 and SYTO 13 to assess the content of nuclear molecules.

Results: Active smoking of one cigarette caused an immediate and significant increase in the numbers of circulating EPCs and MPs of platelet-, endothelial- and leukocyte origin. Levels of MPs containing nuclear molecules were increased, of which the majority were positive for CD41 and CD45 (platelet- and leukocyte origin). CD144 (VE-cadherin) or HMGB1 release did not significantly change during active smoking.

Conclusion: Brief active smoking of one cigarette generated an acute release of EPC and MPs, of which the latter contained nuclear matter. Together, these results demonstrate acute effects of cigarette smoke on endothelial, platelet and leukocyte function as well as injury to the vascular wall.

Editor: Ingo Ahrens, University Hospital Medical Centre, Germany

Funding: These authors have no support or funding to report.

Competing Interests: The authors have declared that no competing interests exist.

* E-mail: fariborz.mobarrez@ki.se

Introduction

According to the World Health Organization, cigarette smoking is a major health hazard, and is associated with increased risk of cardiovascular mortality. At the beginning of 2000, more than 1 billion people worldwide were active smokers [1] and it is estimated that 5 million people lose their lives each year due to tobacco use. Tobacco smoking substasntially increases the risk of venous thrombosis and is considered one of the major risk factors for atherothrombotic disease, including ischemic heart disease and stroke [2].

The endothelium covers the innermost layer of the vascular wall and plays a pivotal role in regulating vascular tone, coagulation, fibrinolysis and inflammation [3]. Cigarette smoke has been shown to impair vascular repair, induce platelet activation and cause endothelial damage [4]. *In vitro* data also suggest that cigarette smoke induces endothelial cell activation and/or apoptosis in human aortic endothelial cells [5].

A key cell type in the regulation of vasculature health is the endothelial progenitor cell (EPC). EPCs are mainly derived from the bone marrow and can mediate the differentiation, regeneration and maintenance of endothelial cells in response to vascular injury or vascular neogenesis [6,7]. EPC levels have been proposed as an important biomarker for endothelial dysfunction. However, the association between levels of EPCs and endothelial dysfunction is still controversial [8]. Several studies have demonstrated that levels of EPCs are inversely correlated to cardiovascular risk factors and that a low EPC count is an independent predictor of cardiovascular events [9,10].

Another possible marker for endothelial function are microparticles (MPs) of endothelial cell origin. Microparticles, are small membrane-bound particles which are between 0.1–1.0 μm in diameter and circulate in the bloodstream. MPs are released from all types of cells, including leukocytes, platelets and endothelial cells, upon activation or apoptosis of the parent cell. These particles can contain various cytokines, growth factors and proteases and display biological activities that connect them to thrombosis, inflammation and immune responses [11]. Recently, it has been shown that MPs also contain nuclear molecules as shown by SYTO 13 labeling of nucleic acids and binding of antibodies to high mobility group box 1 protein (HMGB1), an important alarmin or danger-associated molecular pattern (DAMP) [12,13]. SYTO 13, a member of the SYTO dye group, is cell permeable and has a high fluorescent yield when bound to DNA or RNA [14], providing the basis for sensitive detection of structures containing nucleic acids.

Previous studies have shown that chronic smokers display increased levels of circulating endothelial MPs (EMPs) [15]. However, exposure to cigarette smoke has also been shown to have more immediate effects. Heiss et al studied the responses of healthy non-smokers after a 30 minute exposure to second-hand smoke (SHS) and described higher levels of EMPs and EPCs early in the experiment as well as up to 24 hours after SHS exposure [16].

To elucidate further the effects of smoking on the vasculature, we investigated the acute effects of active smoking of one cigarette on the generation of EPCs and MPs in healthy intermittent smokers. These studies indicate rapid changes in these markers, suggesting effects of even one cigarette on a variety of cell types which may contribute to vascular disease.

Methods

12 young (mean age 26±5 years, 6 males and 6 females) healthy intermittent/sporadic smokers (max 10 cigarettes per month) were included. Intermittent smokers were recruited due to their ability to completely inhale a cigarette without feeling nausea or sickness. All subjects had a normal health declaration. Exclusion criteria were cardiovascular disease, diabetes mellitus, asthma and/or allergy, respiratory infection within 4 weeks of the study. All subjects smoked one cigarette (John Silver) completely for approximately 5 minutes in a specially prepared temperature-controlled room (22°C), where the exhaled smoke was immediately removed through ventilation. Blood was drawn from an antecubital vein at baseline, 1, 4 and 24 hours after exposure following at least 15 minutes of rest in a semi-supine position (Figure 1). To avoid misinterpretation due to a possible daily variation, blood samplings were also collected without smoke exposure, at least one week apart. Research subjects were required to refrain from alcohol, caffeine and heavy exercise at least 24 hours prior to exposure. Tobacco usage (including Swedish moist snuff) was not permitted within 7 days prior to exposure.

Blinded investigators performed all analysis and written informed consent was obtained from all subjects prior to the study. This study was approved of by the Human Research Ethics Committee at Karolinska Institutet, Stockholm (2012/672-31).

Blood sampling

Blood was drawn into test tubes containing 1/10 volume sodium citrate. Platelet free plasma was obtained after centrifugation at 2000 *g* for 20 minutes at room temperature (RT) and stored at −70°C until analysis.

Measurement of endothelial progenitor cells

The numbers of EPCs were measured as $CD34^+$ KDR^+ (KDR: vascular endothelial growth factor receptor 2) double positive cells using a Beckman Gallios flow cytometer (Brea, CA, USA). Briefly, 20 µl of whole blood were incubated with CD34-FITC (Beckman Coulter, Brea, CA, USA) and CD309 (Becton Dickinson, Franklin Lakes, New Jersey, USA). Conjugate isotype-matched immunoglobulin (IgG1-FITC, IgG1-PE) with no reactivity against human antigens was used as a negative control. After 30 minutes of incubation in a dark environment, BD cell-fix was added to fixate the samples. Twenty thousand events of leukocytes were collected (based on classical forward scatter/side scatter (size/granularity) characteristics of blood leukocytes) and results are presented as the number of EPC events.

Measurement of microparticles

Plasma was thawed and centrifuged at 2000 *g* for 20 minutes at RT. The supernatant was re-centrifuged at 13,000 *g* for 2 minutes at RT. Subsequently, 20 µL of sample was incubated for 20 minutes in the dark with phalloidin-Alexa 660 (Invitrogen, Paisley, UK), lactadherin-FITC (Haematologic Technologies, Vermont, USA), CD41-PE or CD41-APC (Platelet-MP (PMP), Beckman Coulter, Brea, CA, USA), CD45-PC7 (Leukocyte-MP (LMP), Beckman Coulter, Brea, CA, USA), CD14-APC (Monocyte-MP, Beckman Coulter, Brea, CA, USA) and CD144-APC ((EMP), AH diagnostics, Stockholm, Sweden). PMPs were also labeled with CD154-PE (CD40 Ligand, abcam, Cambridge, UK) and EMPs with CD62E-APC (E-selectin, Beckman Coulter, Brea, CA, USA). MPs from platelets and monocytes were also labeled with anti-HMGB1-PE (R&D Systems, Minneapolis, USA). Nuclear staining

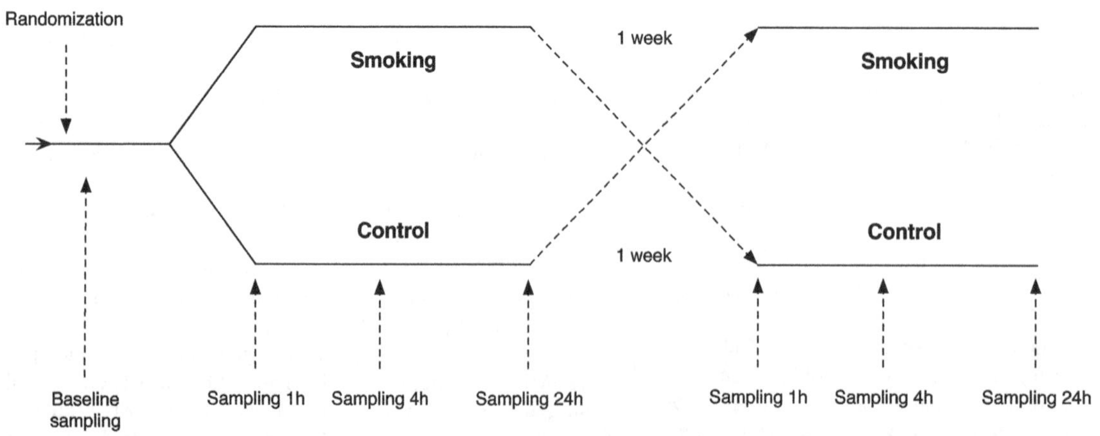

Figure 1. Study design. 12 healthy volunteers were randomized to either smoking or not smoking (control) in a crossover fashion. A time period of at least 1 week separated the experiments. Blood sampling was performed at baseline, 1 h, 4 h and 24 hours.

was performed by labeling samples with SYTO 13 (Invitrogen, Paisley, UK) alone or double stained with anti-HMGB1-PE, CD41-APC, CD144-APC or CD45-PC7. MPs were measured by flow cytometry on a Beckman Gallios instrument. The MP-gate was determined using Megamix beads (BioCytex, Marseille, France), which is a mix of beads with diameters of 0.5 μm, 0.9 μm and 3.0 μm, respectively. MPs were defined as particles less than 1.0 μm in size, negative to phalloidin (in order to exclude cell membrane fragments [17]) and positive to lactadherin or SYTO 13. Conjugate isotype-matched immunoglobulin (IgG1-FITC, IgG1-PE, IgG1-APC and IgG1- PC7) with no reactivity against human antigens was used as a negative control to define the background noise of the cytometric analysis. The absolute number of MPs was calculated by means of the following formula: (MPs counted x standard beads/L)/standard beads counted (FlowCount, Beckman Coulter).

Statistical analysis

Based on previous published data it was estimated that approximately 12 subjects were needed to detect a 30% difference between treatments with a power of 80% at a $p<0.05$ significance level (two sided test). Statistical calculations were performed with Graphpad Prism (5.0c) software using a two-factor (time and exposure) analysis of variance with repeated measures. Skewed data were logarithmically transformed prior to statistical analysis. Statistical significance was taken at $p<0.05$.

Results

Circulating EPCs were measured both during smoking and control visit as $CD34^+$ KDR^+ double positive cells. As shown in Figure 2, active smoking of one cigarette caused a significant increase in the number of circulating EPCs after approximately 1 h and peaked at 4 h (Figure 2).

We next measured MPs to determine more general effects of smoking as MPs can originate from essentially any cell type that undergoes activation or apoptosis. Results of these experiments are presented in Figure 3 and Table 1. The majority of MP subtypes increased significantly following smoking. MPs that are positive for lactadherin (which binds to exposed phosphatidylserine) and cell-specific MPs (platelets, endothelial and leukocyte origin) were all significantly increased after smoking (Figure 3). Interestingly, only EMPs measured as CD62E (E-selectin) were increased, contrasting with results of staining form CD144 (VE-cadherin) (Figure 3B and Table 1). Further phenotyping also revealed a significant increase in PMPs exposing CD62P and CD154 on their surface (Table 1). HMGB1 exposure did not significantly change in monocyte (CD14) or platelet MPs (CD41) (Table 1).

Nuclear content was measured in MPs by assessing SYTO 13 binding (Figure 4A). Data showed a significant increase in all MPs containing nuclear molecules, where the majority were also positive for CD41 and CD45 (platelet and leukocyte origin, Table 1). HMGB1 exposure in SYTO 13^+ MP population was not significantly changed although it showed some tendencies towards higher levels during smoking (Figure 4B). SYTO 13 binding together with CD144 showed no significant changes (Table 1).

Discussion

The present study provides new insights into the effect of smoking on the function of the endothelium as blood cell activation, demonstrating that active smoking of one cigarette causes an immediate increase in the number of circulating EPCs as well as MPs of leukocyte, platelet and endothelial origin. Furthermore, active smoking caused an increase in levels of circulating MPs containing nuclear molecules. Taken together, these results show that smoking as little as just one single cigarette for a short period of time can cause MP-release as well as EPC mobilization. These findings suggest immediate systemic events that can impact on vascular integrity and could promote events important in atherosclerosis.

Following smoking of one cigarette, circulating EPCs measured as $CD34^+$ and KDR^+ were significantly increased (Figure 2). In this study, EPCs were identified as $CD34^+$ and KDR^+ (also known as vascular endothelial growth factor receptor 2). At present, a standardized flow cytometry protocol for EPC measurement is not available [18]. While we could have used additional markers such as CD133 to identify EPCs, our data still show a significant difference between smoking and control visits. This rapid EPC response may seem surprising in terms of known mechanisms for the expression of these cells in the blood. As shown in studies of diabetic mice, EPCs are recruited from the bone marrow in a fashion dependent on endothelial nitric oxide synthase [19]. However, the time frame for this response in the present study suggests that bone marrow recruitment cannot account for the quick increase in EPCs demonstrated less than 1 h after smoking. Animal studies have also demonstrated the presence of EPCs dwelling in the vascular wall as well as in the bronchial wash of mice [20]. Furthermore, in a study by Imaoka et al, EPCs have

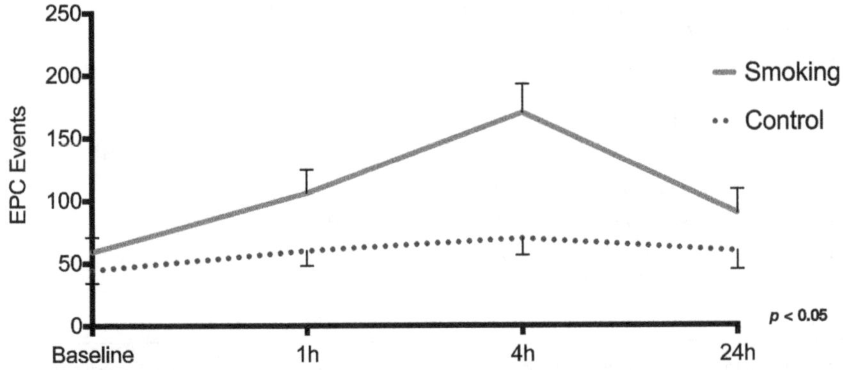

Figure 2. Endothelial progenitor cells during smoking and control. Endothelial progenitor cells were measured as $CD34^+$ KDR^+ double positive cells during smoking and control visit. Data are presented as events of endothelial progenitor cells (mean±SE). Statistical differences (two-factor ANOVA) are indicated in the figure.

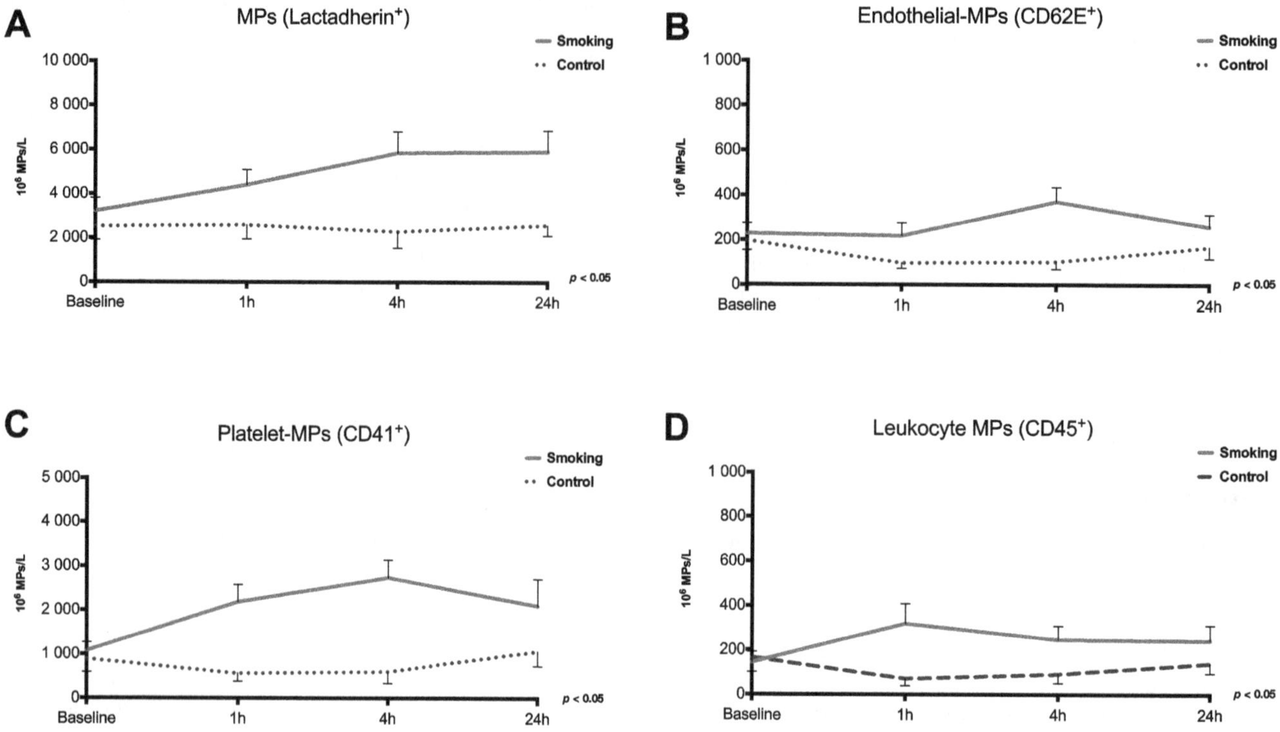

Figure 3. Microparticles during smoking and control. Microparticles were measured by flow cytometry and gated according to size and phosphatidylserine exposure (A) together with cell-specific antigens to determine cellular origin; endothelial-MPs (B), platelet-MPs (C) or leukocyte-MPs (D). Data is presented as mean±SE. Statistical differences (two-factor ANOVA) are indicated for each panel.

Table 1. Microparticles during smoking and control.

Marker	Exposure	Baseline	1 h	4 h	24 h	*p*
Lactadherin⁺ CD41⁺ CD62P⁺	Smoking	268 [51:789]	335 [193:1336]	123 [41:1040]	335 [106:1021]	*<0.05*
	Control	224 [39:639]	138 [19:352]	87 [12:280]	176 [22:615]	
Lactadherin⁺ CD41⁺ CD154⁺	Smoking	84 [12:430]	167 [31:280]	34 [10:321]	72 [31:389]	*<0.05*
	Control	87 [7:135]	41 [1:77]	19 [5:176]	80 [7:203]	
Lactadherin⁺ CD144⁺	Smoking	118 [1:975]	48 [1:1561]	27 [1:1129]	121 [29:1301]	*ns*
	Control	70 [10:1062]	31 [2:333]	22 [2:391]	56 [2:507]	
Lactadherin⁺ CD14⁺ HMGB1⁺	Smoking	80 [10:536]	331 [12:1441]	43 [2:531]	222 [152:921]	*ns*
	Control	130 [43:492]	56 [22:478]	31 [10:929]	70 [10:594]	
Lactadherin⁺ CD41⁺ HMGB1⁺	Smoking	41 [1:106]	22 [1:150]	12 [1:97]	31 [2:101]	*ns*
	Control	19 [2:101]	22 [1:118]	14 [1:191]	31 [1:92]	
SYTO 13⁺ CD41⁺	Smoking	138 [36:536]	331 [12:1441]	43 [2:531]	222 [152:921]	*<0.01*
	Control	130 [43:492]	56 [22:478]	31 [10:929]	70 [10:594]	
SYTO 13⁺ CD45⁺	Smoking	80 [10:536]	188 [12:878]	19 [1:212]	92 [48:425]	*<0.05*
	Control	63 [14:176]	22 [5:169]	5 [1:145]	22 [2:241]	
SYTO 13⁺ CD144⁺	Smoking	7 [1:97]	14 [1:75]	2 [1:46]	24 [7:65]	*ns*
	Control	17 [2:58]	5 [1:46]	2 [1:51]	5 [1:43]	

Microparticles were measured by flow cytometry and gated according to size and phosphatidylserine exposure (lactadherin binding) together with cell-specific antigens CD41 (platelet origin), CD144 (endothelial origin) or CD14 (monocyte origin). Platelet microparticles were also investigated for P-selectin (CD41+CD62P), and CD40 ligand (CD41+CD154) exposure. Furthermore, both platelet (CD41) and monocyte (CD14) microparticles were labeled with anti-HMGB1. To asses nuclear content and origin, microparticles were labeled with SYTO 13 and cell-specific antibodies; CD41 (platelet), CD45 (leukocyte) and CD144 (endothelial). Data is presented as median and interquartiles [25:75]. ns: non significant.

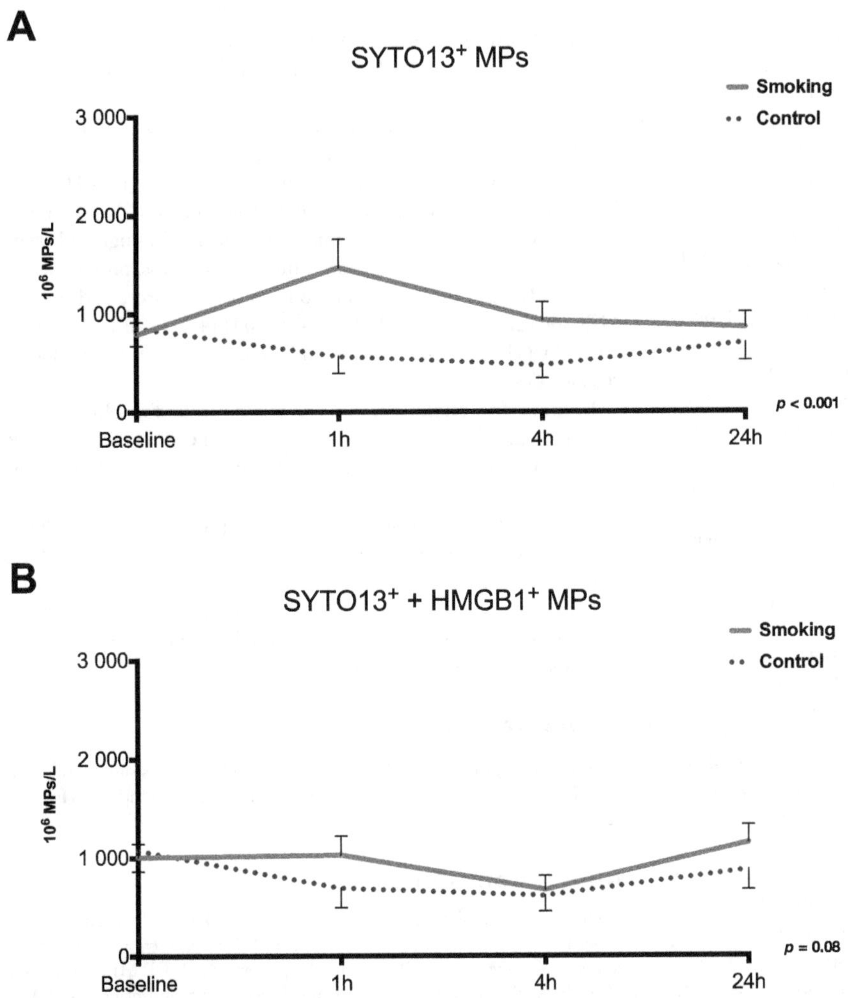

Figure 4. Nuclear molecule content of microparticles after smoking and control. Microparticles were measured by flow cytometry and gated according to size and SYTO 13 binding alone (A) or together with HMGB1 exposure (B). Data is presented as mean±SE. Statistical differences (two-factor ANOVA) are indicated for each panel.

been found in the human lung in patients with asthma [21]. The initial rapid response after active smoking may therefore be explained by a release of EPCs from the bronchial tree and/or the vascular wall rather than bone marrow recruitment.

Cigarette smoke causes increased oxidative stress and reduced levels of nitric oxide (NO) in plasma [22]. Chronic smokers have reduced EPC levels, most likely due to a decrease in NO-bioavailability and resulting reduction in bone marrow recruitment of EPCs [23]. There is an association between low levels of EPCs and conditions characterized by chronic inflammation such as rheumatoid arthritis, systemic lupus erythematosus and ulcerative colitis. Furthermore, circulating EPC-levels are reduced with progression of the disease, implying a gradual depletion of EPCs in the bone marrow [24,25]. In addition to inflammation, these inflammatory diseases are all associated with vascular injury as well as vascular neogenesis [25].

Until recently, it was not clear whether EPCs were released as a part of a systemic inflammatory response or vascular injury. In a study presented by Padfield et al, healthy individuals were exposed to salmonella typhus vaccination; following this exposure, EPC-levels remained unaffected.[26]. Therefore, the authors concluded that EPC mobilization was due to vascular injury rather than systemic inflammation. Hence, it is not unexpected to see an increased number of EPCs following cigarette smoking. This response may be interpreted as a sign of acute vascular injury, which in the long run leads to a depletion of EPC-storages and reduced capability of vascular repair [12].

Results of the present study showed that smoking increased levels of MPs from platelets, endothelial cells and leukocytes, which most likely is due to cell activation in response to cigarette smoke. We observed an increase of platelet-MPs exposing CD40 Ligand (CD154) and CD62P. CD40L is a co-stimulatory molecule expressed mainly on T cells, although it is also present and functionally active on platelets [27]. CD40L on platelets can activate endothelial cells to secrete chemokines, thereby initiating an inflammatory response [28]. CD62P plays an important role in the recruitment of leukocytes by binding to its ligand, P-selectin glycoprotein ligand-1 and can also be expressed on platelets as well as on endothelial cells [29].

The increase in MPs expressing CD45 (leukocyte origin) confirms results in a previous in vitro study by Li et al, in which human monocytes/macrophages exposed to tobacco smoke extract, generated pro-coagulant MPs [30]. Also, type 2 diabetic smokers showed increase in circulating tissue factor after smoking two cigaretts, thus leading to an increase in pro-coagulant state [31]. Circulating tissue factor is believed to be bound to circulating microparticles [32]. As MPs are considered pro-coagulant [33], due to exposed phosphatidylserine or tissue factor, an increase of MPs after one smoked cigarette may offer a mechanistic explanation for the association between cigarette smoke and thrombotic disease. Indeed, smoking is known to be a major risk factor for cardiovascular disease [34] and numerous studies have demonstrated increased levels of MPs in diseases such as acute coronary syndrome and ischemic stroke [35].

EMPs were measured as either CD62E (E-selectin) or CD144 (VE-cadherin)-positive EMPs, of which only $CD62E^+$ MPs increased (Figure 3 and Table 1). CD144 is a large molecule located in tight junctions between endothelial cells [36]. Consequently, more damage may be required to the endothelial cells until $CD144^+$ MPs are released. During exposure to second-hand smoke, both $CD62E^+$ and $CD144^+$ MPs were increased [16]. Whilst the exposure of second hand smoke was 30 minutes, our volunteers only smoked one cigarette for approximately 5 minutes; this difference could influence the findings in the various studies. Results also showed that the amount of HMGB1 exposed on monocytes or platelet MPs was not altered during active smoking. Extracellular HMGB1 is a prototype alarmin that can display pro-inflammatory activity depending on its origin during activation and apoptosis and has previously been found on microparticles [13,37–38]. Interestingly, it has been shown that nicotine can suppress HMGB1 release from macrophages through a nicotinic receptor dependent pathway [39]. Since we only measured exposed HMGB1 on MPs by flow cytometry, we cannot be certain if the nicotine in cigarette smoke has reduced or "masked" a potential effect on HMGB1 levels that may result from other ingredients in smoke or their actions. Soluble HMGB1 can also be measured by conventional ELISA. However, we have previously shown that measurement of MP-bound HMGB1 measured by flow cytometry is more sensitive than ELISA measurement [13].

In addition to a more conventional MP measurement, we also labelled MPs with SYTO 13 together with cell-specific markers or anti-HMGB1 (Figure 4 and Table 1). As previously shown [12], the binding of SYTO 13 by MPs generated from apoptotic cells *in vitro* reflects the presence of both RNA and DNA that likely occurs during translocation of nuclear molecules into particles. Also, LPS, which is known to induce apoptosis, can lead to the release of MPs containing DNA/RNA [13]. In this study levels of all MPs positive for SYTO 13 were significantly altered (Figure 4A) and further phenotyping revealed that the majority of MPs were from platelets and leukocytes (Table 1). Interestingly, platelets lack a nucleus but still contain mitochondrial DNA and mRNA, as well as HMGB1 [40–41]. It is tempting to speculate that these MPs containing nuclear matter were released due to apoptosis, although cell death would be expected to take more time. Nevertheless, an increase in these MPs was noted after only one smoked cigarette. Moreover, MPs measured with SYTO 13 and CD144 as well as SYTO13 and HMGB1 did not significantly change, most likely due to reasons described above.

In summary, smoking as little as one cigarette for a brief period of time can cause an early release of EPCs, as well as MPs containing nuclear molecules, which can have pro-inflammatory activity into the circulation. Because of the origin of MPs, their presence in the blood after smoking suggests important systemic effects in terms of inflammation, impaired endothelial function and vascular injury and repair. Future studies are necessary in order to fully determine the role of biomarkers such as EPCs and MPs, as markers to elucidate both immediate and long-term effects of smoking on the endothelium and blood cells.

Acknowledgments

The authors gratefully acknowledge the technical assistance of Lena Gabrielsson from the Department of Clinical Sciences, Danderyd Hospital, Karolinska Institutet, Stockholm, Sweden.

Author Contributions

Conceived and designed the experiments: FM JB JK ML. Performed the experiments: FM. Analyzed the data: FM ML. Contributed reagents/materials/analysis tools: FM. Wrote the paper: FM JB DP ML. Enrollment of study participants: JK LA. Critically revised the manuscript: FM LA JB DP ML.

References

1. Barnoya J, Glantz SA (2005) Cardiovascular effects of secondhand smoke: nearly as large as smoking. Circulation 111:2684–2698.
2. Jacobs DR, Adachi H, Mulder I, Kromhout D, Menotti A, et al. (1999) Cigarette smoking and mortality risk: twenty-five-year follow-up of the Seven Countries Study. Arch Intern Med 159:733–740.
3. Lerman A, Zeiher AM (2005) Endothelial function: cardiac events. Circulation 111:363–368.
4. Newby DE, Wright RA, Labinjoh C, Ludlam CA, Fox KA, et al. (1999) Endothelial dysfunction, impaired endogenous fibrinolysis, and cigarette smoking: a mechanism for arterial thrombosis and myocardial infarction. Circulation 99:1411–1415.
5. Raveendran M, Wang J, Senthil D, Wang J, Utama B, et al. (2005) Endogenous nitric oxide activation protects against cigarette smoking induced apoptosis in endothelial cells. FEBS Lett 579:733–740.
6. Hibbert B, Olsen S, O'Brien E (2003) Involvement of progenitor cells in vascular repair Trends Cardiovasc Med 13:322–326.
7. Tanaka K, Sata M, Hirata Y, Nagai R (2003) Diverse contribution of bone marrow cells to neointimal hyperplasia after mechanical vascular injuries. Circ Res 93:783–790.
8. Lekakis J, Abraham P, Balbarini A, Blann A, Boulanger CM, et al. (2011) Methods for evaluating endothelial function: a position statement from the European Society of Cardiology Working Group on Peripheral Circulation. Eur J Cardiovasc Prev Rehabil 18:775–789.
9. Vasa M, Fichtlscherer S, Aicher A, Adler K, Urbich C, et al. (2001) Number and migratory activity of circulating endothelial progenitor cells inversely correlate with risk factors for coronary artery disease. Circ Res 89:E1–7.
10. Hill JM, Zalos G, Halcox JPJ, Schenke WH, Waclawiw MA, et al. (2003) Circulating endothelial progenitor cells, vascular function, and cardiovascular risk. N Engl J Med 348:593–600.
11. Martínez MC, Tual-Chalot S, Leonetti D, Andriantsitohaina R. (2011) Microparticles: targets and tools in cardiovascular disease. Trends Pharmacol Sci 32:659–665.
12. Ullal AJ, Reich CF, Clowse M, Criscione-Schreiber LG, Tochacek M, et al. (2011) Microparticles as antigenic targets of antibodies to DNA and nucleosomes in systemic lupus erythematosus. J Autoimmun 36:173–180.
13. Soop AL, Hållström L, Frostell C, Wallén HN, Mobarrez F, et al. (2013) Effect of lipopolysaccharide administration on the number, phenotype and content of nuclear molecules in blood microparticles of normal human subjects. Scand J Immunol 78:205–213
14. Tárnok A (2008) SYTO dyes and histoproteins–myriad of applications. Cytometry A 73:477–479.
15. Gordon C, Gudi K, Krause A, Sackrowitz R, Harvey B-G, et al. (2011) Circulating endothelial microparticles as a measure of early lung destruction in cigarette smokers. Am J Respir Crit Care Med 184:224–232.
16. Heiss C, Amabile N, Lee AC, Real WM, Schick SF, et al. (2008) Brief secondhand smoke exposure depresses endothelial progenitor cells activity and endothelial function: sustained vascular injury and blunted nitric oxide production. J Am Coll Cardiol 51:1760–1771.
17. Mobarrez F, Antovic JP, Egberg N, Hansson M, Jörneskog G, et al. (2010) A multicolor flow cytometric assay for measurement of platelet-derived microparticles. Thromb Res 125:e110–116.
18. Burger D, Touyz RM (2012) Cellular biomarkers of endothelial health: microparticles, endothelial progenitor cells, and circulating endothelial cells. J Am Soc Hypertens. 6:85–99.
19. Gallagher KA, Liu Z-J, Xiao M, Chen H, Goldstein LJ, et al. (2007) Diabetic impairments in NO-mediated endothelial progenitor cell mobilization and homing are reversed by hyperoxia and SDF-1 alpha. J Clin Invest 117:1249–1259.

20. Schniedermann J, Rennecke M, Buttler K, Richter G, Städtler A-M, et al. (2010) Mouse lung contains endothelial progenitors with high capacity to form blood and lymphatic vessels. BMC Cell Biol 11:50.
21. Imaoka H, Punia N, Irshad A, Ying S, Corrigan CJ, et al. (2011) Lung homing of endothelial progenitor cells in humans with asthma after allergen challenge. Am J Respir Crit Care Med 184:771–778.
22. Tsuchiya M, Asada A, Kasahara E, Sato EF, Shindo M, et al. (2002) Smoking a single cigarette rapidly reduces combined concentrations of nitrate and nitrite and concentrations of antioxidants in plasma. Circulation 105:1155–1157.
23. Kondo T, Hayashi M, Takeshita K, Numaguchi Y, Kobayashi K, et al. (2004) Smoking cessation rapidly increases circulating progenitor cells in peripheral blood in chronic smokers. Arterioscler Thromb Vasc Biol 24:1442–1447.
24. Rodríguez-Carrio J, Prado C, de Paz B, López P, Gómez J, et al. (2012) Circulating endothelial cells and their progenitors in systemic lupus erythematosus and early rheumatoid arthritis patients. Rheumatology (Oxford) 51:1775–1784.
25. Grisar J, Aletaha D, Steiner CW, Kapral T, Steiner S, et al. (2007) Endothelial progenitor cells in active rheumatoid arthritis: effects of tumour necrosis factor and glucocorticoid therapy. Ann Rheum Dis 66:1284–1288.
26. Padfield GJ, Tura O, Haeck MLA, Short A, Freyer E, et al. (2010) Circulating endothelial progenitor cells are not affected by acute systemic inflammation. Am J Physiol Heart Circ Physiol 298:H2054–2061.
27. Lievens D, Zernecke A, Seijkens T, Soehnlein O, Beckers L, et al. (2010) Platelet CD40L mediates thrombotic and inflammatory processes in atherosclerosis. Blood 116:4317–4327.
28. Elzey BD, Ratliff TL, Sowa JM, Crist SA (2011) Platelet CD40L at the interface of adaptive immunity. Thromb Res 127:180–183.
29. Guidollet J, Chignier E, Pillot R, Gayet O, MacGregor J, et al. (1999) Enhanced expression of P-selectin (CD62P) by endothelial cells seeded onto synthetic arterial prostheses (PET, Dacron) is correlated with leukocyte interactions. J Biomed Mater Res 44:156–1561.
30. Li M, Yu D, Williams KJ, Liu M-L (2010) Tobacco smoke induces the generation of procoagulant microvesicles from human monocytes/macrophages. Arterioscler Thromb Vasc Biol 30:1818–1824.
31. Sambola A, Osende J, Hathcock J, Degen M, Nemerson Y, et al. (2003) Role of risk factors in the modulation of tissue factor activity and blood thrombogenicity. Circulation 107:973–977.
32. Owens A P, Mackman N (2011) Microparticles in hemostasis and thrombosis. Circ Res. 108:1284–1297.
33. Morel O, Toti F, Hugel B, Bakouboula B, Camoin-Jau L, et al. (2006) Procoagulant microparticles: disrupting the vascular homeostasis equation? Arterioscler Thromb Vasc Biol 26:2594–2604.
34. Go AS, Mozaffarian D, Roger VL, Benjamin EJ, Berry JD (2013) Heart disease and stroke statistics–2013 update: a report from the American Heart Association. Circulation 127:e6–e245.
35. Viera AJ, Mooberry M, Key NS (2012) Microparticles in cardiovascular disease pathophysiology and outcomes. J Am Soc Hypertens 6:243–252.
36. Harris ES, Nelson WJ (2010) VE-cadherin: at the front, center, and sides of endothelial cell organization and function. Curr Opin Cell Biol 22:651–658.
37. Maugeri N, Franchini S, Campana L, Baldini M, Ramirez GA, et al. (2012) Circulating platelets as a source of the damage-associated molecular pattern HMGB1 in patients with systemic sclerosis. Autoimmunity 45:584–587.
38. Maugeri N, Rovere-Querini P, Baldini MM, Baldissera E, Sabbadini MG, et al. (2013) Oxidative stress elicits platelet/leukocyte inflammatory interactions via HMGB1: a candidate for microvessel injury in sytemic sclerosis. Antioxid Redox Signal. Sep 26 [Epub ahead of print].
39. Wang H, Liao H, Ochani M, Justiniani M, Lin X, et al. (2004) Cholinergic agonists inhibit HMGB1 release and improve survival in experimental sepsis. Nat Med 10:1216–1221.
40. Soslau G (1983) De novo synthesis of DNA in human platelets. Arch Biochem Biophys. 226:252–256.
41. Rouhiainen A, Imai S, Rauvala H, Parkkinen J (2000) Occurrence of amphoterin (HMG1) as an endogenous protein of human platelets that is exported to the cell surface upon platelet activation. Thromb Haemost. 84:1087–1094.

8

Respiratory Syncytial Virus Infections Enhance Cigarette Smoke Induced COPD in Mice

Robert F. Foronjy[1], Abdoulaye J. Dabo[1], Clifford C. Taggart[2], Sinead Weldon[2], Patrick Geraghty[1]*

1 St. Luke's Roosevelt Hospital, Mount Sinai Health System, Division of Pulmonary and Critical Care Medicine, New York, New York, United States of America, **2** Centre for Infection and Immunity, School of Medicine, Dentistry and Biomedical Sciences, Queen's University Belfast, Belfast, Northern Ireland, United Kingdom

Abstract

Respiratory syncytial viral (RSV) infections are a frequent cause of chronic obstructive pulmonary disease (COPD) exacerbations, which are a major factor in disease progression and mortality. RSV is able to evade antiviral defenses to persist in the lungs of COPD patients. Though RSV infection has been identified in COPD, its contribution to cigarette smoke-induced airway inflammation and lung tissue destruction has not been established. Here we examine the long-term effects of cigarette smoke exposure, in combination with monthly RSV infections, on pulmonary inflammation, protease production and remodeling in mice. RSV exposures enhanced the influx of macrophages, neutrophils and lymphocytes to the airways of cigarette smoke exposed C57BL/6J mice. This infiltration of cells was most pronounced around the vasculature and bronchial airways. By itself, RSV caused significant airspace enlargement and fibrosis in mice and these effects were accentuated with concomitant smoke exposure. Combined stimulation with both smoke and RSV synergistically induced cytokine (IL-1α, IL-17, IFN-γ, KC, IL-13, CXCL9, RANTES, MIF and GM-CSF) and protease (MMP-2, -8, -12, -13, -16 and cathepsins E, S, W and Z) expression. In addition, RSV exposure caused marked apoptosis within the airways of infected mice, which was augmented by cigarette smoke exposure. RSV and smoke exposure also reduced protein phosphatase 2A (PP2A) and protein tyrosine phosphates (PTP1B) expression and activity. This is significant as these phosphatases counter smoke-induced inflammation and protease expression. Together, these findings show for the first time that recurrent RSV infection markedly enhances inflammation, apoptosis and tissue destruction in smoke-exposed mice. Indeed, these results indicate that preventing RSV transmission and infection has the potential to significantly impact on COPD severity and progression.

Editor: Navneet K. Dhillon, University of Kansas Medical Center, United States of America

Funding: This work was supported by grants made available to P.G. (Flight Attendant Medical Research Institute (YCSA 113380)) (http://www.famri.org/intro/) and to R.F. (US National Institutes of Health 5R01HL098528-04) (http://www.nih.gov/). The funders had no role in study design, data collection and analysis, decision to publish, or preparation of the manuscript.

Competing Interests: The authors have declared that no competing interests exist.

* E-mail: pgeraghty@chpnet.org

Introduction

Chronic obstructive pulmonary disease (COPD) is the third leading cause of death in the US [1] and a foremost cause of morbidity. Indeed, those with the disease have difficulty performing simple daily tasks such as walking, bathing and feeding themselves. The economic costs of COPD are substantial both in terms of healthcare expenditures and lost productivity [2,3]. Acute exacerbations of COPD, defined as a sudden worsening of COPD symptoms (shortness of breath, quantity and color of phlegm) that typically lasts for several days, are a major contributor to disease morbidity and mortality [4,5]. Indeed, those with 3 or more exacerbations over a five-year time period had a survival rate of 30% compared to a survival rate of 80% for those without an exacerbation [6]. In the Perception of Exacerbations of Chronic Obstructive Pulmonary Disease (PERCEIVE) survey, 89% of COPD subjects experienced at least one exacerbation in the past year and 21% of these exacerbations resulted in hospital admission [7]. These findings show that exacerbations are common in COPD and impact significantly on the natural history of the disease. Thus, these studies underscore the importance of determining the etiologic factors underlying COPD exacerbations.

Infectious agents, such as viral infections, have been implicated in the pathogenesis of COPD exacerbations [8,9]. Rhinovirus, influenza and respiratory syncytial virus (RSV) are frequently detected in the respiratory tract of COPD patients [10]. It is estimated that almost everyone has experienced at least one RSV infection as an infant [11] but immunity against RSV infections is uncommon. RSV infections are frequently reported in infants, the elderly and immunocompromised patients but also in healthy adults [12,13]. RSV is detected in stable COPD patients [14] but whether RSV plays a role in COPD progression is undetermined. RSV readily infects the airway epithelium [11], which could significantly contribute to inflammation and airway disease progression. In fact, infection with RSV is associated with airway inflammation and an accelerated decline in FEV1 in COPD patients [15]. Moreover, the presence of RSV infection worsens outcomes in COPD patients hospitalized for disease exacerbations [16]. Once infected, RSV can persist in the lungs of COPD patients by antagonizing antiviral cytokines, mimicking chemokines, escaping detection through antigenic drift and by entering immune-privileged cells such as pulmonary neurons [17]. Though cigarette smoke impairs antiviral responses that clear RSV [18,19], the consequence of persistent RSV infection on key disease parameters and outcomes in COPD has yet to be determined and larger clinical studies are need to identify if smoke exposure is a risk factor for increased RSV infections in COPD patients [20].

Few studies have examined the effects of cigarette smoking and viral infections *in vivo* and the subsequent impact on lung morphology [21,22]. Environmental tobacco smoke has been associated with increased RSV infection and hospitalization in children [23], however little is known about the clinical implications in COPD, a disease that RSV frequently colonizes [15,24]. Therefore this study aimed to examine how combined RSV infections and smoke exposure would impact on airway inflammation, protease production, apoptosis, lung tissue destruction and phosphatase activity. We hypothesized that dual stimulation could lead to excessive inflammation and an enhanced disease state closer to human COPD. We show that RSV infection enhances cigarette smoke induced immune cell infiltration, cytokine and protease production and airway remodeling. Collectively, these data demonstrate that viral infection alone or in combination with smoke exposure can significantly contribute to airway remodeling and disease progression.

Methods

Ethics Statement

All animal procedures performed in this study are in accordance with Institutional Animal Care and Use Committee (IACUC) guidelines, and have been approved by St. Luke's Roosevelt's Hospital IACUC at Mount Sinai School of Medicine.

RSV Culture

Human RSV strain A2 (ATCC, Manassas, VA; #VR-1540) was infected at a multiplicity of 0.1 into Hep2 cells. The virus was allowed to grow for 5 days at 37°C in a 5% CO_2 atmosphere. The infected Hep2 monolayers were collected and the virus was released by sonication. Cell debris was removed by centrifugation at 2500 g for 5 minutes at 4°C. Virus was collected by centrifuging the supernatant for 2 hours at 22000×g at 4°C. Virus were suspended in culture media and snap frozen and maintained at −80°C. Infectious virus titers were determined on Hep2 cells by performing serial dilutions of the RSV stocks and counting infected cells stained for indirect immunofluorescence with an RSV F-specific monoclonal antibody (Abcam, Cambridge, MA). Additionally, plaque assays were performed as previously described [25] on Hep2 cells using methyl cellulose overlay media (R&D Systems) and staining with 0.5 mg/ml thiazolyl blue tetrazolium bromide (MTT; Sigma Aldrich) solution in PBS for 3 hours at 37°C. Non-infected Hep2 cell cultures were processed in the same manner as RSV infected cells and the resulting sample collection was used as a mock control.

Cigarette Smoke Exposure and RSV Infection

C57BL/6J mice were purchased from the Jackson Laboratory (Bar Harbor, ME). All mice were maintained in a specific pathogen-free facility at St. Luke's Roosevelt's Hospital. 12-week-old mice were used at the initiation point for all experiments and each experimental parameter had 12 animals per group. Mice were anesthetized by intraperitoneal injection of a mixture of ketamine and xylazine. Mice were exposed to cigarette smoke in a chamber (Teague Enterprises, Davis, CA) for four hours a day, 5 days per week at a total particulate matter concentration of 80 mg/m^3. Smoke exposure was continued for 6 months with RSV dosing or mock administered 2 weeks after initiation of smoke exposures and continued monthly. RSV was intranasally administered at a dose of 1×10^6 pfu. RSV infected animals were housed separately from non-infected animals. Animals were monitored for discomfort, weight loss and any notable unusual behavior. Body weight and survival were measured every 5 days, for 6 months. Animals were sacrificed 12 hours after the last smoke exposure, which was 10 days after the last RSV or mock administration. The lungs underwent pressure-fixation and morphometric analysis in accordance with our previously published protocol [26] and in accordance with the ATS/ERS issue statement on quantitative assessment of lung structure [27]. Bronchoalveolar lavage fluid (BALF) isolation was performed on the mice. All mouse experiments were carried in strict accordance with institutional protocols.

Lung Titers and RSV N Copy Number

Lungs of infected mice were excised 10 days post the last RSV infection and homogenized using a mechanical homogenizer (Kinematica, Bohemia, NY, USA). The viral titers in the homogenates were quantified by plaque assay on Hep2 cells. The concentration of RSV N (pg) was determined by PCR based on a standard curve. The following primers were used at 100 pmol each: 5′-TGG GAG AGG TAG CTC CAG AA-3′ and 5′-AGA ATC TGT CCC CTG CTG CTA-3′. Ct was plotted against known RSV standards. A Ct-value of 45 was chosen as the cut-off value for sample infection positive. Results are represented as natural log pico grams (pg).

Histological Analysis

Fixed tissue was H&E stained for inflammation and fibrosis scoring and mean linear intercept (MLI) determination. Matrix accumulation was assessed on fixed tissue with trichrome evaluations using a commercial available kit (Abcam; ab150686). Histological analysis of H&E stained slides were used to determine perivascular vascular inflammation (PVI) and bronchial inflammation using a modified quantification schema [28,29]. Briefly, the intensity of perivascular or bronchial inflammation was scored on a scale of 1 to 9. 0, was no inflammation; 1–3, was scant cells but not forming a defined layer; 4–6, one to three layers of cells surrounding the vessel; 7–9, four or greater layers of cells surrounding the vessel or bronchial. Every vascular vessel and bronchus was measured on multiple lung lobes from 3 different depths of sectioned tissue. The validated semiquantitative Ashcroft score was used to score pulmonary fibrosis; scoring from 0 (normal lung) to 8 (total fibrous obliteration of the field) under 100X magnification using trichrome stained sections [30,31]. Each histology analysis was performed on 12 animals per treatment group.

Protease and Cytokine Measurements

MMP, cathepsin and cytokine gene expression was performed by qPCR using validated Taqman probes (Life technologies/Applied Biosystems, Carlsbad, CA). RNA was isolated using Qiagen RNeasy kit following tissue homogenizing and cDNA was reverse transcribed using the Applied Biosystems high capacity cDNA kit. qPCR was performed on the Bio-Rad CFX384 real time system. No cDNA template, no reverse transcriptase treated samples and no DNA polymerase controls were examined for each qPCR throughout this study. Exogenous (human targets) and endogenous (Actin) positive controls were also monitored for each assay. All qPCR results are represented as relative quantification (RQ) compared to the mock and room air treated animals and corrected to actin levels. Several MMP and cytokine levels were measured in BALF using a beads assay (EMD Millipore, Billerica, MA) with the BioRad Bio-Plex 200 system (BioRad, Hercules, CA). Cathepsin S activity assays were performed on BALF as

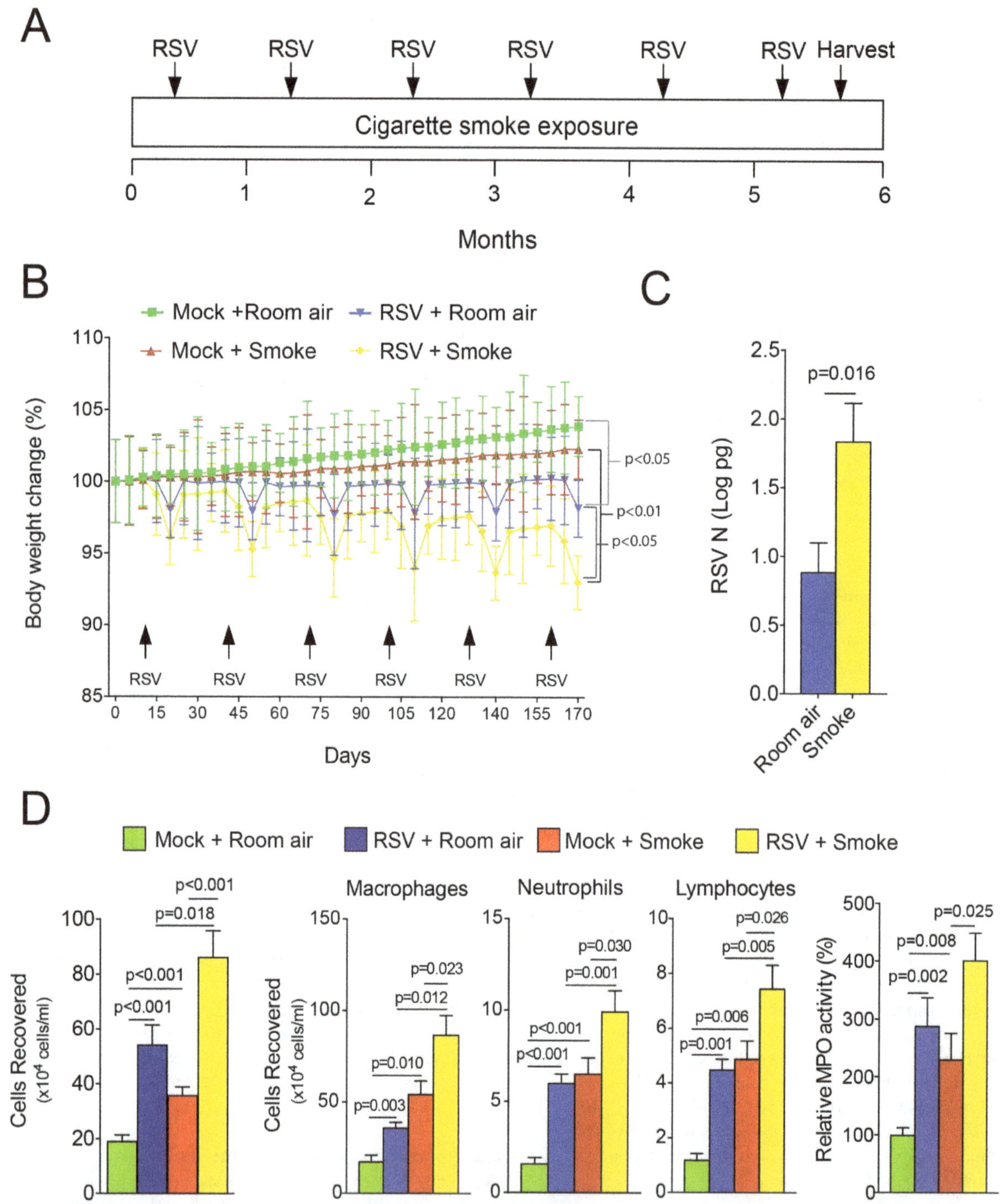

Figure 1. Chronic cigarette smoke exposure enhances RSV pathology in mouse airways. (A) Protocol for administering A2 RSV strain and cigarette smoke to C57BL/6J mice. C57BL/6J mice (n = 12 animals/group) were infected with monthly RSV infections in combination with 6 months of smoke exposure. (B) Changes in body weight of each treatment group of C57BL/6J mice, represented as a percentage of initial weight of mock and room air treated mice at the beginning of this study. p values shown, comparing both groups by 2-way ANOVA. (C) RSV N copy number was determined 10 days post final infection in the lungs of C57BL/6J mice infected with 1×10^6 pfu of RSV A2 strain and exposed to either room air or cigarette smoke for 6 months. Absolute RSV N concentration was represented as natural log pg. (D) BALF immune cellularity was measured and changes were observed following repeat monthly RSV infections in combination with 6 months of smoke exposure on total immune cell number, macrophages, neutrophils and lymphocytes. Graphs are represented as mean ± S.E.M., where each measurement was performed 3 times on 12 animals/group. p values shown, comparing both treatments connected by a line.

previously described [32]. BALF collagenase activity was determined by a colorimetric ninhydrin method, as previously described [33]. Results of enzyme activity are expressed as a relative percentage of activity compared of the mock and room air treated animal group. BALF gelatinase activity was determined by gelatin zymography as described previously [34].

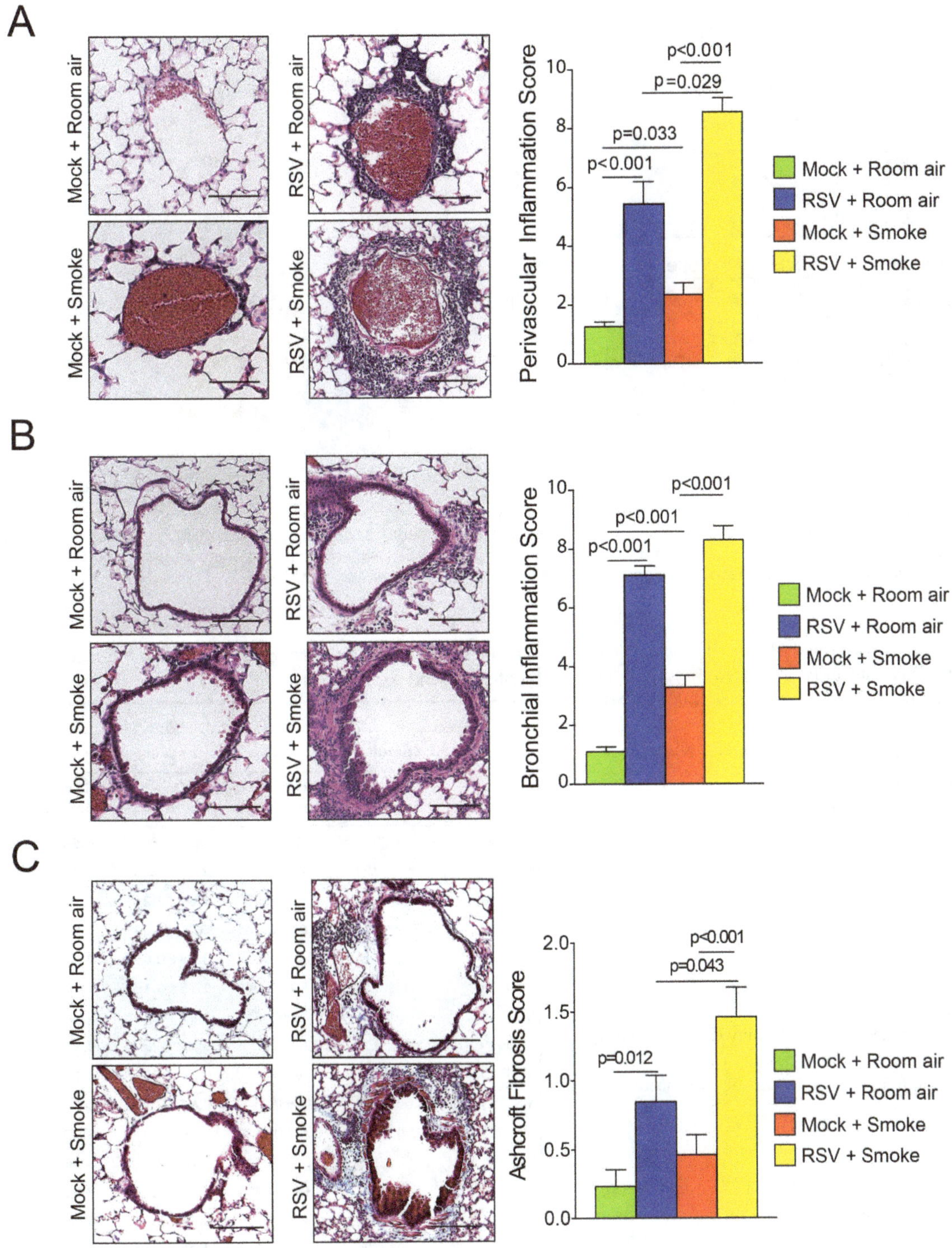

Figure 2. RSV infections enhance cigarette smoke induced airway enlargements and fibrosis. (A) Perivascular and (B) bronchial inflammation was recorded in mice exposed to cigarette smoke and RSV for 6 months and their corresponding controls. (C) Matrix accumulation was assessed with trichrome staining in each mouse group and quantified by the Ashcroft fibrosis score. Representative images of mice lungs from each group are presented here (scale bar = 20 μM; left panels). Fibrosis and inflammation scores were calculated for each treatment group (right panels where n = 12 animals/group). Each graph is represented as mean ± S.E.M. where each measurement was performed on 12 animals/group. p values shown, comparing both treatments connected by a line.

Intracellular Signaling

Lung tissue protein from mice was homogenized in RIPA buffer, centrifuged at 13,000×*g* for 10 minutes and supernatants collected. Immunoblots were conducted to determine levels of cathepsin E, S, G, K, W, Z (all cathepsin antibodies from Santa Cruz Biotechnology, Paso Robles, CA), MMP-28 (EMD Millipore) and actin (Cell Signaling Technologies, Danvers, MA). Chemiluminescence detection was performed using the Bio-Rad Laboratories Molecular Imager ChemiDoc XRS+ imaging

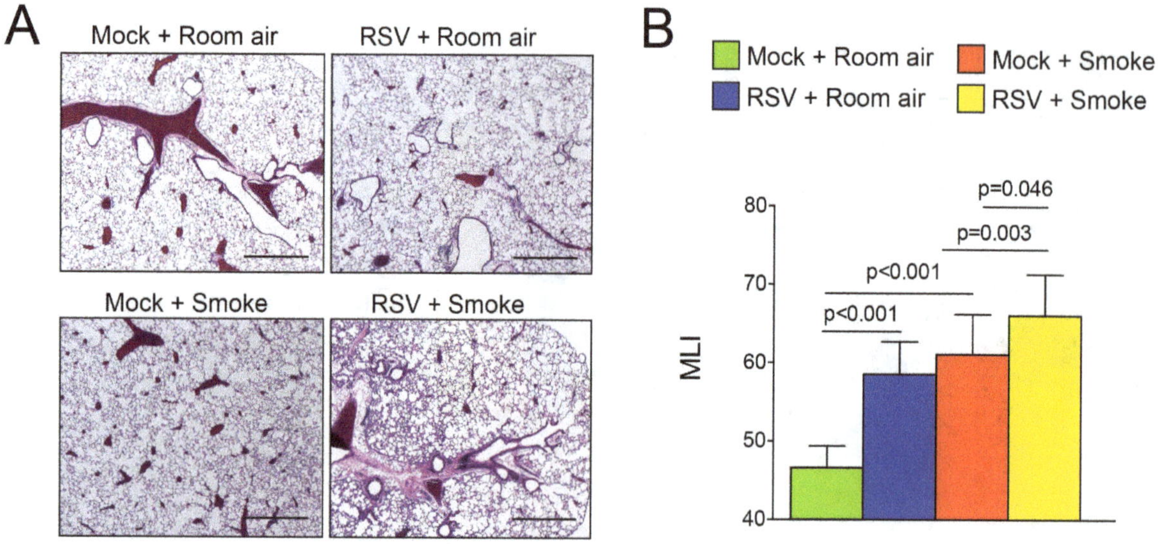

Figure 3. RSV infections enhance cigarette smoke induced airway enlargements. Lung morphology was determined in mice exposed to cigarette smoke and RSV for 6 months and their corresponding controls. (A) Representative images (scale bar = 50 μM) and (B) mean linear intercepts (MLI) of mice lungs from each group are presented here. Graph is represented as mean ± S.E.M., where each measurement was performed on 12 animals/group. p values shown, comparing both treatments connected by a line.

system. Densitometry was performed on each target and represented as a ratio of pixel intensity compared to actin, using Bio-Rad Laboratories Image Lab software (version 4.0, build 16).

Terminal Deoxynucleotidyl Transferase dUTP Nick End-labeling (TUNEL) Analysis

Apoptosis was determined on paraffin-embedded tissue by the TUNEL in situ cell death detection kit AP (Roche Diagnostics), using the instructions provided by the manufacturer. At least 10 random sections were obtained from each lung from 3 different depths of sectioned tissue. After staining, a minimum of 1000 cells was visually evaluated in each section. The labeled cells were expressed as a percentage of total nuclei.

Phosphatase Levels

PP2A and PTP1B activities were determined as previously described [35]. qPCR was performed for PTP1B and the A subunit of PP2A using Taqman probes, under the same criteria as described above.

Statistical Analyses

Data are expressed as means ± S.E.M. We determined statistical significance by Student t-tests (two tailed) using GraphPad Prism Software (Version 5 for Mac OS X). Two-tailed ANOVA repeat measure analysis was employed to determine the changes in animal body weight over time. All data sets are represented as mean +/− standard error.

Results

Cigarette Smoke Enhances RSV Infection

Mice were administered a monthly dose of RSV either in combination with daily cigarette smoke or room air, as depicted in Figure 1A. Animals were sacrificed 10 days after receiving the final dose of RSV, to eliminate a saturation of inflammation persisting from the viral infection. Mice exposed to cigarette smoke gained less weight over the study, which was amplified by repeated RSV

Table 1. RSV infections alter cigarette smoke induced airway protease gene expressions.

	Stimuli			
Target	**Mock/ Room air**	**Mock/ Smoke**	**RSV/ Room air**	**RSV/ Smoke**
MMP-2	1.00±0.13	1.21±0.17	1.65±0.30	**4.54±0.41**#
MMP-8	1.00±0.21	**2.73±0.38***	**3.45±0.83***	**3.82±0.75**#
MMP-9	1.00±0.05	**1.93±0.26***	**1.81±0.24***	1.23±0.15
MMP-12	1.00±0.13	**1.87±0.24***	**6.76±1.04***	**7.85±1.56**#
MMP-13	1.00±0.26	0.74±0.11	**3.93±0.63***	**4.38±0.60**#
MMP-14	1.00±0.13	**1.59±0.04***	**1.75±0.16***	1.81±0.16
MMP-16	1.00±0.11	0.72±0.18	**1.57±0.20***	**1.88±0.11**#
MMP-19	1.00±0.13	0.78±0.07	1.12±0.20	**1.36±0.17**#
MMP-20	1.00±0.31	0.49±0.16	0.95±0.30	**1.74±0.40**#
MMP-23	1.00±0.19	0.99±0.08	**0.47±0.10***	0.75±0.29
MMP-28	1.00±0.23	0.75±0.14	1.22±0.39	**1.89±0.27**#
Cathepsin A	1.00±0.29	1.02±0.04	0.51±0.07	**0.55±0.16**#
Cathepsin E	1.00±0.43	**3.99±0.78***	**5.82±1.15***	**7.53±1.16**#
Cathepsin F	1.00±0.12	0.80±0.12	**0.54±0.02***	0.87±0.19
Cathepsin G	1.00±0.26	**2.75±0.52***	**3.90±0.34***	4.93±0.76
Cathepsin K	1.00±0.19	1.32±0.25	0.82±0.13	**0.71±0.15**#
Cathepsin L1	1.00±0.06	**0.81±0.02***	**0.70±0.10***	0.90±0.01
Cathepsin M	1.00±0.16	**1.89±0.19***	**1.79±0.23***	2.12±0.43
Cathepsin S	1.00±0.11	**1.67±0.12***	**5.08±0.84***	**7.13±1.42**#
Cathepsin W	1.00±0.03	0.91±0.14	**5.35±1.41***	**6.05±0.70**#
Cathepsin Z	1.00±0.16	0.73±0.07	**1.62±0.05***	**1.65±0.12**#

Values are represented as mean ± S.E.M., where each measurement was performed 3 times on 12 animals/group. Bold numbers denoted by *represents a p value less than 0.05 compared to mock and room air treated mice. #denotes a p value less than 0.05 compared to either smoke or RSV treated mice.

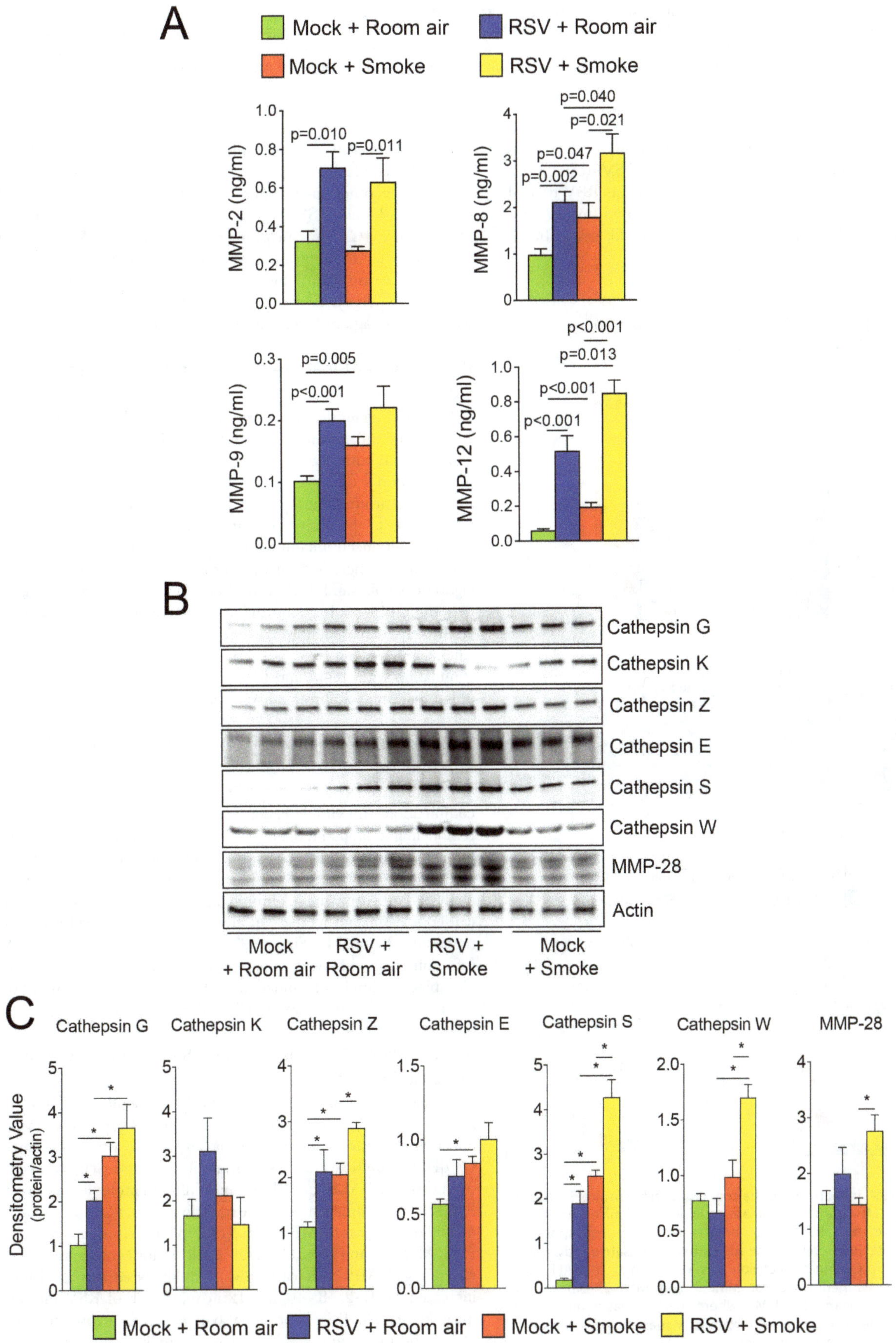
A
Mock + Room air
RSV + Room air
Mock + Smoke
RSV + Smoke
MMP-2 (ng/ml)
p=0.010
p=0.011
MMP-8 (ng/ml)
p=0.040
p=0.021
p=0.047
p=0.002
MMP-9 (ng/ml)
p=0.005
p<0.001
MMP-12 (ng/ml)
p<0.001
p=0.013
p<0.001
p<0.001
B
Cathepsin G
Cathepsin K
Cathepsin Z
Cathepsin E
Cathepsin S
Cathepsin W
MMP-28
Actin
Mock + Room air
RSV + Room air
RSV + Smoke
Mock + Smoke
C
Cathepsin G
Cathepsin K
Cathepsin Z
Cathepsin E
Cathepsin S
Cathepsin W
MMP-28
Densitometry Value (protein/actin)
Mock + Room air
RSV + Room air
Mock + Smoke
RSV + Smoke

Figure 4. RSV infections enhance cigarette smoke induced airway protease response. (A) BALF MMP (-2, -8, -9 and -12) levels were determined by multiplex analysis in the BALF of mice exposed to cigarette smoke and RSV for 6 months and their corresponding controls. Cathepsin G, K, Z, E, S, W and MMP-28 lung protein expression levels were analyzed by (B) immunoblotting and (C) densitometry. Graphs are represented as mean ± S.E.M., where each measurement was performed 2 times on 12 animals/group. p values shown, comparing both treatments connected by a line.

infections (Figure 1B). Significant differences in body weight loss were initially found between mock controls and RSV treated mice after 140 days ($p<0.05$), between smoke and smoke/RSV treated mice after 45 days ($p<0.01$) and between RSV and smoke/RSV treated mice after 140 days ($p<0.05$). RSV was still detectable in the lungs of mice 10 days post infection, by qPCR (Figure 1C) but was undetectable by plaque assay (data not shown) as similarly observed by other investigators [25]. Cigarette smoke exposed mice had a higher RSV N copy number than room air exposed mice (Figure 1C). Not surprisingly, exposure to RSV or smoke alone lead to an infiltration of macrophages, neutrophils and lymphocytes into the lung (Figure 1D). Interestingly, smoke exposure synergistically enhanced RSV induced inflammation, with macrophages, neutrophils and lymphocytes.

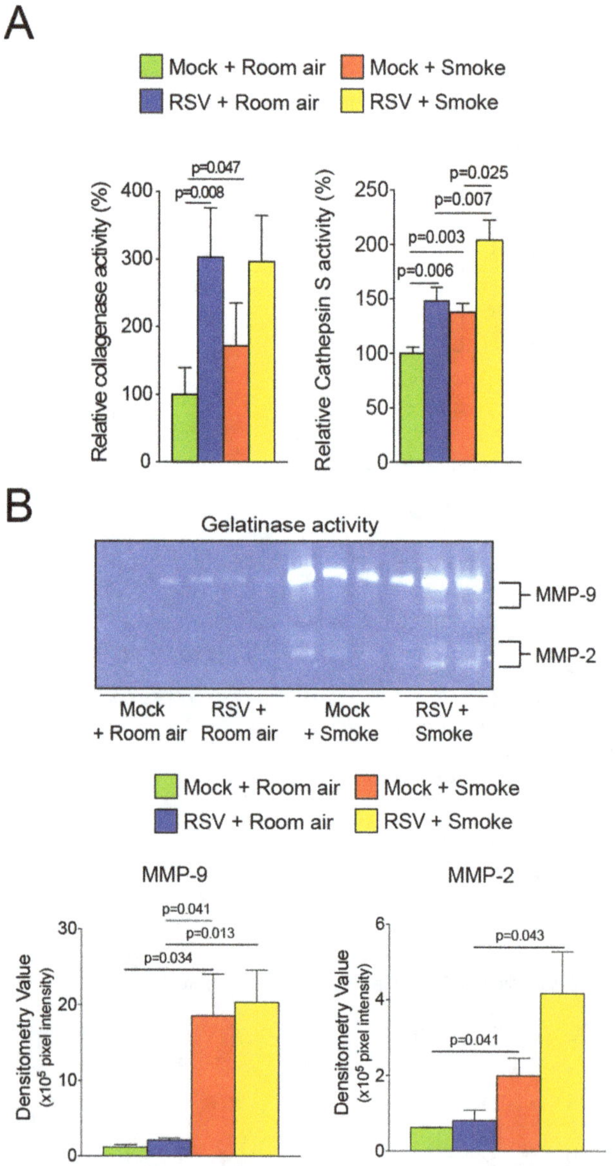

Figure 5. RSV infections enhance cigarette smoke induced cathepsin S activity. BALF protease activity was of mice exposed to cigarette smoke and RSV for 6 months and their corresponding controls. (A) Total BALF collagenase and cathepsin S relative activity was determined. (B) Gelatinase activity was determined in BALF and densitometry was performed for MMP-9 and MMP-2. Graphs are represented as mean ± S.E.M., where each measurement was performed 3 times on 12 animals/group. p values shown, comparing both treatments connected by a line.

RSV Enhances Cigarette Smoke Inflammation and Fibrosis

RSV and cigarette smoke-exposed mice exhibited perivascular lymphocytic inflammation, which was additionally augmented by exposure to both RSV and cigarette smoke (Figure 2A). An inflammation score was also performed on the inflammatory cell infiltration around the bronchial airways and the results were comparable to the perivascular inflammation, with RSV enhancing smoke-induced inflammation (Figure 2B). Trichrome staining demonstrated increased airway fibrosis in mice exposed to both cigarette smoke and RSV infections (Figure 2C), with collagen deposition observed around the airways. Ashcroft fibrosis scoring confirmed increased fibrosis in mice exposed to both cigarette smoke and repeat RSV infection (Figure 2C). Therefore, dual stimulation with smoke and RSV infection lead to an exaggerated inflammation and fibrotic airway remodeling response.

RSV Infections Enhance Cigarette Smoke Induced Airway Remodeling

Others have demonstrated that short term smoke exposure in combination with viral infection or poly (i:c) could enhance airway remodeling in animal models [21,36]. To investigate the long-term impact of combined smoke exposure and multiple viral infections on lung remodeling, we examined airway remodeling by MLI analysis. Not surprisingly, chronic cigarette smoke exposure alone caused a significant increase in alveolar size determined morphometrically by MLI (Figure 3). Interestingly, repeated RSV infection also enhanced airspace enlargement (Figure 3A–B). Combined stimuli of smoke and RSV induced a synergistic enhancement of airway remodeling (Figure 3A–B).

RSV Infections Alter the Cigarette Smoke Induced Airway Protease Response

Increased protease levels have been frequently observed in human airway diseases [33,37]. The influence of exposures to viral infection on smoke induced protease expression was investigated by qPCR, multiplex analysis, immunoblots and activity assays from tissue or BALF. C57BL/6J mice infected multiple times with RSV have significant gene expression increases for matrix metalloproteinases (MMP) -8, -9, -12, -13, -14, -16 and cathepsins E, G, M, S, W and Z (Table 1; see Table S1 for gene expression of remaining MMPs and cathepsins). Multiplex assays confirmed increased MMP-2, -8, -9 and -12 in the BALF of RSV infected mice (Figure 4A). RSV exposure also increased tissue protein levels of cathepsin G, S and Z (Figure 4B–C). Smoke exposure induced significant gene expression increases for MMP-8, -9, -12, -14 and

Table 2. RSV infections alter cigarette smoke induced airway cytokine release.

Cytokine (pg/ml)	Mock/Room air	RSV/Room air	Mock/Smoke	RSV/Smoke
IL-1α	2.07±0.36	**30.11±9.63***	1.11±0.25	**74.35±8.62#**
IL-1β	59.09±6.20	**78.75±5.32***	55.73±3.76	75.60±8.40
IL-3	27.91±0.83	**22.77±0.98***	**24.82±0.91***	21.76±0.80
IL-5	4.68±0.09	**4.07±0.20***	**4.16±0.13***	4.37±0.36
IL-6	3.78±0.44	**9.631±3.81***	4.568±0.38	9.147±2.75
IL-10	61.43±9.92	**76.45±12.60***	**35.49±2.98***	59.78±18.34
IL-13	48.41±2.44	**29.61±3.50***	40.23±1.77	**33.59±2.65#**
IL-17	43.66±5.06	**64.17±6.72***	**81.62±10.70***	**122.40±7.52#**
IFN-γ	12.15±0.72	**35.47±11.26***	15.49±1.30	**80.15±12.02#**
RANTES	12.41±0.84	**107.30±11.7***	12.38±1.03	129.1±11.73
TNF-α	524.90±41.34	438.80±55.48	**609.10±29.10***	**508.4±58.42#**
MIP-2	10.51±0.27	**9.10±0.18***	**9.31±0.29***	9.53±0.34
GM-CSF	39.72±2.99	**30.49±1.30***	35.00±2.00	33.88±2.64
CXCL1/KC	6.79±1.34	**18.94±2.13**	**12.83±1.85**	**21.59±1.82**

Values are represented as mean ± S.E.M., where each measurement was performed 3 times on 12 animals/group. Bold numbers denoted by *represents a p value less than 0.05 compared to mock and room air treated mice.
#denotes a p value less than 0.05 compared to either smoke or RSV treated mice.

cathepsins E, G, M and S (Table 1). Multiplex assays confirmed increased MMP-8, -9 and -12 in the BALF of smoke exposed mice (Figure 4A) and immunoblotting confirmed that smoke induced cathepsin G, Z, E and S levels in tissue (Figure 4C). Combined RSV infection and smoke exposure induced enhanced gene expression of MMP-2, -8, -12, -13, -16, -19, -20, -28 and cathepsins E, S, W and Z (Table 1). Multiplex assays confirmed that smoke enhanced RSV-induced MMP-8 and -12 in the BALF (Figure 4A). Tissue protein levels of cathepsin G, S and W were also synergistically enhanced by smoke (Figure 4B–C). MMP-3 BALF protein levels were also examined to confirm qPCR data of a protease that was unaltered by either stimuli and was confirmed to be unchanged in all mouse groups (Figure S1 and Table S1). Protease activities were also altered within the BALF of mice, with repeat RSV or smoke exposure increasing collagenase, gelatinase and cathepsin S activity in BALF of mice (Figure 5). Repeat RSV exposure enhanced smoke induced cathepsin S activity in BALF of mice but did not appear to enhanced total BALF collagenase activity (Figure 5A). Interestingly, smoke alone increased MMP-9 gelatinase activity levels more so than RSV infection, which varied from the qPCR and multiplex data (Figure 5B). Therefore, RSV infections impacts on smoke associated protease production, which may contribute to the airway remodeling observed in this animal model.

Table 3. RSV infections alter cigarette smoke induced airway cytokine gene expressions.

	Stimuli			
Target	Mock/ Room air	RSV/ Room air	Mock/ Smoke	RSV/ Smoke
IL-1β	1.00±0.08	**2.92±0.30***	2.04±0.18	2.890±0.43
IL-6	1.00±0.25	**3.08±0.64***	2.00±0.14	2.43±0.09
IL-10	1.00±0.37	**3.42±0.68***	2.12±0.63	2.00±0.34
IL-13	1.00±0.43	**6.57±1.55***	**14.01±2.71***	**17.17±3.70#**
IL-17	1.00±0.28	**3.61±0.66***	**2.69±0.40***	**6.69±1.45#**
IL-27	1.00±0.21	**2.66±0.53***	1.41±0.21	**3.95±1.42#**
CXCL1/KC	1.00±0.14	**1.85±0.24***	**2.61±0.23***	**3.42±0.31#**
CXCL9	1.00±0.29	**14.47±1.01***	**5.69±1.43***	**17.75±2.35#**
CXCL10	1.00±0.42	**4.88±0.62***	**2.65±0.24***	2.86±0.22
CXCL11	1.00±0.09	**6.64±1.35***	**3.47±0.88***	4.25±1.22
RANTES/ CCL5	1.00±0.19	**13.44±2.59***	**2.99±1.02***	**19.04±5.40#**
MIF	1.00±0.14	**0.49±0.04***	0.87±0.08	**1.43±0.05#**
GM-CSF	1.00±0.11	1.60±0.20	1.59±0.30	**2.44±0.36#**
G-CSF	1.00±0.40	**2.11±0.65***	1.20±0.53	1.07±0.19
IFN-α	1.00±0.25	**3.81±0.91***	**4.15±1.05***	2.87±1.17
IFN-β	1.00±0.15	**4.71±0.83***	**2.33±0.38***	2.88±0.65
IFN-γ	1.05±0.30	**14.61±2.23***	**2.64±0.62***	**20.10±3.61#**

Values are represented as mean ± S.E.M., where each measurement was performed 3 times on 12 animals/group. Bold numbers denoted by *represents a p value less than 0.05 compared to mock and room air treated mice.
#denotes a p value less than 0.05 compared to either smoke or RSV treated mice.

RSV Infections Alter Cigarette Smoke Induced Airway Cytokine Release

Microbial infection in the airways can contribute to disease exacerbations, which have been associated with cytokine and chemokine release from lung-residential cells [21]. C57BL/6J mice infected multiple times with RSV have significant BALF increases for IL-1α, IL-1β, IL-6, IL-10, IL-17, IFN-γ, RANTES and KC (Table 2; see Table S2 for cytokines unaltered by RSV or smoke), determined by multiplex assays. Gene expression analysis also identified increased IL-13, IL-27, CXCL9, CXCL10, CXCL11, G-CSF, IFN-α and IFN-β in the tissue of RSV infected mice (Table 3; see Table S3 for gene expression cytokines unaltered by RSV or smoke). Smoke exposure alone-induced increased BALF protein levels of IL-17, TNF-α and KC (Table 2).

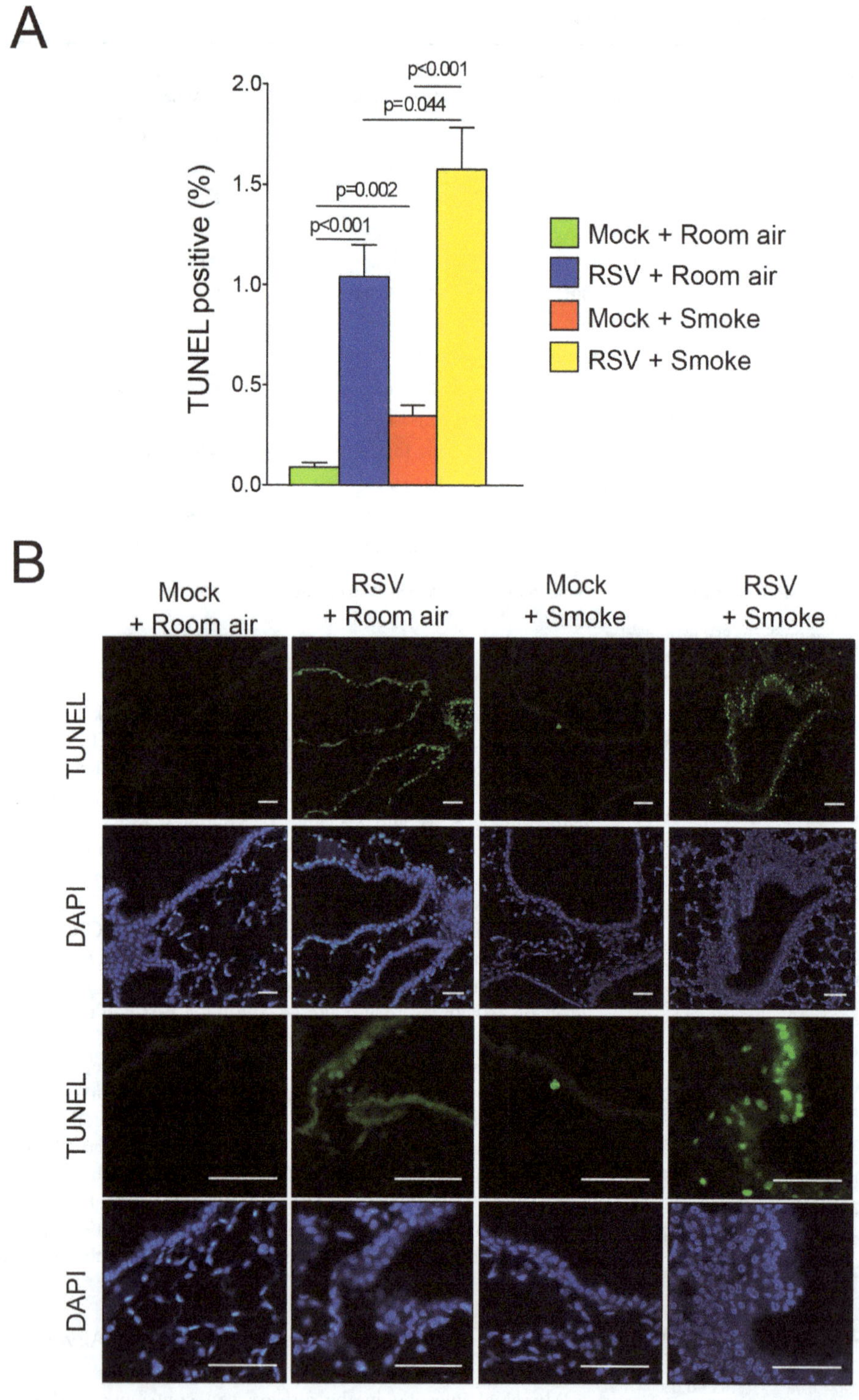

Figure 6. RSV infections enhance cigarette smoke induced airway cell death. (A) TUNEL analysis was performed on lung tissue from mice exposed to cigarette smoke and RSV for 6 months and their corresponding controls. Graph represented as mean ± S.E.M., where each measurement was performed on 12 animals/group. p values shown, comparing both treatments connected by a line. (B) Representative images of TUNEL staining of mice lungs from each group are presented here (scale bar = 50 μM).

Increased gene expressions of IL-13, CXCL9, CXCL10, CXCL11, RANTES, IFN-α, IFN-β and IFN-γ were observed after 6 months of smoke exposure (Table 3). Combined smoke and RSV infection lead to an enhanced induction of IL-1α, IL-17, IFN-γ and KC in the BALF and IL-13, IL-27, CXCL9, RANTES, MIF and GM-CSF by qPCR (Table 2 and Table 3). Therefore, combined exposure to cigarette smoke and RSV can synergistically enhance certain immune responses. Equally, trend decreases in several BALF cytokines were observed following dual stimulation of smoke and RSV infection, such as IL-2, IL-3, IL-5,

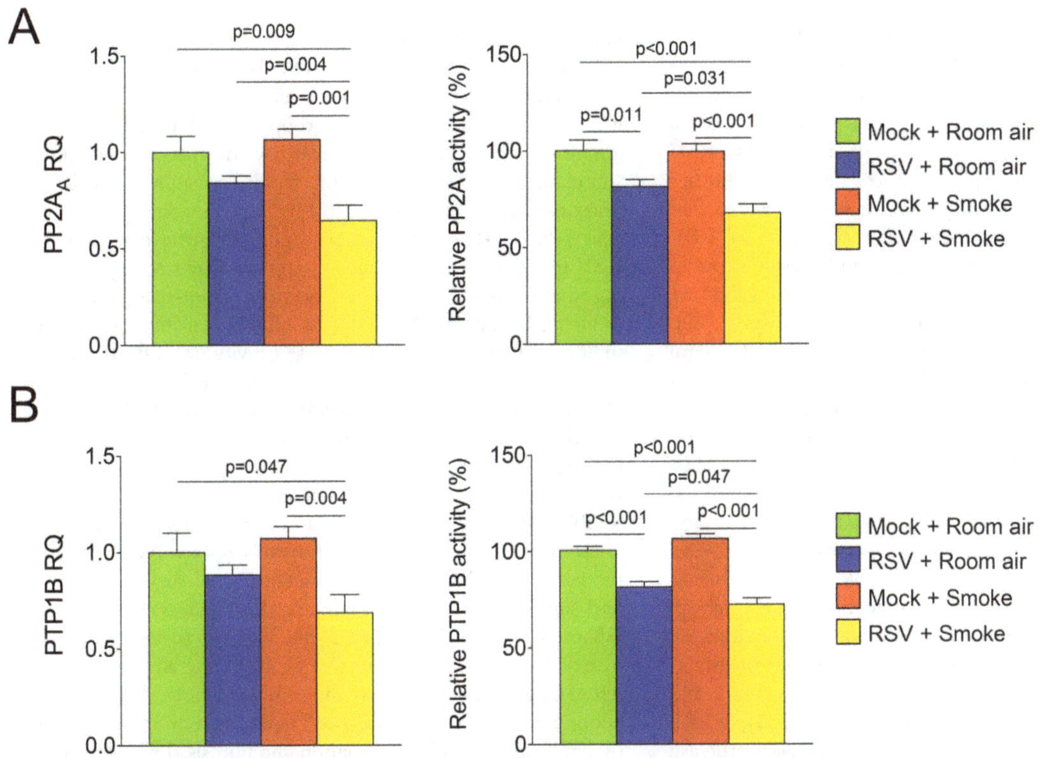

Figure 7. Smoke enhances RSV inhibition of PTP1B and PP2A activities. Lung tissue from C57BL/6J mice was examined for gene expression and phosphatase activity for (A) PP2A and (B) PTP1B. Graphs are represented as mean ± S.E.M., where each measurement was performed on 12 animals/group. p values shown, comparing both treatments connected by a line.

IL-7, IL-9, IL-10, IL-12p70, IL-13, TNF-α, VEGF, MIP1α, and MIP1β (Tables 2 and S2). Altered cytokine levels were probably not dependent on AP-1 or NF-κB activation, as dual exposure did not enhance activity of either transcription factor (Figure S2). However, additional studies are required to fully confirm this observation.

RSV Infections Enhance Cigarette Smoke Induced Airway Cell Death

Studies were undertaken to evaluate the impact of RSV and smoke exposure on cell death responses in the mouse lung. In cell culture, cigarette smoke causes necrosis rather than virus-induced apoptosis [38]. Our *in vivo* analysis demonstrated that administration of either smoke or RSV to mice caused significant increases in the number of cells that were undergoing apoptosis (Figure 6). RSV caused significant increase in the number of TUNEL positive cells. Smoke alone induced a modest induction of TUNEL positive cells within the lung. However, the combined exposure to smoke and RSV induced the most impressive changes with the detection of many TUNEL positive cells (Figure 6). An increase in the number of TUNEL-positive cells was seen in the bronchial airways of smoke exposed mice that were treated with RSV (Figure 6B).

RSV Infection Subdued PTP1B and PP2A Expressions and Activities

Chronic cigarette smoke exposure subdues the PTP1B and PP2A anti-inflammation response [35,39] and viruses can prevent PP2A activity [40]. Therefore, we investigated whether dual exposure to smoke and RSV infections could enhance inflammation by preventing the inductions of airway PTP1B and PP2A. As observed before [35,39], chronic smoke exposure did not induce PTP1B and PP2A activity (Figure 7). RSV inhibited PP2A and PTP1B activities, which was further enhanced by smoke exposure (Figure 7). Exposure to both smoke and RSV significantly reduced gene expression of both phosphatases (Figure 7).

Discussion

An exacerbation is a seminal event in the life of a COPD patient that frequently marks the transition from relative stability to a more rapid decline in lung function. Given the importance of exacerbations in the severity and progression of the disease, it is critical to establish the mechanisms by which an exacerbation leads to a decline in lung function. It has long been observed that RSV infections are frequently detected in the lungs of COPD patients during an exacerbation [16]. Moreover, RSV is known to persist in the lung even after an exacerbation has appeared to resolve [17]. What this study shows is that the presence of RSV infection exacerbates the underlying inflammatory, proteolytic and apoptotic responses triggered by cigarette smoke exposure in the lung. Indeed, RSV exposure significantly enhanced lung tissue destruction in smoke exposed mice. This study is also the first study to examine the impact of repeat viral infections in animals actively exposed to smoke throughout the study and suggests that inhibition of phosphatase activities may contribute to the inflammation observed in COPD viral exacerbations. Furthermore, these results indicate the specific strategies aimed at preventing and treating RSV infection would have a significant impact on COPD development.

RSV exposure exacerbated the protease/anti-protease imbalance in the lungs of the smoke-exposed mice. This finding was not altogether surprising as RSV induces MMP-3 and -10 expression in nasal epithelial cells [41,42], MMP-9 expression in human bronchial epithelial cells [43,44] and MMP-9 and -2 in a BALB/c mouse model [45]. However, the diversity of proteases that were regulated by RSV was impressive and this likely has a wide-ranging biological impact on the lung. Certainly, the role of proteases in emphysema is well established [46,47] and RSV induced emphysematous changes in mice that were further exacerbated by cigarette smoke exposure. It is conceivable that the proteolytic response may mediate the clearance of RSV infections from the lung. Indeed, collagen and elastin peptides exert chemotactic effects that draw in inflammatory cells that are needed for the elimination of viral infections in the lung [48]. However, it is also possible that proteases may delay viral clearance by degrading proteins that bind RSV and eliminate it from the lung. In fact, proteases degrade surfactant protein A [49], which clears RSV from the lung [50], as well as secretory leukoprotease inhibitor (SLPI), elafin and SerpinB1, which have been reported to exert antiviral effects [51,52]. Whether all of the proteases identified in this study are present in human viral exacerbations or contribute to disease progression or viral clearance is yet to be determined but the role of each protease in COPD progression represents many potential future topics of interest. The mechanism by which RSV enhances smoke induced proteases also represents an important area for future investigation. Smoke and RSV have several common targets that could impact on protease production, such as TLR4 [53,54], TLR9 [53], RIG-I [21]. We have previously observed increased protease induction in the absence of PP2A [39] and PTP1B [35] expression. Loss of phosphatase responses could play a major part on the proteases expressed in this study. Equally, phosphatases can regulate cytokine production, which may also contribute to the protease production observed in this study.

The induction of cytokines is necessary to clear viral infections like RSV that contribute to lung injury and disease progression. Many of the cytokines induced by RSV exposure in our model have also been linked with apoptosis, protease expression, mucus metaplasia and lung tissue destruction in COPD [55,56]. Virus-associated exacerbations have greater loss in lung function and increased CCL5, CXCL10, and CXCL11 [57], which were also observed in our mouse model. COPD patients have increased IFN-γ in BALF fluid [32], possibly from smoke induced CD8+ T cells that are a key regulator of the inflammation response in COPD [58]. IFN-γ primes cytotoxic T cell responses against RSV infection that are important for eliminating the virus from the lung. However, persistent or repeated viral infections, as occurred in our model, leads to chronic upregulation of IFN-γ in the lung, which induces protease expression, apoptosis and emphysema in mice [55] and is associated with disease severity in humans. Loss of PTP1B expression leads to increased smoke induced IFN-γ and IL-17 in the lungs of mice [35]. IL-17, which was induced in our model, modulates airway hyperreactivity and emphysema formation in mice [59]; however, the expression of IL-17 is required for the clearance of bacterial and viral infections in the lung. Indeed, there is some data to suggest that deficient cytokine responses could impair viral clearance from the lung [60], which based on our findings would exacerbate inflammatory and emphysematous changes in the lung. NF-κB and interferon stimulatory response element (ISRE) have been associated with smoke enhanced RSV stimulated cytokines [61]. We do not see a synergistic enhancement of NF-κB activation but we specifically examined animals at the end of the infection. Perhaps smoke may alter NF-κB earlier during the infection. This and the role of ISREs in viral and smoke responses will be an area of future investigation.

Large increases in TUNEL positive epithelial cells were detected in our RSV infected mice and this increase was further enhanced by smoke exposure. This is significant as there have been conflicting reports about the role of RSV in airway epithelial cell death and survival. One group showed that RSV inhibits apoptosis and prolongs survival by downregulating p53 or stimulating epidermal growth factor receptor (EGFR) and phosphatidylinositol 3-kinase (PI3K) signaling in lung epithelial cells [62,63,64]. On the other hand, others have reported that RSV sensitizes the epithelium to apoptosis by strongly upregulating the expression of tumor necrosis factor-related apoptosis-inducing ligand (TRAIL) [65] or CD95 (fas) [66,67]. Emphysematous airways are extremely sensitivity to TRAIL-mediated apoptosis [68], which may account for the increased apoptosis observed in our study following smoke and RSV exposures. TRAIL receptors are overexpressed in human emphysema patients [69] and their expression is sensitive to oxidative stress such as H_2O_2 stimulation. RSV infections coincide with increased soluble TRAIL levels in the BALF of respiratory failure patients [70]. Equally, RSV has been shown to reduce NRF2 in animal models [71]. NRF2 regulates numerous cell survival genes [72] and anti-oxidants [71] that are key players in mediating inflammation [35,73]. PTP1B and PP2A activities are sensitive to oxidation [35] and inhibition of PP2A increases sensitivity to TRAIL signaling [74]. It is interesting to note that the intense apoptotic responses in the airways in this study were accompanied by significant airway inflammation and fibrosis. Thus, determining how epithelial cell death leads to airway fibrosis would shed important insights in the pathophysiologic changes that occur in this disease.

Little clinical data is available on RSV susceptibility and inflammatory markers in COPD patients. However other viruses can give us a potential depiction of the human airway responses to RSV. Experimental rhinovirus studies in humans confirm that viral load correlates strongly with inflammatory markers [60]. BALF cells from COPD patients infected *ex vivo* with rhinovirus have deficient IFN-β induction, which coincides with reduced IFN-stimulated gene CXCL10 [60]. However, others have reported enhanced inflammation in tracheobronchial cells from COPD patients compared to healthy donor cells [75]. Our *in vivo* model observed enhanced inflammation from BALF and lung tissue after RSV infection. Future clinical studies will be required to determine how RSV infection impacts on the inflammatory responses in COPD.

The role of RSV in the progression of COPD has been debated as the virus is detected in up to a third of stable COPD subjects [17]. However, our findings affirm that RSV is not merely a colonizer of the lung but rather a key etiologic factor driving cytokine, protease and apoptotic responses that lead to air space enlargement and airway fibrosis. In fact, RSV exposure by itself induced biological and structural changes that were at least as severe as cigarette smoke exposure. Whether smoke exposure is enhancing RSV inflammation synergistically or accumulatively still remains to be determined but our data suggests that synergistic inhibition of phosphatase activities may be playing a major role in COPD exacerbations. These results provide a clear rationale for developing better RSV prevention and treatment strategies as a means of countering the progression and severity of this disease. This data indicates that the detecting RSV may help identify those subjects who are likely to experience a clinical deterioration over time.

Supporting Information

Figure S1 RSV infections and cigarette smoke had no impact on MMP-3 BALF levels. BALF MMP-3 levels were determined by multiplex analysis in the BALF of mice exposed to cigarette smoke and RSV for 6 months and their corresponding controls. Graph is represented as mean ± S.E.M., where each measurement was performed 2 times on 12 animals/group.

Figure S2 AP-1 and NF-κB activities following RSV and smoke stimuli. Transcription factor (AP-1 and NF-κB) activation was examined in the lungs of mice exposed to cigarette smoke and RSV for 6 months and their corresponding controls. Graphs are represented as mean ± S.E.M., where each measurement was performed 2 times on 12 animals/group. p values shown, comparing both treatments connected by a line.

Table S1 Protease gene responses in airways to RSV infections and cigarette smoke exposure.

Table S2 Cytokine release in airways to RSV infections and cigarette smoke exposure.

Table S3 Cytokine gene responses in airways to RSV infections and cigarette smoke exposure.

Methods S1 NFB and AP1 activation.

Acknowledgments

The authors would like to thank the James P. Mara Center for Lung Disease of the Pulmonary Division of St. Luke's Roosevelt Hospital for their support and Dr. Edward Eden and Dr. Gerard Turino.

Author Contributions

Conceived and designed the experiments: RF PG. Performed the experiments: RF AD CT SW PG. Analyzed the data: RF CT SW PG. Contributed reagents/materials/analysis tools: RF CT PG. Wrote the paper: RF PG.

References

1. Miniño AM, Xu J, Kochanek KD (2010) Deaths: Preliminary Data for 2008. National Vital Statistics Reports 59: 1–72.
2. Sin DD, Stafinski T, Ng YC, Bell NR, Jacobs P (2002) The impact of chronic obstructive pulmonary disease on work loss in the United States. Am J Respir Crit Care Med 165: 704–707.
3. DiBonaventura M, Paulose-Ram R, Su J, McDonald M, Zou KH, et al. (2012) The impact of COPD on quality of life, productivity loss, and resource use among the elderly United States workforce. COPD 9: 46–57.
4. Langsetmo L, Platt RW, Ernst P, Bourbeau J (2008) Underreporting exacerbation of chronic obstructive pulmonary disease in a longitudinal cohort. Am J Respir Crit Care Med 177: 396–401.
5. Donaldson GC, Seemungal TA, Bhowmik A, Wedzicha JA (2002) Relationship between exacerbation frequency and lung function decline in chronic obstructive pulmonary disease. Thorax 57: 847–852.
6. Soler-Cataluna JJ, Martinez-Garcia MA, Roman Sanchez P, Salcedo E, Navarro M, et al. (2005) Severe acute exacerbations and mortality in patients with chronic obstructive pulmonary disease. Thorax 60: 925–931.
7. Miravitlles M, Anzueto A, Legnani D, Forstmeier L, Fargel M (2007) Patient's perception of exacerbations of COPD–the PERCEIVE study. Respir Med 101: 453–460.
8. Wedzicha JA (2001) Airway infection accelerates decline of lung function in chronic obstructive pulmonary disease. Am J Respir Crit Care Med 164: 1757–1758.
9. Mallia P, Johnston SL (2005) Mechanisms and experimental models of chronic obstructive pulmonary disease exacerbations. Proc Am Thorac Soc 2: 361–366; discussion 371–362.
10. Sajjan US (2013) Susceptibility to viral infections in chronic obstructive pulmonary disease: role of epithelial cells. Curr Opin Pulm Med 19: 125–132.
11. Zhang L, Peeples ME, Boucher RC, Collins PL, Pickles RJ (2002) Respiratory syncytial virus infection of human airway epithelial cells is polarized, specific to ciliated cells, and without obvious cytopathology. J Virol 76: 5654–5666.
12. Falsey AR, Hennessey PA, Formica MA, Cox C, Walsh EE (2005) Respiratory syncytial virus infection in elderly and high-risk adults. N Engl J Med 352: 1749–1759.
13. (2004) Respiratory syncytial virus activity–United States, 2003–2004. MMWR Morb Mortal Wkly Rep 53: 1159–1160.
14. Seemungal T, Harper-Owen R, Bhowmik A, Moric I, Sanderson G, et al. (2001) Respiratory viruses, symptoms, and inflammatory markers in acute exacerbations and stable chronic obstructive pulmonary disease. Am J Respir Crit Care Med 164: 1618–1623.
15. Wilkinson TM, Donaldson GC, Johnston SL, Openshaw PJ, Wedzicha JA (2006) Respiratory syncytial virus, airway inflammation, and FEV1 decline in patients with chronic obstructive pulmonary disease. Am J Respir Crit Care Med 173: 871–876.
16. Cody SH (2013) Editorial Commentary: Rapid Detection and Investigation of an Outbreak of Escherichia coli O157:H7 Infections: Shoe-leather Epidemiology on and Around the Strawberry Farm. Clin Infect Dis 57: 1135–1137.
17. Sikkel MB, Quint JK, Mallia P, Wedzicha JA, Johnston SL (2008) Respiratory syncytial virus persistence in chronic obstructive pulmonary disease. Pediatr Infect Dis J 27: S63–70.
18. Modestou MA, Manzel LJ, El-Mahdy S, Look DC (2010) Inhibition of IFN-gamma-dependent antiviral airway epithelial defense by cigarette smoke. Respir Res 11: 64.
19. Robbins CS, Dawe DE, Goncharova SI, Pouladi MA, Drannik AG, et al. (2004) Cigarette smoke decreases pulmonary dendritic cells and impacts antiviral immune responsiveness. Am J Respir Cell Mol Biol 30: 202–211.
20. Mehta J, Walsh EE, Mahadevia PJ, Falsey AR (2013) Risk factors for respiratory syncytial virus illness among patients with chronic obstructive pulmonary disease. COPD 10: 293–299.
21. Kang MJ, Lee CG, Lee JY, Dela Cruz CS, Chen ZJ, et al. (2008) Cigarette smoke selectively enhances viral PAMP- and virus-induced pulmonary innate immune and remodeling responses in mice. J Clin Invest 118: 2771–2784.
22. Bauer CM, Zavitz CC, Botelho FM, Lambert KN, Brown EG, et al. (2010) Treating viral exacerbations of chronic obstructive pulmonary disease: insights from a mouse model of cigarette smoke and H1N1 influenza infection. PLoS One 5: e13251.
23. DiFranza JR, Masaquel A, Barrett AM, Colosia AD, Mahadevia PJ (2012) Systematic literature review assessing tobacco smoke exposure as a risk factor for serious respiratory syncytial virus disease among infants and young children. BMC Pediatr 12: 81.
24. Lee N, Lui GC, Wong KT, Li TC, Tse EC, et al. (2013) High morbidity and mortality in adults hospitalized for respiratory syncytial virus infections. Clin Infect Dis 57: 1069–1077.
25. Boukhvalova MS, Yim KC, Prince GA, Blanco JC (2010) Methods for monitoring dynamics of pulmonary RSV replication by viral culture and by real-time reverse transcription-PCR in vivo: Detection of abortive viral replication. Curr Protoc Cell Biol Chapter 26: Unit26 26.
26. Foronjy RF, Mirochnitchenko O, Propokenko O, Lemaitre V, Jia Y, et al. (2006) Superoxide dismutase expression attenuates cigarette smoke- or elastase-generated emphysema in mice. Am J Respir Crit Care Med 173: 623–631.
27. Hsia CCW, Hyde DM, Ochs M, Weibel ER and on behalf of the ATS/ERS Joint Task Force on the Quantitative Assessment of Lung Structure (2010) An Official Research Policy Statement of the American Thoracic Society/European Respiratory Society: Standards for Quantitative Assessment of Lung Structure. Am J Respir Crit Care Med 181: 394–418.
28. Ford JG, Rennick D, Donaldson DD, Venkayya R, McArthur C, et al. (2001) Il-13 and IFN-gamma: interactions in lung inflammation. J Immunol 167: 1769–1777.
29. Mehra D, Geraghty PM, Hardigan AA, Foronjy R (2012) A comparison of the inflammatory and proteolytic effects of dung biomass and cigarette smoke exposure in the lung. PLoS ONE 7: e52889.
30. Ashcroft T, Simpson JM, Timbrell V (1988) Simple method of estimating severity of pulmonary fibrosis on a numerical scale. J Clin Pathol 41: 467–470.
31. De Langhe E, Vande Velde G, Hostens J, Himmelreich U, Nemery B, et al. (2012) Quantification of lung fibrosis and emphysema in mice using automated micro-computed tomography. PLoS One 7: e43123.
32. Geraghty P, Greene CM, O'Mahony M, O'Neill SJ, Taggart CC, et al. (2007) Secretory leucocyte protease inhibitor inhibits interferon-gamma-induced cathepsin S expression. J Biol Chem 282: 33389–33395.
33. D'Armiento JM, Goldklang MP, Hardigan AA, Geraghty P, Roth MD, et al. (2013) Increased matrix metalloproteinase (MMPs) levels do not predict disease severity or progression in emphysema. PLoS ONE 8: e56352.
34. Geraghty P, Rogan MP, Greene CM, Boxio RM, Poiriert T, et al. (2007) Neutrophil elastase up-regulates cathepsin B and matrix metalloprotease-2 expression. J Immunol 178: 5871–5878.
35. Geraghty P, Hardigan AA, Wallace AM, Mirochnitchenko O, Thankachen J, et al. (2013) The glutathione peroxidase 1-protein tyrosine phosphatase 1B-protein

phosphatase 2A axis. A key determinant of airway inflammation and alveolar destruction. Am J Respir Cell Mol Biol 49: 721–730.
36. Zhou Y, Kang MJ, Jha BK, Silverman RH, Lee CG, et al. (2013) Role of ribonuclease L in viral pathogen-associated molecular pattern/influenza virus and cigarette smoke-induced inflammation and remodeling. J Immunol 191: 2637–2646.
37. Geraghty P, Rogan MP, Greene CM, Brantly ML, O'Neill SJ, et al. (2008) Alpha-1-antitrypsin aerosolised augmentation abrogates neutrophil elastase-induced expression of cathepsin B and matrix metalloprotease 2 in vivo and in vitro. Thorax 63: 621–626.
38. Groskreutz DJ, Monick MM, Babor EC, Nyunoya T, Varga SM, et al. (2009) Cigarette smoke alters respiratory syncytial virus-induced apoptosis and replication. Am J Respir Cell Mol Biol 41: 189–198.
39. Wallace AM, Hardigan A, Geraghty P, Salim S, Gaffney A, et al. (2012) Protein phosphatase 2A regulates innate immune and proteolytic responses to cigarette smoke exposure in the lung. Toxicol Sci 126: 589–599.
40. Collison A, Hatchwell L, Verrills N, Wark PA, de Siqueira AP, et al. (2013) The E3 ubiquitin ligase midline 1 promotes allergen and rhinovirus-induced asthma by inhibiting protein phosphatase 2A activity. Nat Med 19: 232–237.
41. Hirakawa S, Kojima T, Obata K, Okabayashi T, Yokota SI, et al. (2013) Marked induction of matrix metalloproteinase-10 by respiratory syncytial virus infection in human nasal epithelial cells. J Med Virol.
42. Schuurhof A, Bont L, Hodemaekers HM, de Klerk A, de Groot H, et al. (2012) Proteins involved in extracellular matrix dynamics are associated with respiratory syncytial virus disease severity. Eur Respir J 39: 1475–1481.
43. Elliott MB, Welliver RC Sr, Laughlin TS, Pryharski KS, LaPierre NA, et al. (2007) Matrix metalloproteinase-9 and tissue inhibitor of matrix metalloproteinase-1 in the respiratory tracts of human infants following paramyxovirus infection. J Med Virol 79: 447–456.
44. Yeo SJ, Yun YJ, Lyu MA, Woo SY, Woo ER, et al. (2002) Respiratory syncytial virus infection induces matrix metalloproteinase-9 expression in epithelial cells. Arch Virol 147: 229–242.
45. Li W, Shen HH (2007) Effect of respiratory syncytial virus on the activity of matrix metalloproteinase in mice. Chin Med J (Engl) 120: 5–11.
46. Shapiro SD (2003) Proteolysis in the lung. Eur Respir J Suppl 44: 30s–32s.
47. Zheng T, Kang MJ, Crothers K, Zhu Z, Liu W, et al. (2005) Role of cathepsin S-dependent epithelial cell apoptosis in IFN-gamma-induced alveolar remodeling and pulmonary emphysema. J Immunol 174: 8106–8115.
48. Houghton AM, Quintero PA, Perkins DL, Kobayashi DK, Kelley DG, et al. (2006) Elastin fragments drive disease progression in a murine model of emphysema. J Clin Invest 116: 753–759.
49. Schochett P, Mora R, Mark L, Butler M, Ingenito EP (1999) Calcium-dependent degradation of surfactant protein A by activated neutrophils due to serine proteases. Exp Lung Res 25: 595–616.
50. LeVine AM, Gwozdz J, Stark J, Bruno M, Whitsett J, et al. (1999) Surfactant protein-A enhances respiratory syncytial virus clearance in vivo. J Clin Invest 103: 1015–1021.
51. Drannik AG, Nag K, Sallenave JM, Rosenthal KL (2013) Antiviral activity of trappin-2 and elafin in vitro and in vivo against genital herpes. J Virol 87: 7526–7538.
52. Gong D, Farley K, White M, Hartshorn KL, Benarafa C, et al. (2011) Critical role of serpinB1 in regulating inflammatory responses in pulmonary influenza infection. J Infect Dis 204: 592–600.
53. Nadigel J, Prefontaine D, Baglole CJ, Maltais F, Bourbeau J, et al. (2011) Cigarette smoke increases TLR4 and TLR9 expression and induces cytokine production from CD8(+) T cells in chronic obstructive pulmonary disease. Respir Res 12: 149.
54. Geraghty P, Dabo AJ, D'Armiento J (2011) TLR4 protein contributes to cigarette smoke-induced matrix metalloproteinase-1 (MMP-1) expression in chronic obstructive pulmonary disease. J Biol Chem 286: 30211–30218.
55. Wang Z, Zheng T, Zhu Z, Homer R, Riese RJ, et al. (2000) Interferon Gamma Induction of Pulmonary Emphysema in the Adult Murine Lung. J Exp Med 192: 1587–1599.
56. Zheng T, Zhu Z, Wang Z, Homer RJ, Ma B, et al. (2000) Inducible targeting of IL-13 to the adult lung causes matrix metalloproteinase- and cathepsin-dependent emphysema. J Clin Invest 106: 1081–1093.
57. Bafadhel M, McKenna S, Terry S, Mistry V, Reid C, et al. (2011) Acute exacerbations of chronic obstructive pulmonary disease: identification of biologic clusters and their biomarkers. Am J Respir Crit Care Med 184: 662–671.
58. Maeno T, Houghton AM, Quintero PA, Grumelli S, Owen CA, et al. (2007) CD8+ T Cells are required for inflammation and destruction in cigarette smoke-induced emphysema in mice. J Immunol 178: 8090–8096.
59. Murdoch JR, Lloyd CM (2010) Resolution of allergic airway inflammation and airway hyperreactivity is mediated by IL-17-producing {gamma}{delta}T cells. Am J Respir Crit Care Med 182: 464–476.
60. Mallia P, Message SD, Gielen V, Contoli M, Gray K, et al. (2011) Experimental rhinovirus infection as a human model of chronic obstructive pulmonary disease exacerbation. Am J Respir Crit Care Med 183: 734–742.
61. Castro SM, Kolli D, Guerrero-Plata A, Garofalo RP, Casola A (2008) Cigarette smoke condensate enhances respiratory syncytial virus-induced chemokine release by modulating NF-kappa B and interferon regulatory factor activation. Toxicol Sci 106: 509–518.
62. Monick MM, Cameron K, Staber J, Powers LS, Yarovinsky TO, et al. (2005) Activation of the epidermal growth factor receptor by respiratory syncytial virus results in increased inflammation and delayed apoptosis. J Biol Chem 280: 2147–2158.
63. Thomas KW, Monick MM, Staber JM, Yarovinsky T, Carter AB, et al. (2002) Respiratory syncytial virus inhibits apoptosis and induces NF-kappa B activity through a phosphatidylinositol 3-kinase-dependent pathway. J Biol Chem 277: 492–501.
64. Groskreutz DJ, Monick MM, Yarovinsky TO, Powers LS, Quelle DE, et al. (2007) Respiratory syncytial virus decreases p53 protein to prolong survival of airway epithelial cells. J Immunol 179: 2741–2747.
65. Kotelkin A, Prikhod'ko EA, Cohen JI, Collins PL, Bukreyev A (2003) Respiratory syncytial virus infection sensitizes cells to apoptosis mediated by tumor necrosis factor-related apoptosis-inducing ligand. J Virol 77: 9156–9172.
66. O'Donnell D R, Milligan L, Stark JM (1999) Induction of CD95 (Fas) and apoptosis in respiratory epithelial cell cultures following respiratory syncytial virus infection. Virology 257: 198–207.
67. van den Berg E, van Woensel JB, Bos AP, Bem RA, Altemeier WA, et al. (2011) Role of the Fas/FasL system in a model of RSV infection in mechanically ventilated mice. Am J Physiol Lung Cell Mol Physiol 301: L451–460.
68. Morissette MC, Parent J, Milot J (2011) The emphysematous lung is abnormally sensitive to TRAIL-mediated apoptosis. Respir Res 12: 105.
69. Morissette MC, Vachon-Beaudoin G, Parent J, Chakir J, Milot J (2008) Increased p53 level, Bax/Bcl-x(L) ratio, and TRAIL receptor expression in human emphysema. Am J Respir Crit Care Med 178: 240–247.
70. Bem RA, Bos AP, Wosten-van Asperen RM, Bruijn M, Lutter R, et al. (2010) Potential role of soluble TRAIL in epithelial injury in children with severe RSV infection. Am J Respir Cell Mol Biol 42: 697–705.
71. Hosakote YM, Jantzi PD, Esham DL, Spratt H, Kurosky A, et al. (2011) Viral-mediated inhibition of antioxidant enzymes contributes to the pathogenesis of severe respiratory syncytial virus bronchiolitis. Am J Respir Crit Care Med 183: 1550–1560.
72. Niture SK, Jaiswal AK (2012) Nrf2 protein up-regulates antiapoptotic protein Bcl-2 and prevents cellular apoptosis. J Biol Chem 287: 9873–9886.
73. Foronjy R, Mirochnitchenko O, Lemaitre V, Jia Y, Inouye M, et al. (2005) Transgenic Expression of Human CuZn Superoxide Dismutase Prevents Cigarette Smoke-Induced Inflammation and Emphysema Formation American Thoracic Society. San Diego, California.
74. Yang H, Chen X, Wang X, Li Y, Chen S, et al. (2013) Inhibition of PP2A Activity Confers a TRAIL-sensitive Phenotype During Malignant Transformation. Mol Cancer Res.
75. Schneider D, Ganesan S, Comstock AT, Meldrum CA, Mahidhara R, et al. (2010) Increased cytokine response of rhinovirus-infected airway epithelial cells in chronic obstructive pulmonary disease. Am J Respir Crit Care Med 182: 332–340.

9

The Burden Attributable to Mental and Substance Use Disorders as Risk Factors for Suicide: Findings from the Global Burden of Disease Study 2010

Alize J. Ferrari[1,2]*, Rosana E. Norman[1,3], Greg Freedman[4], Amanda J. Baxter[1,2], Jane E. Pirkis[5], Meredith G. Harris[1,2], Andrew Page[6], Emily Carnahan[4], Louisa Degenhardt[5,7], Theo Vos[1,4], Harvey A. Whiteford[1,2]

1 University of Queensland, School of Population Health, Herston, Queensland, Australia, **2** Queensland Centre for Mental Health Research, Wacol, Queensland, Australia, **3** Queensland Children's Medical Research Institute, University of Queensland, Herston, Queensland, Australia, **4** Institute for Health Metrics and Evaluation, University of Washington, Seattle, Washington, United States of America, **5** Melbourne School of Population and Global Health, University of Melbourne, Melbourne, Australia, **6** School of Science and Health, University of Western Sydney, Campbelltown, New South Wales, Australia, **7** National Drug and Alcohol Research Centre, University of New South Wales, Sydney, Australia

Abstract

Background: The Global Burden of Disease Study 2010 (GBD 2010) identified mental and substance use disorders as the 5th leading contributor of burden in 2010, measured by disability adjusted life years (DALYs). This estimate was incomplete as it excluded burden resulting from the increased risk of suicide captured elsewhere in GBD 2010's mutually exclusive list of diseases and injuries. Here, we estimate suicide DALYs attributable to mental and substance use disorders.

Methods: Relative-risk estimates of suicide due to mental and substance use disorders and the global prevalence of each disorder were used to estimate population attributable fractions. These were adjusted for global differences in the proportion of suicide due to mental and substance use disorders compared to other causes then multiplied by suicide DALYs reported in GBD 2010 to estimate attributable DALYs (with 95% uncertainty).

Results: Mental and substance use disorders were responsible for 22.5 million (14.8–29.8 million) of the 36.2 million (26.5–44.3 million) DALYs allocated to suicide in 2010. Depression was responsible for the largest proportion of suicide DALYs (46.1% (28.0%–60.8%)) and anorexia nervosa the lowest (0.2% (0.02%–0.5%)). DALYs occurred throughout the lifespan, with the largest proportion found in Eastern Europe and Asia, and males aged 20–30 years. The inclusion of attributable suicide DALYs would have increased the overall burden of mental and substance use disorders (assigned to them in GBD 2010 as a direct cause) from 7.4% (6.2%–8.6%) to 8.3% (7.1%–9.6%) of global DALYs, and would have changed the global ranking from 5th to 3rd leading cause of burden.

Conclusions: Capturing the suicide burden attributable to mental and substance use disorders allows for more accurate estimates of burden. More consideration needs to be given to interventions targeted to populations with, or at risk for, mental and substance use disorders as an effective strategy for suicide prevention.

Editor: Bernhard T. Baune, University of Adelaide, Australia

Funding: AJF, AJB, MGH and HAW are associated with the Queensland Centre for Mental Health Research which acquires funding from the Queensland Department of Health. REN, GF, EC and TV received funding for the Global Burden of Disease project from the Bill and Melinda Gates Foundation. LD is supported by an Australian National Health and Medical Research Council (NHMRC) Principal Research Fellowship. The National Drug and Alcohol Research Centre at the University of NSW is supported by funding from the Australian Government under the Substance Misuse Prevention and Service Improvements Grants Fund. The funders had no role in study design, data collection and analysis, decision to publish, or preparation of the manuscript

Competing Interests: The authors have declared that no competing interests exist.

* E-mail: alize_ferrari@qcmhr.uq.edu.au

Introduction

There has been growing recognition of the importance of mental and substance use disorders as contributors to health loss in all countries. The Global Burden of Disease Study 2010 (GBD 2010) is the largest and most recent effort to quantify this by systematically integrating years of life lost (YLLs) and years of life with disability (YLDs) into disability adjusted life years (DALYs) for diseases, injuries and risk factors [1–7].

GBD 2010 presented age-, sex-, year-, country-, and region-specific DALYs for 291 diseases and injuries as well as for 67 risk factors [1–7]; using improved methodology compared to previous GBD studies [8,9]. Mental and substance use disorders explained 7.4% (95% uncertainty interval: 6.2–8.6%) of total DALYs in 2010, confirming them as the leading disease category of YLDs, and the 5th leading category of DALYs globally [10–12]. This estimate reflects 'direct burden' where mental and substance use disorders are the direct cause of health loss, but excludes the excess (attributable) burden resulting from the increased risk of mortality and disability due to subsequent health outcomes captured elsewhere in the mutually exclusive disease and injury categories in GBD 2010. Jointly considering the direct and the attributable burden of mental and substance use disorders provides an estimation of the putative causal relationship between the disorders and other health outcomes. This is of clinical and policy relevance as it clearly delineates the disability and mortality that potentially can be modified by interventions to prevent and treat mental and substance use disorders.

Here, we expand on the published GBD 2010 findings by estimating the additional burden attributable to mental and substance use disorders as risk factors for suicide. Suicide, defined as deaths caused by intentional, self-inflicted poisoning or injury [13], was the 13th leading cause of YLLs worldwide in 2010 [1,6]. Nearly 1 million people complete suicide every year with over 50% aged between 15 and 44 years [14,15]. Over 80% of suicides occur in low to middle income countries and close to 50% occur in India and China alone [15,16]. Suicide from firearms, car exhaust and poisoning are more common in high income countries and suicide from pesticide poisoning, hanging and self-immolation are more common in low to middle income countries [17]. It is important to consider these differences in the global epidemiology of suicide while quantifying the suicide burden attributable to mental and substance use disorders.

The link between mental and substance use disorders and suicide is well documented [14–20] and authors such as Prince and colleagues argued [14] that failure to include suicide as part of mental and substance use disorder estimates in the previous GBD studies [8,9] led to an underestimate of the extent of the burden. A literature review and meta-analysis by Harris and Barraclough showed that of the 249 studies and 44 mental disorders assessed, 36 disorders were associated with an increased risk of suicide [19]. Li and collaborators also found that the risk of suicide was 7.5 (6.2–9.0) times higher in males and 11.7 (9.7–14.1) times higher in females with a mental or substance use disorder compared to males and females with no disorder. Depression and bipolar disorder accounted for the highest risk [20]. Even when other risk factors such as adverse marital effects, employment and socio-economic status were considered, mental and substance use disorders remain strongly associated with suicide [20,21].

Quantifying the suicide burden attributable to mental and substance use disorders also corrects for the low burden from premature mortality (YLLs) directly attributed to mental and substance use disorders in GBD 2010. Although mental and substance use disorders were identified as a leading cause of global burden, YLDs contributed to 95% of DALYs [5,10]. In spite of evidence of excess mortality attributable to many mental and substance use disorders, only substance use disorders, anorexia nervosa, and schizophrenia are recognized as underlying causes of death in the International Classification of Diseases (ICD-10) cause of death guidelines [13] used in GBD 2010. Even for those disorders, few deaths were captured in the vital registrations used in the estimation of YLLs, as this typically involves the cumbersome task of disentangling the effect of multiple mental, substance and physical disorders to identify primary cause of death.

Investigating mental and substance use disorders as risk factors for fatal outcomes like suicide allows us to circumvent this problem by making use of GBD 2010's comparative risk analysis (CRA) methodology [7]. Rather than rely on certification and coding practices in mortality registration systems, this method allows quantification of the difference in population health in a counterfactual with a theoretical minimum level of exposure [7]. We make use of this method here to calculate the suicide burden attributable to mental and substance use disorders, and examine variations by region, country, age, year and disorder.

Methods

The suicide burden attributable to mental and substance use disorders was estimated by comparing the current health status with a theoretical-minimum-risk exposure defined as the counter-factual status of the absence of mental and substance use disorders. Population attributable fractions (PAFs) were determined from the prevalence of exposure to each disorder and the relative-risk (RR) of suicide [7]. For each disorder this involved:

1. Reviewing the strength of the evidence for a causal relationship between the disorder and suicide.
2. Expanding on existing systematic reviews of the literature quantifying the effect size for the disorder as a risk factor for suicide. The preferred metric was population-representative RR estimates.
3. Pooling all RR estimates using meta-analysis.
4. Combining the pooled RR estimate with GBD 2010 prevalence estimates to generate PAFs by age, sex, country, and year.
5. Adjusting PAFs for global differences in suicide attributable to mental and substance use disorders versus differences attributable to other causes.
6. Multiplying PAFs by suicide YLLs reported in GBD 2010 to estimate attributable burden.

Case definition

GBD methods suggest that for each risk factor-outcome pairing, there should be (1) sufficient data to enable estimation of relative effect sizes as well as (2) sufficient evidence for a causal effect [7]. A literature review by Baxter and collaborators [22] as well as other studies summarised in the previous section [14–20] investigating mental and substance use disorders as risk factors for other health outcomes found sufficient evidence to meet these two conditions for suicide.

Mental and substance use disorders investigated were those included in GBD 2010 for which there was evidence of an increased risk of suicide [10,19,20]. These were major depressive disorder (MDD), bipolar disorder, schizophrenia, anxiety disorder, anorexia nervosa, alcohol dependence, amphetamine dependence, cocaine dependence and opioid dependence. All disorders were defined using the Diagnostic and Statistical Manual of Mental disorders (DSM) [23] or ICD diagnostic criteria [13]. Suicide was defined as cases meeting ICD-10 cause of death codes for intentional self-inflicted poisoning or injury (X60–X84) [13]. In some countries a large proportion of injury-related deaths are coded as 'underdetermined intent' for cultural, religious or medico-legal reasons. GBD 2010 developed a method to redistribute these deaths to specific underlying causes, including suicide [6]. Although GBD 2010 also considered the effects of attempted suicide as 'non-fatal self-harm' [5], this was not investigated in this paper.

Literature search to identify relative-risk estimates

We used data sources from recent and methodologically comparable systematic reviews of the association between suicide and mental and substance use disorders [20,24–27], specifically affective disorders, anxiety disorders, schizophrenia (14 studies from these 3 disorder groups) [20], cocaine, opioid, and amphetamine dependence (24 studies) [24–26] and alcohol dependence (12 studies) [27]. We expanded the Li and collaborators systematic review and replicated the literature search [20] to collect data for bipolar disorder and MDD separately (rather than affective disorders combined), and anorexia nervosa which was not included in the original review. The search strategy used was in keeping with the Preferred Reporting Items for Systematic Reviews and Meta-analyses (PRISMA) statement [28] (See Text S1 in File S1 for the PRISMA checklist and flow diagram). Electronic databases (Medline and Embase) were searched between 1966 and 2010. A secondary search of reference lists and the grey literature was also conducted. Studies were included that; (1) considered mental and substance use disorders as a risk factor associated with suicide; (2) reported a RR with 95% uncertainty, or provided sufficient information for these to be calculated; (3) were individual-level case-control or cohort studies where a clear temporal association between exposure and outcome could be determined; (4) had a minimum follow up period of 1 year and; (5) included disorders based on ICD [13] or DSM [23] nomenclature to ensure consistency in case definitions. Sex-specific data were preferred but non sex-specific estimates were included (e.g. for substance use disorders) where data were sparse. For each study, information on study methodology, quality and findings were extracted into a Microsoft Excel spreadsheet. See Table S1 in File S1 for a summary of the study variables extracted.

Meta-analysis of relative-risk estimates

For each disorder (except alcohol dependence for which a pooled estimate was available [27]), MetaXL software, an add-in for Microsoft Excel [29], was used to pool RR estimates from different studies. This was done for males and females separately and also combined. RR estimates were pooled using a random effects model, and if there was sufficient data to do so, a quality effects model [30]. Pooled RRs from the quality-effects model were preferred as these gave greater weight to studies of high quality versus studies of lesser quality, and avoided the anomaly of random effects models which revert to equal weighting regardless of sample size if heterogeneity is large [30–32]. Study quality was assessed using a quality index which scored studies based on sampling design and representativeness and also the availability of age- and gender-specific estimates. It was limited to these items to reduce potential subjectivity within and between quality scores. To prevent inter-rater bias, all studies were rated by one researcher and a random sample of scores was checked by an independent researcher. See Table S1 in File S1 for the quality index and scores.

Prevalence of mental and substance use disorders

We obtained the prevalence distribution of each mental and substance use disorder from the epidemiological disease models used in the calculation of direct burden (i.e. YLDs) in GBD 2010 [10,12]. These were based on a separate literature review (presented in greater detail elsewhere [33–38]) conducted between 1980 to 2010 to capture studies reporting prevalence, incidence, remission, duration and all cause-excess mortality associated with mental and substance use disorders. Point (current or past month) prevalence estimates of DSM/ICD defined disorders were required. Twelve-month prevalence estimates were accepted to maximize inclusion but adjusted towards the level of point prevalence using study-level covariates. Lifetime prevalence was excluded as it is more likely than point or period prevalence to be affected by recall bias [39,40]. GBD 2010's DisMod-MR, a Bayesian meta-regression tool, was used to integrate these estimates into an epidemiological disease model. From the epidemiological inputs, DisMod-MR generated prevalence by sex and age for 187 countries, 21 world regions and 1990, 2005 and 2010 [2,41]. Prevalent cases for each disorder have been summarised in previous publications [2,10,12].

Population attributable fractions

PAFs were calculated from the DisMod-MR prevalence output (P) for each disorder and the pooled RR of suicide given exposure to the disorder. PAFs were calculated by age, sex, country, year and disorder (consistent with the format of GBD 2010 estimates) using the following formula [42]:

$$PAF = \frac{p(RR-1)}{p(RR-1)+1}$$

Given the presence of comorbidity between mental and substance use disorders, disorder-specific PAFs cannot be summed to obtain the 'joint effect' of combined mental and substance use disorders on suicide. Instead, a joint PAF was estimated using the multiplicative method of adjusting for comorbidity between disorders [43]. This can be understood as calculating the complement of the product of the complements of each individual PAF. The following formula was used where i is the individual risk factor, and n is the total number of risk factors [7];

$$Joint\, PAF = 1 - \prod_{i=1}^{n} (1 - PAF_i)$$

Ceiling values for joint population attributable fractions

Although studies from high income countries have consistently shown that up to 90% of suicides occur as a result of an underlying mental or substance use disorder [18,21,44], there is also evidence to suggest that this proportion is substantially lower in China, Taiwan and India; where symptoms of 'dysphoric affect' and 'impulsivity' (which do not constitute a mental and substance use disorder) are expressed through more lethal methods of self-harming such as pesticide poisoning and self-immolation [45–48]. This in turn, increases the number of completed suicides occurring from self-harm behaviours (characteristically instigated as impulsive acts, without the presence of a mental and substance use disorder or a clear intent to die) in these countries which would have resulted in an "attempted suicide" had such methods not been available [46,47].

So as not to overestimate the total proportion of suicide burden attributable to mental and substance use disorders, we first portioned out global differences in suicide attributable to mental and substance use disorders from differences attributable to other causes. More specifically, the total proportion of suicide cases attributable to mental and substance use disorders in different countries was calculated and used to set a ceiling value (or upper threshold) for the joint PAFs. We examined reference lists of existing reviews for psychological autopsy studies [18,21,44] and conducted a supplementary literature search to capture additional data sources up to 2010. The psychological autopsy method is a retrospective assessment of causes of death which involves canvassing the views of individuals closest to the deceased and substantiating evidence from sources such as hospital and police records [49]. The overall number of suicide cases attributable to mental and substance use disorders was extracted from these studies if DSM/ICD diagnostic criteria [13,23] were used and the number of attributable suicide cases was reported for mental and substance use disorders as a group rather than for individual disorders. If gender was not recorded we also accepted combined estimates for males and females. Given that there were insufficient data to calculate ceiling values individually for each country or region, we pooled estimates into 2 broad categories based on the percentage of suicide cases reported to be due to mental and substance use disorders. Meta-analyses based on quality effects models were used to generate separate pooled proportions for Group 1: China, India and Taiwan and Group 2: all other countries.

These calculated proportions of suicide cases due to mental and substance use disorder were used to set the ceiling value of joint PAFs. All quantities of interest in GBD 2010 were calculated a thousand times in order to incorporate all sources of uncertainty. Similarly, we created a thousand draws of the 'ceiling values' based on the pooled estimates of mean and standard error. When estimating the joint PAFs of suicide attributed to all mental and substance use disorders we did not allow PAF estimates in any of the one thousand draws to exceed the ceiling value in the corresponding draw. For draws that did exceed the ceiling, we scaled down each of the component mental and substance use disorder PAFs by the ratio of the ceiling to the combined PAF.

Attributable burden

The final step was to multiply PAFs by the corresponding GBD 2010 YLLs for suicide [5,6] to calculate attributable burden. Since only completed suicides were considered in our analyses, only YLLs were included in attributable DALY estimates. To quantify 95% uncertainty around our final burden estimate we calculated attributable YLLs and DALYs at the one thousand draw level and bounded the 95% uncertainty interval by the 2.5 and 97.5 centile values. All reporting of DALYs by region and country is based on age-standardised estimates using direct standardization to the global standard population proposed by the World Health Organization (WHO) in 2001 [50].

Results

Pooled relative-risk estimates

Our search culminated in a dataset of 40 studies and 85 RR estimates covering 14 countries (Table S1 in File S1 summarizes included studies). There was a statistically significant increased risk of suicide for all selected mental and substance use disorders (table 1). The greatest risk was seen in MDD followed by schizophrenia, and alcohol dependence. The 95% confidence intervals around each pooled RR indicated high levels of uncertainty with statistical heterogeneity (as measured by the I^2 statistic) of up to 90%. A statistically significant sex difference was only observed for alcohol dependence (Table S2 in File S1 summarizes sex-specific pooled RRs) hence the overall pooled proportions for both sexes combined were used in PAF calculations. Given that the one RR estimate for amphetamine dependence was not statistically different (i.e. occurred within overlapping 95% uncertainty) to the three estimates for cocaine dependence, we combined them to calculate a pooled RR for all psychostimulants. This was used to calculate PAFs for both disorders.

Ceiling values for joint PAFs

Out of 166 psychological autopsy studies reviewed, 43 studies and 57 estimates covering 20 countries were used to calculate ceiling value for joint PAFs (Table S3 in File S1 summarizes included studies). In China, India and Taiwan (group 1), 68.3% (55.2%–80.0%) of suicide cases was due to mental and substance use disorders which was lower than in all other countries (group 2), where 84.5% (78.6%–89.6%) of suicide cases were due to mental and substance use disorders. These two pooled proportions were used as the ceiling values for joint PAFs from China, India and Taiwan (Group 1) and all other countries (Group 2) respectively. Note that there was considerable heterogeneity between studies. As we found no statistically significant sex difference, the overall pooled proportions were used in PAF calculations (Table S4 in File S1 summarizes sex-specific pooled proportions).

Attributable burden

Mental and substance use disorders were responsible for 22.5 million (14.8–29.8 million) of the 36.2 million (26.5–44.3 million) DALYs allocated to suicide in 2010, amounting to 62.1% (43.8%–75.3%) of total suicide DALYs. The proportion of attributable suicide DALYs in 1990 was almost identical to that in 2010 (62.1% (44.5%–75.4%)). The remainder of this section focuses on 2010 estimates with 1990 estimates summarised in Table S5 in File S1.

There were twice as many mental and substance use disorders attributable suicide DALYs for males (14.9 million (9.5–20.1 million)) compared to females (7.6 million (4.4–10.6 million)). For all disorders, this sex difference was consistent throughout the lifespan. Attributable suicide DALYs were apparent from those aged ≥5 years, with the highest proportion occurring between those aged 20–30 years (Figure 1).

The proportion of suicide DALYs explained by mental and substance use disorders was reasonably consistent between regions and within the range of the ceiling values presented in the previous section. When considered in terms of absolute DALYs, Asia South and Asia East had the highest burden attributable to mental and substance use disorders, given their large population size. In terms of age-standardized rates, Europe Eastern had the highest burden (almost 3 times higher than the global mean) and Sub-Saharan Africa West the lowest (6 times lower than the global mean) (Figure 2 and Table S5 in File S1 summarize attributable DALYs by disorder, region, age and sex).

There were also differences in attributable suicide DALYs across countries (plot 1, figure 3). Attributable DALY rates were highest in Kazakhstan and lowest in Saudi Arabia, however many of the country level differences presented in plot 1 were within overlapping ranges of uncertainty (plot 2, figure 3). Except for Guyana, Suriname and Zimbabwe, all countries with statistically higher attributable DALY rates than the global mean were from Eastern Europe and South Asia. Countries with statistically lower DALY rates than the global mean included those from South America, Oceania, Africa and the Middle East and parts of Asia.

Of the suicide DALYs attributable to mental and substance use disorders, MDD was responsible for the largest proportion (46.1% (28.0%–60.8%)), followed by alcohol dependence (13.25% (12.0%–15.0%)), anxiety disorder (7.4% (3.0%–12.7%)), bipolar disorder (5.4% (1.8%–10.7%)), schizophrenia (4.7% (4.1%–5.3%)), amphetamine dependence (2.4% (0.9%–4.6%)), opioid dependence (1.9% (1.1%–2.9%)), cocaine dependence (0.9% (0.3%–1.8%)) and anorexia nervosa (0.2% (0.02%–0.5%)) (figure 4). MDD explained the most suicide DALYs and anorexia nervosa the least across all age groups, sex and regions although most of the age and regional differences between disorders remained within wide and overlapping confidence intervals (Table S6 in File S1).

The additional burden attributable to suicide for each mental and substance use disorder (over and above the DALYs assigned to them as a direct cause) is also illustrated in figure 4. The inclusion of attributable suicide burden increased the fatal burden (YLLs)

Table 1. Pooled relative-risk of suicide in those diagnosed with a mental or substance use disorder.

Disorder	Number of studies	Pooled relative risk (95% UI)
Major depressive disorder	4	19.9 (9.5–41.7)
Anxiety disorder	7	2.7 (1.7–4.3)
Schizophrenia	4	12.6 (11.0–14.5)
Bipolar disorder	4	5.7 (2.6–12.4)
Anorexia nervosa	9	7.6 (2.2–25.6)
Alcohol dependence[b]	12	9.8 (9.0–10.7)
Opioid dependence	21	6.9 (4.5–10.5)
Psychostimulant dependence	4	8.2 (3.9–16.9)
Amphetamine dependence[a]	1	4.5(1.1–9.03)
Cocaine dependence[a]	3	16.9(6.01–47.2)

Note. 95% UI: 95% uncertainty interval;
[a]*Due to lack of data, simultaneously pooled cocaine and amphetamine relative-risk estimates into an overall estimate for psychostimulants which was applied to both disorders;*
[b]*Used reported pooled standardised mortality ratios from Wilcox et al [27] for alcohol dependence.*

due to mental and substance use disorders from 0.5% (0.4%–0.7%) (assigned to them as a direct cause) to 1.8% (1.4%–2.2%) of global YLLs and the overall burden (DALYs) of mental and substance use disorders from 7.4% (6.2%–8.6%) to 8.3% (7.1%–9.6%) of global DALYs. Out of the 10 leading classes of diseases included in GBD 2010 [5], mental and substance use disorders increased from the 5th to the 3rd leading class of disease burden once the burden attributable to suicide was considered; exceeding the burden due to neoplasms (7.6% (7.0%–8.2%) of global DALYs) and neonatal conditions (8.1% (7.3%–9.0%) of global DALYs) but not cardiovascular and circulatory diseases (11.9% (11.1%–12.7%) of global DALYs) and diarrhea, LRI, meningitis, and other common infectious diseases (11.4% (10.4%–12.8%) of global DALYs). The global DALY ranking of individual disorders (as presented in GBD 2010's publication series [5]) also increased when attributable suicide burden was included (table 2). Although within overlapping ranges of uncertainty, the ranking for alcohol dependence increased the most, from the 35th (29th–45th) to the 28th (26th–37th) leading cause of burden.

Discussion

Mental and substance use disorders are associated with an increased risk of suicide, a finding that is well established in the literature [19,20,27] but until now, not quantified in terms of a global comparison of disease burden. DALY rankings in GBD 2010 were based on a classification of mutually exclusive disease and injury categories [5,10]. Considering the additional burden due to mental and substance use disorders as a risk factor for suicide elevated mental and substance use disorders from the fifth to the third leading disease category of global burden in 2010. Few mental and substance use disorders are recognized as a primary cause of death in mortality registrations, and those that are recognised are often under-represented. The data presented here provide a more comprehensive insight into the magnitude of the burden due to these disorders.

Mental and substance use disorders were the cause of two-thirds of all suicide DALYs reported in GBD 2010. Aside from emphasising these as a debilitating group of disorders, our findings highlight the importance of prioritising the prevention, early detection and effective management of mental and substance use disorders – particularly MDD – as a key suicide prevention strategy. Presenting the differences in attributable burden between regions and countries also provides a beginning for developing policies or intervention strategies that are applicable at the national level. Such interventions can be described as 'selective', in the sense that they target subgroups of the population whose members have yet to manifest suicidal behaviours, but exhibit risk factors (in this case, mental and substance use disorders) that predispose them to do so in the future. These can be contrasted with 'universal' interventions, which target whole populations with the aim of favorably shifting proximal and distal risk (and protective) factors across the entire population, and 'indicated interventions' which are designed for individuals already exhibiting suicidal behaviours [51].

Typically, countries that have put in place national suicide prevention strategies have funded a range of universal, selective and indicated interventions, in recognition of the variety of risk and protective factors associated with suicide [52]. However our findings suggest that a relatively greater emphasis on selective interventions targeting individuals with mental and substance use disorders may be applicable. By way of example, equipping general practitioners to detect, diagnose and manage MDD is likely to have benefits, particularly because many individuals with MDD will receive care from a general practitioner rather than a specialist mental health provider. This was one of the few interventions for which there was good evidence of effectiveness as a suicide prevention strategy in a recent review by Mann and colleagues [53]. That said, ensuring that care from general practitioners is evidence-based requires further consideration, given findings that rates of minimally adequate treatment for depression are lower among patients treated solely by general practitioners or in the general medical care sector, compared to those treated by specialist mental health providers [54,55].

However universal and indicated interventions have their place, particularly in low and middle income countries where mental and substance use disorders were associated with a lesser proportion of the burden of suicide. In these countries, universal interventions for example restricting access to means (e.g., pesticides) is worth pursuing given that they are relatively cheap to implement, can have a broad community reach and are known to be effective [53].

Although within overlapping bounds of uncertainty, we found that attributable suicide DALY rates among young people aged 15–19 years were approaching those of the adult age groups.

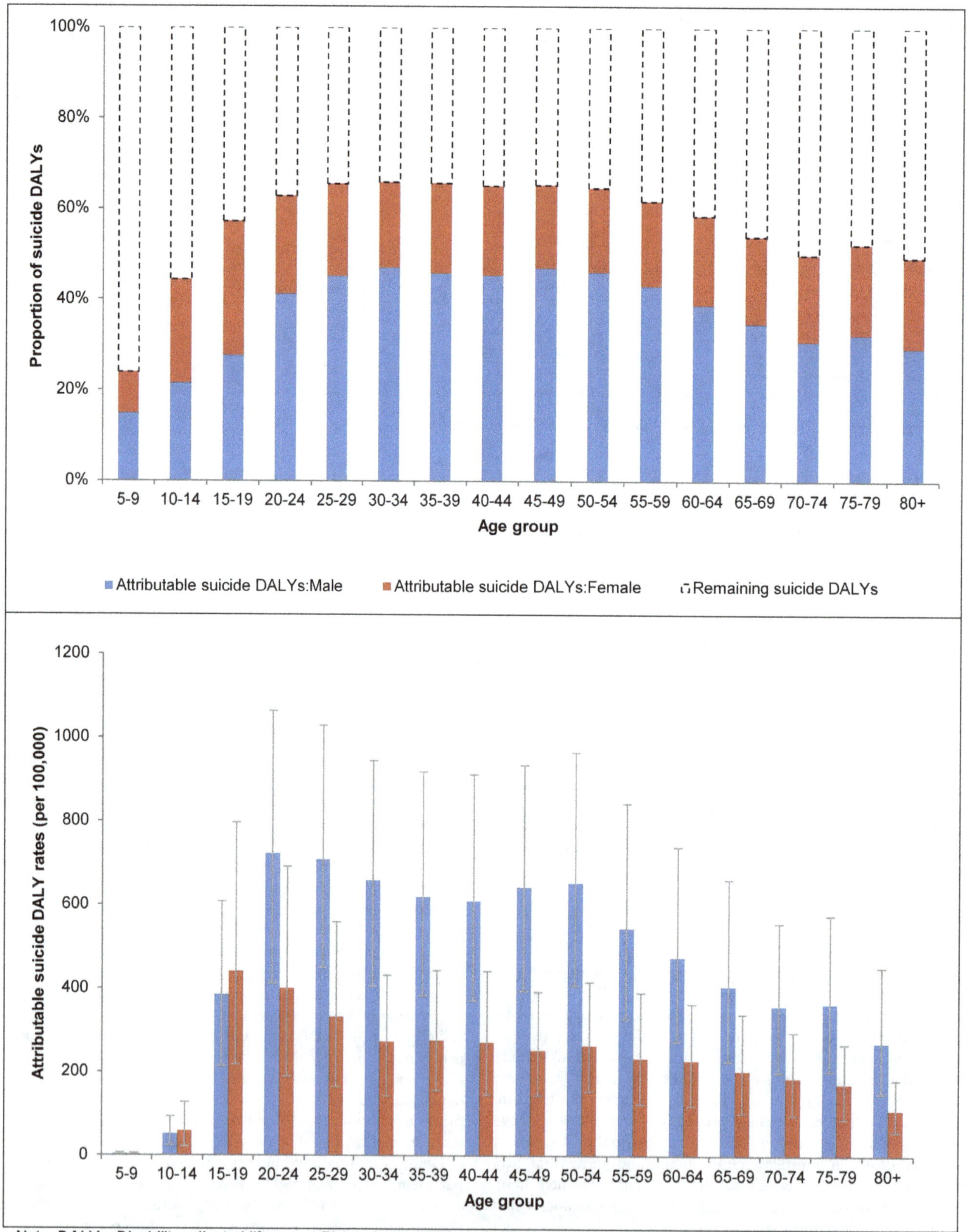

Note. DALYs: Disability adjusted life years. Plot 1 shows attributable DALYs as proportion of suicide DALYs. Plot 2 shows attributable DALYs as a rate per 100,000

Figure 1. Suicide DALYs attributable to mental and substance use disorders by age and sex, in 2010.

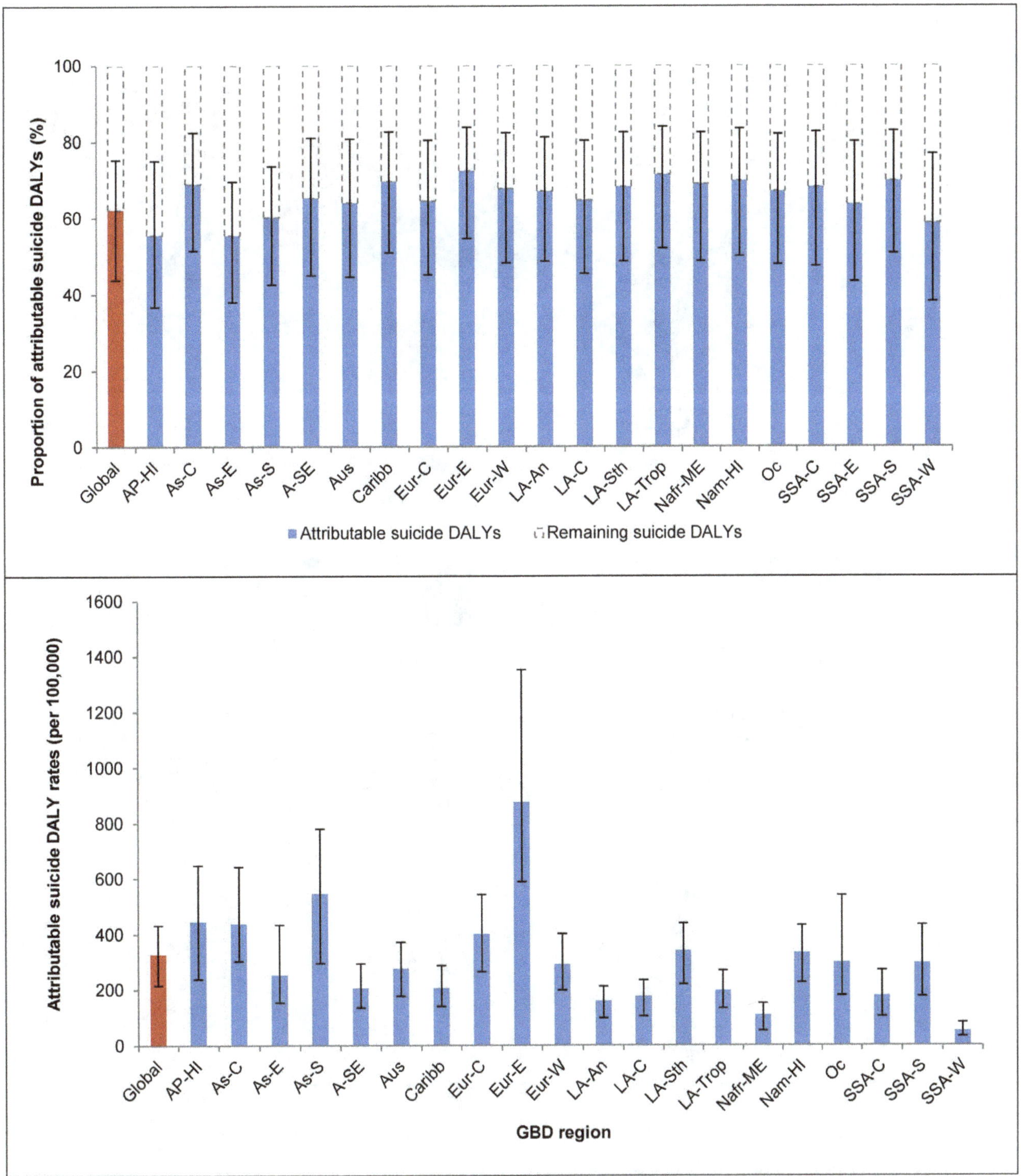

Note. DALYs: Disability adjusted life years; Plot 1 shows attributable DALYs as proportion of suicide DALYs. Plot 2 shows attributable DALYs as a rate per 100,000; AP-HI: Asia Pacific, High Income, As-C: Asia Central, AS-E: Asia East, AS-S: Asia South, A-SE: Asia Southeast, Aus: Australasia, Caribb: Caribbean, Eur-C: Europe Central, Eur-E: Europe Eastern, Eur-W: Europe Western, LA-An: Latin America, Andean, LA-C: Latin America, Central, LA-Sth: Latin America, Southern, LA-Trop: Latin America, Tropical, Nafr-ME: North Africa/Middle East, Nam-HI: North America, High Income, Oc: Oceania, SSA-C: Sub-Saharan Africa, Central, SSA-E: Sub-Saharan Africa, East, SSA-S: Sub-Saharan Africa Southern, SSA-W: Sub-Saharan Africa, West.

Figure 2. Suicide DALYs attributable to mental and substance use disorders by region, in 2010.

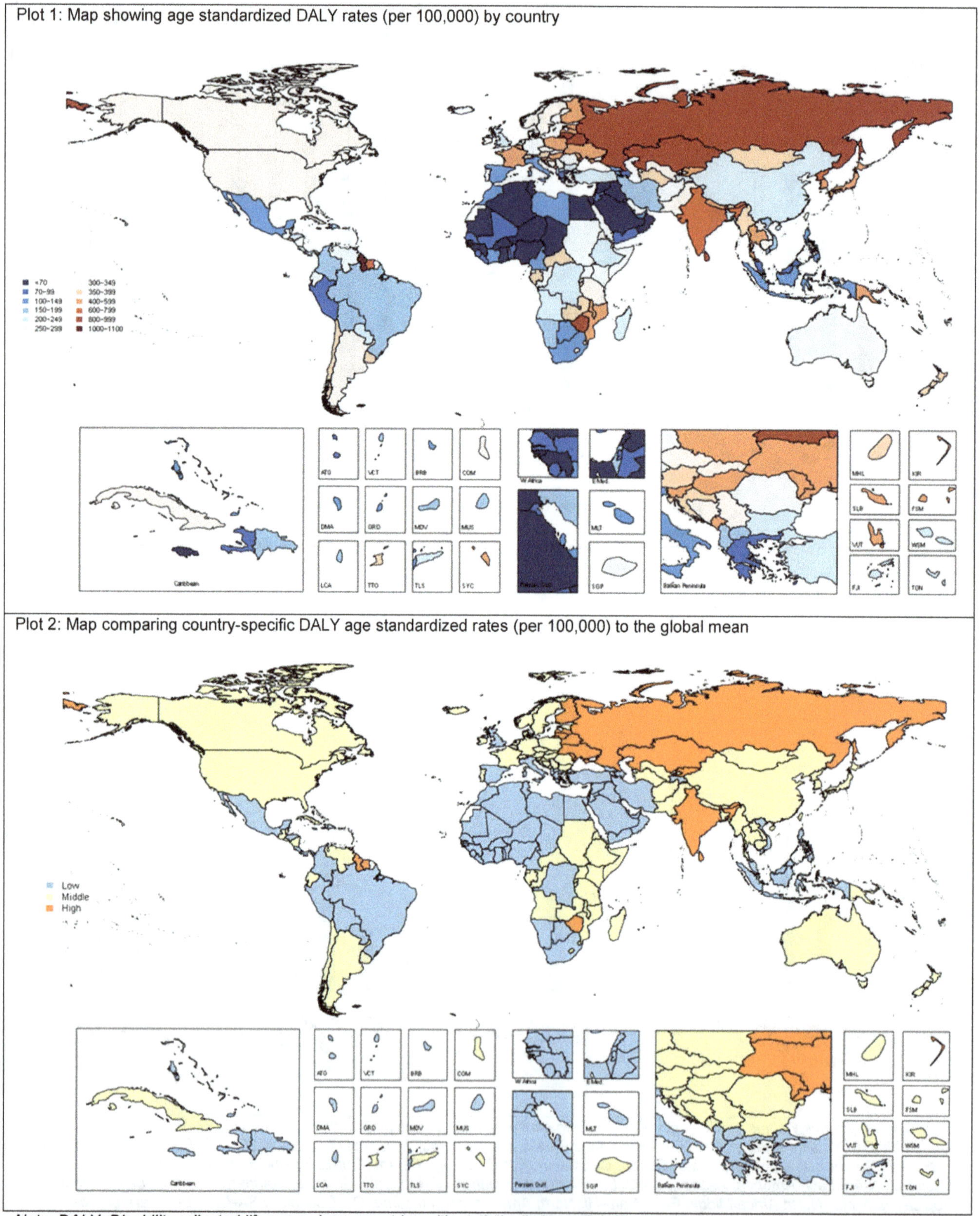

Note: DALY: Disability adjusted life years; Low: countries with statistically lower DALY rates than the global mean; middle: countries with statistically similar DALY rates to the global mean; high: countries with statistically higher DALY rates than the global mean.

Figure 3. Suicide DALYs (rates per 100,000) attributable to mental and substance use disorders by country, in 2010.

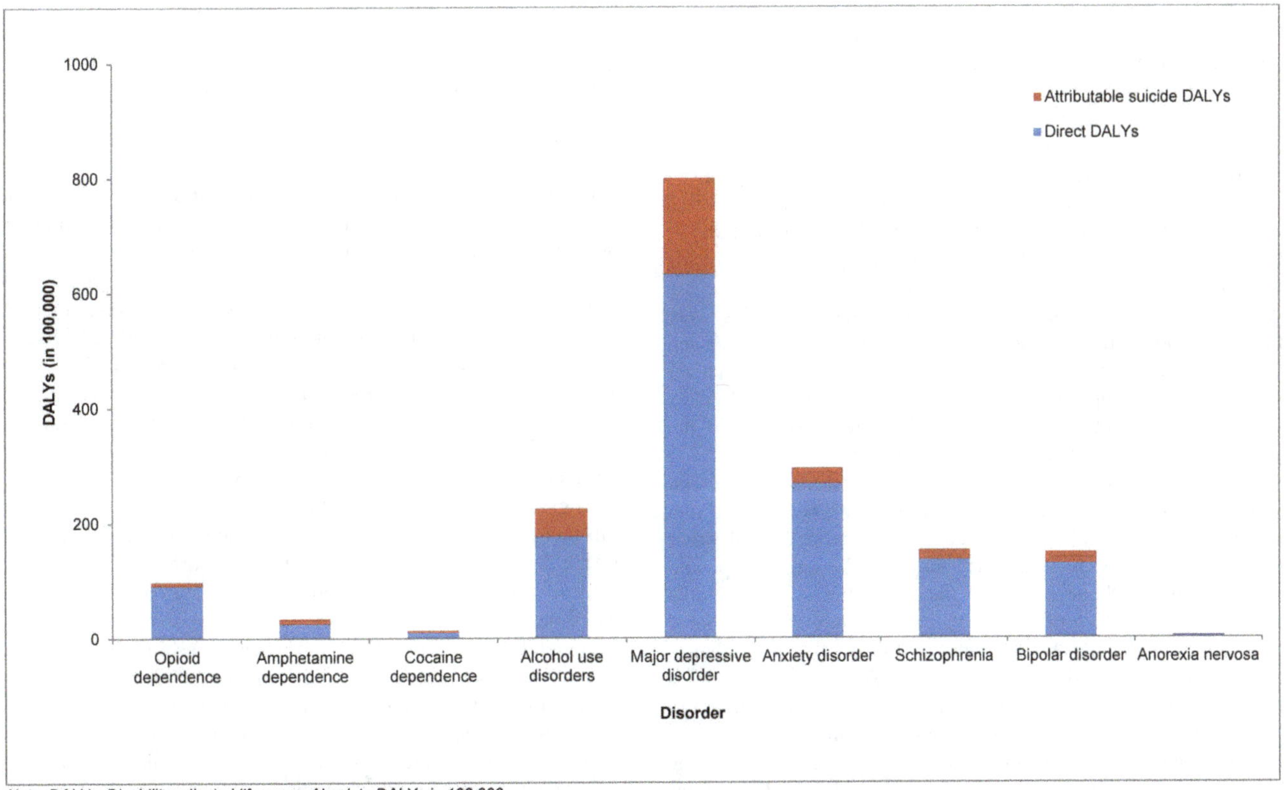

Note. DALYs: Disability adjusted life years; Absolute DALYs in 100,000.

Figure 4. Suicide DALYs attributable to mental and substance use disorders by disorder, in 2010.

Although males had higher rates of attributable burden in most age groups, female rates were higher between the ages of 10 and 19 years. These age-related findings support the importance of school-based prevention programs which include a focus on mental health targeted to at-risk adolescents. The sex-difference in attributable burden also needs to be considered when formulating prevention strategies for this age group. Although evidence of a reduction in suicide behaviours has not been demonstrated, there is evidence for the effectiveness of school-based programs in reducing the effect of risk factors such as depression [52,56]. A recent systematic review of interventions targeting adolescents or young adults at risk of suicide identified individual cognitive behavioral therapy-based interventions and attachment-based family therapy as promising interventions, requiring further investigation [57].

As there was insufficient data to (1) obtain pooled RR estimates for all countries or regions included in GBD 2010 and (2) clearly detect differences in RR estimates between all countries/regions,

Table 2. Global DALY proportions and rankings before and after the addition of attributable suicide burden, in 2010.

Disorder	After addition of attributable suicide burden (95% UI)			
	Direct DALYs	Mean rank	Direct plus attributable DALYs	Mean rank
	As a proportion of total DALYs		As a proportion of total DALYs	
Major depressive disorder[a]	2.5% (1.9%–3.3%)	11 (7–14)	3.2% (2.5%–4.0%)	8 (4–11)
Anxiety disorder[a]	1.1% (0.8%–1.5%)	26 (19–33)	1.2% (0.9%–1.6%)	25 (17–30)
Alcohol dependence[a]	0.7% (0.5%–0.9%)	35 (29–45)	0.9% (0.7%–1.1%)	28 (26–37)
Schizophrenia[a]	0.6% (0.4%–0.7%)	43 (36–57)	0.7% (0.5%–0.9%)	39 (30.5–50)
Bipolar disorder[a]	0.5% (0.3%–0.8%)	46 (35–59)	0.6% (0.4%–0.8%)	44 (31–56)
Mental and substance use disorders combined[b]	7.4% (6.2%–8.6%)	5 (3–6)	8.3% (7.1%–9.6%)	3 (3–6)

Note. DALYs: Disability adjusted life years; 95% UI: 95% uncertainty interval;
[a]Global ranking of direct burden for each disorder was from the official GBD 2010 disease ranking for 2010 [5]. Illicit drug use disorders have not been included here as the GBD 2010 official disease ranking investigated drug use disorders as group (rather than by specific drug types). Similarly, the ranking for anorexia nervosa was presented in addition to bulimia nervosa;
[b]The global ranking of direct burden of mental and substance use disorders as a group compares the direct burden of the 11 main classes of diseases in GBD 2010 [10].

the pooled RR estimates used to estimate PAFs were assumed to be constant across age, sex and country. Instead, the variation in attributable DALYs across countries was driven by (a function of both) the prevalence of mental and substance use disorders and the amount of burden accounted for by suicide in each country. In addition, given evidence for differences in the underlying causes of suicide in China, India and Taiwan [45–48], where it has been well documented that the ease of availability of particularly lethal means of self-harm such as pesticides may influence patterns of suicide, we constrained the maximum proportion of suicide attributable to mental and substance use disorders to a ceiling value of 68.3%. In spite of this, some Asian countries were amongst those with the highest rates of attributable suicide burden due to the high rates of suicide in those countries. This emphasizes the fact that although there may be other risk factors for suicide, the prioritisation of mental and substance use disorders in the prevention of suicide remains a global priority.

The maximum proportion of suicide attributable to mental and substance use disorders in all other countries was constrained to a ceiling value of 84.5%. The studies categorized as "all other countries" were mainly from North America, Western Europe and Australia and, although we had data for three low to middle income countries (Colombia, Pakistan and Indonesia), this pooled proportion might not be appropriate for use in Sub-Saharan Africa where we found no data. It is possible that these countries have a different distribution of suicides attributable to mental and substance use disorders but more cross-national RR data are required before we can incorporate this in our findings. Islamic countries, for instance from North Africa/Middle East, were amongst the countries with the lowest proportion of attributable burden, despite being allocated the higher ceiling value of 84.5%. In contrast to the high rates of depression in the Middle East, rates of suicide were low. The lowest rate of suicide recorded in GBD 2010 was from Saudi Arabia. Stigma around suicide due to religious beliefs and legislative prohibition (i.e. suicide being considered as a criminal offence) can lead to fewer cases of suicide being recorded as a cause of death in countries from the Middle East. For similar reasons, the degree of psychopathology underpinning suicide cannot be as clearly assessed in these countries [58,59]. These issues may have biased our estimates of attributable burden. The large bounds of uncertainty presented reflect this to some extent; however, more data are required on the distribution and aetiology of suicide in these countries to improve estimates.

Like all population-based analyses, a number of methodological limitations need to be considered here. The ceiling values for suicide attributable to mental and substance use disorders were derived from psychological autopsy studies. As these collect retrospective data after the individual had died, they are limited by the accuracy of coroners' reports and systematic bias from interviewees [49]. Although the pooled RR estimates used were derived from more representative population-based prospective cohort studies, there were only a few estimates available for most disorders. We applied the same pooled RR across all countries, sex and age groups for each disorder to reduce errors in estimates as a result of paucity in the data. It is possible that this masked differences in the distribution of attributable suicide DALYs. More representative population cohort studies are now emerging from low and middle income countries such as India [16]. We hope that the scrutiny of data presented here will encourage more and better quality data collection for mental and substance use disorders as risk factors for suicide. Until then, it is important to consider the uncertainty around our final estimates in interpreting these findings.

CRA methodology assumes a causal relationship between the exposure and outcome [7]. In support for this, the RR estimates used here showed that mental and substance use disorders were significantly associated with suicide risk, even when other risk factors such as socio-economic factors (e.g. adverse marital, employment and socio-economic status) were considered [20,21]. Another assumption was that the proportion of suicide burden attributable to mental and substance use disorders was estimated while holding all other independent risk factors constant. We estimated the joint effect of all mental and substance use disorders on suicide while adjusting for comorbidity between these disorders, the next step would be to explore the joint effect of mental and substance use disorder with other risk factors of suicide. Finally, PAF calculations were sensitive to the exposure distribution used. Here we used DisMod-MR to pool the prevalence of each disorder based on the raw epidemiological data that were available [10,38]. Although this provided consistent prevalence estimates by country, region, age, sex, and year, in some cases DisMod-MR was required to adjust for considerable heterogeneity in the raw data. This was, to some extent, incorporated in our analyses through the 95% uncertainty intervals around all prevalence estimates propagated to the final attributable burden estimates.

Conclusions

Mental and substance use disorders were responsible for two thirds of the suicide burden in 2010, adding a further 22 million DALYs to their global burden. More consideration needs to be given to interventions targeted to populations with, or at risk for, mental and substance use disorders as an effective strategy for suicide prevention.

Acknowledgments

We would like to acknowledge members of the mental and illicit drug use expert group and other international collaborators for their assistance with the methodology used in this paper. We would like to specifically thank Abraham D. Flaxman, Institute of Heath Metrics and Evaluation, University of Washington, for his assistance with the DisMod-MR modeling of mental and substance use disorders and suicide and Chiara Stone, National Drug and Alcohol Research Centre, University of New South Wales for her assistance with the literature review for illicit drug use disorders.

Author Contributions

Conceived and designed the experiments: AJF TV HAW. Analyzed the data: AJF REN GF EC TV. Wrote the paper: AJF REN GF AJB JEP MGH AP EC LD TV HAW. Wrote the first draft of the manuscript: AJF. Contributed to consequent drafts: REN GF AJB JEP MGH AP EC LD TV HAW.

References

1. Wang H, Dwyer-Lindgren L, Lofgren KT, Rajaratnam JK, Marcus JR, et al. (2012) Age-specifi c and sex-specifi c mortality in 187 countries, 1970–2010: a systematic analysis for the Global Burden of Disease Study 2010. Lancet 380: 2071–2094.

2. Vos T, Flaxman AD, Naghavi M, Lozano R, Michaud C, et al. (2012) Years lived with disability (YLDs) for 1160 sequelae of 289 diseases and injuries 1990–2010: a systematic analysis for the Global Burden of Disease Study 2010. Lancet 380: 2163–2196.
3. Salomon JA, Wang H, Freeman MK, Vos T, Flaxman AD, et al. (2012) Healthy life expectancy for 187 countries, 1990–2010: a systematic analysis for the Global Burden Disease Study 2010. Lancet 380: 2144–2162.
4. Salomon JA, Vos T, Hogan DR, Gagnon M, Naghavi M, et al. (2012) Common values in assessing health outcomes from disease and injury:disability weights measurement study for the Global Burden of Disease 2010 Lancet 380: 2129–2143.
5. Murray CJL, Vos T, Lozano R, Naghavi M, Flaxman AD, et al. (2012) Disability-adjusted life years (DALYs) for 291 diseases and injuries in 21 regions, 1990–2010: a systematic analysis for the Global Burden of Disease Study 2010. Lancet 380: 2197–2223.
6. Lozano R, Naghavi M, Foreman K, Lim S, Shibuya K, et al. (2012) Global and regional mortality from 235 causes of death for 20 age groups in 1990 and 2010: a systematic analysis for the Global Burden of Disease Study 2010. Lancet 380: 2095–2128.
7. Lim SS, Vos T, Flaxman AD, Danaei G, Shibuya K, et al. (2012) A comparative risk assessment of burden of disease and injury attributable to 67 risk factors and risk factor clusters in 21 regions, 1990–2010: a systematic analysis for the Global Burden of Disease Study 2010. Lancet 380: 2224–2260.
8. Murray CJL, Lopez AD, editors (1996) The Global Burden of Disease: a comprehensive assessment of mortality and disability from diseases, injuries, and risk factors in 1990 and projected to 2020. Cambridge, MA: Published by the Harvard School of Public Health on behalf of the World Health Organization and the World Bank ; Distributed by Harvard University Press.
9. World Health Organization (2008) The Global Burden of Disease: 2004 update. Switzerland.
10. Whiteford HA, Degenhardt L, Rehm J, Baxter AJ, Ferrari AJ, et al. (2013) The Global Burden of Mental and Substance Use Disorders, 2010. The Lancet Published online August 28. Available: http://www.sciencedirect.com/science/article/pii/S0140673613616116.
11. Ferrari AJ, Charlson FJ, Norman RE, Patten SB, Murray CJL, et al. (2013) Burden of depressive disorders by country, sex, age and year: Findings from the Global Burden of Disease Study 2010. PloS Medicine In press.
12. Degenhardt L, Whiteford HA, Ferrari AJ, Baxter AJ, Charlson FJ, et al. (2013) The global burden of disease attributable to illicit drug use: Results from the GBD 2010 study. The Lancet Published online August 28. Available: http://dx.doi.org/10.1016/S0140-6736(13)61530-5.
13. World Health Organization (1992) The ICD-10 Classification of Mental and Behavioural Disorders. Clinical descriptions and diagnostic guidelines Geneva: World Health Organisation.
14. Prince M, Patel V, Saxena S, Maj M, Maselko J, et al. (2007) No health without mental health. Lancet 370: 859–877.
15. Phillips MR, Cheng HG (2012) The changing global face of suicide. Lancet 379: 2318–2319.
16. Patel V, Ramasundarahettige C, Vijayakumar L, Thakur JS, Gajalakshmi V, et al. (2012) Suicide mortality in India: a nationally representative survey. Lancet 379: 2343–2351.
17. Vijayakumar L (2005) Suicide and mental disorders in Asia. International Review of Psychiatry 17: 109–114.
18. Arsenault-Lapierre G, Kim C, Turecki G (2004) Psychiatric diagnoses in 3275 suicides: a meta-analysis. BMC Psychiatry 37: 1–11.
19. Harris EC, Barraclough B (1997) Suicide as an outcome for mental disorders: A meta-analysis. British Journal of Psychiatry 170: 205–228.
20. Li Z, Page A, Martin G, Taylor R (2011) Attributable risk of psychiatric and socio-economic factors for suicide from individual-level, population-based studies: a systematic review. Soc Sci Med 72: 608–616.
21. Yoshimasu K, Kiyohara C, Miyashita K (2008) Suicidal risk factors and completed suicide: meta-analyses based on psychological autopsy studies. Environmental Health and Preventive Medicine 13: 243–256.
22. Baxter AJ, Charlson FJ, Somerville AJ, Whiteford HA (2011) Mental disorders as risk factors: assessing the evidence for the global burden of disease study. BMC Medicine 9: 1–7.
23. American Psychiatric Association (2000) Diagnostic and Statistical Manual of Mental Disorders (DSM-IV-TR). Washington DC: American Psychiatric Association.
24. Degenhardt L, Bucello C, Mathers B, Briegleb C, Ali H, et al. (2011) Mortality among problematic users of heroin and other illicit opioids: A systematic review and meta-analysis. Addiction 106: 32–51.
25. Degenhardt L, Singleton J, Calabria B, McLaren J, Kerr T, et al. (2011) Mortality among cocaine users: A systematic review of cohort studies. Drug and Alcohol Dependence 113: 88–95.
26. Singleton J, Degenhardt L, Hall W, Zabransky T (2009) Mortality among people who use amphetamines: A systematic review of cohort studies. Drug & Alcohol Dependence 105: 1–8.
27. Wilcox HC, Conner KR, Caine ED (2004) Association of alcohol and drug use disorders and completed suicide: an empirical review of cohort studies. Drug Alcohol Depend 76 Suppl: S11–19.
28. Moher D, Liberati A, Tetzlaff J, Altman DG, The PG (2009) Preferred reporting items for systematic reviews and meta-analyses: the PRISMA Statement. PLoS Med 6: e1000097.
29. Epigear (2012) MetaXL
30. Doi SA, Thalib L (2008) A quality-effects model for meta-analysis. Epidemiology 19: 94–100
31. Barendregt JJ, Doi SA (2010) MetaXL User Guide: Version 1.0. Wilston, Australia: EpiGear International Pty Ltd.
32. Doi SA, Barendregt JJ, Mozurkewich EL (2011) Meta-analysis Of heterogenous clinical trials: An empirical example. . Contemporary Clinical Trials 32: 288–298.
33. Baxter AJ, Scott K, Vos T, Whiteford HA (2012) Global prevalence of anxiety disorders: A systematic review and meta-regression Psychological Medicine 43: 897–910.
34. Degenhardt L, Bucello C, Calabria B, Nelson P, Roberts A, et al. (2011) What data are available on the extent of illicit drug use and dependence globally? Results of four systematic reviews. Drug Alcohol Depend 117: 85–101.
35. Ferrari AJ, Baxter AJ, Whiteford HA (2010) A systematic review of the global distribution and availability of prevalence data for bipolar disorder. Journal of Affective Disorders 34: 1–13.
36. Ferrari AJ, Somerville AJ, Baxter AJ, Norman R, Patten SB, et al. (2013) Global variation in the prevalence and incidence of major depressive disorder: A systematic review of the epidemiological literature. Psychological Medicine 43: 471–481.
37. Saha S, Chant D, Welham J, McGrath J (2005) A systematic review of the prevalence of schizophrenia. PLoS Medicine 2: e141.
38. Whiteford HA, Ferrari AJ, Baxter AJ, Charlson FJ, Degenhardt L (2013) How did we arrive at burden of disease estimates for mental and illicit drug use disorders in the Global Burden of Disease Study 2010? Current Opinion in Psychiatry 26: 376–383.
39. Kruijshaar ME, Barendregt J, Vos T, de Graaf R, Spijker J, et al. (2005) Lifetime prevalence estimates of major depression: An indirect estimation method and a quantification of recall bias. European Journal of Epidemiology 20: 103–111.
40. Moffitt TE, Caspi A, Taylor AJ, Kokaua J, Milne BJ, et al. (2010) How common are common mental disorders? Evidence that lifetime prevalence rates are doubled by prospective versus retrospective ascertainment. Psychological Medicine 40: 899–909.
41. Flaxman AD, Vos T, Murray CJL, editors (2013) An integrative metaregression framework for descriptive epidemiology. Washington: University of Washington Press, In press.
42. Bonita R, Beaglehole R, Kjellstrom T (2006) Basic epidemiology. Geneva World Health Organization.
43. Haagsma JA, van Beeck EF, Polinder S, Toet H, Panneman M, et al. (2011) The effect of comorbidity on health-related quality of life for injury patients in the first year following injury: comparison of three comorbidity adjustment approaches. Popul Health Metr 9: 10.
44. Cavanagh JT, Carson AJ, Sharpe M, Lawrie SM (2003) Psychological autopsy studies of suicide: a systematic review. Psychological Medicine 33: 395–405.
45. Conner KR, Phillips MR, Meldrum S, Knox KL, Zhang Y, et al. (2005) Low-planned suicides in China. Psychol Med 35: 1197–1204.
46. Phillips MR (2010) Rethinking the role of mental illness in suicide. Am J Psychiatry 167: 731–733.
47. Yang GH, Phillips MR, Zhou MG, Wang LJ, Zhang YP, et al. (2005) Understanding the unique characteristics of suicide in China: national psychological autopsy study. Biomed Environ Sci 18: 379–389.
48. Zhang J, Xiao S, Zhou L (2010) Mental disorders and suicide among young rural Chinese: A case-control psychological autopsy study. American Journal of Psychiatry 167: 773–781.
49. Isometsa ET (2001) Psychological autopsy studies – a review. European Psychiatry 16: 379–385.
50. Ahmad OB, Boschi-Pinto C, Lopez AD, Murray CJL, Lozano R, et al. (2001) Age standardization of rates: A new WHO standard. WHO.
51. Silverman MM, Maris RW (1995) The prevention of suicidal behaviors: an overview. Suicide Life Threat Behav 25: 10–21.
52. Scott A, Guo B (2012) For which strategies of suicide prevention is there evidence of effectiveness? Copenhagen: World Health Organization.
53. Mann JJ, Apter A, Bertolote J, Beautrais A, Currier D, et al. (2005) Suicide prevention strategies: a systematic review. JAMA 294: 2064–2074.
54. Briffault X, Morvan Y, Rouillon F, Dardennes R, Lamboy B (2010) [Use of services and treatment adequacy of major depressive episodes in France]. Encephale 36 Suppl 2: D48–58.
55. Gabilondo A, Rojas-Farreras S, Rodriguez A, Fernandez A, Pinto-Meza A, et al. (2011) Use of primary and specialized mental health care for a major depressive episode in Spain by ESEMeD respondents. Psychiatr Serv 62: 152–161.
56. Katz C, Bolton SL, Katz LY, Isaak C, Tilston-Jones T, et al. (2013) A Systematic Review of School-Based Suicide Prevention Programs. Depress Anxiety.
57. Robinson J, Hetrick SE, Martin C (2011) Preventing suicide in young people: systematic review. Aust N Z J Psychiatry 45: 3–26.
58. Khan MM (2005) Suicide prevention and developing countries. J R Soc Med 98: 459–463.
59. Pritchard C, Amanullah S (2007) An analysis of suicide and undetermined deaths in 17 predominantly Islamic countries contrasted with the UK. Psychol Med 37: 421–430.

10

Tobacco Smoking, Alcohol Drinking, Diabetes, Low Body Mass Index and the Risk of Self-Reported Symptoms of Active Tuberculosis: Individual Participant Data (IPD) Meta-Analyses of 72,684 Individuals in 14 High Tuberculosis Burden Countries

Jayadeep Patra[1,2]*, Prabhat Jha[1,2], Jürgen Rehm[2,3], Wilson Suraweera[1]

1 Centre for Global Health Research, St Michael's Hospital, Toronto, Canada, **2** Dalla Lana School of Public Health, University of Toronto, Toronto, Canada, **3** Centre for Addiction and Mental Health, Toronto, Canada

Abstract

Background: The effects of multiple exposures on active tuberculosis (TB) are largely undetermined. We sought to establish a dose-response relationship for smoking, drinking, and body mass index (BMI) and to investigate the independent and joint effects of these and diabetes on the risk of self-reported symptoms of active TB disease.

Methods and Findings: We analyzed 14 national studies in 14 high TB-burden countries using self-reports of blood in cough/phlegm and cough lasting $>=3$ weeks in the last year as the measures of symptoms of active TB. The random effect estimates of the relative risks (RR) between active TB and smoking, drinking, diabetes, and BMI$<$18.5 kg/m^2 were reported for each gender. Floating absolute risks were used to examine dyads of exposure. Adjusted for age and education, the risks of active TB were significantly associated with diabetes and BMI$<$18.5 kg/m^2 in both sexes, with ever drinking in men and with ever smoking in women. Stronger dose-response relationships were seen in women than in men for smoking amount, smoking duration and drinking amount but BMI$<$18.5 kg/m^2 showed a stronger dose-response relationship in men. In men, the risks from joint exposures were statistically significant for diabetics with BMI$<$18.5 kg/m^2 (RR = 6.4), diabetics who smoked (RR = 3.8), and diabetics who drank alcohol (RR = 3.2). The risks from joint risk factors were generally larger in women than in men, with statistically significant risks for diabetics with BMI$<$18.5 kg/m^2 (RR = 10.0), diabetics who smoked (RR = 5.4) and women with BMI$<$18.5 kg/m^2 who smoked (RR = 5.0). These risk factors account for 61% of male and 34% of female estimated TB incidents in these 14 countries.

Conclusions: Tobacco, alcohol, diabetes, and low BMI are significant individual risk factors but in combination are associated with triple or quadruple the risk of development of recent active TB. These risk factors might help to explain the wide variation in TB across countries.

Editor: Madhukar Pai, McGill University, Canada

Funding: This study is supported by grants from the US National Institutes of Health (R01-TW05991-01 and TW07939-01), Canadian Institutes of Health Research (IEG-53506), and the Bill & Melinda Gates Foundation (57350). The funders had no role in study design, data collection and analysis, decision to publish, or preparation of the manuscript.

Competing Interests: The authors have declared that no competing interests exist.

* E-mail: patraj@smh.ca

Introduction

The World Health Organization (WHO) estimated that 8·6 million people developed new tuberculosis (TB) infection and close to 1 million died of it in 2012 [1]. Over 95% of TB deaths occur in low- and middle-income countries (LMIC), and 22 high burden countries account for 82% of annual new cases globally [1].

Various studies and meta-analyses of published studies [2–6] have shown a strong association between tobacco smoking and TB infection, active TB disease or TB mortality. A smaller number of meta-analyses have noted the association between active TB disease and alcohol drinking [7,8], diabetes mellitus [9], and low Body Mass Index (BMI) [10]. These risk factors may help predict the wide variation in TB prevalence and mortality across countries [11]. However, these meta-analyses have not explored the effects of multiple exposures on active TB disease. For example, many adult males in LMICs smoke tobacco and drink alcohol. These interactions can be measured using individual patient data (IPD), but not easily from summary measures from published studies. Nationally representative studies enable reliable projections for an entire country of the proportion of TB attributed to these various risk factors. We conducted IPD meta-analyses of standardized national surveys in 14 high-TB burden countries to establish a dose-response relationship for smoking, drinking, and BMI and to

Table 1. Background characteristics of respondents in World Health Surveys among high TB- burden countries, 2002-4 (18–54 years)*.

Country†	Population in 2010 (10^3)	# people surveyed	Currently married, %		Less than primary, %		Rural residence, %		Smoking, %		Drinking, %		Low BMI (<18.5), %		Diabetes, %		TB£, %	
			M	W	M	W	M	W	M	W	M	W	M	W	M	W	M	W
India	1 224 614	8205	74·0	82·5	30·6	55·6	90·3	89·1	49·6	13·5	19·3	1·5	30·5	35·6	2·7	1·7	2.2	1.2
China	1 341 335	2511	81·9	86·3	6·8	13·8	69·8	68·6	59·5	1·4	44·7	9·2	4·9	10·5	0·9	1·4	0.2	0.3
South Africa	50 133	2031	40·1	33·1	16·0	18·4	39·2	47·4	40·4	14·5	42.0	17·3	25·3	26·9	5·1	8·7	1.3	1.5
Pakistan	173 593	5437	68·4	81·3	43·7	72·8	68·4	63·9	31·9	5·1	0·4	0.0	13·3	16·1	1·4	2·4	1.2	1.3
Bangladesh	148 692	4697	76·0	83·6	50·5	61·5	69·8	77·5	63·2	25·2	14·4	0·4	17·8	17·4	3·2	3·3	1.7	1.3
Philippines	93 261	8509	64·9	71·0	16·3	11·9	39·4	37·8	60.0	10·8	75·6	29·6	10·9	17·6	2·8	3.0	1.3	1.6
Ethiopia	82 950	4160	68·9	68·6	48·8	68·5	85·4	83·3	8·9	0·5	38·6	33·2	11.0	15·7	0·3	0·1	2·5	2·3
DR Congo	65 966	2196	26·8	30·2	17·3	23·9	5·1	6·0	15·6	2·1	41·4	34·2	6·7	8·7	1·5	1·4	0.8	0.6
Viet Nam	87 848	2957	78·0	78·3	13·3	19·6	80·0	76·2	57·3	2.0	64·4	4·4	16.0	27.0	0·3	0·4	0.4	0.1
Myanmar	47 963	4710	58·1	61·7	34·6	44·1	72·1	69·9	49·9	13·1	34·4	2·1	13·7	16·3	0·5	0·3	0.3	0.2
Russia	142 958	2525	54·2	54·1	0·5	0·3	13·9	11·6	59·9	19·1	88·9	77·7	1.0	4.0	1.0	1·1	0.3	0.5
Kenya	40 513	3675	60·9	66·9	28·0	41·8	81·9	82·2	27·8	1·6	39·6	11.0	14·3	10·1	0·8	1.0	1.8	1.0
Brazil	194 946	3901	45·3	43·4	21·5	21·0	17·0	16·3	28·4	20·2	88·4	71·8	2·9	6·9	3·2	5·3	2.0	1.9
Zimbabwe	12 571	3419	58·9	65·1	12·4	25·9	62·5	65·6	24·4	1·7	42·1	6·3	4·8	4·5	0·8	1.0	2.4	2.4
14 HBCs ¶	**3 707 343**	**58 933**	**72·9**	**77·4**	**21·2**	**33·9**	**70·9**	**68·3**	**50·6**	**9.0**	**36·8**	**14·2**	**15·2**	**19·6**	**1·9**	**2·2**	**1.4**	**1.2**

* Samples were nationally representative except in China, India, and the Russian Federation, where the survey was carried out in geographically limited regions;

†Countries are ranked by TB incidence.

£ Presence of symptoms of active TB disease was based on self-reports of blood in cough or phlegm and self-reports of coughs lasting more than 3 weeks in last 12 months.

¶Proportions are gender specific weighted average using respective population; M: men; W: women.

investigate the independent and joint effects of tobacco, alcohol use, diabetes and BMI<18.5 kg/m^2 on the risk of self-reported symptoms of active TB disease.

Methods

Ethics

An ethics statement was not required for this work.

Data

WHO implemented the World Health Surveys (WHS) between 2002 and 2004 in 70 countries [12] including 14 of the 22 high-TB burden countries (India, China, South Africa, Pakistan, Bangladesh, Philippines, Ethiopia, Democratic Republic of Congo, Viet Nam, Myanmar, Russia, Kenya, Brazil, Zimbabwe; ranked by no of TB cases), which collectively cover about 70% of estimated global annual new TB cases. WHS household samples were drawn from nationally representative sampling frames [13] except in China, India, and in Russia, where the surveys were done in specific regions. One adult aged 18+ years was randomly selected from each eligible household. We focused on ages 18–54 years, during which about two-thirds of all global TB cases or TB mortality occur [1].

The main outcome was the presence of self-reported symptoms of active TB disease, as defined by a positive answer to two questions 'Over the last 12 months, have you coughed blood or had blood in your phlegm?' and 'Over the last 12 months, have you coughed that lasted for 3 weeks or longer?'. Four exposures were studied. Current smoking was defined as daily or occasional smoking. Most smoked products were of cigarettes, except in South Asia, where bidis were more common. As cessation is uncommon in most of these countries [14], current smoking approximated ever smoking in most countries. Among current smokers, daily consumption was classified as 1–10, 11–20, 21+ times per day, and the duration as 1–10, 11–20, and 21+ years of daily smoking. Drinking was defined as ever versus never drinkers. Drinkers were asked how many standard drinks (12 grams of pure alcohol was used as one standard drink) were consumed per day in the last week from which we defined the dose of drinking as 1–2, 3+ standard drinks per day. Diabetes was defined as those individuals who reported yes to either of two questions: 'Have you ever been diagnosed with diabetes (high blood sugar)?' and 'Have you ever had any treatment or medications or attended a program for diabetes?' BMI was calculated from self-reported body weight and height. Low BMI was defined as <18.5 kg/m^2 with dose-response analysis examining BMI scores of <16·0 kg/m^2, 16·0–16·99 kg/m^2, 17–18·49 kg/m^2.The WHS did not include mycobacterial culture or sputum smear microscopy confirmation or any biological testing to confirm diabetes or smoking status.

Statistical analysis

We used logistic regression to relate the odds ratios, as an approximation of the relative risk (RR) and the corresponding 99% confidence intervals (CI) for self-reported symptoms of active TB disease. Analyses were stratified by gender and adjusted for age (in linear years), completed years of education (none, 1–5, 6–10, or 11+ years), and where relevant, ever/never smoking or alcohol use, presence of diabetes and BMI<18.5 kg/m^2. We used floating absolute risks to compare more than two categories of the various dyads of exposures. Floating absolute risks do not change the RRs, but the confidence intervals are assigned an appropriate standard error (the coefficient of variation of the RR) to the logRR estimates including reference category with RR = 1 to capture each level's random variation [15].

For dose-response estimates, where available, we used the midpoint of the following categories: duration of smoking, number of cigarettes or bidis or pipes, number of standard drinks and BMI score (cut off scores of 15 to 60 kg/m^2). Sensitivity analyses compared pooled summary estimates for subgroups stratified on quality-associated study characteristics Including Directly Observed Therapy – Short course (DOTS) coverage over 75% and step by step adjustments for age, education, and where applicable smoking, alcohol use, diabetes and BMI<18.5 kg/m^2.

To estimate gender specific alcohol-, tobacco-, diabetes- and BMI<18·5 kg/m^2-attributable new TB incident cases in 14 HBCs, the Population Attributable Fractions (PAF) were applied to WHO's estimation of new TB cases in each country for 2012 [1]. PAF was calculated as $P(RR-1)/(1+P(RR-1))$. R refers to pooled RR based on 14 countries derived from the current meta-analysis and P refers to the prevalence in each country, drawn from independent surveys of tobacco [16,17], alcohol use [16,18], diabetes [19], and BMI <18·5 kg/m^2 [16,20]. Where independent surveys were not available, we used age and gender specific WHS survey prevalence [21] among those not reporting a history of active TB symptoms.

The DerSimonian and Laird random-effects method was used to combine the natural logarithm of the adjusted odds ratios across countries. Where a survey provided dose-response analysis data (e.g., smoking, drinking and BMI), the risk estimates for each category were pooled using the inverse variance weighted method to derive a single estimate for each range of dose. We conducted a meta-regression using linear as well as first-order and second-order fractional polynomials to estimate the best fitting curve. Statistical heterogeneity between studies was assessed using I^2 statistic. All analyses were done using STATA12·1.

Results

A total of 72,684 respondents aged 18+ years were included from 14 countries (Table 1) of which 58,933 respondents were age 18–54 years (Men: 27,102; Women: 31,831). More women (34%) than men (21%) had less than primary education. Among men, 50% smoked tobacco, 37% drank alcohol, 15% had BMI < 18·5 kg/m^2 and 2% reported diabetes; among women, 9% smoked tobacco, 14% drank alcohol, 20% had <18·5 kg/m^2 and 2% reported diabetes. About 1·4% of men and 1·2% of women self-reported symptoms of active TB disease in the last year. Inexplicably, women surveyed in India and Bangladesh reported much higher prevalences of smoking than reported in recent nationally-representative surveys [17]. The gender-specific prevalences of drinking alcohol, diabetes and BMI <18·5 kg/m^2 were generally consistent with those reported from global reviews of the country-specific data [16,18,19,22,23].

Risks and Quality assessment

Ever smoking, ever drinking, diabetes history, or BMI< 18·5 kg/m^2 were each independently associated with the risks of self-reported symptoms of active TB (Table 2). Adjusted for age and education, the risks of self-reported symptoms of active TB were significantly associated in men for diabetes (RR = 2.9), followed by BMI<18·5 kg/m^2 (RR = 2·3), ever drinking (RR = 1·3), and non-significantly associated with ever smoking (RR = 1·2). Among women, the corresponding risks were significantly associated for diabetes (RR = 2·7), then BMI<18·5 kg/m^2 (RR = 2·3), ever smoking (RR = 2·0) and ever drinking (RR = 1·5). These risks showed little downward attenuation after additional adjustment for the other risk factors. A history of diabetes in men, which showed increased risk with adjustment. The risks for the

Table 2. Quality assessment and stratification: tobacco smoking, alcohol use, diabetes, low Body Mass Index (BMI) and risk of self-reported symptoms of active Tuberculosis (TB) disease in HBCs, 18–54 years.

Risk factors	Adjustments	Men					Women				
		Exposed TB+/ Total	Non-exposed TB+/Total	Pooled Est.	99% CI	I^2 (surveys)	Exposed TB+/ Total	Non-exposed TB+/Total	PooledEst.	99% CI	I^2 (surveys)
Ever smoking	A	178/11,690	209/15,058	1.09	0.71–1.89	0.0% (14)	59/2434	336/29,079	2.14	1.71–3.48	0.3% (9)
	A+E			1.16	0.64–2.13	0.0% (14)			2.02	1.52–3.11	0.0% (9)
	A+E+Alc			1.07	0.74–1.87	0.0% (14)			1.93	1.35–2.70	0.0% (9)
	A+E+Alc+DM+LBMI			1.14	0.72–1.91	0.0% (14)			2.11	1.43–3.40	0.0% (8)
Ever drinking	A	174/11,302	211/15,146	1.28	1.03–1.81	0.0% (13)	97/6094	296/25,169	1.31	0.91–1.96	25.1% (10)
	A+E			1.26	1.01–1.73	0.0% (13)			1.50	1.10–2.24	17.1% (10)
	A+E+Alc			1.19	0.95–1.62	0.0% (13)			1.31	0.88–1.89	10.3% (10)
	A+E+T+DM+LBMI			1.11	0.81–1.67	0.0% (12)			1.28	0.78–1.67	2.2% (10)
Diabetes	A	18/513	370/26,483	2.59	1.51–5.80	0.0% (8)	19/679	376/31,055	2.41	1.46–4.12	0.0% (8)
	A+E			2.87	1.44–5.69	0.0% (8)			2.68	1.35–5.32	0.0% (8)
	A+E+Alc+T			3.11	1.51–6.37	18.2% (8)			2.31	1.31–4.32	0.0% (8)
	A+E+Alc+T+LBMI			3.78	1.82–7.56	17.1% (8)			2.54	1.56–5.39	0.0% (7)
Low BMI	A	85/3106	213/18,637	2.30	1.64–3.23	0.0% (13)	76/4138	197/19,567	2.44	1.61–3.31	0.0% (12)
	A+E			2.27	1.61–3.20	0.0% 13)			2.32	1.55–2.91	0.0% (12)
	A+E+Alc+T			2.29	1.63–3.23	0.0% 13)			2.18	1.60–3.26	0.0% (12)
	A+E+Alc+T+DM			2.35	1.67–3.34	0.0% 13)			2.28	1.56–3.45	0.0% (12)

TB[+] referred to active TB disease; A: Age; E: Education, Alc: ever alcohol use, T: current tobacco smoking; DM: Self-reported diabetes; LBMI: Low BMI.

Table 3. Dose-response relationship between current smoking, current alcohol drinking, Body Mass Index (BMI) and risk of self-reported symptoms of active TB disease in HBCs, 18-54 years.

Category*	Exposure level	Men					Women				
		TB^+/Total	TB Prev.	Pooled Est.¶	99% CI	I^2	TB^+/Total	TB Prev.	Pooled Est.¶	99% CI	I^2
Duration of current daily smoking†	Never smoker	209/15,058	1.4%	1·00	0·81–1·23	*0·0%*	316/28,298	1.1%	1.00	0·83–1·20	*0·0%*
	1–10 years	71/4817	1.5%	*1.06*	*0.74–1.52*	*0·0%*	37/1315	2.8%	*2.78*	*1.65–4.70*	*0·0%*
	11–20 years	45/2804	1.6%	*1.16*	*0.76–1.78*	*3.1%*	9/648	1.4%	*1.38*	*0.53–3.57*	*0·0%*
	>=21 years	34/1574	2.2%	*1.57*	*1.00–2.54*	*0·0%*	13/471	2.8%	*2.04*	*0.82–5.08*	*0·0%*
Test for trend of odds:			**χ2 = 7.1, p<0·008**					**χ2 = 10.5, p<0·002**			
Daily no. of cigarettes/pipes†	Never smoker	209/15,058	1.4%	1.00	0·87–1·21	*0·0%*	316/28,298	1.1%	1.00	0·81–1·23	*0·0%*
	1–10	84/5673	1.4%	*1.09*	*0.62–1.93*	*0·0%*	45/1971	2.3%	*1.71*	*1.12–2.61*	*17·0%*
	11–20	38/2685	1.4%	*1.09*	*0.57–2.09*	*32.4%*	11/383	2·9%	*2.52*	*1.13–5.63*	*71.5%*
	>=21	28/837	3.3%	*2.19*	*1.08–4.44*	*0·0%*	3/80	3.8%	*2.96*	*0.64–13.62*	*0·0%*
Test for trend of odds:			**χ2 = 10.1, p<0·002**					**χ2 = 13.5, p<0·0001**			
Daily no. of standard drinks‡	Abstainer	211/15,126	1.4%	1.00	0·82–1·23	*0·0%*	296/25,155	1.2%	1.00	0·86–1·16	*0·0%*
	1–2 std. drinks/day	150/9896	1.5%	*1.25*	*0.94–1.66*	*34.1%*	91/5906	1.5%	*1.58*	*1.08–2.31*	*0·0%*
	3+ std. drinks/day	24/1459	1.6%	*1.31*	*0.74–2.30*	*0·0%*	7/213	3.3%	*3.16*	*0.84–11.89*	*23·0%*
Test for trend of odds:			**χ2 = 3·9, p<0·01**					**χ2 = 9.3, p<0·003**			
BMI (kg/m²)	18.5 and over	204/18,469	1.1%	1.00	0·79–1·19	*0·0%*	192/19,357	1.0%	1.00	0·79–1·17	*0·0%*
	17.0–18.49	37/1855	2.0%	1.65	1.01–2.67	*0·0%*	35/2371	1.5%	1.51	0.93–2.45	*0·0%*
	16.0–16.99	22/566	3.9%	3.40	1.95–5.94	*0·0%*	14/774	1.8%	1.78	0.86–3.68	*0·0%*
	<16.0	26/674	3.9%	3.47	1.91–6.30	*0·0%*	26/961	2.7%	2.66	1.53–4.63	*0·0%*
Test for trend of odds:			**χ2 = 70.8, p<0·001**					**χ2 = 29·6, p<0·001**			

* adjusted for age and level of education; self-reported alcohol use†, current smoking‡, diabetes, and BMI<18.5 kg/m² were additionally adjusted in the respective model;
¶99% CIs shown in the reference categories indicate floating absolute risks (FARs).

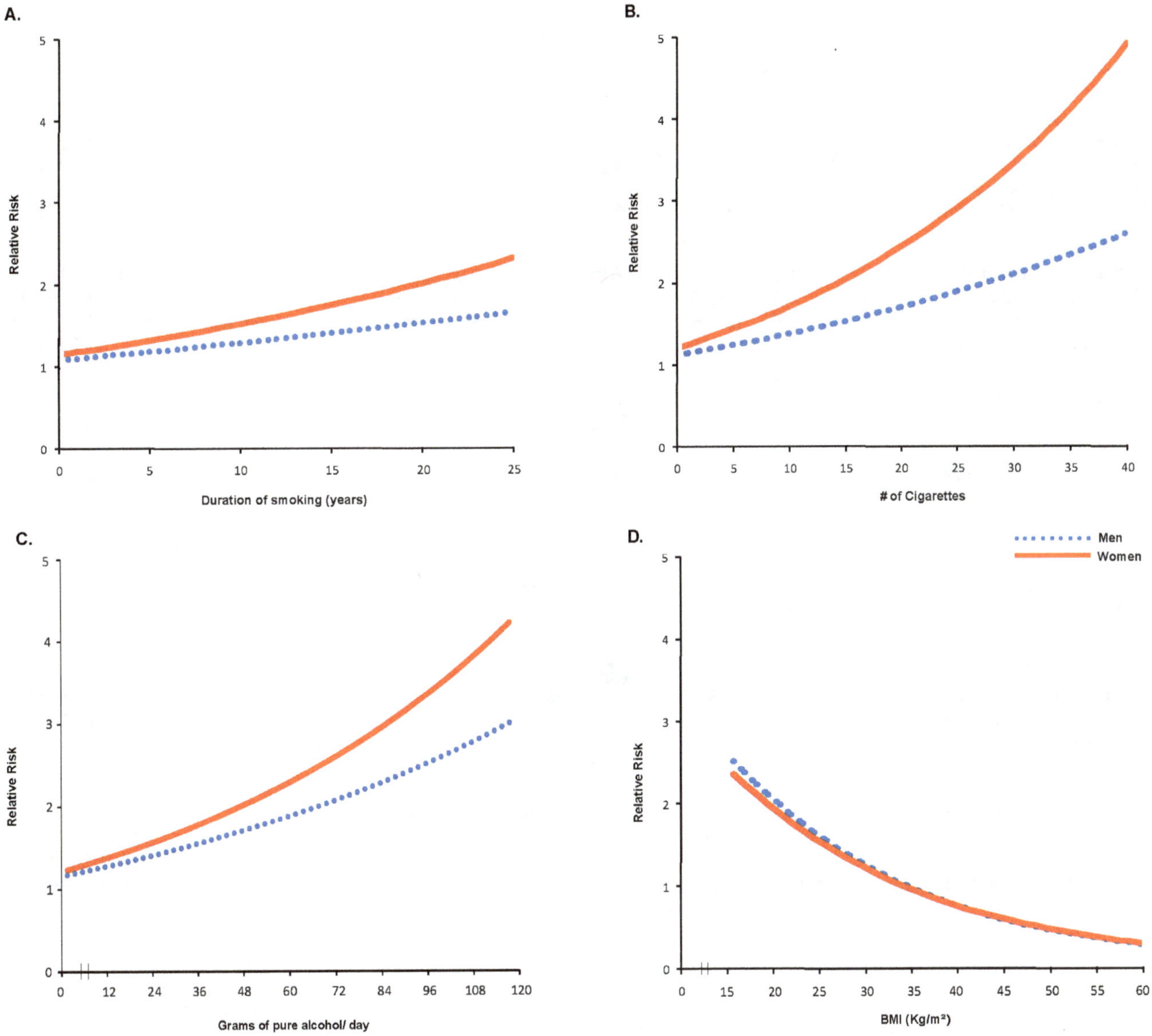

Figure 1. Dose-response relationships of (A) duration of smoking, (B) quantity of smoking, (C) quantity of alcohol consumption, and (D) BMI with self-reported symptoms of active TB disease by gender.

four exposures were comparable in settings where DOTS coverage surpassed 75% and was below 75%. Risks were slightly greater for those reporting a history of diabetes than those reporting treatment for diabetes in men, but were similar in women. The heterogeneity of the risks across countries (as defined by the I^2 statistic) was below 20%, with the exception of ever drinking among women.

Dose-response relationships

After adjustment for confounders, smoking amount, smoking duration and drinking amount showed a stronger dose response relationship in women than in men; however BMI<18·5 kg/m^2 showed a stronger dose-response relationship in men (Table 3). Substantial risks of self-reported symptoms of active TB were seen in men and especially in women for 21 or more years of smoking (Men RR = 1·6; Women RR = 2·0), 21 or more cigarettes per day (Men RR = 2·2, Women RR = 3·0), for 3 or more standard drinks (Men RR = 1·3, Women RR = 3.2) and for BMI<16·0 kg/m^2 (Men RR = 3.5, Women RR = 2.7). Use of linear units to measure smoking and alcohol quantity showed similar findings to the categorical results with a weaker association for the duration of smoking. Smoking amount, smoking duration, and drinking amount showed a steeper dose-response relationships in women than in men (Figure 1). By contrast, BMI<17·0 kg/m^2 showed similar yet stronger (RR>2·1) relationships in both men and women. The heterogeneity of the risks across countries was below 20%, with the exception of number of cigarettes per day and number of standard drinks in both men and women.

Interactions of smoking, drinking, diabetes and low BMI

Drinking and smoking were closely correlated in men; about 38% of the control men (6,288/16,352) without any history of self-reported symptoms of active TB reported both drinking alcohol and smoking tobacco. Among women, reported drinking and

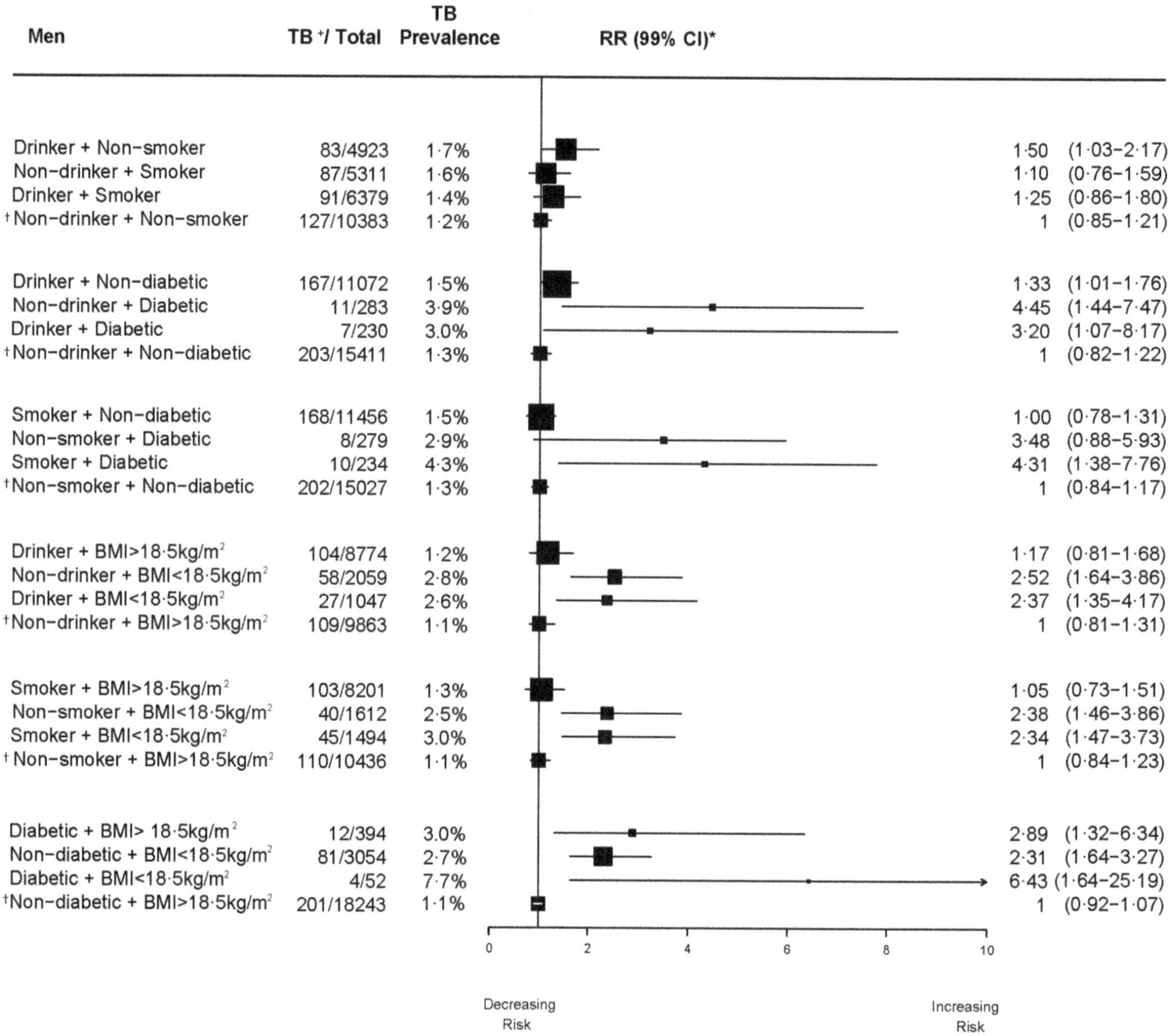

Figure 2. Independent and joint effects of risk factors on self-reported symptoms of active TB disease, 18–54 years in men.

smoking was less common (14%; 1,112/8,021; Figure 2). By contrast the other dyads of diabetes, drinking, smoking, and BMI<18·5 kg/m^2 were less common in men and women. The floating absolute risks of the six dyads of exposure, comparing independent and interactive relative risks (smoking, drinking, diabetes, and BMI<18·5 kg/m^2), were adjusted for age and education (see Figures 2 & 3). In men, the risks of self-reported symptoms of active TB for individual risk factors were statistically significant for those reporting a history of diabetes who did not drink alcohol (RR = 4.5), diabetics who did not smoke tobacco (RR = 3.5), diabetics with BMI> = 18·5 kg/m^2 (RR = 2.9; but with large heterogeneity across the countries), and those with BMI<18·5 kg/m^2 who did not drink alcohol (RR = 2.5) (Figure 2). In men, the risks from joint exposures were statistically significant diabetics with BMI<18·5 kg/m^2 (RR = 6.4), for diabetics who smoked (RR = 4.3, with large heterogeneity across countries), and diabetics who drank alcohol (RR = 3·2). Much lower individual and joint risks were seen for smoking or drinking in men. The numbers of cases in men and women were small for the dyads related to diabetes and BMI<18·5 kg/m^2, and the confidence intervals were wide. Similarly, the small number of cases precluded the ability to detect statistically significant interactions of joint exposures.

In women, the risks of self-reported symptoms of active TB for individual risk factors were generally lower than for men, with the exception of smoking among women who did not drink alcohol (Figure 3). In women, the most notable individual risks for self-reported symptoms of active TB were for diabetics who did not drink alcohol (RR = 2.7), diabetics with BMI> = 18·5 kg/m^2 (RR = 2·2), smokers with BMI>18·5 kg/m^2 (RR = 2·2), diabetics who did not smoke (RR = 2·0), or women with BMI<18·5 kg/m^2 who did not drink alcohol (RR = 2.0). The risks from joint risk factors were generally larger in women than in men, with the greatest risks for diabetics with BMI<18·5 kg/m^2 (RR = 10.0), diabetics who smoked (RR = 5.4) and those with BMI<18·5 kg/m^2 who smoked (RR = 5.0). There was little heterogeneity in these individual and joint risks across countries for women.

Women	TB⁺/ Total	TB Prevelence	RR (99% CI)*
Drinker + Non-smoker	67/4952	1·4%	1.45 (1·00–2·08)
Non-drinker + Smoker	49/2073	2·4%	1.82 (1·20–2·77)
Drinker + Smoker	30/1142	2·6%	2.85 (1·71–4·76)
†Non-drinker + Non-smoker	249/23567	1·1%	1 (0·87–1·19)
Drinker + Non-diabetic	90/5918	1·5%	1.55 (1·13–2·14)
Non-drinker + Diabetic	12/503	2·4%	2.71 (1·00–4·46)
Drinker + Diabetic	7/176	4.0%	4.24 (1·54–11·69)
†Non-drinker + Non-diabetic	286/25137	1·1%	1 (0·79–1·51)
Smoker + Non-diabetic	72/3101	2·3%	1·92 (1·36–2·72)
Non-smoker + Diabetic	12/565	2·1%	1·98 (1·00–4·28)
Smoker + Diabetic	7/114	6·1%	5·40 (1·94–15·02)
†Non-smoker + Non-diabetic	304/27954	1·1%	1 (0·85–1·11)
Drinker + BMI>18·5kg/m²	58/4335	1·3%	1·68 (1·11–2·54)
Non-drinker + BMI<18·5kg/m²	65/3671	1·8%	1·96 (1·30–2·85)
Drinker + BMI<18·5kg/m²	11/467	2·4%	2·94 (1·30–6·67)
†Non-drinker + BMI>18·5kg/m²	139/15232	0·9%	1 (0·81–1·15)
Smoker + BMI>18·5kg/m²	38/1797	2·1%	2·20 (1·37–3·54)
Non-smoker + BMI<18·5kg/m²	56/3679	1·5%	1·71 (1·13–2·54)
Smoker + BMI<18·5kg/m²	20/459	4·4%	4·95 (2·31–8·19)
†Non-smoker + BMI>18·5kg/m²	159/17770	0·9%	1 (0·80–1·21)
Diabetic + BMI> 18·5kg/m²	10/447	2·2%	2·23 (1·00–5·34)
Non-diabetic + BMI<18·5kg/m²	70/4075	1·7%	1·73 (1·20–2·50)
Diabetic + BMI<18·5kg/m²	6/63	9·5%	10·00 (3·24–20·87)
†Non-diabetic + BMI>18·5kg/m²	187/19120	1.0%	1 (0·81–1·22)

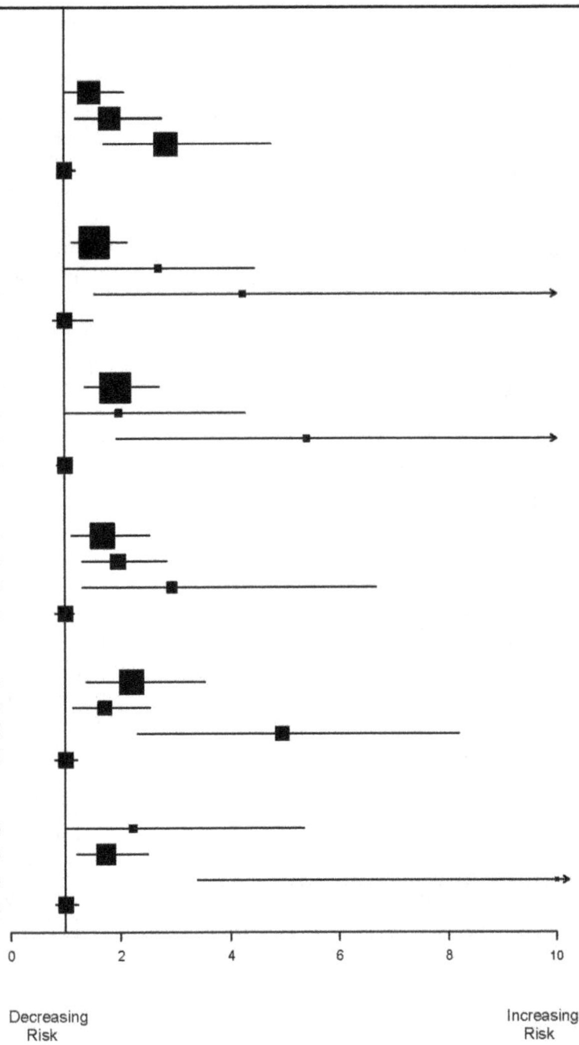

Figure 3. Independent and joint effects of risk factors on self-reported symptoms of active TB disease, 18–54 years in women.

Risk factor contribution to TB incidence in 14 high-burden TB countries

These relative risks, adjusted for age and education might be causally important for prevalent active TB (although the reverse causality of TB causing low BMI cannot be excluded). If these measured risks are causally important, then it is possible to estimate indirectly their contribution to WHO's estimate of incidence cases occurring in these 14 high-burden TB countries. Incident TB cases are estimated to be 3·9 and 2 million in men and women, respectively in these countries in 2012 (Table 4). Among men, BMI<18·5 kg/m^2 accounted for 17% of incident TB cases (653,000/year), followed by daily smoking (16%; 629,000/year), drinking of 40+ grams/day of alcohol (15%; 569,000/year), and diabetes (13%; 508,000/year), and. Among women, BMI<18·5 kg/m^2 accounted for 15% of incident TB cases (304,000/year), followed by diabetes (11%; 221,000/year), daily smoking (5%; 102,000/year) and drinking of 20+ grams/day (2%; 65,000/year). In these 14 high TB burden countries, all 4 risk factors combined contributed more than one-third of global TB burden (See Table S1 for country-wise estimates).

Discussion

Our pooled analyses of individual participant data from standardized surveys in 14 LMIC find that smoking, heavy alcohol use, diabetes, and BMI<18·5 kg/m^2 are individual risk factors but combined together can triple or quadruple the risk of development of recent active TB disease. A clear dose-response relationship of increased TB risks was noted with increasing amounts of tobacco and alcohol consumption, increasing smoking duration and with decreasing BMI. Unlike previous meta-analyses, we were able to explore the joint and independent effects of various exposures. Notwithstanding the wide confidence intervals, the greatest elevated risks of self-reported symptoms of active TB for both genders, particularly for women were seen consistently with diabetes or BMI<18·5 kg/m^2. Even within sub-groups of those who smoked or drank alcohol diabetes and BMI<18·5 kg/

Table 4. Smoking, drinking, diabetes, BMI<18.5 kg/m^2 attributable new TB incident cases among men and women (18+ years) in 14 High-Burden Countries (HBCs), 2012.

Sex	New cases in HBC	Smoking*, %		Drinking†, %		Diabetes ‡, %		BMI<18.5 kg/m^2¶, %	
Men	3,893,910	629,304	16	569,304	15	508,066	13	652,534	17
Women	2,045,090	102,076	5	65,111	3	221,011	11	303,614	15
M+W	**5,939,000**	**731,380**	**12**	**634,415**	**11**	**729,077**	**12**	**956,148**	**16**

*Sources of prevalence for daily smoking were taken from Global Adult Tobacco Survey (GATS) [17], Demographic and Health Survey (DHS) [16], World Health Survey (WHS) [21]; RR men = 1·71 (99% CI:1·20–2·70) and RR women = 2·44 (99% CI:1·54–4·17) were taken from our continuous dose-response meta-regression model.
†Prevalences for daily alcohol drinking (men: 40+ grams/day; women: 20+ grams/day) were taken from WHS [21] and where data on large nationally representative surveys were available [16,18]; RR men = 1·84 (99% CI:1·32–2·83) and RR women = 1·61 (99% CI:1·11–2·49) were taken from our continuous dose-response meta-regression model.
‡Prevalence on diabetes were taken from International Diabetes Federation (2011) [19]; RR men = 2.87 (99%CI:1·44–5.69) and RR women = 2·68 (99% CI: 1·35–5.32) were taken from our D-L meta analysis.
¶Prevalence on low BMI (<18·5 kg/m^2) were taken from DHS [16]; RR men = 2·12 (99% CI: 1·41–3.31) and RR women = 2·00 (99% CI: 1·43–3·24) were taken our continuous dose-response meta-regression model.

m^2 significantly raised risks of self-reported symptoms of active TB.

Causal mechanisms

WHO estimates that about one-third of the people in the world are infected with *Mycobacterium tuberculosis* [24] with 90% being asymptomatic latent TB infections [25]. Smoking, drinking, diabetes and low BMI might each plausibly enable progression from latent to active TB disease. Possible mechanisms for smoking include the impaired clearance of secretions on the tracheobronchial mucosal surface [26], reduced phagocytic function of pulmonary alveolar macrophages [27], decreased production of tumor necrosis factor in pulmonary macrophages [28], and increased iron overload in pulmonary macrophages [29]. Chronic alcohol use has been shown to reduce macrophage response to immune system modifiers raising the risk of acquiring disease [30,31]. Experimental studies find that hyperglycemia may affect the host immune response to TB [32,33]. BMI<18·5 kg/m^2 is a possible marker for under-nutrition [34,35], which can reduce host protective immune response either by interfering in the interaction between monocyte-macrophages and T-lymphocytes and their cytokines [36], or by secondary immunodeficiency that increases the host susceptibility to infection [37].

These risk factors account for 61% of male and 34% of female estimated incident TB cases in these 14 countries. The consistency of the relative risks suggests that worldwide, these risk factors might play an important role in explaining the wide country-specific variation in TB. Notably, the inter-relation of low BMI and tobacco use might well help to explain the high levels of TB infection and mortality in India [38]. A joint effect of tobacco use and BMI has already been reported for all-cause mortality [39] in India. The cross-sectional nature of the analysis cannot exclude if TB infection leads to low BMI, even though earlier longitudinal studies have shown that low BMI increased subsequent risk of developing active TB [35,40]. Micronutrient intake has also been shown to decrease the risk of reversion of sputum culture to positivity after initial conversion in the first month in both HIV-infected and non-infected patients [41]. A randomized trial found that nutritional counseling with provision of supplements in TB patients produced a short term increase in body weight, lean mass, and physical function [42].

About 1·4% of men and 1·3% of women without self-reported symptoms of active TB reported having both diabetes and BMI< 18·5 kg/m^2, consistent with some reports in LMICs [43,44]. By contrast, in most high income countries diabetes is associated with high BMI (and prolonged adiposity can be a cause of diabetes [45]). Adiposity and diabetes prevalences are rising overall in many LMICs [46,47], and their possible interaction with smoking or heavy alcohol drinking on active TB disease is of concern.

Limitations and Strengths

The study results are broadly representative of many countries where TB infection remains common and are based on standardized methods. Results showed consistency across countries with little attenuation with adjustment for possible confounding variables, and clear dose-response relationships. There are, however, a few potential limitations to this study. First, confounding by variables might be associated with each of the exposures. Stratification by quality of study indicators, and adjustment for education found only slight reductions in the risks, except diabetes in men, which increased with adjustment. Second, microbiological confirmation of TB was not possible as the WHS did not include mycobacterial culture or sputum smear microscopy. An affirmative response to questions on bloody cough or phlegm might indicate those with pneumonia or lung cancer, although lung cancer would tend to occur at older ages than our specified range of 18–54 years. The ongoing Million Death Study [48] in India found that the vast proportion of those reporting a history of blood in phlegm had a final diagnosis of tuberculosis, with far less due to pneumonia and even fewer due to lung cancer. Although not every participant with these TB symptoms will have microbiologically confirmed TB case, yet studies show self-reported TB has a sensitivity between 65 to 70% and specificity between 55 to 75% in comparison to sputum testing [49,50]. Third, the assessment of risk factors were also based on self-reports only. For example, diabetes was not measured on test of fasting-plasma glucose. However, earlier studies suggest sensitivity and specificity of these with self-reported diabetes are between 65 to 85% and 95 to 99%, respectively, compared with biochemical markers, with overall Kappa coefficients above 0·80 [51,52]. The assessment of tobacco smoking, drinking alcohol or height/weight measurements relied on self-reported behavior, which may not have been accurate due to recall or reporting bias, especially among those who consider smoking or drinking to be socially prohibitive or stigmatizing, such as women in some cultural settings. However, this would tend to make our estimates more conservative. The prevalence of smoking among those self-reporting bloody cough/phlegm and chronic cough was lower than that reported in other studies of tuberculosis disease [4–6]. This might reflect under-reporting of smoking by those with recent symptoms of active active TB. Indeed higher prevalences of smoking are reported among TB deaths by living household respondents [53] from whom under-reporting of smoking is less likely than from self-reports.

Implications

TB patients generally lack access to smoking cessation services, and smoking is associated with worse outcomes for TB treatment [54,55]. Most smoking-related immunologic abnormalities appear to be reversible within weeks of cessation. Thus, cessation might yield substantial positive effects on TB treatment outcomes, relapse and future lung disease [56,57]. Our findings suggest that TB control programs might consider targeting patients with diabetes for interventions such as active case finding and the treatment of latent TB and, conversely, those efforts to diagnose, detect, and treat diabetes may have a beneficial impact on TB control [58]. The TB control programs in China and India recently introduced bidirectional screening of TB and diabetes [59,60].

These findings suggest the need to adopt stricter health policies, most notably higher taxation to reduce smoking and heavy drinking in various populations where TB infection, disease and mortality remain common [61,62]. Prospective studies are required to document if these risk factors account for the wide variation in TB disease across various countries.

Acknowledgments

Disclaimer: The opinions expressed in this Article are those of the authors and do not necessarily represent those of the institutions with which they are affiliated. This study is supported by grants from the US National Institutes of Health (R01-TW05991-01 and TW07939-01), Canadian Institutes of Health Research (IEG-53506), and the Bill & Melinda Gates Foundation (57350). We thank Cindy Gauvreau for her helpful comments.

Author Contributions

Conceived and designed the experiments: JP PJ. Performed the experiments: JP PJ WS. Analyzed the data: JP WS. Contributed reagents/materials/analysis tools: JP PJ. Wrote the paper: JP PJ JR.

References

1. WHO (2013) Global tuberculosis control: WHO report 2013. Geneva, WHO Press.
2. Bothamley GH (2005) Smoking and tuberculosis: a chance or causal association? Thorax 60:527–28.
3. Pai M, Mohan A, Dheda K, Leung CC, Yew WW, et al. (2007) Lethal interaction: the colliding epidemics of tobacco and tuberculosis. Expert Rev Anti Infect Ther 5:385–91.
4. Bates MN, Khalakdina A, Pai M, Chang L, Lessa F, et al. (2007) Risk of Tuberculosis From Exposure to Tobacco Smoke. Arch Intern Med 167:335–42.
5. Lin H, Ezzati M, Murray C (2007) Tobacco Smoke, Indoor Air Pollution and Tuberculosis: A Systematic Review and Meta-Analysis. PLoS Med 4:173–89.
6. Slama K, Chiang C-Y, Enarson DA, Hassmiller K, Fanning A, et al. (2007) Tobacco and tuberculosis: a qualitative systematic review and meta-analysis. Int J Tuberc Lung Dis 11:1049–61.
7. Rehm J, Samokhvalov AY, Neuman MG, Room R, Parry C, et al. (2009) The association between alcohol use, alcohol use disorders, and tuberculosis (TB). A systematic review. BMC Public Health 9:450.
8. Lönnroth K, Williams BG, Staldlin S, Jaramillo E, Dye C (2008) Alcohol use as a risk factor for tuberculosis – a systematic review. BMC Public Health 8:289.
9. Jeon CY, Murray MB (2008) Diabetes Mellitus Increases the Risk of Active Tuberculosis: A Systematic Review of 13 Observational Studies. PLoS Med 5:e152.
10. Lönnroth K, Williams BG, Cegielski P, Dye C (2010) A consistent log-linear relationship between tuberculosis incidence and body mass index. Int J Epidemiol 9:149–55.
11. Lönnroth K, Gastro KG, Chakaya JM, Chauhan LS, Floyd K, et al. (2010) Tuberculosis control and elimination 2010-50: cure, care, and socail development. Lancet 375:1814–29.
12. Ustun TB, Chatterji S, Mechbal A, Murray C (2003) Health systems performance assessment debates, methods and empiricisms. In: Murray C, Evans DB, eds. The World Health Surveys. Geneva: World Health Organization; 797–808.
13. Andreotti A, Minicuci N, Kowal P, Chatterji S (2009) Multidimensional Profiles of Health Status: An Application of the Grade of Membership Model to the World Health Survey. Plos One 4.
14. World Health Organization (2007) A WHO/The Union monograph on TB and tobacco control: joining efforts to control two related global epidemics. Geneva: WHO.
15. Plummer M (2004) Improved estimates of floating absolute risk. Stat Med 23:93–104.
16. ICF International (2012) Demographic and Health Surveys 2004-1012. Calverton, Maryland: ICF International.
17. Giovino G, Mirza S, Samet J, Gupta PC, Jarvis MJ, et al. (2012) Tobacco use in 3 billion individuals from 16 countries: an analysis of nationally representative cross-sectional household surveys. Lancet 380:668–79.
18. Millwood I, Li L, Smith M, Guo Y, Yang L, et al. (2013) Alcohol consumption in 0.5 million people from 10 diverse regions of China: prevalence, patterns and socio-demographic and health-related correlates. Int J Epidemiol 42:816–27.
19. International Diabetes Federation (2009) International Diabetes Federation Diabetes Atlas, 2010 estimates: 2009. Brussels, IDF.
20. Razak F, Corsi D, Subramaniam S (2013) Change in the Body Mass Index Distribution for Women: Analysis of Surveys from 37 Low- and Middle-Income Countries. PLoS Med 10.
21. World Health Organization. World Health Survey, 2003-2005. Geneva, WHO.
22. International Institute for Population Sciences (2007) National Family Health Survey (NFHS-3), 2005-06. Mumbai, India: International Institute for Population Sciences, Mumbai, IIPS.
23. Lim S, Vos T, Flaxman A, Danaei G, Shibuya K, et al. (2012) A comparative risk assessment of burden of disease and injury attributable to 67 risk factors and risk factor clusters in 21 regions, 1990—2010: a systematic analysis for the Global Burden of Disease Study 2010. Lancet 380:2224–60.
24. Raviglione MC, Snider DE, Kochi A (1995) Global epidemiology of tuberculosis. Morbidity and mortality of a worldwide epidemic. JAMA 273:220–226.

25. Comstock GW (1982) Epidemiology of tuberculosis. Am Rev Respir Dis 125:8–15.
26. Houtmeyers E, Gosselink R, Gayan-Ramirez G, Decramer M (1999) Regulation of mucociliary clearance in health and disease. Eur Respir J 13:1177–88.
27. Sopori M (2002) Effects of cigarette smoke on the immune system. Nat Rev Immunol 2:372–77.
28. Wang H, Yu M, Ochani M, Amella CA, Tanovic M, et al. (2003) Nicotinic acetylcholine receptor alpha7 subunit is an essential regulator of inflammation. Nature 421:384–88.
29. Boelaert JR, Gomes MS, Gordeuk VR (2003) Smoking, iron, and tuberculosis. Lancet 362:1243–44.
30. Mason CM, Dobard E, Zhang P, Nelson S (2004) Alcohol exacerbates murine pulmonary tuberculosis. Infect Immun 72:2556–63.
31. Szabo G (2012) Alcohol and susceptibility to tuberculosis. Alcohol Health Res World 21:30–41.
32. Rayfield EJ, Ault MJ, Keusch GT, Brothers MJ, Nechemias C, et al. (1982) Infection and diabetes: The case for glucose control. Am J Med 72:439–50.
33. Stalenhoef JE, Alisjahbana B, Nelwan EJ, van der Ven-Jongejrijg J, Ottenhoff T, et al. (2008) The role of interferon-gamma in the increased tuberculosis risk in type 2 diabetes mellitus. Eur J Clin Microbiol Infect Dis 27:97–103.
34. British Association for Parenteral and Enteral Nutrition Malnutrition Advisory Group (2000) Guidelines for Detection and Management of Malnutrition: 2000. Reddich, Worcs. BAPEN.
35. Cegielski JP, Arab L, Cornoni-Huntley J (2012) Nutritional Risk Factors for Tuberculosis Among Adults in the United States, 1971–1992. Am J Epidemiol 176:409–22.
36. Rook GA, Hernamndez-Pando R (1996) The pathogenesis of tuberculosis. Annu Rev Microbiol 50:258–84.
37. Chan J, Tanaka KE, Mannion C, Carroll D, Tsang MS, et al (1997) Effects of protein calorie malnutrition on mice infected with BCG. I Nutr Immunol 5:11–19.
38. Pednekar MS, Hakama M, Gupta PC (2012) Tobacco Use or Body Mass – Do They Predict Tuberculosis Mortality in Mumbai, India? Results from a Population-Based Cohort Study. Plos One 7:e39443.
39. Pednekar MS, Gupta PC, Hebert JR, Hakama M (2008) Joint effect of tobacco use and body mass on all-cause mortality in Mumbai, India: Results from a population-based cohort study. Am J Epidemiol 167:330–40.
40. Tverdal A (1986) Body mass index and incidence of tuberculosis. Eur J Respir Dis 69:355–62.
41. Villamore E, Mugusi F, Urassa W, Bosch RJ, Saathoff E, et al. (2008) A trial of the effect of micronutrient supplementation on treatment outcome, T cell counts, morbidity, and mortality in adults with pulmonary tuberculosis. J Infect Dis 197:1499–1505.
42. Paton NI, Chua YK, Earnest A, Chee CB (2004) Randomized controlled trial of nutritional supplementation in patients with newly diagnosed tuberculosis and wasting. Am J Clin Nutr 80:460–65.
43. Thompson KH, Godin DV (1995) Micronutrients and antoixidants in the progression of diabetes. Nutr Res 15:1377–1410.
44. Rao RH (1984) The role of undernutrition in the pathogenesis of diabetes mellitus. Diabetes Care 7:595–601.
45. Meisinger C, Doring A, Thorand B, Heier M, Lowel H (2006) Body fat distribution and risk of type 2 diabetes in the general population: are there differences between men and women? The MONICA/KORA Augsburg cohort study. Am J Clin Nutr 84:483–89.
46. Finucane MM, Stevens GA, Cowan MJ, Danaei G, Lin JK, et al. (2011) National, regional, and global trends in body-mass index since 1980: systematic analysis of health examination surveys and epidemiological studies with 960 country-years and 9·1 million participants. Lancet 377:557–67.
47. Danaei G, Finucane MM, Lu Y, Singh GM, Cowan MJ, et al. (2011) National, regional, and global trends in fasting plasma glucose and diabetes prevalence since 1980: systematic analysis of health examination surveys and epidemiological studies with 370 country-years and 2·7 million participants. Lancet 378:31–40.
48. Jha P, Gajalaxmi V, Gupta P, Kumar R, Mony P, et al. (2006) Prospective Study of One Million Deaths in India: Rationale, Design, and Validation Results. PLoS Med 3:e18.
49. Ayles H, Schaap A, Nota A, Sismanidis C, Tembwe R, et al. (2009) Prevalence of tuberculosis, HIV and respiratory symptoms in two Zambian communities: implications for tuberculosis control in the era of HIV. Plos One 4.
50. Rosen MJ (2006) Chronic cough due to tuberculosis and other infections: ACCP evidence-based clinical practice guidelines. Chest 129:197S–201S.
51. Goldhaber-Fiebert JD, Jeon CY, Cohen T, Murray MB (2011) Diabetes mellitus and tuberculosis in countries with high tuberculosis burdens: individual risks and social determinants. Int J Epidemiol 40:417–28.
52. Okura Y, Urban LH, Mahoney DW, Jacobsen SJ, Rodeheffer RJ (2004) Agreement between self-report questionnaires and medical record data was substantial for diabetes, hypertension, myocardial infarction and stroke but not for heart failure. J Clin Epidemiol 57:1096–1103.
53. Gajalaxmi V, Peto R (2009) Smoking, drinking and incident tuberculosis in rural India: population-based case–control study. Int J Epi 38:1018–25.
54. Wang J, Shen H (2009) Review of cigarette smoking and tuberculosis in China: intervention is needed for smoking cessation among tuberculosis patients. BMC Public Health 9:292–300.
55. Thomas A, Gopi PG, Santha T, Chandrasekaran V, Subramani R, et al. (2005) Predictors of relapse among pulmonary tuberculosis patients treated in a DOTS programme in South India. Int J Tuberc Lung Dis 9:556–61.
56. Lavigne M, Rocher I, Steensma C, Brassard P (2006) The impact of smoking on adherence to treatment for latent tuberculosis infection. BMC Public Health 66.
57. Anderson JE, Jorenby DE, Scott WJ, Fiore MC (2002) Treating tobacco use and dependence: an evidence-based clinical practice guideline for tobacco cessation. Chest 121:932–41.
58. Jeon CY, Harries AD, Baker MA, Hart JE, Kapur A, et al. (2010) Bi-directional screening for tuberculosis and diabetes: a systematic review. Trop Med Int Health 15:1300–14.
59. Li L, Lin Y, Mi F, Du J, Dong Y, et al. (2012) Screening of patients with tuberculosis for diabetes mellitus in China. Trop Med Int Health 17:1301.
60. Indian Diabetes Mellitus - Tuberculosis Study Group, India (2013) Screening of patients with tuberculosis for diabetes mellitus in India. Trop Med Int Health 18:636–45.
61. Jha P, Peto R (2014) Global effects of smoking, of quitting, and of taxing tobacco. N Eng J Med 370:60–68.
62. Anderson P, Chisholm D, Fuhr DC (2009) Effectiveness and cost-effectiveness of policies and programmes to reduce the harm caused by alcohol. Lancet 373:2234–46.

11

Mouse *Protocadherin-1* Gene Expression Is Regulated by Cigarette Smoke Exposure *In Vivo*

Henk Koning[1,2,4], Antoon J. M. van Oosterhout[2,4], Uilke Brouwer[2,4], Lisette E. den Boef[2,4], Renée Gras[2,4], Marjan Reinders-Luinge[3,4], Corry-Anke Brandsma[3,4], Marco van der Toorn[2,4], Machteld N. Hylkema[3,4], Brigitte W. M. Willemse[1,4], Ian Sayers[4], Gerard H. Koppelman[1,4]*, Martijn C. Nawijn[2,4]

1 Pediatric Pulmonology and Pediatric Allergology, Beatrix Children's Hospital, University of Groningen, University Medical Center Groningen (UMCG), Groningen, the Netherlands, **2** Laboratory of Allergology and Pulmonary Diseases, Department of Pathology and Medical Biology, University of Groningen, University Medical Center Groningen (UMCG), Groningen, the Netherlands, **3** Department of Pathology and Medical Biology, University of Groningen, University Medical Center Groningen (UMCG), Groningen, the Netherlands, **4** GRIAC research institute, University of Groningen, University Medical Center Groningen (UMCG), Groningen, the Netherlands, **5** Division of Therapeutics and Molecular Medicine, Nottingham Respiratory Biomedical Research Unit, University of Nottingham, Queen's Medical Centre, Nottingham, United Kingdom

Abstract

Protocadherin-1 (*PCDH1*) is a novel susceptibility gene for airway hyperresponsiveness, first identified in families exposed to cigarette smoke and is expressed in bronchial epithelial cells. Here, we asked how mouse Pcdh1 expression is regulated in lung structural cells *in vivo* under physiological conditions, and in both short-term cigarette smoke exposure models characterized by airway inflammation and hyperresponsiveness and chronic cigarette smoke exposure models. *Pcdh1* gene-structure was investigated by Rapid Amplification of cDNA Ends. Pcdh1 mRNA and protein expression was investigated by qRT-PCR, western blotting using isoform-specific antibodies. We observed 87% conservation of the *Pcdh1* nucleotide sequence, and 96% conservation of the Pcdh1 protein sequence between men and mice. We identified a novel *Pcdh1* isoform encoding only the intracellular signalling motifs. Cigarette smoke exposure for 4 consecutive days markedly reduced *Pcdh1* mRNA expression in lung tissue (3 to 4-fold), while neutrophilia and airway hyperresponsiveness was induced. Moreover, *Pcdh1* mRNA expression in lung tissue was reduced already 6 hours after an acute cigarette-smoke exposure in mice. Chronic exposure to cigarette smoke induced loss of Pcdh1 protein in lung tissue after 2 months, while Pcdh1 protein levels were no longer reduced after 9 months of cigarette smoke exposure. We conclude that *Pcdh1* is highly homologous to human *PCDH1*, encodes two transmembrane proteins and one intracellular protein, and is regulated by cigarette smoke exposure *in vivo*.

Editor: Thomas H. Thatcher, University of Rochester Medical Center, United States of America

Funding: This study was supported by research grants from the Netherlands' Lung Foundation (project NAF 3.2.09.055), the Stichting Astmabestrijding (SAB 2010/043) and the EU-funded FP6 project Gabriel (a multidisciplinary study to identify the genetic and environmental causes of asthma). GHK has received grant support from the University Medical Center Groningen. The funders had no role in study design, data collection and analysis, decision to publish, or preparation of the manuscript.

Competing Interests: The authors have declared that no competing interests exist.

* Email: g.h.koppelman@umcg.nl

Introduction

Asthma is a complex disease caused by gene-gene and gene-environment interactions [1]. Many asthma susceptibility genes have been identified, several of which are expressed in the airway epithelium [2]. The airway epithelium in asthma has a disrupted barrier function [3] and an impaired repair response upon injury [4,5] that might contribute to airway remodelling. In addition, the airway epithelium of asthmatics shows an enhanced immune response towards harmful agents (allergens or viruses) by secreting increased amounts of pro-inflammatory mediators such as IL-33, CCL20, GM-CSF or TSLP [6–9]. Polymorphisms in asthma susceptibility genes expressed by airway epithelial cells, affecting the level or regulation of their expression [10], might therefore contribute to both altered barrier function of airway epithelial cells and to enhanced induction of an immune response upon airway epithelial injury [11].

Previously, we identified protocadherin-1 (*PCDH1*) as a novel susceptibility gene for airway hyperresponsiveness (AHR) in asthma families [12]. Interestingly, a strong linkage signal of *PCDH1* with asthma and AHR was observed in families exposed to environmental tobacco smoke (ETS). *PCDH1* encodes for two main isoforms: a 3 exon and a 5 exon isoform that are expressed in the airway epithelium [12]. In addition a putative third isoform was identified that lacks exon 1 and part of exon 2 [13]. Both main isoforms encode a protein containing an extracellular domain with seven cadherin repeats, a transmembrane domain, and an intracellular domain containing several Serine and Tyrosine residues, that have been found to be subject to phosphorylation [14,15]. The third isoform only contains two extracellular cadherin repeats and the shared intracellular domain. In addition, both isoforms 2 and 3 encode an additional intracellular domain containing three intracellular conserved motifs (CM1–CM3), of which CM3 is the binding motif for protein phosphatase 1 alpha

(PP1α) [16,17]. We previously reported complex splicing patterns of *PCDH1* regarding the expression of intracellular conserved motifs, and observed a marked upregulation of PCDH1 during mucociliary differentiation of primary bronchial epithelial cells [13].

In mouse, *Pcdh1* mRNA expression was identified in several adult tissues (brain, kidney, heart, lung and uterus), but highest expression was observed in lung [18]. During mouse embryogenesis, *Pcdh1* mRNA expression in lung was restricted to mesenchyme and blood vessels, and was not detected in the bronchial epithelium. Similar to the human situation, two main transcripts were identified in the mouse, as well as a variant displaying variation in expression of conserved motifs [16].

As *PCDH1* was originally identified as a susceptibility gene for AHR in families exposed to cigarette smoke and encodes an adhesion molecule that is expressed in the airway epithelium, we hypothesize that environmental exposures such as cigarette smoke may affect PCDH1 levels or function in the airways. Currently, detailed knowledge about Pcdh1 expression in lung structural cells and its regulation by environmental exposures *in vivo* is unknown. Therefore, we aimed to investigate the expression and regulation of Pcdh1 under basal conditions *in vivo* and in both short-term and chronic cigarette smoke exposure mouse models.

Materials and Methods

Animal Models

BALB/c and A/J mice (6 to 8 weeks, n = 61 for BALB/c and n = 28 for A/J in total) were purchased from Charles River Laboratories (L'Arbresle-Cedex, France), housed in individually ventilated cages, kept under specific pathogen-free conditions and maintained on a 12 h light-dark cycle, with food and water ad libitum. Experiments were approved by the Institutional Animal Care and Use Committee of the University of Groningen (The Netherlands), and carried out following (inter-)national welfare regulations.

Sub-chronic and acute cigarette smoke (CS) exposure models.

BALB/c mice were exposed to gaseous-phase CS from Kentucky 3R4F research reference cigarettes (Tobacco Research Institute, University of Kentucky, Lexington, USA). Each cigarette was smoked without filter in 5 minutes at a rate of 5 L/hr in a ratio with 60 L/hr air using whole body exposure. Gaseous-phase CS was directly distributed inside 6-liter perspex boxes. In this study we employed two whole-body CS-exposure models:

Sub-chronic CS exposure model: Female mice (n = 8 per group) were exposed to CS of 1–5 cigarettes for 5 days or filtered air each morning and afternoon, using a peristaltic pump as described previously [19]. Mice were sacrificed 2 h after the last CS exposure. The results were replicated in a second independent experiment (n = 8 per group) that was performed in the same way, with the exception that no Bronchial Alveolar Lavage (BAL)-fluid was isolated. In total 32 mice were used for these two independent experiments.

Acute CS exposure model: Male mice were exposed to CS of 10 cigarettes (n = 8) in 1.5 h or filtered air (n = 5), and were sacrificed 6 h after the last CS exposure. This experiment was performed once, with 13 mice in total.

From all mice, BAL-fluid was isolated and the smallest lung lobe was stored at −80°C for RNA or protein isolation. BAL was obtained, by lavaging through a tracheal cannula with five 1 ml aliquots of saline of 37°C. Differential BAL cell counts (3 times 100 cells) were obtained from cytospin preparations stained with Diff-Quick (Merz & Dade A.G., Dudingen, Switzerland).

Airway responsiveness (AHR) was assessed in a separate group of sub-chronic CS exposed mice at day 5, by omitting the final smoke exposure (n = 8 per group, 16 mice in total). AHR was determined by measuring airway resistance in response to i.v. administration of increasing doses of methacholine (acetyl-b-methylcholine chloride, Sigma-Aldrich, St. Louis, MO), using a computer-controlled small-animal ventilator (Flexivent; SCIREQ, Montreal, Quebec, Canada) as described previously [20].

Chronic CS exposure model:

Female A/J mice were exposed to cigarette smoke from 2R1 reference cigarettes twice daily (2 cigarettes/session, 10 puffs/cigarette), 5 days per week by nose-only exposure as described previously [32]. After 2 or 9 months of cigarette smoke exposure, mice were sacrificed. The right lung lobe was snap frozen for further analyses.

RNA purification, Rapid amplification of cDNA ends (RACE) and quantitative (q)RT-PCR

RNA was isolated from 50–100 mg of mouse lung tissue homogenized in 1 ml of TriReagent (MRC, Cincinnati, OH). gDNA traces were removed enzymatically, followed by purification using RNeasy Mini Kit (QIAGEN). RNA concentration and integrity was determined by Nanodrop measurements (ND-1000 spectrophotometer, Isogen Lifesciences, de Meern, Netherlands).

RACE was performed on RNA purified from lung tissue according to the manufacturer's instructions (GeneRacer-RLM-RACE Kit, Invitrogen, Carlsbad, USA), and as described previously [13] using the primers described in Table 1. RACE was performed from *Pcdh1* exon 1 for 5′ transcripts and from exon 3 for 3′transcripts. Furthermore, additional 5′RACE experiments from exon 3 were performed in order to identify a homolog of the putative human isoform 3 [13]. PCR products were TOPO-cloned and *Pcdh1* transcripts were sequenced (StarSEQ, Mainz, Germany) as described previously [13]. Pcdh1 mRNA and protein sequences were compared to human PCDH1 using ClustalW (http://www.ebi.ac.uk/Tools/msa/clustalw2/).

Expression levels of *Pcdh1* transcripts were determined by qRT-PCR as described previously [13], using ABI primer-probe sets. In brief, two microgram of RNA was reverse transcribed in 20 µl reaction volume using Omniscript™ reverse transcriptase (QIAGEN Benelux BV, Venlo, the Netherlands). *Pcdh1* exon 1–2 (Mm01264041_m1, Applied Biosystems Europe BV, Nieuwekerk A/D IJssel, the Netherlands), *Pcdh1* exon 3–4 and *Pcdh1* exon m-1B (Custom assays, Applied Biosystems, Table 1 for primer sequences) expression was determined relative to the most stable combination of four housekeeping genes (*HPRT1* (Mm01545399_m1), *Pgk1* (Mm01225301_m1), *B2m* (Mm00437762_m1), *Ipo8* (Mm01255158_m1), Applied Biosystems). Data was analyzed using SDS2.3 software by applying the ΔΔCt-method (Applied Biosystems User Bulletin 2). As four house-keeping genes were used, for normalization the best combination of house-keeping genes was determined by using the Normfinder applet [21]. We calculated relative expression levels as follows: First the cycle threshold value (Ct-value) of the average of the combination of most stable house-keeping genes was subtracted from the Ct-values of our *Pcdh1*-assays (formula 1). Next, we converted the ΔCt-value to expression level (EL; formula 2), and normalized the expression levels relative to the average of the control group (formula 3). In formulas: 1). $\Delta Ct_{Pcdh1} = Ct_{Pcdh1} - Ct_{HKG\text{-}average}$, 2). $EL_{Pcdh1} = 2^{-\Delta Ct\,Pcdh1}$; 3). Relative $EL = EL_{Pcdh1}/EL_{Pcdh1\text{-}control}$.

Table 1. Pcdh1 RACE and qPCR primer sequences.

Pcdh1 RACE primer	Sequence (5′-3′)	Corresponding GeneRacer primer	Sequence (5′-3′)
5′RACE 301Rev	GAGGTCTCTGTGGTGAAAATGTCT	GeneRacer 5′ primer	CGACTGGAGCACGAGGACACTGA
5′RACE 162Rev	GTTCCTCTGGCACCTTGTATACTACC	GeneRacer 5′ nested primer	GGACACTGACATGGACTGAAGGAGTA
3′RACE FW1	GCCCAGGAGCTGCAGGATCCAT	GeneRacer 3′ primer	GTCGTCAACGATACGCTACGTAACG
3′RACE FW2	GAAACACCCTCTAGCAAGTCATCCT	GeneRacer 3′ nested primer	CGCTACGTAACGGCATGACAGTG
5′RACE Ex3 Rev3	GCTGTGATGGATCCTGCAGCTCCT	GeneRacer 5′ primer	CGACTGGAGCACGAGGACACTGA
5′RACE Ex3 Rev2	ACTGGTGGCCGAGAAGGTGACA	GeneRacer 5′ nested primer	GGACACTGACATGGACTGAAGGAGTA
qPCR assay	Forward (5′-3′)	Probe (FAM-NFQ labelled)	Reverse (5′-3′)
M-1B–Ex1	CTCAGCATGCGCAGAAGAAAA	ACTGTTCTCCTGATTCTGG	CCTCAGAGGCCCCATCCT
Ex2-Ex3	GAGCAGTACTCCGACTACAG	CCAGCAAGCAGTTACCTCAC	TAGAGGGTGTTTCCGATTCC

Ex = exon; Rev = reverse; FW = Forward.

Cloning and overexpression of Pcdh1 isoform 3 in BEAS2B bronchial epithelial cells

Cloning: The human cDNA sequence corresponding to the mouse isoform 3 sequence obtained by RACE PCR experiments was amplified from the isoform 2 plasmid (pCMV-XL6-iso2, TC109554, Origene, Rockville, USA) with forward primer CCGCGAATTCATTCTCTTTGGTGTGGTGG and reverse primer CACTGGAGTGGCAACTTC by using Phusion™ High Fidelity PCR Kit (F-553S, Finnzymes, Fisher Scientific, Landsmeer, The Netherlands), followed by subcloning of the PCR product into the pCMV-XL6 expression vector (Origene, USA). The resulting pCMV-XL6-Pcdh1-Iso3 plasmids were sequenced (StarSeq Sequencing, Mainz, Germany).

Overexpression: BEAS2B cells were grown as described previously [22], seeded into 24-well plates, and transfected at a confluency of 60–80% with 0.5 µg of eGFP (expression control, pEGFP-C1, Westburg BV, Leusden, The Netherlands), full-length Isoform 2 (pCMV-XL6-Pcdh1-iso2), or Isoform 3 plasmid (pCMV-XL6-Pcdh1-iso3), using Fugene HD transfection reagent according to the manufacturer's procedures (Roche Diagnostics, Almere, the Netherlands). Cells were harvested 48 h after transfection using leammli buffer (2x leammli: 4% SDS; 20% glycerol; 10% β-mercaptoethanol; 0.004% bromphenol blue; 0.125 M Tris HCl; pH 6.8), boiled for 5 min, and analysed for PCDH1 protein expression by western blotting using the antibody specific for the intracellular domain encoded by exon 4 (EP76, Figure 1A) [13].

Detection of Pcdh1 protein expression levels by western blotting

Protein isolation: Frozen lungs were homogenized in 5 µl/mg lysis buffer (1% Triton-X 100, 150 mM NaCl, 5 mM $MgCl_2$, 10 mM HEPES, 1:500 Protease Inhibitor Cocktail (P8340, Sigma-Aldrich, Zwijndrecht, the Netherlands)) using a tissue homogenator (T10 basic, ULTRA-TURRAX, IKA, Staufen, Germany). Subsequently lung homogenates were boiled for 10 minutes with 2x laemmlli buffer and stored at −80°C.

Western blotting: Lung tissue homogenates were separated on 7.5% acrylamide SDS-page gels (Bio-Rad Laboratories BV, Veenendaal, the Netherlands). Detection of Pcdh1 protein was performed using antibodies that were designed against isoform-specific peptide sequences in the intracellular tail of both human *PCDH1* variants as described previously [13] (Figure 2A). These antibodies showed cross-reactivity with mouse *Pcdh1* due to high homology of the immunizing peptide sequences: (QPFQLSTPQPLPHPYH, EP78, 86% conserved; SPSPPEDRNTKTAPV, EP76, 100% conserved) (See Figure 1A for binding sites of antibodies). Antibodies were affinity column purified against immunizing peptides (Eurogentec, Liege, Belgium), and were validated by blocking experiments using a pre-incubation period of 30 min at 37°C with 10x molar excess of immunizing peptides or H_2O.

Pcdh1 bands on western blots were visualized using Goat-anti-Rabbit-Peroxidase (GARPO, Daco, Heverlee, Belgium) as secondary antibody, and as tertiary step Rabbit-anti-Goat-Peroxidase (RAGPO, Dako, Heverelee, Belgium) was used. Next, blots were incubated with Luminol-reagent, and subsequently analysed using Fuji Medical X-Ray films (Fuji Photo Film Gmbh, Germany), followed by densitometric analysis using Quantity One Software v4.6.2 (Bio-Rad), relative to the β-actin loading control (sc-47778, Santa-Cruz Biotechnology, Heidelberg, Germany).

Statistical analysis

Differences in mRNA or protein expression levels were statistically tested by Mann-Whitney tests (GraphPad v4.0, La Jolla, USA). Experimental outliers were determined by using the Grubbs analysis (http://www.graphpad.com/quickcalcs/Grubbs1.cfm). Differences in airway hyperresponsiveness between smoke- and air-exposed mice were determined by testing for differences in the area under the curve (AUC) using GraphPad software.

Results

Pcdh1 expression in the mouse lung

To allow an accurate investigation of *Pcdh1* expression regulation in the mouse lung, we first determined the *Pcdh1* gene-structure by RACE experiments. Compared to the published mouse *Pcdh1* gene-structure [16], we detected two novel exons on the 5′ end of *Pcdh1* (exon m-1b and m-1c, Figure 1A), two novel exons on the 3′ end (exon 3b and exon 5), as well as major variation in exon 4, containing the conserved CM2-domain and PDZ-BS motifs (Figure 1A). Exon 3b is a short 39 basepair exon encoding a premature stop codon, which is completely conserved between men and mice (See Table 2 for corresponding Genbank accession numbers). Remarkably, mouse *Pcdh1* exons had high homology to human exons resulting in a 87% homology at the nucleotide level (Figure 1A) and a 96% homology on protein level (Figure S1). Previously we detected an isoform lacking several extracellular domains in human bronchial epithelial cells [13]. We therefore performed 5′RACE experiments from exon 3 in mouse

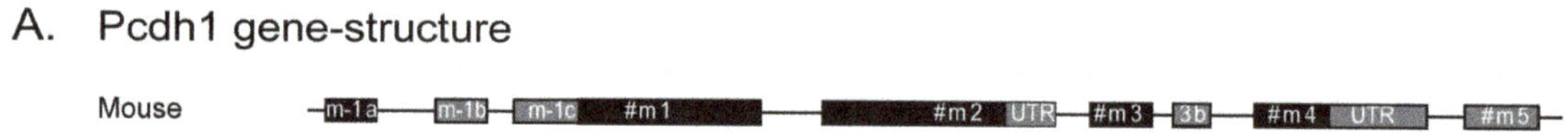

Homology

Mouse exons	m-1a	m-1b	m-1c	1	2cds	2+UTR	3	3b	4cds	4+UTR	5
Size (basepair)	182	153	211	863	2280	2835	220	39	398	1055	100
Human exons	1a	Na	1e/1f	1	2cds	2+UTR	3	3b	4cds	4+UTR	5
Size (basepair)	180	Na	195	863	2280	2776	220	39	395	1063	146
Homology (%)	87	Na	73	87	89	86	89	100	96	87	97

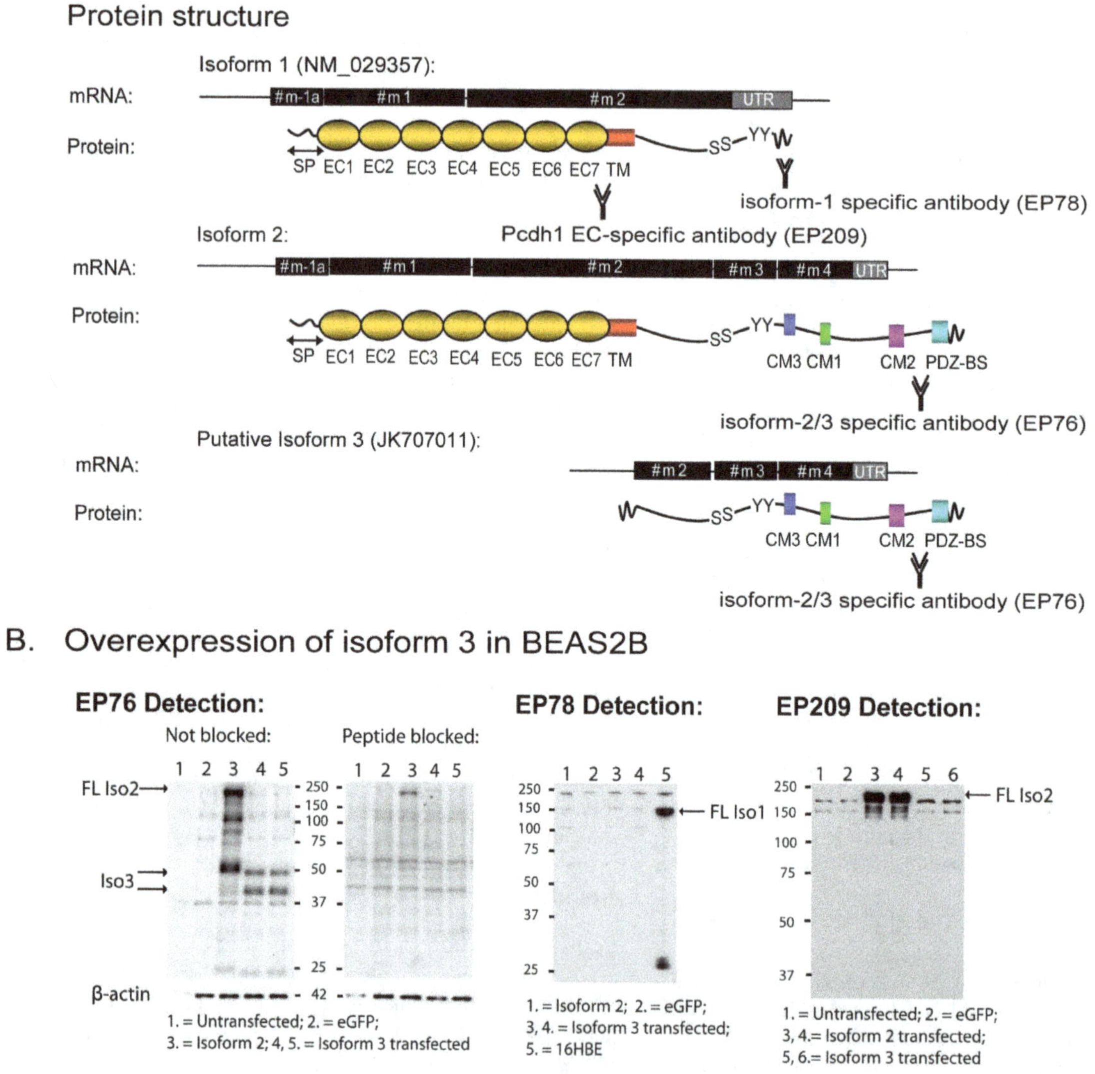

Figure 1. Pcdh1 gene-structure and isoforms. (A) Two novel exons were detected at the 5'end of PCDH1, and one novel exon on the 3'end of Pcdh1. Mouse Pcdh1 exons share high homology with human PCDH1 exons. Corresponding isoforms (isoforms 1, 2 and putative isoform 3) and their protein structures are depicted. Only isoform 2 and putative isoform 3 contain evolutionary conserved motifs (CM1–3). Two antibodies were generated against sequences in the intracellular tail of both isoform 1 (EP78) and isoform 2 (EP76) of Pcdh1. An antibody directed against the extracellular domains of Pcdh1 (EP209) was generated previously [12]. (B) Western blot of lysates of BEAS2B cells overexpressing the open reading frame of Pcdh1 isoform 3, using antibody EP76 for detection as indicated (left hand panel) including a pre-incubation with the immunizing peptide ('Peptide blocked') as a control for specificity (right hand panel). Western blots using EP78 and EP209 antibodies for detection are also included as indicated. cds = coding sequence; UTR = Untranslated region; SP = Signal peptide (amino-acid (aa) 1–57); EC = Extracellular Cadherin domain; TM = Transmembrane domain; CM = Conserved Motif; PDZ-BS = PDZ-domain Binding Site; S = Serine residue; Y = Tyrosine residue; EP209 = Binding site for antibody directed against the extracellular domain of Pcdh1; EP78 = Binding site for antibody directed against a specific intracellular sequence of isoform 1, encoded by exon 2; EP76 = Binding site for antibody directed against the intracellular domain present in isoforms 2 and 3 and encoded by exon 4; FL = full length. Genbank accession numbers of novel transcripts are provided in Table 2.

Table 2. Genbank accession numbers of novel *Pcdh1* transcripts.

RACE reaction	*Protocadherin-1* Sequence	GenBank Accession number
Mm 5′RACE exon 1	Exon m-1b - 1	JK707005
Mm 5′RACE exon 1	Exon m-1c - 1	JK707006
Mm 5′RACE exon 1	Exon m-1c - 1 (short exon)	JK707007
Mm 3′RACE exon 3	Exon 3-3b-4	JK707008
Mm 3′RACE exon 3	Exon 4 including gap	JK707009
Mm 3′RACE exon 3	Exon 4-5	JK707010
Mm 5′RACE exon 3	Exon 2-3 (Isoform 3)	JK707011
Hs 3′RACE exon 3	Exon 3-3b-4–5	JK707004

Mm = Mus musculus; Hs = Homo sapiens.

lung. Interestingly, we identified an additional transcript starting from within exon 2, containing a CTG Kozak-sequence (isoform 3, Genbank accession JK707011), and putatively encoding a protein product with an in-frame translation initiation site at amino-acid no 870 of the full-length Pcdh1 isoform 2 protein (Genbank accession NP_115796). Overexpression of the corresponding 5′-truncated open reading frame in BEAS2B cells induced 40- and 50 kD Pcdh1 proteins. Both protein products were specifically detected by the EP76-antibody as intensity of these bands clearly diminished after blocking with immunizing peptide, and were not detected with the EP78 and EP209 antibodies (Figure 1B). These results show that in mouse lung a third, intracellular Pcdh1 isoform is expressed that does not contain the extracellular and transmembrane domains, but retains all intracellular domains also present in Pcdh1 isoform 2 (Figure 1A).

We next investigated basal expression of *Pcdh1* mRNA and protein levels in mouse lung tissue. We observed very low levels of *Pcdh1* using the exon m-1b/exon-1 specific qRT-PCR assay, while much higher expression levels of *Pcdh1* were detected using exon 1–2 and exon 3–4 specific assays (Figure 2A). On western blot of whole mouse lung homogenate, we observed one specific band of 150 kD and a non-specific band of 140 kD, using an antibody generated against the intracellular tail of the PCDH1 isoform 1 (EP78, Figure 2B). In contrast, we observed a 50 kD and 170 kD bands using a specific antibody generated against the intracellular tail present in PCDH1 isoforms 2 and 3 (EP76, Figure 2B).

Short term smoke exposure down regulates Pcdh1 expression levels

Given the initial linkage of *PCDH1* to AHR and asthma in cigarette smoke exposed families defined by a significant smoking history of the asthma proband of more than 5 packyears [12], we investigated whether *Pcdh1* expression was regulated in a sub-chronic (5 days) smoke exposure model (Figure 3A). This model induced a neutrophillic influx into the airways (Figure 3A), a feature of sub-chronic smoke exposure models [19,23], as well as a trend towards AHR to methacholine ($p = 0.056$, Figure 3A).

In CS-exposed mice, we observed significantly lower expression of *Pcdh1* transcripts encoding exon 1–2 (3.9 fold, $p = 0.0003$) and exon 3–4 (3.3-fold, $p = 0.0003$) in total lung (Figure 3B, left panel). Next, we investigated whether this was reflected at the protein level in total mouse lung homogenate. No differences in Pcdh1 isoform 1 protein levels were found, but a trend towards lower levels of the 170 kd Pcdh1 isoform 2 protein band ($p = 0.052$, Figure 3C and 3D, left panels) was observed by western blot after 5 days of smoke exposure.

In order to evaluate the reproducibility of our results, we performed an independent replication of the sub-chronic smoke exposure model. One RNA sample of the air-exposed group was excluded due to insufficient RNA quality. We detected one outlier in the smoke exposed group, both for exon 1–2 and exon 3–4 expression and tested for differences between smoke and air exposed mice with and without outliers. We observed a trend towards lower *Pcdh1* exon 1–2 expression ($p = 0.16/p = 0.39$;

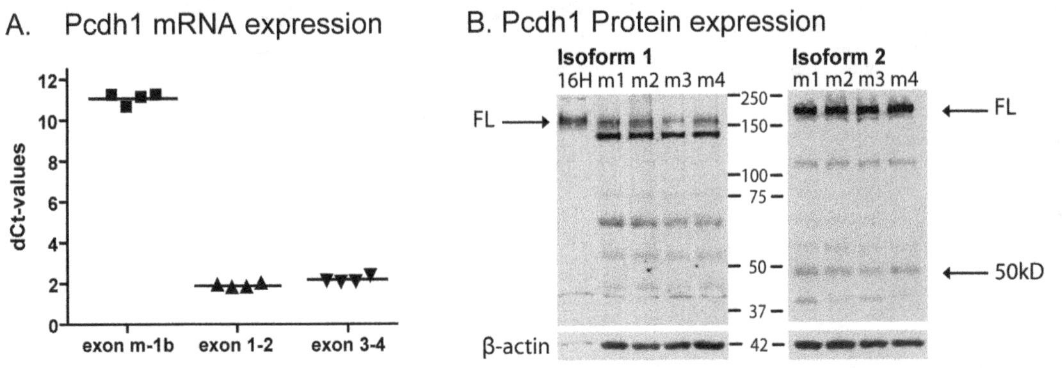

Figure 2. Basal Pcdh1 mRNA and protein expression in lung. (A) mRNA expression levels of exon m-1b, exon 1–2 and exon 3–4 containing transcripts in naive mouse lung of four mice. (B) Western blot of mouse lung homogenate using the antibody directed against the intracellular domain of Pcdh1 isoform 1 (EP78), and the antibody directed against the intracellular domain encoded by exon 4 of Pcdh1 (isoform 2, EP76) (see arrows for the Pcdh1 specific bands), with β-actin as loading control. m1 = lung homogenate of mouse number 1; FL = full length.

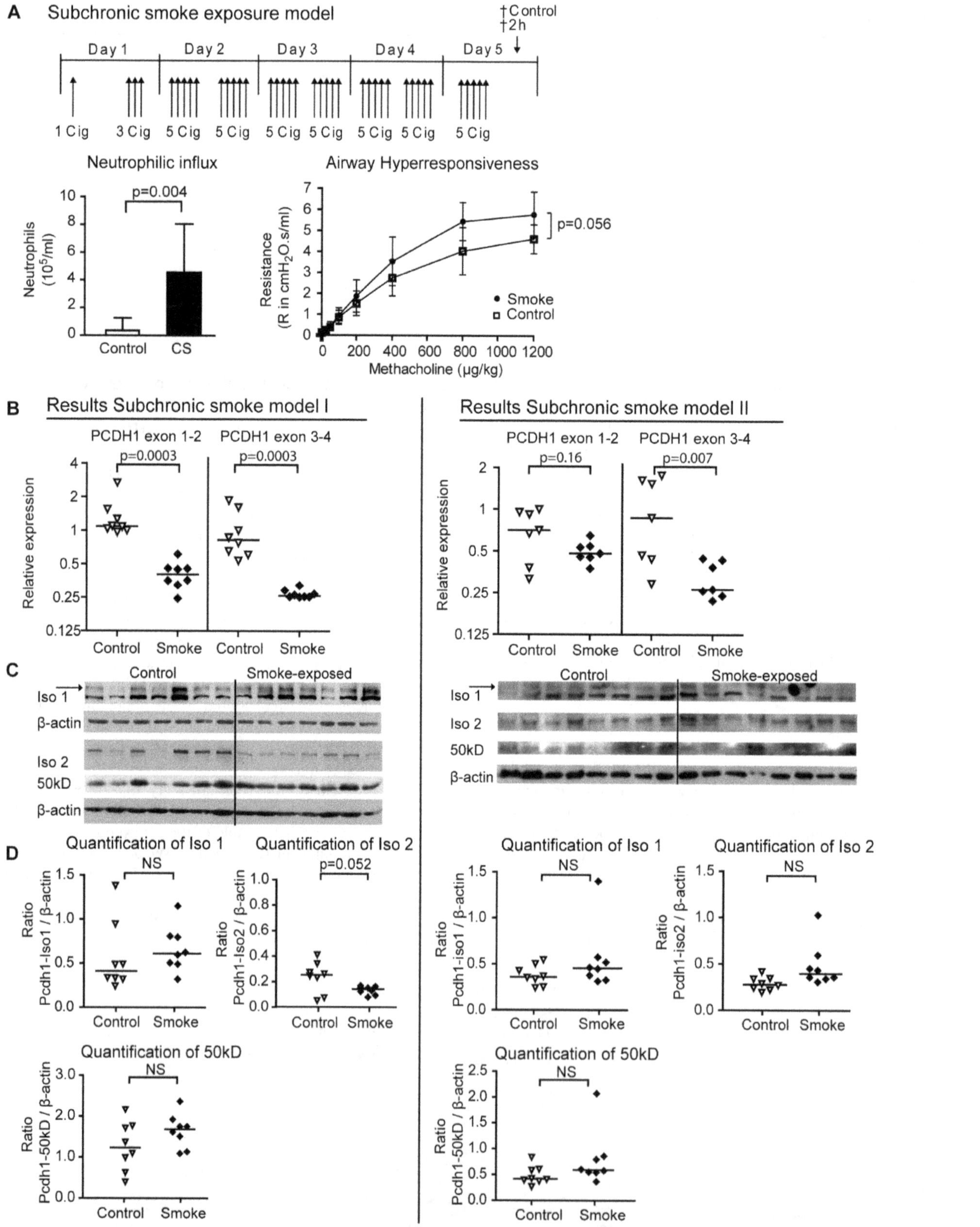

Figure 3. Pcdh1 mRNA expression levels decrease after sub chronic smoke exposure. (A) In the sub chronic smoke exposure model, mice were exposed to 1 and 3 cigarettes or air at day 1, followed by 5 cigarettes at day 2–5 or air. 2 h after the last cigarette both smoke and air exposed mice were sacrificed. Neutrophils in the bronchoalveolar lavage fluid, and airway hyperresponsiveness to methacholine were determined. Error bars show Standard Deviation. Two independent experiments are shown individually. (B) Pcdh1 exon 1–2 and 3–4 transcript levels were determined in lungs of air exposed (open symbols) and smoke exposed (closed symbols) mice. (C) Pcdh1 protein levels were determined by western blot of lung homogenate of air (control) and smoke exposed mice. Pcdh1 isoform 1 (arrow indicates the specific band; EP78-antibody), full-length isoform 2

(EP76-antibody) and 50 kD (EP76-antibody) levels are shown, with β-actin as loading control. (D) Densitometric quantification of Pcdh1 expression levels of full-length isoform 1 and 2, and the 50 kD fragment, relative to β-actin. Cig = cigarette; † = time-point at which mice are sacrificed.

without/with outliers) and clearly replicated the decrease of *Pcdh1* exon 3–4 expression after smoke exposure ($p = 0.007/p = 0.04$; without/with outliers; results without outliers are shown in Figure 3B, right panel). When we combined the two experiments we observed very significantly reduced expression of *Pcdh1* exon 1–2 ($p = 0.0015$) and *Pcdh1* exon 3–4 ($p < 0.0001$) mRNA. We were not able to replicate the trend towards lower isoform 2 protein expression, as we did not detect a difference in protein levels of all Pcdh1 isoforms in the replication experiment (Figure 3C and 3D, right panels).

To test whether the down regulation of *Pcdh1* mRNA expression levels was a direct effect of CS-exposure, we also analyzed *Pcdh1* expression shortly after an acute CS-exposure, in which no significant neutrophilic influx was observed (Figure 4A). Remarkably, already 6 hours after CS-exposure, a 2-fold ($p = 0.006$) decrease in exon 1–2 expression levels and a 1.6-fold ($p = 0.03$) decrease in exon 3–4 expression levels was observed (Figure 4B), suggesting that *Pcdh1* expression indeed is directly regulated by CS-exposure. This difference was not paralleled by a reduced lung Pcdh1 protein expression at this time-point (Figure 4C and 4D).

Chronic smoke exposure down regulates Pcdh1 protein levels after 2 months

Next, we aimed to test whether the observed effects of CS exposure on Pcdh1 isoform 2 expression levels in lung tissue were retained after chronic smoke exposure. To this end, we analyzed lung tissue of A/J mice exposed for 5 days a week to cigarette smoke for 2 months and 9 months, compared to air-treated control mice (Figure 5). Here, we find that both the 150 kd full-length ($p = 0.011$) and the 50 kd band ($p = 0.049$) of Pcdh1 isoform 2 were significantly reduced in lung tissue after 2 months of CS exposure compared to control treatments (Figure 5A, B) while after 9 months of CS exposure, no differences in Pcdh1 protein levels in lung tissue could be detected compared to air control-treatment (Figure 5A, C).

Discussion

In this study, we provide a full characterization of the expression pattern of Pcdh1, the murine homologue of PCDH1, a novel AHR susceptibility gene identified in families exposed to environmental cigarette smoke. We assessed Pcdh1 expression in the mouse lung and its regulation *in vivo* in both short-term and chronic CS exposure models. Here, we show that the mouse and human genes for *Protocadherin-1* are highly homologous, both at the nucleotide and at the amino-acid level, validating the mouse as a relevant model to study Pcdh1 function. In addition to the two annotated isoforms of Pcdh1 that differ in their cytoplasmic signalling domains, we observed expression of a novel Pcdh1 isoform, characterized by the lack of extracellular and transmembrane domains, whilst containing all of the intracellular domains also present in isoform 2. Exposure of mice to cigarette smoke induced a rapid and strong reduction of Pcdh1 mRNA expression in lung tissue within 6 hours. Moreover, exposure of mice to CS for 5 days induced a strongly reduced level of *Pcdh1* mRNA expression in the lung, which in one out of two experiments performed was also observed at the protein level for Pcdh1 isoform 2. The reduced protein levels of Pcdh1 isoform2 are retained in chronic CS exposure models after 2 months, but are no longer observed after 9 months of CS exposure.

When comparing the gene-structure of *Pcdh1* to human *PCDH1* [13], we observed a striking homology between the two; with 87% at the nucleotide level and 96% at the amino-acid level (Figure 1A, Figure S1). Moreover, the low expression levels of alternative 5′exons (exon m-1b), the gap in exon 4 [13,16] resulting in deletion of conserved CM2-domains, and the novel exon 5 are also conserved between man and mouse [13]. In addition to the high level of conservation we obtained evidence for a third *Pcdh1* isoform that initiates transcription from within exon 2 and contains a CTG start-codon [24] within a conserved KOZAK sequence (Figure 1A). Overexpression of this isoform induced expression of 40-and 50 kD PCDH1 proteins that were only detected by the antibody generated against the intracellular domain encoded by exon 4 also present in isoform 2 (EP76-antibody). These results suggest that in mouse lung a third Pcdh1 protein isoform is expressed containing intracellular domains, but not extracellular cadherin repeats. Its function may involve cell signalling rather than cell adhesion, which will be subject of future investigations. We were not able to identify the exact cell-types that express this novel isoform, using the combination of approaches employed by us. The 16HBE bronchial epithelial cell-line however, was shown to display a 50 kd band on Western blot that could correspond to this novel isoform [13], but it might also represent a posttranslational modification of the full-length isoform 2 protein as has been observed for other protocadherins [25].

PCDH1 was first identified as a susceptibility gene for AHR in families exposed to environmental tobacco smoke [12]. The human chromosomal region 5q31–33, containing *PCDH1*, was previously linked to AHR and asthma in 95 ETS exposed families. In this study, ETS exposure was defined by a significant smoking history of the proband of the asthma family. Associations of *PCDH1* gene-variants with AHR were further investigated in four populations of children exposed to ETS *in utero* or in early life. *PCDH1* gene-variant rs3822357 was associated with AHR in ETS exposed children in one population only [12]. The effect of genetic variation of the AHR susceptibility gene *PCDH1* on its expression and the putative interaction with cigarette smoke exposure as an environmental factor is currently unknown.

In the current study, we analyzed the regulation of Pcdh1 expression in experimental mouse models of cigarette smoke exposure. We observed that CS-exposure strongly reduced *Pcdh1* mRNA expression levels, as determined in whole lung homogenate. Since loss of *Pcdh1* expression is already observed as early as 6 hours after CS-exposure, *Pcdh1* expression might in fact be regulated directly by CS-exposure as this time-point precedes significant influx of inflammatory cells in the airways. Importantly, we replicated the reduction of *Pcdh1* mRNA expression levels after 4 days CS exposure, and we were able to detect down-regulation of Pcdh1 isoform 2 protein levels in lung tissue in this sub-chronic CS exposure model in one out of two experiments. Importantly, the observed down-regulation of Pcdh1 isoform 2 protein levels was retained after 2 months of chronic CS exposure.

Remarkably, in some cases we detect altered expression levels of Pcdh1 mRNA in absence of altered Pcdh1 protein levels. This apparent lack of consistent results between mRNA and protein data for the effect of CS exposure on Pcdh1 expression levels in lung tissue might be the result of differences in sensitivity between the qRT-PCR assay used to detect mRNA levels and the western blot assay used to detect protein levels. Alternatively, posttrans-

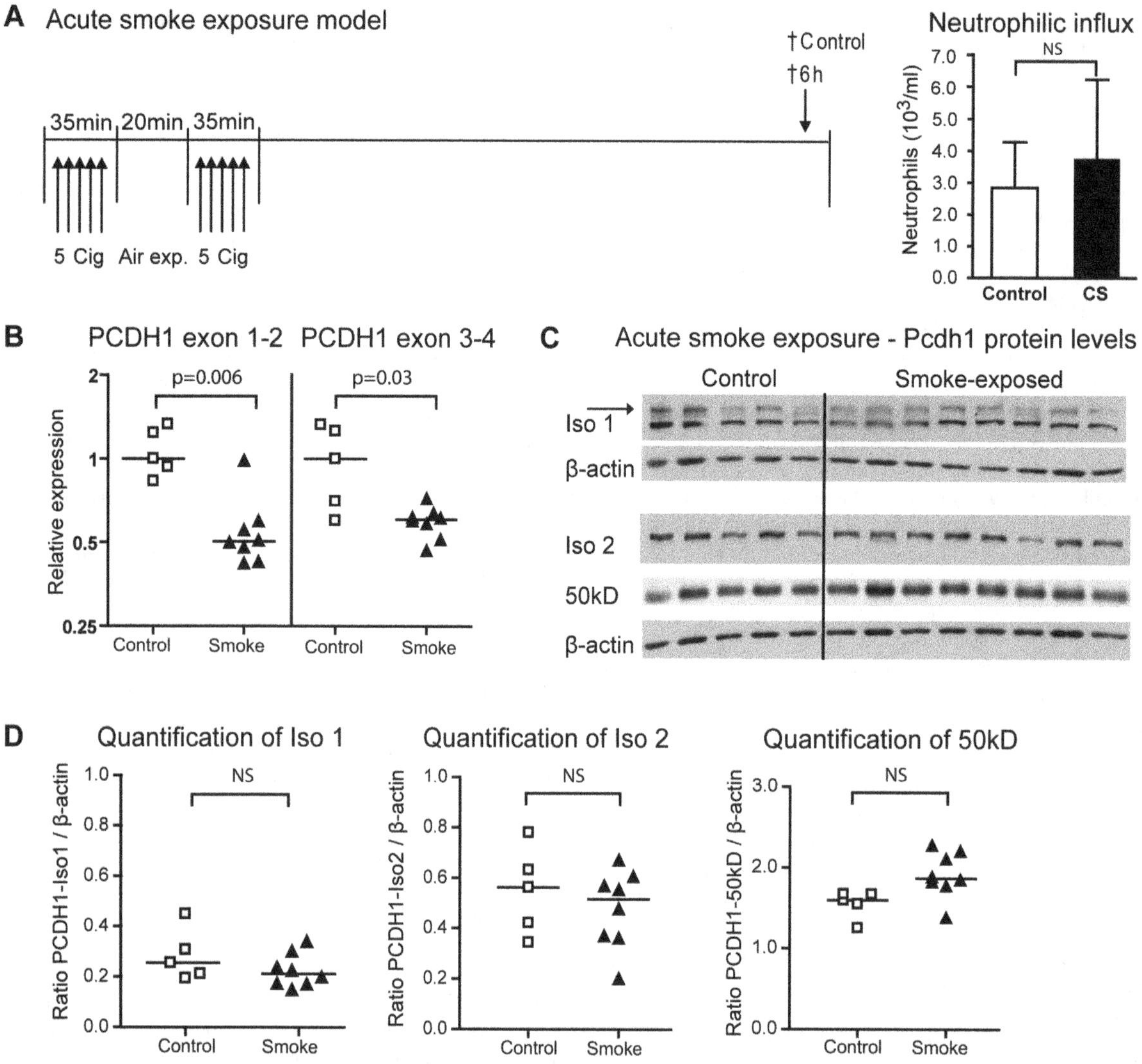

Figure 4. Pcdh1 mRNA expression levels decrease after acute smoke exposure. (A) In the acute smoke exposure model, mice were exposed to 10 cigarettes, with a 20 min rest period in between two sessions of 5 cigarettes, or to air as a control. Low numbers of neutrophils were observed in the lung, 6 h the last exposure. (B) Pcdh1 exon 1–2 and 3–4 mRNA expression levels were determined in the cigarette smoke exposed group (closed symbols) and compared to the air-exposed group (open symbols). (C) Western blot of Pcdh1 isoform 1 (iso 1, EP78-antibody, specific band indicated with an arrow), isoform 2 (iso 2, EP76-antibody) and the 50 kD fragment (EP76-antibody) in lung homogenate of mice exposed to cigarette smoke (smoke) or air (control). (D) Densitometric quantification of Pcdh1 expression levels of full-length isoform 1 and 2, and the 50 kD fragment, relative to β-actin. Cig = cigarette; † = time-point at which mice are sacrificed; CS = cigarette smoke.

lational modifications of the Pcdh1 protein might affect protein stability, resulting in a half-life that significantly exceeds that of the mRNA, indicating that changes in mRNA levels might only translate into altered protein levels at a relatively late time-point. All-in-all, the fact that CS exposure reproducibly induces loss of Pcdh1 expression in all three short-term exposure models and in the 2 months chronic CS exposure model presented here does indicate that CS exposure is a relevant environmental factor acting on Pcdh1 expression levels. These data are very relevant to the interpretation of the original identification of PCDH1 as an AHR gene in families exposed to environmental cigarette smoke [12]. Given our results, it is of interest to test whether in human lung tissue, too, PCDH1 expression levels are affected by CS exposure, and whether this is a function of the *PCDH1* polymorphisms identified in the original study. Moreover, studies addressing a putative role for PCDH1 gene polymorphisms in AHR in COPD patients might also be of considerable interest.

Remarkably, the differences in Pcdh1 isoform 2 protein levels in lung tissue between smoke- and air-exposed mice were no longer found after 9 months of CS exposure. Comparing the relative levels of Pcdh1 isoform 2 protein between the two time-points of the chronic CS exposure models indicates that this might be due to a loss of Pcdh1 protein expression over time in the air-control treated lungs, rather than a restoration of Pcdh1 protein levels in lungs of CS exposed mice (Figure 5B, C). Further research will need to disentangle whether progressive loss of Pcdh1 in occurring in aging lungs or whether any CS-induced regulation of Pcdh1 protein levels is lost at this late time-point.

Mice sub chronically exposed to cigarette smoke showed a trend towards hyperresponsiveness to methacholine in our experiments, an effect that was also observed in other studies in smoke exposed

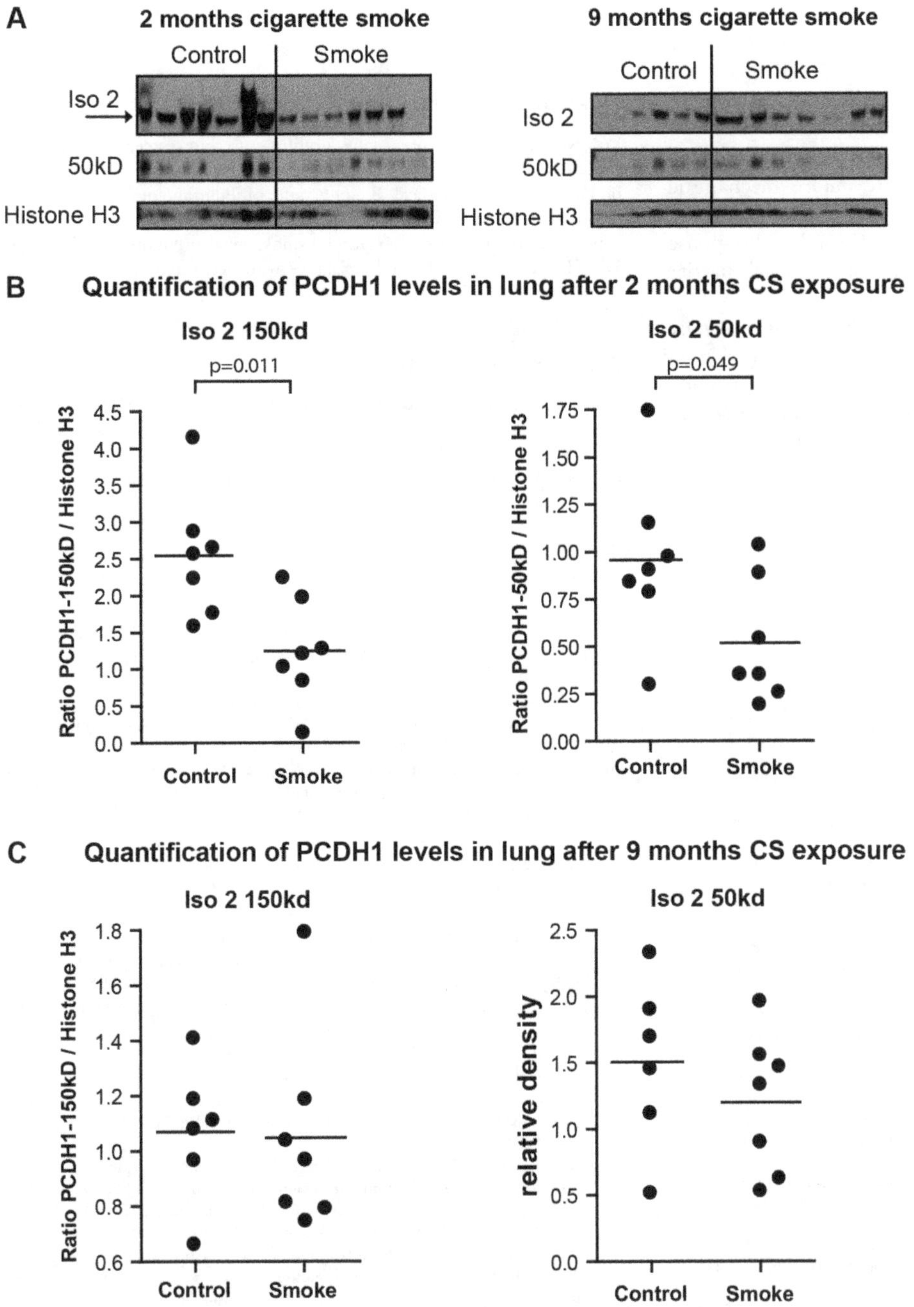

Figure 5. Pcdh1 protein levels are reduced after 2 months of cigarette smoke exposure. (A) Western blot of Pcdh1 isoform 2 (iso 2, EP76-antibody) and the 50 kD fragment (EP76-antibody) in lung homogenate of mice exposed to cigarette smoke (smoke) or air (control) for 2 months (left panel) or 9 months (right panel). (B) Densitometric quantification of Pcdh1 protein levels of full-length 2 and the 50 kD fragment, relative to Histone H3, after 2 months of CS exposure. (C) Densitometric quantification of Pcdh1 protein levels of full-length 2 and the 50 kD fragment, relative to Histone H3, after 9 months of CS exposure. Cig = cigarette; † = time-point at which mice are sacrificed; CS = cigarette smoke.

mice [26] and guinea pigs [27]. While PCDH1 was identified as a susceptibility gene for AHR originally, our data are merely associative: reduced Pcdh1 expression levels are associated with a trend towards AHR to methacholine, but no role for Pcdh1 in the regulation of AHR can be inferred from these data. Nevertheless, it will be of interest to test in future mechanistic experiments whether Pcdh1 protein has a direct protein-protein interaction with other epithelial proteins involved in the regulation of AHR, or whether loss of Pcdh1 induces a transcriptional response that induces an increased responsiveness to methacholine inhalation, for instance through decreased epithelial barrier function. CS is known to impair the epithelial barrier function, and thereby induces permeability of airway epithelium, as evidenced by a decrease in electrical [28] or trans-epithelial [3] resistance. Epithelial cells are interconnected by tight-junctions (TJ) and adherens junctions (AJ). CS exposure has been observed to delocalize the TJ adaptor molecule ZO-1 [29], and down-regulates several AJ adhesion molecules, including E-cadherin

[30]. The resulting loss of TJ- and AJ stability may subsequently lead to loss of barrier function of the epithelium. As *PCDH1* was previously reported to have a role in cell-cell adhesion [31], we hypothesize that CS-induced decrease in Pcdh1 levels might contribute to the reduced epithelial barrier function after CS exposure. Since we only provide data on the association of reduced Pcdh1 expression levels after CS exposure, future mechanistic studies in for instance Pcdh1 knock-out mice will need to address whether Pcdh1 has any functional role in the CS-induced response by the airway epithelium, including loss of epithelial barrier function.

In conclusion, our data show that Pcdh1 is strongly conserved between mouse and man. Furthermore, our data are the first to show that *Pcdh1* mRNA expression is strongly regulated by CS-exposure, both in acute and chronic exposure models. Future studies on the function of Protocadherin-1, using novel knockout and/or transgenic approaches, and its interaction with environmental factors such as CS exposure are required to provide novel insights into the origins of airway hyperresponsiveness.

Acknowledgments

We would like to express our gratitude to our esteemed colleagues professors Wim Timens, Dirkje Postma and Huib Kerstjens (Departments of Pathology and Medical Biology, and of Pulmonology, University of Groningen, University Medical Center Groningen, the Netherlands) for supervision of the long-term cigarette smoke exposure mouse models (WT, DP, HK) and for advice and assistance with performing and interpreting immunohistochemistry (WT).

Author Contributions

Conceived and designed the experiments: HK AO MH GK MN. Performed the experiments: HK UB LB RG MT MR CB BMW IS. Analyzed the data: HK UB AO IS MH GK CB BMW MN. Wrote the manuscript: HK GK MN. Critically reviewed the manuscript: HK AO UB LB RG MR CB MT MH BW IS GK MN.

References

1. Koppelman GH (2006) Gene by environment interaction in asthma. Curr Allergy Asthma Rep. 6: 103–111.
2. Ober C, Yao TC (2011) The genetics of asthma and allergic disease: A 21st century perspective. Immunol Rev 242: 10–30.
3. Xiao C, Puddicombe SM, Field S, Haywood J, Broughton-Head V, et al. (2011) Defective epithelial barrier function in asthma. J Allergy Clin Immunol. 128: 549–556.
4. Davies DE (2009) The role of the epithelium in airway remodeling in asthma. Proc Am Thorac Soc. 6: 678–682.
5. Kicic A, Hallstrand TS, Sutanto EN, Stevens PT, Kobor MS, et al. (2010) Decreased fibronectin production significantly contributes to dysregulated repair of asthmatic epithelium. Am J Respir Crit Care Med 181: 889–898.
6. Prefontaine D, Nadigel J, Chouiali F, Audusseau S, Semlali A, et al. (2010) Increased IL-33 expression by epithelial cells in bronchial asthma. J Allergy Clin Immunol 125: 752–754.
7. Pichavant M, Charbonnier AS, Taront S, Brichet A, Wallaert B, et al. (2005) Asthmatic bronchial epithelium activated by the proteolytic allergen der p 1 increases selective dendritic cell recruitment. J Allergy Clin Immunol 115: 771–778.
8. Hackett TL, Singhera GK, Shaheen F, Hayden P, Jackson GR, et al. (2011) Intrinsic phenotypic differences of asthmatic epithelium and its inflammatory responses to RSV and air pollution. Am J Respir Cell Mol Biol 45: 1090–1100.
9. Uller L, Leino M, Bedke N, Sammut D, Green B, et al. (2010) Double-stranded RNA induces disproportionate expression of thymic stromal lymphopoietin versus interferon-beta in bronchial epithelial cells from donors with asthma. Thorax 65: 626–632.
10. Ierodiakonou D, Postma DS, Koppelman GH, Boezen HM, Gerritsen J, et al. (2011) E-cadherin gene polymorphisms in asthma patients using inhaled corticosteroids. Eur Respir J 38: 1044–1052.
11. Nawijn MC, Hackett TL, Postma DS, van Oosterhout AJ, Heijink IH (2011) E-cadherin: Gatekeeper of airway mucosa and allergic sensitization. Trends Immunol 32: 248–255.
12. Koppelman GH, Meyers DA, Howard TD, Zheng SL, Hawkins GA, et al. (2009) Identification of PCDH1 as a novel susceptibility gene for bronchial hyperresponsiveness. Am J Respir Crit Care Med 180: 929–935.
13. Koning H, Sayers I, Stewart CE, de Jong D, Ten Hacken NH, et al. (2012) Characterization of protocadherin-1 expression in primary bronchial epithelial cells: Association with epithelial cell differentiation. FASEB J 26: 439–448.
14. Dephoure N, Zhou C, Villen J, Beausoleil SA, Bakalarski CE, et al. (2008) A quantitative atlas of mitotic phosphorylation. Proc Natl Acad Sci U S A 105: 10762–10767.
15. Rush J, Moritz A, Lee KA, Guo A, Goss VL, et al. (2005) Immunoaffinity profiling of tyrosine phosphorylation in cancer cells. Nature Biotechnol 23: 94–101.
16. Vanhalst K, Kools P, Staes K, van Roy F, Redies C (2005) Delta-protocadherins: A gene family expressed differentially in the mouse brain. Cell Mol Life Sci. 62: 1247–1259.
17. Yoshida K, Watanabe M, Kato H, Dutta A, Sugano S (1999) BH-protocadherin-c, a member of the cadherin superfamily, interacts with protein phosphatase 1 alpha through its intracellular domain. FEBS Lett 460: 93–98.
18. Redies C, Heyder J, Kohoutek T, Staes K, Van Roy F. (2008) Expression of protocadherin-1 (Pcdh1) during mouse development. Dev Dyn. 237: 2496–2505.
19. Vlahos R, Bozinovski S, Jones JE, Powell J, Gras J, et al. (2006) Differential protease, innate immunity, and NF-kappaB induction profiles during lung inflammation induced by subchronic cigarette smoke exposure in mice. Am J Physiol Lung Cell Mol Physiol. 290: L931–45.
20. Post S, Nawijn MC, Hackett TL, Baranowska M, Gras R, et al. (2011) The composition of house dust mite is critical for mucosal barrier dysfunction and allergic sensitisation. Thorax 67: 488–495.
21. Andersen CL, Jensen JL, Orntoft TF (2004) Normalization of real-time quantitative reverse transcription-PCR data: A model-based variance estimation approach to identify genes suited for normalization, applied to bladder and colon cancer data sets. Cancer Res 64: 5245–5250.
22. Heijink IH, Brandenburg SM, Noordhoek JA, Postma DS, Slebos DJ, et al. (2010) Characterisation of cell adhesion in airway epithelial cell types using electric cell-substrate impedance sensing. Eur Respir J 35: 894–903.
23. Botelho FM, Gaschler GJ, Kianpour S, Zavitz CC, Trimble NJ, et al. (2010) Innate immune processes are sufficient for driving cigarette smoke-induced inflammation in mice. Am J Respir Cell Mol Biol 42: 394–403.
24. Lock P, Ralph S, Stanley E, Boulet I, Ramsay R, et al. (1991) Two isoforms of murine hck, generated by utilization of alternative translational initiation codons, exhibit different patterns of subcellular localization. Mol Cell Biol 11: 4363–4370.
25. Haas IG, Frank M, Veron N, Kemler R (2005) Presenilin-dependent processing and nuclear function of gamma-protocadherins. J Biol Chem 280: 9313–9319.
26. Seymour BW, Schelegle ES, Pinkerton KE, Friebertshauser KE, Peake JL, et al. (2003) Second-hand smoke increases bronchial hyperreactivity and eosinophilia in a murine model of allergic aspergillosis. Clin Dev Immunol 10: 35–42.
27. Matsumoto K, Aizawa H, Inoue H, Koto H, Takata S, et al. (1998) Eosinophilic airway inflammation induced by repeated exposure to cigarette smoke. Eur Respir J 12: 387–394.
28. Heijink IH, Brandenburg SM, Postma DS, van Oosterhout AJ (2012) Cigarette smoke impairs airway epithelial barrier function and cell-cell contact recovery. Eur Respir J 39: 419–428.
29. Petecchia L, Sabatini F, Varesio L, Camoirano A, Usai C, et al. (2009) Bronchial airway epithelial cell damage following exposure to cigarette smoke includes disassembly of tight junction components mediated by the extracellular signal-regulated kinase 1/2 pathway. Chest 135: 1502–1512.
30. Shaykhiev R, Otaki F, Bonsu P, Dang DT, Teater M, et al. (2011) Cigarette smoking reprograms apical junctional complex molecular architecture in the human airway epithelium in vivo. Cell Mol Life Sci 68: 877–892.
31. Sano K, Tanihara H, Heimark RL, Obata S, Davidson M, et al. (1993) Protocadherins: A large family of cadherin-related molecules in central nervous system. EMBO J 12: 2249–2256.
32. van der Strate BW, Postma DS, Brandsma CA, Melgert BN, Luinge MA, et al. (2006) Cigarette smoke-induced emphysema: A role for the B cell? Am J Respir Crit Care Med 173: 751–758.

12

The Experimental Autoimmune Encephalomyelitis Disease Course Is Modulated by Nicotine and Other Cigarette Smoke Components

Zhen Gao[1,2], Jillian C. Nissen[1], Kyungmin Ji[1], Stella E. Tsirka[1,2*]

1 Department of Pharmacological Sciences, School of Medicine, Stony Brook University, Stony Brook, New York, United States of America, **2** Program in Neuroscience, School of Medicine, Stony Brook University, Stony Brook, New York, United States of America

Abstract

Epidemiological studies have reported that cigarette smoking increases the risk of developing multiple sclerosis (MS) and accelerates its progression. However, the molecular mechanisms underlying these effects remain unsettled. We have investigated here the effects of the nicotine and the non-nicotine components in cigarette smoke on MS using the experimental autoimmune encephalomyelitis (EAE) model, and have explored their underlying mechanism of action. Our results show that nicotine ameliorates the severity of EAE, as shown by reduced demyelination, increased body weight, and attenuated microglial activation. Nicotine administration after the development of EAE symptoms prevented further disease exacerbation, suggesting that it might be useful as an EAE/MS therapeutic. In contrast, the remaining components of cigarette smoke, delivered as cigarette smoke condensate (CSC), accelerated and increased adverse clinical symptoms during the early stages of EAE, and we identify a particular cigarette smoke compound, acrolein, as one of the potential mediators. We also show that the mechanisms underlying the opposing effects of nicotine and CSC on EAE are likely due to distinct effects on microglial viability, activation, and function.

Editor: Guadalupe Mengod, IDIBAPS, Spain

Funding: This work was supported by National Multiple Sclerosis Society awards CA1044A1 and PP181, National Aeronautics and Space Administration NNA14AB04A and National Institutes of Health R01NS42168 (ST), and National Institutes of Health K12GM102778 to JN. The funders had no role in study design, data collection and analysis, decision to publish, or preparation of the manuscript.

Competing Interests: Co-author Stella E. Tsirka is a PLOS ONE Editorial Board member. This does not alter the authors' adherence to PLOS ONE Editorial policies and criteria.

* Email: styliani-anna.tsirka@stonybrook.edu

Introduction

Cigarette smoking has emerged as a major risk factor for multiple sclerosis (MS) [1], an autoimmune disease of the central nervous system (CNS) that affects over 2.5 million people worldwide (National Multiple Sclerosis Society). Compared with non-smoking MS patients, smokers develop more severe symptoms and have more aggressive secondary progression. A dose-response relationship exists for cigarette smoking and MS severity, and the incidence of MS increases with prolonged smoking exposure [2–4]. However, the mechanism by which cigarette smoking promotes MS remains unclear.

Nicotine has been suggested to contribute to cigarette smoking's detrimental effects in the context of MS. As nicotine increases microvascular blood flow [5] and the permeability of the blood brain barrier (BBB) [6], these effects could suffice to promote significant BBB leakage, an event important in the initiation of MS [7]. Nicotinic acetylcholine receptors (nAChRs) are expressed by immune cells that play critical roles in MS, including T cells [8], macrophages/microglia [9] and dendritic cells [10], raising the possibility that nicotine might stimulate immunomodulatory pathways that initiate or accelerate MS progression. However, recent studies suggested that nicotine did not promote more severe symptoms during EAE -, but rather inhibited disease development [11]. Moreover, evidence supported the idea that the use of tobacco moist snuff is not associated with increased MS risk [12,13]. Since the use of moist snuff resulted in similar serum levels of nicotine to cigarette smoking, this suggested that components other than nicotine in cigarettes might actually underlie the adverse effects of cigarette smoking in MS.

Microglia are the resident macrophage-like immune cells in the CNS. They play critical roles during MS and its corresponding animal model (experimental autoimmune encephalomyelitis – EAE). Microglial activation is an early event in MS/EAE and persists throughout the course of the disease [14,15]. MS/EAE is characterized by predominance of pro-inflammatory (M1) microglia, although both M1 and anti-inflammatory (M2) microglia modulate MS/EAE progression [16]. Inhibition of microglial activation by either the tripeptide macrophage/microglial inhibitory factor MIF (TKP) or minocycline ameliorates EAE symptoms [17–19]. Moreover, we have shown that shifting microglial activation towards an M2 state leads to a corresponding shift of T cells towards immunoprotective phenotypes, resulting in improved EAE outcomes [20]. Therefore, microglia have key roles in determining MS/EAE pathogenic outcomes, and pharmacological fine-tuning of their function could greatly affect disease progression.

The findings we described above were paradoxical in that cigarette smoking has been identified as a risk factor for MS, while nicotine has been described as having beneficial effects during the EAE disease course [1–4,11]. We thus set out to examine whether the non-nicotine components of cigarette smoke underlay the linkage to MS/EAE development. In this study, we investigated and compared the roles of nicotine and non-nicotine components of cigarette smoke in EAE. Our results demonstrate that nicotine improves EAE symptoms, whereas cigarette smoke condensate (CSC), which contains the non-nicotine components of cigarette smoke but only 3% nicotine [21], worsens EAE severity during early stages of this model system, correlating with the presence of M1 microglia. These findings suggest that the non-nicotine components in cigarettes contribute to the detrimental effects to MS/EAE, while nicotine has strong potential as an MS therapeutic.

Materials and Methods

Animals

C57BL/6 (wild-type) mice were purchased from Jackson Laboratory and bred in-house under pathogen-free conditions on a 12-hour light/dark cycle. Access to food and water was *ad libitum*. All experimental procedures were in accordance to NIH guidelines and protocols approved by Stony Brook University Institutional Animal Care and Use Committee (IACUC) and the Division of Laboratory Animal Research.

EAE induction and evaluation

EAE was actively induced by subcutaneous injection of MOG_{35-55} peptide (MEVGWYRSPFSRVVHLYRNGK) as previously described [17,22]. Briefly, 8–10 week-old female wild-type mice were anesthetized with intra-peritoneal injection of atropine (0.6 mg/kg body weight) and 2.5% avertin (0.02 ml/g body weight). 300 μg MOG was emulsified in complete Freund's adjuvant (CFA, DIFCO) supplemented with 500 μg of heat-inactivated Mycobacterium tuberculosis (DIFCO) and injected into the mouse hind-flank on day 0. On day 7, mice were boosted with injection of 300 μg of MOG into the other flank. 500 ng pertussis toxin (List Biologicals) was injected intra-peritoneally on day 0 and 2. The MOG_{35-55} peptide was purchased from Quality Controlled Biochemicals, Inc and from the Yale University Peptide Synthesis Facility.

EAE clinical symptoms were scored blindly starting on day 3 on a scale of 0 to 5 with gradations of 0.5 for intermediate symptoms. 0, no detectable symptoms; 1, loss of tail tone; 2, hindlimb weakness or abnormal gait; 3, complete paralysis of the hindlimbs; 4, complete hindlimb paralysis with forelimb weakness or paralysis; 5, moribund or death. Weights were measured weekly starting from day 0.

Quantification of Cotinine

The serum levels of cotinine, a metabolite of nicotine, were used as an indicator of nicotine levels in mice after nicotine and CSC delivery [23]. Blood samples were collected using sterile tubes without anticoagulants and left at room temperature for 30 minutes or until the blood was clotted. The tubes were then centrifuged at 3000 rpm for 10 minutes and the serum collected and stored at −80°C. Cotinine levels were measured using the Calbiotech cotinine direct ELISA kit following the manufacturer's protocol.

Drug delivery

The amount and concentration of the nicotine solution administered *in vivo* was adapted from the literature (Shi et al., 2009). 200 mg/ml nicotine ditartrate solution in saline was freshly prepared and loaded into mini-osmotic pumps (14-day or 28-day, infusion rate of 0.25 μL/h, Alzet), as previously described (Shi et al., 2009). Pumps were incubated in saline at 37°C overnight (14-day pumps) or for at least 40 hours (28-day pumps) to ensure a steady pump rate (0.25 μl/hr) and then implanted subcutaneously in the back of the mice. At 14 or 28 days of infusion, the serum cotinine levels were measured at 83.8 ng/ml (14-day infusion) and 85.7 ng/ml (28-day infusion), which is comparable to that found in heavy smokers (80–100 ng/ml) [24]. The preparation of CSC is at 40 mg/ml in DMSO (Murty Pharmaceuticals). Since DMSO can be delivered effectively by osmotic pumps only when it is diluted in water/saline (up to 50%), the pump-delivered working concentrations of CSC were 20 mg/ml and 10 mg/ml for the two types of pumps. After 14 days of infusion, the serum cotinine levels in mice with CSC pumps (20 mg/ml) were measured at 1.54 ng/ml. Control mice received pumps containing vehicle (saline or DMSO). We compared clinical scores of DMSO- and saline-treated mice. There was no difference between these two groups (Figure S1). This result is in agreement with results described in the literature [25]. Depending on experimental design, the pumps were implanted either immediately after, 14 days after, or 14 days before the first injection of MOG.

Tissue processing

Mice were deeply anesthetized with intra-peritoneal injection of 2.5% avertin (0.02 ml/g body weight) and then transcardially perfused using PBS (pH 7.4) followed by 4% paraformaldehyde (PFA)/PBS (pH 7.4). Spinal cords were isolated, post-fixed in 4% PFA/PBS at 4°C overnight, and dehydrated in 30% sucrose at 4°C until the samples sank. After the meninges were removed, the spinal cord was cut into equal sections, embedded in optimal cutting temperature compound (Tissue Tek), frozen and stored at −80°C until use.

Immunofluorescence

Coronal sections (25 μm) were prepared with a cryostat (Leica). Spinal cord sections were blocked in 3% BSA in PBS-T (0.3% TritionX-100 in PBS) and incubated with primary antibodies (rabbit anti-Iba1 1:500, Wako; mouse anti-iNOS 1:500, BD Biosciences; mouse anti-Arg1 1:500, BD Biosciences; rabbit anti-Caspase-3, 1:1000, R&D systems; rat anti-Mac2 1:1000, Cedarlane; rat anti-CD45, 1:1000, BD systems) overnight at 4°C. Incubation with fluorescence-conjugated secondary antibody at 1:1000 was performed for 1 hour at room temperature, followed by washing with PBS and mounting using Fluoromount-G with DAPI (Southern Biotech). 4–8 spinal cord sections in the lumbar region were imaged per biological replicate. In each section, 1–2 fields in the dorsal white matter and 5–6 fields in the ventral white matter (WM) were captured for analysis. ImageJ (NIH) was used to quantify the intensity of the fluorescent signals.

To quantify iNOS/Arg1 staining of spinal cords, images were taken at seven selected locations throughout the white matter that were consistent among all samples. For Iba1 intensity, images encompassing the entirety of a coronal section were taken, with seven images taken per animal. Values were quantified using ImageJ software by multiplying the staining intensity by the cell count, divided by the total tissue area. All quantification was non-blind.

For cell culture staining, primary microglia were seeded onto coverslips. After treatments, cells were stained using the protocol described above. Four fields selected at random per biological replicate were captured for imaging and quantification.

Eriochrome cyanine staining and measure of demyelination

Slides were incubated with acetone for 5 min, air-dried at room temperature for 30 minutes, stained in eriochrome cyanine (EC) solution (0.2% eriochrome cyanine RS (Sigma), 0.5% H_2SO_4 (Sigma), 0.4% iron alum (Sigma) in distilled water) for 30 min, sequentially differentiated in 5% iron alum (Sigma) for 10 minutes and in borax-ferricyanide solution (1% borax (Sigma), 1.25% potassium ferricyanide (Sigma), in distilled water) for 5 min, dehydrated through graded ethanol solutions and mounted using Permount (Fisher Scientific).

6–9 spinal cord sections in the lumbar region were imaged per biological replicate. ImageJ (NIH) was used to measure the demyelinated and total areas of WM. The final % value for demyelination was calculated using equation listed below:

$$Demyelinated\ area\ (\%) = \frac{Demyelinated\ area\ in\ white\ matter}{Total\ white\ matter\ area} * 100\%$$

Fluoromyelin staining

Slides were rehydrated in PBS for 5 minutes, incubated with fluromyelin staining solution (1:300) for 20 minutes at room temperature, washed, and mounted with Fluoromount-G (Southern Biotech). The ImageJ freeware (NIH) was used to measure the demyelinated and total areas of WM as described above.

Mixed cortical and primary microglia cultures

Mixed cortical cultures were prepared as previously described [26,27]. Briefly, newborn pups (d0–d2) of wild-type mice were decapitated and the cortices freed from meninges, hippocampi and midbrain and kept in HBSS (Cellgro) on ice. The cortical tissue was digested in 0.25% Trypsin/EDTA (Cellgro) at 37°C for 20 min and triturated mechanically. After filtration, the cell suspension was plated in mixed cortical medium (DMEM, 10% FBS, 1mM sodium pyruvate, 40 μg/ml Gentamycin) onto poly-D-lysine coated tissue culture dishes (37°C, 5 μg/ml PDL). Medium was changed 3 days after plating.

Microglia were harvested 10 days after plating by adding lidocaine (15 mM, Sigma) into the medium for 15 minutes at room temperature. The medium containing the floating microglia was collected and centrifuged at 1500 rpm for 5 min. The cell pellet was then resuspended in an appropriate volume of microglia medium (DMEM, 1% FBS) and the cell number counted. The purity of the microglial cultures was>98% as described previously [26,27]. The microglia were used for experiments after 24–48 hours of culture.

Primary hippocampal neuronal culture

Mouse hippocampi of newborn pups (P0) were dissected, digested (0.25% trypsin in HBSS) at 37°C for 20 minutes and then triturated to form single cell suspensions. The cell suspension was filtered and the cells plated in neuronal medium (Neurobasal with B27 supplements, 0.5 mM L-glutamine) at a density of 100,000 cells/well on PDL-coated 12-well plates. AraC (10 μM) was added to the medium on day 2 of the culture to inhibit glial growth and the media replaced on day 4. After being cultured for 12 days, the neurons were treated with 100 μM glutamate for 24 hours and the medium collected and kept at −80°C until use.

ELISA

Protein concentrations were measured using the Bio-Rad protein assay kit. Mouse TNF-α/IL-10 ELISA kit (eBioscience) was measured according to the manufacturer's instructions. In brief, a 96-well plate was coated overnight with capturing antibody. The antibody was then blocked with assay diluent for 1 hour at room temperature. 100 μl of samples or cytokine standards diluted in assay diluent were added and incubated for 2 hours at room temperature. Biotin-conjugated detection antibody, Avidin-HRP reagent, substrate solution and stop solution were then added into the wells sequentially and incubated for specific time-periods as per the protocol. Extensive washes were performed after each step. Absorbance at 450 nm was measured immediately by microplate reader after adding stop solution. Cytokine release was calculated using the equation below and the values normalized to neuronal conditioned medium (NCM)-treated samples.

$$Cytokine\left(\frac{pg}{mg}\right) = \frac{Re\ ading\ value\ from\ ELISA\ assay\left(\frac{pg}{ml}\right)}{protein\ concentration\left(\frac{mg}{ml}\right)}$$

Live/dead assay

Live/dead assay (Life Technologies) was conducted following manufacturer's instruction. Calcein AM (1:2000) and ethidium homodimer-1 (1:500) were added to the culture medium to label live and dead cells, respectively. Imaging was performed 10 minutes later; 4 fields were captured per biological replicate for quantification.

Analysis

Results are presented as an average with error bars indicating the standard error of the mean (Mean ± SEM). Two-way ANOVA was performed for multiple comparisons in clinical score and weight changes results. For other experiments, two-tailed *t*-test was used for comparisons between two groups. One-way ANOVA was performed for comparisons between multiple groups. Significance is indicated by $*p<0.05$, $**p<0.01$, $***p<0.001$.

Results

Non-nicotine components of cigarette smoke worsen EAE clinical symptoms, whereas nicotine attenuates the symptoms

To examine whether the non-nicotine components of cigarette smoke underlie the linkage to MS/EAE development, cigarette smoke condensate (CSC), a complex mixture of compounds that includes nicotine, was infused into mice using osmotic mini-pumps. The amount of nicotine in CSC is quite small, only approximately 2–3% of the total particulate matter (TPM). We first infused 10 or 20 mg/ml of CSC into EAE mice starting from day 0 of the protocol (the day when MOG was injected to initiate EAE) for 28 days. In the control (50% DMSO vehicle-treated) group, the clinical symptoms began around day 7, increased gradually, reached their peak between days 21–23, and then subsided (Fig. 1A). CSC infusion starting from day 0 resulted in similar EAE clinical symptoms (Fig. 1A). Since prior history as a smoker predisposes individuals to MS [4], we performed the experiment again using mice that were exposed to CSC for 14 days prior to MOG injection, in addition to infusion during the disease course. Using this paradigm, 20 mg/ml CSC significantly worsened EAE clinical scores during the early phase of the disease (day 12–15). For example, on day 13 the clinical score of CSC-treated mice was 2.31±0.69 as opposed to 1.38±0.25 for the vehicle-treated mice (Fig. 1B). However, it is possible that the effect of CSC on these animals was blunted by the presence of atropine used as pre-anesthetic. Atropine is a potent antagonist of muscarinic acetylcholine inhibitors, which have been shown to be expressed on a variety of immune cells. Further, studies have shown that atropine may have an effect on the immune system through suppressing inflammation [8]. Nevertheless, CSC application did not significantly change the peak or the cumulative score of EAE mice with the sample group sizes used in this experiment (Fig. 1D, E).

To assess nicotine's effect on EAE, a 200 mg/ml solution was infused into mice using osmotic mini-pumps. This dosage achieved steady-state serum levels of cotinine, a nicotine metabolite, at 83.8 ng/ml, which is comparable to the cotinine levels found in heavy smokers (80–100 ng/ml) [11,24]. Drug delivery started on day 0 of the experiment and lasted for 28 days. Our results showed that the mice treated with nicotine became symptomatic with a similar temporal pattern as saline vehicle-treated mice, but exhibited a significantly milder course of disease (Fig. 1C). The effects of nicotine on mean EAE scores achieved significance on individual days during the early stages (days 11, 12, and 14, and 17), at the peak (day 21), and beyond (Fig. 1C). The average peak score for the control mice in nicotine experiments was 3.2±0.2, meaning that these mice exhibited total paralysis of hindlimbs accompanied by weakness of forelimbs (Fig. 1D). In contrast, the average peak score for the nicotine-treated mice was 2.5±0.5, equating to paralysis in one leg or severe weakness of both legs but without paralysis. More generally, the nicotine-treated EAE mice exhibited a significantly lower cumulative score (30.7±3.3) in comparison to the vehicle-treated EAE mice (42.0±2.9), indicating an overall attenuation of the disease severity (Fig. 1E). Infusion of either 5 mg/ml or 10 mg/ml nicotine via osmotic pump, a concentration higher than the one found in CSC (calculated at 0.48 mg/ml in the 20 mg/ml CSC dose) [28], had no effect on disease scores (Figure S2), suggesting that the effect of the nicotine present in CSC is negligible. Taken together, the non-nicotine components in CSC worsened EAE scores during early stages, while nicotine administration significantly attenuated EAE severity.

Weight loss is another important hallmark of MS patients and EAE animals. Body weights of the vehicle-treated EAE mice were measured weekly. As expected, we observed that, while control vehicle-injected non-EAE mice steadily increased in weight during the 28 days, the EAE mice lost weight relative to controls as they became strongly symptomatic, and then gained weight during the recovery phase (Fig. 2A, B). CSC-treated EAE mice did not show differences from vehicle-treated animals on weight change during the experiment (Fig. 2A).

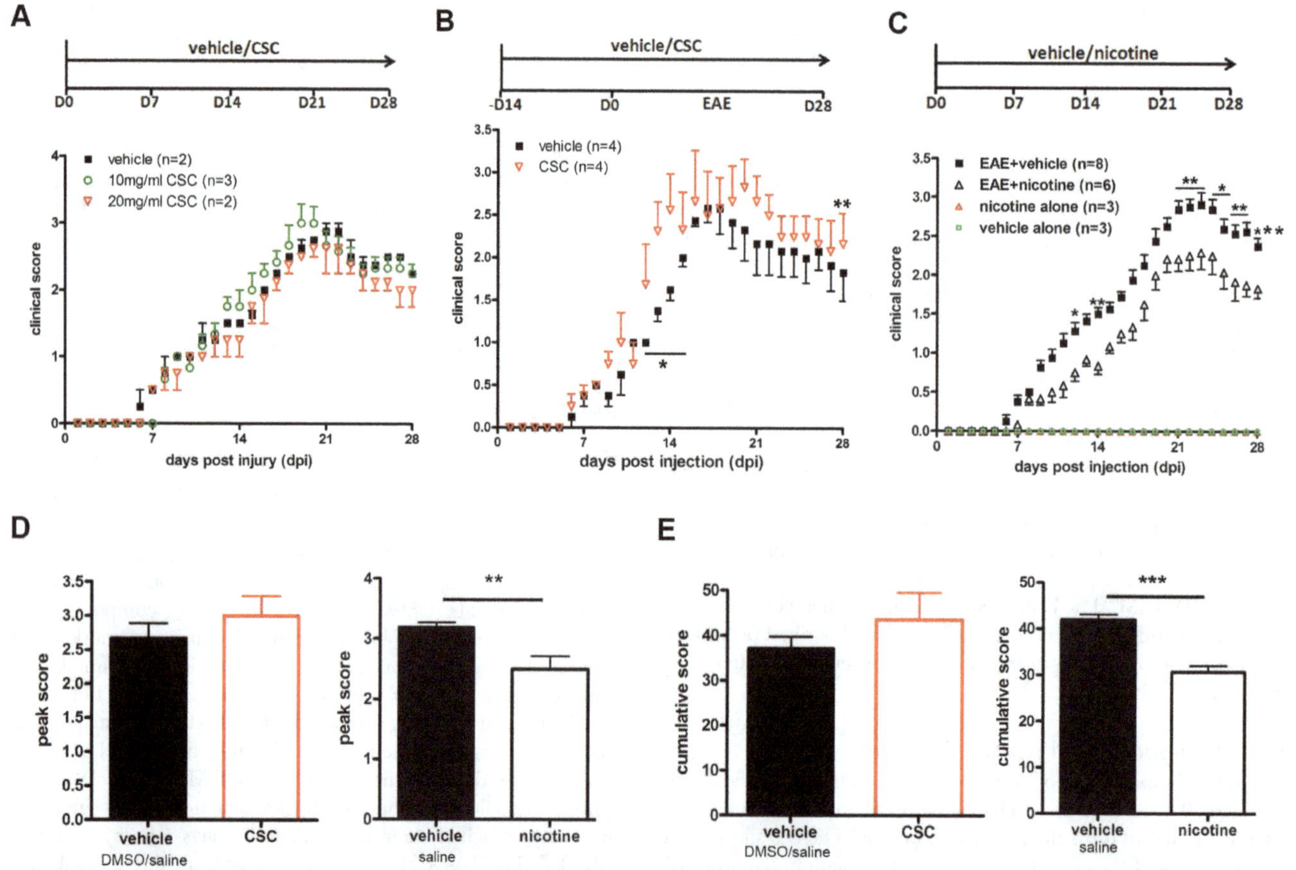

Figure 1. Effects of nicotine and non-nicotine components of cigarette smoke on EAE severity. EAE was induced by injection of MOG_{35-55} in CFA and pertussis toxin. **(A)** CSC was infused at 10 or 20 mg/ml into EAE mice starting at day 0 of EAE for 28 days, with DMSO as vehicle. **(B)** 20 mg/ml CSC was infused into the mice from 14 days prior to EAE induction through day 28, with 50% DMSO as vehicle. **(C)** Nicotine (200 mg/ml) was infused into EAE mice starting at Day 0 of EAE for 28 days, with saline as vehicle. Peak score **(D)** and cumulative score **(E)** were compared between CSC (n = 3)/nicotine (n = 6) and control mice (n = 8). (*** p<0.001; **p<0.01; *p<0.05).

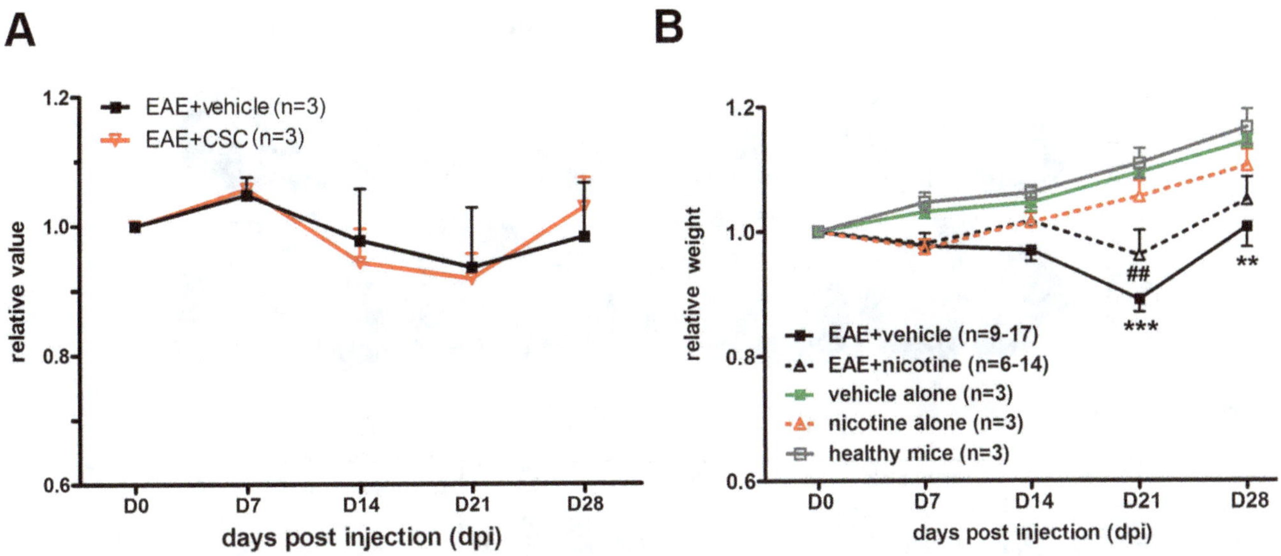

Figure 2. Weight changes of CSC- or nicotine-treated EAE animals. Weight changes were recorded and compared between vehicle (DMSO, n = 3 at all time points) and CSC- **(A)** or nicotine-treated **(B)** mice. In **(B)**, * denote significance compared to mice treated with vehicle (saline) alone (n = 3 at all time points). #: significance compared to mice treated with nicotine alone (n = 3 at all time points). Weights were plotted as a ratio over day 0 weights. (*** $p<0.001$; ** $p<0.01$; ## $p<0.01$). On day 28 there were n = 9 mice in the EAE+vehicle group and n = 6 in the EAE+nicotine group. On day 21 there were n = 12 mice in the EAE+vehicle group and n = 11 in the EAE+nicotine group. On days 0, 7 and 14 there were n = 17 mice in the EAE+vehicle group and n = 14 in the EAE+nicotine group.

Nicotine and non-nicotine components have distinct effects on EAE-induced spinal cord demyelination

EAE is characterized by focal demyelination of the spinal cord, which can be assessed by staining spinal cord sections with fluoromyelin or eriochrome cyanine (EC), which adheres to myelin, creating either fluorescent or intense blue coloration; demyelination thus presents as sites of hypo-colorization. Spinal cords analyzed from vehicle-treated EAE mice displayed no areas of focal demyelination at day 0 (the day of injection of MOG to induce EAE) and only infrequent sites at day 14, but had many foci of demyelination at days 21 and 28 (Fig. 3A, B), correlating with the peak severity of symptoms. In contrast, the areas of focal demyelination were less frequent and smaller in the nicotine-treated EAE mice. Quantitatively, equivalent amounts of demyelination (about 3.3–3.8%) were observed in vehicle- and nicotine-treated EAE mice at day 14, which correlated with only mild symptomology, but the demyelination became extensive in the vehicle-treated mice at days 21 (13.3±7.59% of the WM) and 28 (12.9±6.05%), whereas little additional demyelination was observed in the nicotine-treated EAE mice (5.1±3.07% on day 21 or 2.9±4.40 on day 28) (Fig. 3C).

In CSC-treated EAE samples, the demyelination at day 14 (6.33±0.83%), was three fold higher than the demyelination observed in control samples (2.16±0.4%, Fig. 4A, B). However, no significant difference in myelination was found between CSC- and vehicle-treated samples at day 28 (Fig. 4B). These results correlated with symptomology showed in clinical scores.

Taken together, our results indicate that the non-nicotine cigarette components in CSC have adverse effects on EAE severity, as evidenced by a higher clinical score and increased spinal cord demyelination. We also confirmed that nicotine does have protective effects on EAE outcomes, through reduced disease score, loss in body weight, and demyelination.

Nicotine and non-nicotine components have opposite effects on microglial activation during early EAE

As immune cell function is an essential component of disease progression and resolution in EAE, the immunomodulatory functions of nicotine could underlie the nicotine-induced protective effects described thus far. Microglia express most of the nicotine receptors that have been linked to immune-regulatory functions [29].

We have previously reported that changing the timing or decreasing the extent of microglial activation affects the outcome of EAE [17]. To evaluate whether nicotine and non-nicotine components in cigarette smoke affect microglial activation, anti-Iba1 antibody was used to visualize microglial morphology in the experimental settings previously described. Microglia in spinal cord sections prepared from control animals on day 0 of the experimental protocol exhibited the ramified morphology characteristic of non-activated, "resting" microglia (arrow, Fig. 5A). By day 14 of the EAE induction protocol, large numbers of microglia were clustered at the periphery of the WM in spinal cords from vehicle-treated mice and they exhibited an activated morphology characterized by enlarged cell bodies and retracted cell processes. However, CSC infusion into the spinal cord resulted in extensive peripheral clustering and widespread microglial activation and differentiation into amoeboid morphology (Fig. 5B), which characterized the highest levels of activation. In contrast, peripheral WM clustering of microglia was not observed in spinal cords sections prepared from the EAE mice treated with nicotine at this time point, and the microglia observed were predominantly still ramified, or had undergone only partial activation. By day 28 of EAE, microglia in both the vehicle and nicotine-treated spinal cord sections had begun to reverse their activation process while microglia in CSC-treated samples still remained activated.

Quantification of the anti-Iba1 staining intensity as a measure of microglial/macrophage number and activation revealed an increase in the EAE vehicle-treated sections at day 14 of the protocol but no increase in the nicotine-treated sections (quanti-

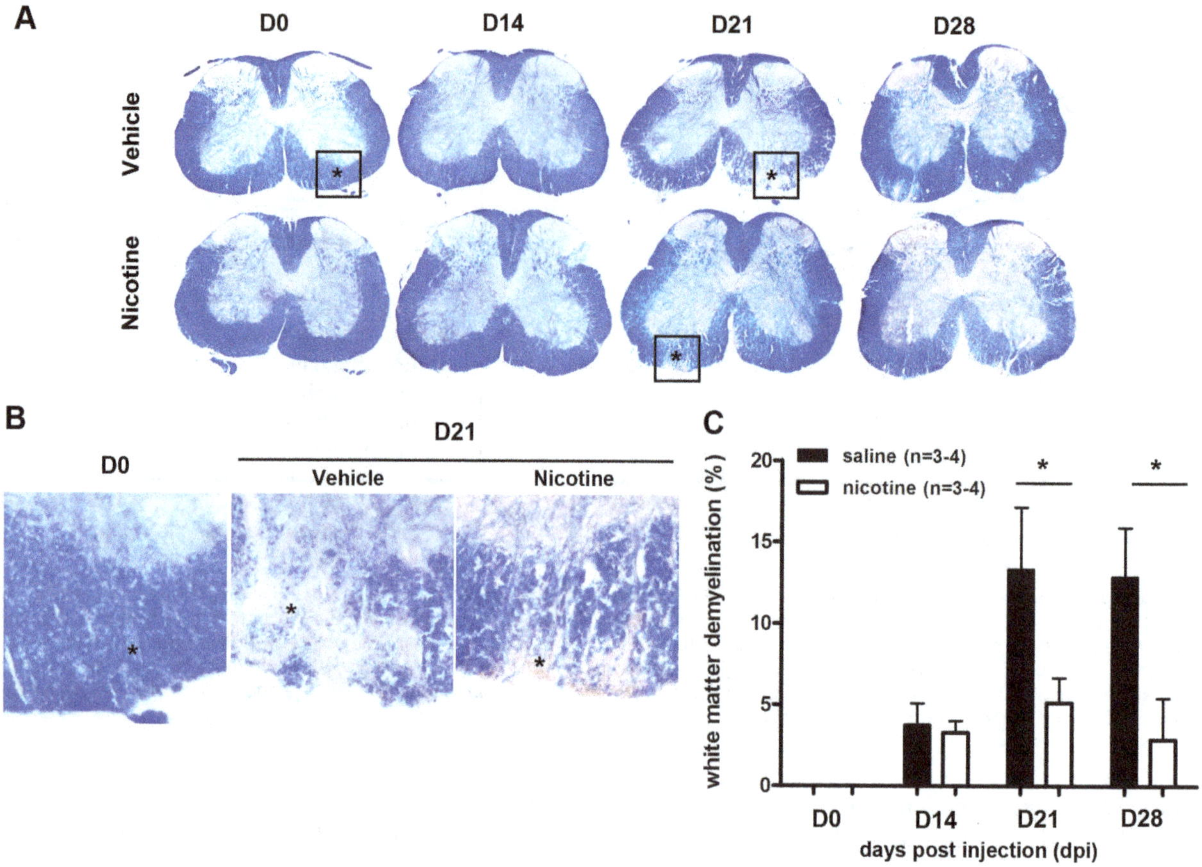

Figure 3. Decreased demyelination in nicotine-treated mice during EAE. (A) Frozen sections of spinal cords were isolated from vehicle (saline) and nicotine-treated mice at different time points during EAE. Eriochrome cyanine (EC) was used to visualize demyelination. Intact white matter (WM) is indicated by the blue staining and demyelination is revealed by diminished color. Areas of demyelination are indicated by asterisks; boxed regions are shown at higher magnification. **(B)** Demyelinated areas were measured using ImageJ and calculated based on equation listed in Methods. (n = 3–4, $^{*}p<0.05$).

fications in the graph). In contrast, Iba1+ immunofluorescence was almost 3 fold higher in CSC-treated animals at day 14 than in control sections (quantification in the graph), either due to increased microglial activation/proliferation or macrophage infiltration. These results demonstrate that non-nicotine components of cigarette smoke exacerbate microglial/macrophage activation at early time points of EAE while nicotine attenuates their activation.

Nicotine and non-nicotine components have opposing effects on the M1 microglial subpopulation in the white matter at early stages in EAE

Resting microglia differentiate into pro-inflammatory M1 microglia starting at the onset of EAE and remain detectable throughout the course of disease [16]. Differentiation of resting microglia into anti-inflammatory M2 microglia occurs less quickly and less efficiently, resulting in a predominance of M1 microglia and a pro-inflammatory milieu [15,30]. We showed above that microglial activation during EAE is stimulated by non-nicotine components in CSC, but suppressed by nicotine administration; here we address whether these distinct effects of nicotine and non-nicotine components of cigarette smoke are due to the different extent of their effect on microglial subtypes.

Microglia in the spinal cord white matter were generally found to express low levels of both M1 (iNOS) and M2 (Arg1) markers in the absence of disease; these cells were defined as M0 resting microglia (Fig. 6A). A small number of microglia with a predominantly resting phenotype expressed iNOS at high levels, but none were observed to express Arg1. Induction of EAE and microglial activation resulted in substantial increases in both M1 and M2 microglia (Fig. 6A, day 14 Vehicle), but the majority were of an M1 phenotype. ~73.2% of the microglia were activated at day 14 (Fig. 6D). Of these, 61.4±9.5% were iNOS+ (Fig. 6B) and 11.9±9.2% were Arg1+ (Fig. 6C).

CSC treatment did not significantly modify the ratios of iNOS+ M1 microglia (68.8±7.2, Fig. 6A, B) to Arg1+ M2 cells (12.1±3.8, Fig. 6A, C). In total, there was an increase in microglial activation after CSC treatment (80.9%, Fig. 6D, 5C). In contrast, only ~23.2% of the microglia in nicotine-treated samples became activated (Fig. 6A, D), primarily due to a reduction in M1 microglia (15.8±20.0%, Fig. 6B). There was also a decrease in M2 microglia after nicotine treatment (Fig. 6C); however, the effect on the M2 microglia was smaller and not significant.

Therefore, both nicotine and non-nicotine components in cigarette smoke regulate microglial activation by affecting the M1 microglial/macrophage subpopulation. CSC slightly enhances the M1 markers assessed, which leads to a pro-inflammatory environment in the CNS and a faster disease progression. In contrast, nicotine application significantly suppresses the M1 markers examined, including MHCII and CD86 (data not shown),

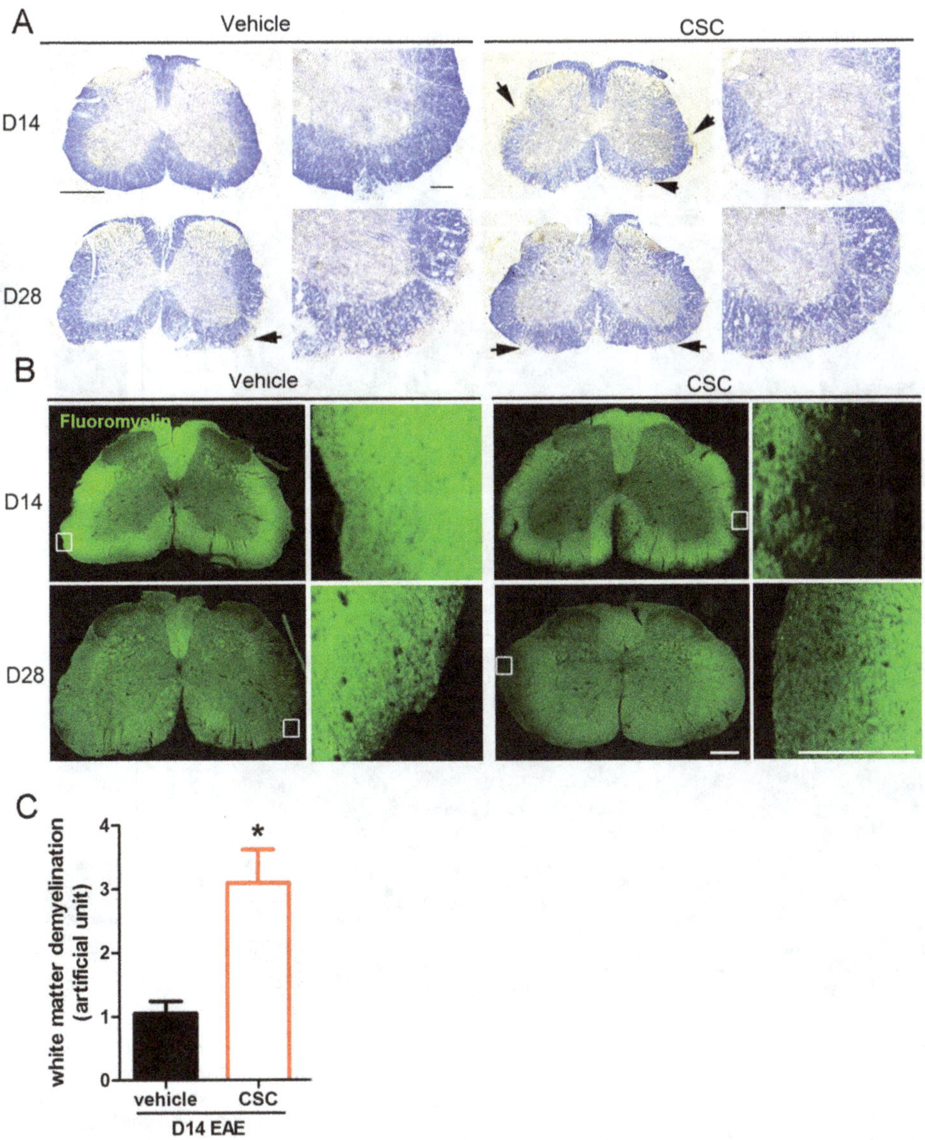

Figure 4. Increased demyelination in CSC-treated mice at day 14. Frozen sections of spinal cords were isolated from vehicle (saline/DMSO) and CSC-treated mice at day 14 and day 28 of EAE. Eriochrome cyanine **(A)** or fluoromyelin **(B)** was used to visualize demyelination. Areas of demyelination are indicated by diminished fluorescence; boxed regions are shown at higher magnification. **(C)** Demyelinated areas from **(B)** were measured using ImageJ and calculated based on equation listed in Methods (n = 4, $*p<0.05$). The levels of demyelination at day 14 in saline- or nicotine-infused spinal cords are also shown for comparison.

decreasing the M1 predominance, presumably creating a relatively anti-inflammatory environment and outcome.

Non-nicotine components in CSC have cytotoxic effects on microglia

To extend the findings above, we examined the effect of CSC on microglial activation and morphology *in culture*. At all concentrations used, CSC induced the microglia to change from a ramified morphology to the amoeboid state (arrows), while the same concentration of nicotine (approximately 40-fold greater than the nicotine found in CSC) did not have any effect (Fig. 7). Shrunken cell bodies were observed after CSC treatment (arrowheads, Fig. 7), suggesting that CSC might potentially be cytotoxic for microglia. This was found to be the case, as total cell death for microglia was increased with exposure to CSC but not nicotine (Fig. 8A), and this finding was even more dramatic for apoptosis, which increased more than 5-fold in the presence of CSC (Fig. 8B). These results were surprising, as *in vivo* administration of CSC promoted an increase in microglial activation (Fig. 5) and M1 polarization (Fig. 6). This could potentially be attributed to the fact that *in vitro* the CSC is acting exclusively on microglial cells, in the absence of other cell types. On the other hand, in the animal there are many more targets for CSC as well as a variety of interactions between microglia and other CNS cells, most likely astrocytes, which may be able to neutralize CSC-induced oxidative death. The drastic difference in microenvironment may be able to explain the difference between these experiments. The concentration of nicotine in CSC we applied was ~2–3%. To examine whether this low level of nicotine in CSC may contribute to any cytotoxic effects, nicotine (0.3 μg/ml nicotine for 10 μg/ml CSC and 1.2 μg/ml nicotine for

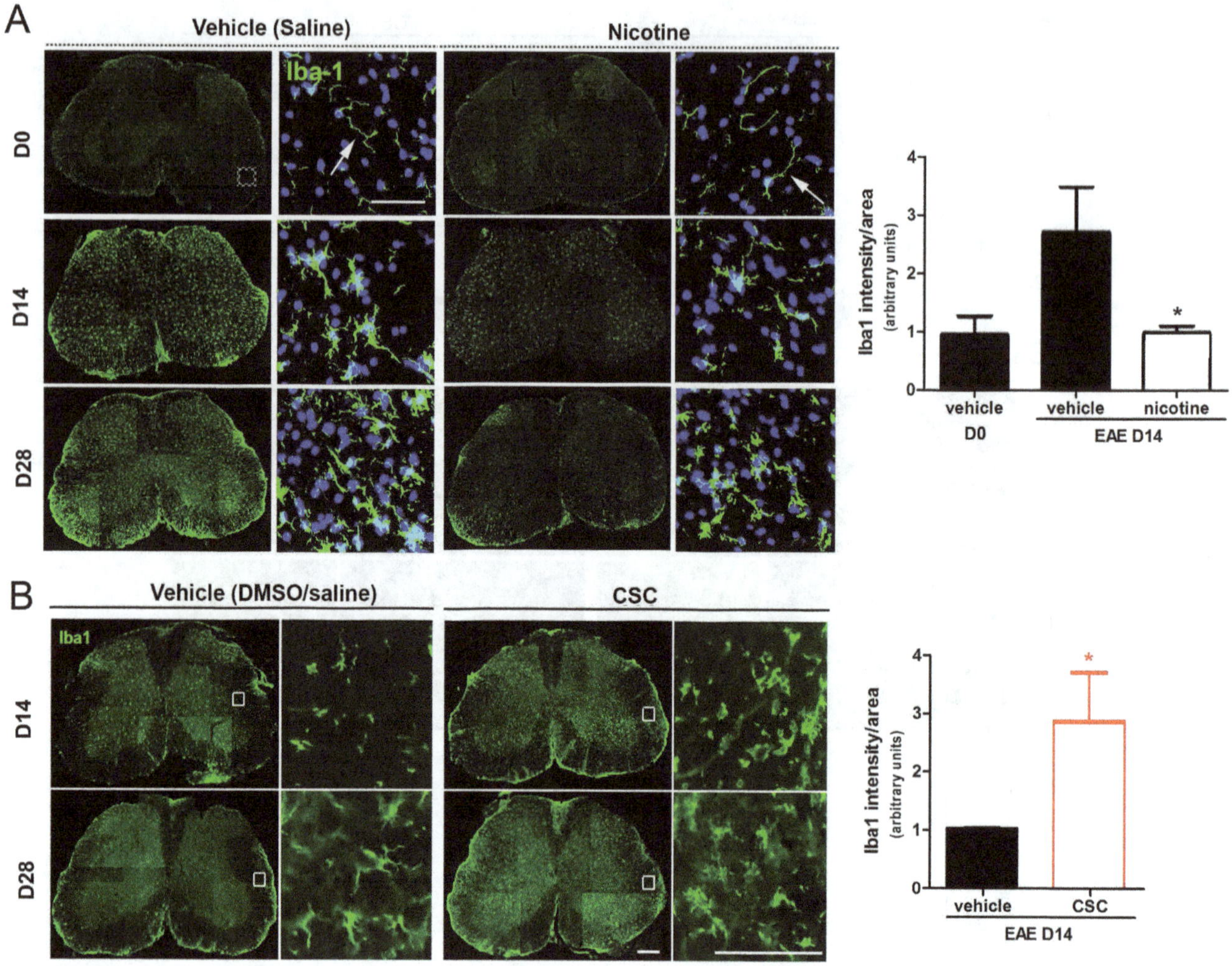

Figure 5. Effects of nicotine and non-nicotine components of cigarette smoke on microglia/macrophage activation during EAE. (A) Iba1 staining (green) was used to detect microglia in vehicle (saline), CSC-treated and nicotine-treated samples collected at D0, D14 and D28 during EAE. DAPI is indicated by blue fluorescence. Higher magnifications show morphologies of microglia in white matter (the box in D0 vehicle indicates the location of the high magnification images). **(B)** Iba1 staining (green) was used to detect microglia in vehicle (saline/DMSO) and CSC-treated samples collected at D14 and D28 during EAE. Quantification of Iba1 signals at days 0 and 14 of EAE after vehicle and nicotine (n = 3–4), or day14 CSC treatment (n = 4). Bar = 20 μm. *$p<0.05$.

40 μg/ml CSC) was added to the culture medium of primary microglia. Cell viability was not affected by nicotine (Figure S3), suggesting that non-nicotine components in CSC led to death of microglia. CSC showed a trend towards higher TNF levels released from the microglia, but this increase did not reach significance (Fig. 8C). Taken together, these findings again suggest that the non-nicotine components in CSC are responsible for the detrimental effects of cigarette smoke on microglial activation/ function and EAE outcome.

Acrolein contributes to the cytotoxic effects of CSC on microglia

Candidate compounds potentially responsible for the cytotoxic effects of CSC were explored. Acrolein, a volatile component of cigarette smoke, is a product of oxidative stress and lipid peroxidation, and increased expression of acrolein-lysine is found in EAE samples [31]. Inhibition of acrolein by hydralazine (an acrolein scavenger) has been reported to significantly improve behavioral outcomes for EAE [31]. We applied acrolein to microglia *in culture* to examine whether it could recapitulate the cytotoxic effects of CSC. Concentrations higher than 1 μg/ml killed all of cells (data not shown). Being treated with acrolein even at lower concentrations (0.1 μg/ml and 0.4 μg/ml) for 24 hours sufficed to elicit cell death to a significant extent (Fig. 9). These concentrations of acrolein are equal or lower than that contained in the CSC used in Fig 7. We calculated the concentration of acrolein as 0.18 μg/ml or 3.2 μM in the 40 μg/ml CSC (0.091 μg/ml in the 20 μg/ml and 0.045 μg/ml in the 10 μg/ml CSC). The calculation was based on the amount of total particulate matter (TPM) per 3R4F cigarette (which is 11 mg), and the amount of acrolein per cigarette (approximately 50 μg) [32–35]. Further, we observed that CSC elicited cell death in microglia at even higher levels than acrolein alone. However, when acrolein in CSC was inhibited through treatment with hydralazine, as previously described [36,37], this effect was significantly attenuated, although not completely reduced to control levels (Figure S4). Thus, our findings suggest that acrolein may, at least in part, mediate the cytotoxic effects of CSC. As acrolein can promote oxidative microglial cell death *in vitro*, we

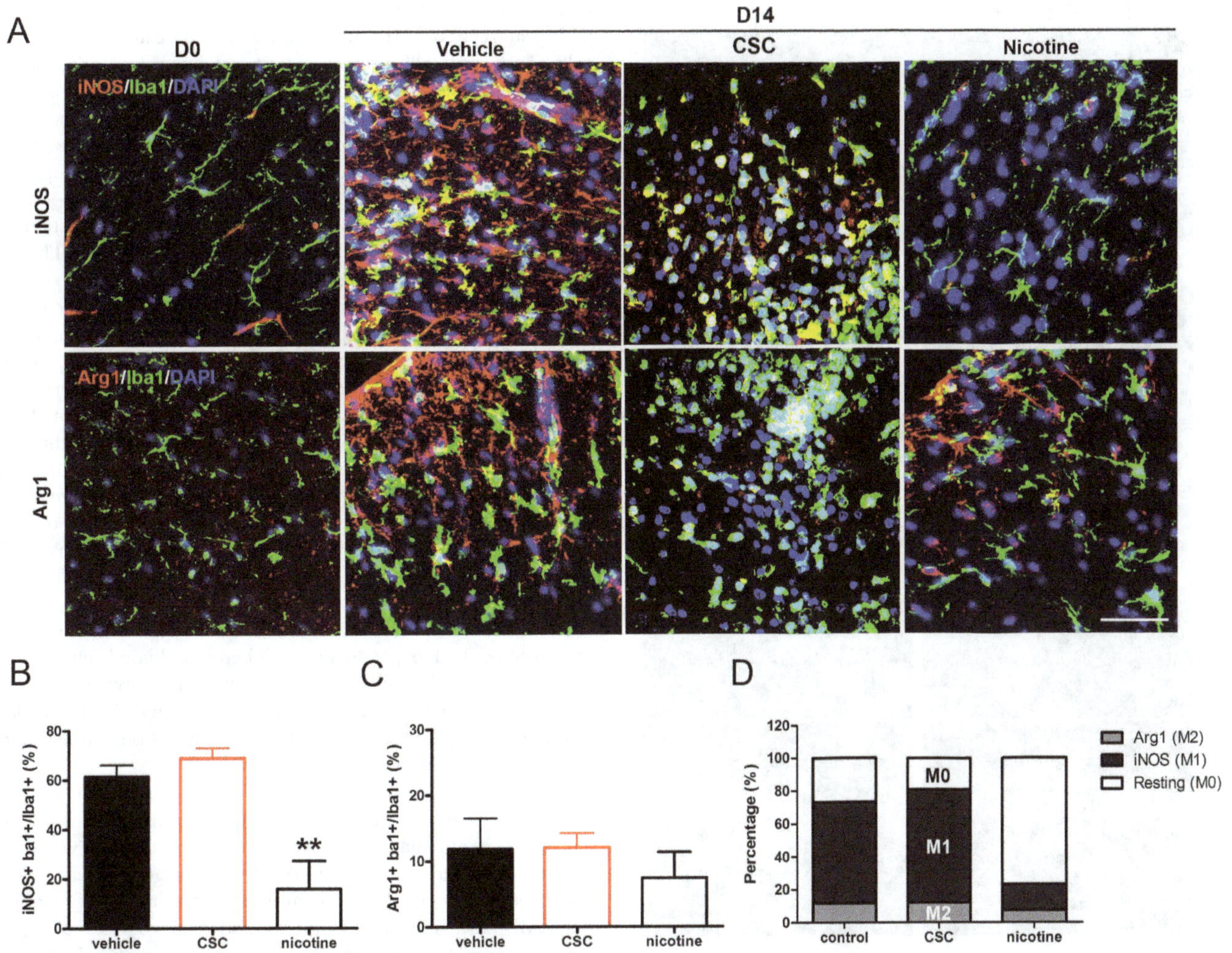

Figure 6. Non-nicotine components of cigarette smoke and nicotine have opposite effects on microglial state during early stages of EAE. (**A**) Resting Iba1+ (M0), pro-inflammatory (M1) and anti-inflammatory (M2) microglia were identified by labeling with anti-iNOS/Iba1 and anti-Arg1/Iba1, respectively. iNOS^{+}/Iba1^{+} (**B**) and Arg1^{+}/Iba1^{+} (**C**) cells were counted and compared between vehicle (pooled DMSO/saline samples) (n = 4) and CSC (n = 3)/nicotine-treated (n = 3) samples. Percentages of each population after treatment are indicated in (**D**). Bar = 50 μm (**p<0.01).

evaluated whether such oxidative damage also occurred *in vivo*. Spinal cords from mice treated with CSC or DMSO control were stained for nitrotyrosine, an indicator of oxidative stress. There was notable induction of nitrotyrosine in CSC-infused animals compared to controls, which suggests that acrolein has a similar mechanism during EAE (Figure S5). Taken together, these results provide one mechanism to potentially rationalize how CSC aggravates EAE, in particular in the earlier phases of the disease.

Nicotine has an anti-inflammatory function under MS/EAE relevant conditions in culture

The effect of nicotine on microglial activation was further examined using cell cultures. Glutamate excitotoxicity-induced neurodegeneration has been described in MS and observed in the EAE model [38,39]. To mimic the microglial microenvironment in MS/EAE, we treated primary microglia with neuronal conditioned medium (NCM) and measured the level of pro-inflammatory cytokine TNF-α in the microglial medium. As shown in Fig. 10A, nicotine supplementation decreased TNF-α release from NCM-stimulated microglia and the nicotine effect was dose-dependent, confirming that nicotine has an anti-inflammatory function under MS/EAE relevant conditions. Nicotine alone did not induce demyelination, inflammation or cell death, *in vivo* (Fig. 10B) or *in vitro* (Fig. 8).

Therapeutic nicotine administration attenuates EAE symptoms

Since nicotine confers benefits in EAE when provided during the initiation phase, we next assessed the possibility of using nicotine therapeutically, i.e., after the mice become symptomatic. Nicotine pumps were implanted in the backs of EAE mice at day 14, at which point the mice had developed mild clinical signs of disease (Fig. 11A). Although nicotine was not provided until after EAE initiation, when the mice were symptomatic, it still had a beneficial effect in that the symptom progression was halted (peak score of 2.25±0.25 as opposed to 2.80±0.30 for the vehicle-infused mice, Fig. 11A, B). Cumulative scores (32.3±3.3 versus 26.3±2.4, Fig. 11C) and body weights (Fig. 11D) were similarly different between the control and treatment groups. Therefore, nicotine could potentially be used as a therapeutic option if its utility in EAE is predictive for MS.

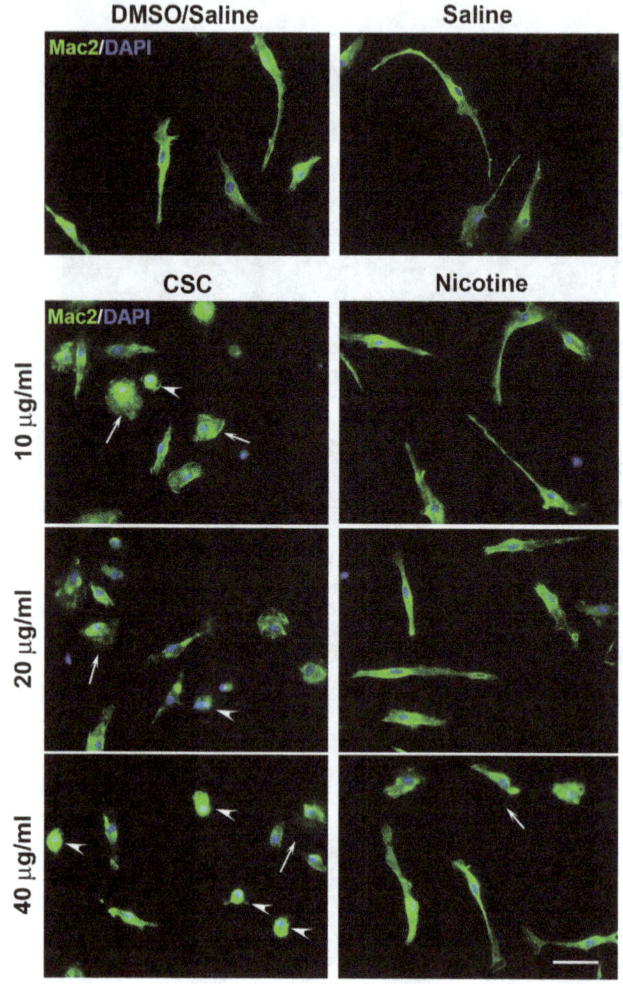

Figure 7. CSC exposure induces ameboid morphology in microglia. Primary microglia were treated with different concentrations of CSC and nicotine for 24 hours and cell morphology visualized by staining with Mac2 antibody. Arrows point to enlarged cell bodies and retracted cell processes. Arrowheads point to cell shrinkage after CSC treatment. (Bar = 20 μm, n = 4).

Discussion

It is well accepted that cigarette smoking increases susceptibility to MS and worsens the disease [1,40]. However, definition of the component(s) in cigarettes that mediate these effects has not been undertaken. In this study, we assessed the effects of nicotine and non-nicotine components of cigarette smoke on EAE. We found that nicotine significantly ameliorated EAE symptoms, including clinical score, demyelination, and microglial activation. In contrast, non-nicotine components worsened the disease severity at early stages of disease, including disease onset, demyelination and microglial activation, consistent with results from previous epidemiological studies showing that MS progressed faster in patients who smoked [4]. Our results suggest that the non-nicotine components could be responsible for the detrimental effects of cigarette smoking on MS, whereas nicotine may confer benefit.

Multiple factors could possibly contribute to nicotine's positive effects on EAE/MS, since nAChRs are found expressed on different cell populations, including neurons, microglia/macrophages [9], T cells [41], dendritic cells [10], and even oligodendrocyte progenitors [42] and endothelial cells [43]. Type 1 T helper cells (Th1) and Type 17 T helper cells (Th17) are the main pathogenic cells of EAE. Anti-inflammatory Th2 and regulatory T cells (Treg) normally protect against autoimmunity by inducing tolerance of self-antigens, however, their functions are impaired during the early stages of disease [44]. Nicotine has been shown to suppress the reactivity of pro-inflammatory T helper cells (Th1) and increase that of anti-inflammatory Th2 and immunosuppressive Treg cells in the CNS during EAE [11]. Moreover, as shown by Nizri *et al.*, *in vitro* nicotine exposure reduces production of Th1 and Th17 cytokines and induces a shift towards Th2 in response to an encephalitogenic antigen [45].

In this study, we focused on nicotine's effect on microglial functions during EAE. We previously demonstrated that changing the timing and extent of activation [17] or the differentiation path [22] of microglia changed the outcomes of EAE. Here, we examined nicotine's effect on microglia in the context of these states and found that nicotine significantly delayed and inhibited microglial activation during EAE, and that this inhibition primarily proceeded through suppression of M1 (iNOS$^+$) microglial differentiation. In culture, nicotine decreased TNF-α release from NCM-stimulated microglia. Previous studies demonstrated that M1 microglia promote T cell differentiation toward Th1 and Th17 fates [46], induce neurodegeneration [38] and impair remyelination [47]. These effects of M1 microglia were mediated primarily by TNF-α [38,46,48,49]. Therefore, biased suppression of M1 microglia through nicotine administration supports an anti-inflammatory environment, possibly re-balancing T cell populations, protecting neurons and myelin sheaths from insults, and promoting recovery of the tissues.

It was reported that nicotine inhibited microglia/macrophage activation primarily through binding to α7nAChRs [50,51]. Nevertheless, attenuation of EAE outcomes by nicotine was only partially reversed in α7-/- mice, which suggested that other nAChRs subunits might also contribute to the impact of nicotine on EAE [29]. Ohnishi *et al.* showed that, besides α7, β2-containing nAChRs were involved in nicotine's effects on thrombin-activated microglia [52]. In addition, α5 subunits contributed to immune regulatory functions, because the absence of α5 increased severity of experimental colitis [53]. Taken together, nicotine could potentially regulate microglia functions and EAE outcomes through targeting multiple nAChRs pathways.

In contrast, we demonstrated that CSC had a detrimental effect on EAE progression. However, the significant effect was only achieved during early stages of EAE. This might be due to the fact that the inflammation in mice due to ongoing EAE is more severe than the inflammatory effects mediated by this concentration of CSC. The highest concentration of CSC that we could use *in vivo* was 20 mg/ml, which contains only 2–3% of nicotine. If we had been able to deliver significantly higher concentrations of CSC, then more severe EAE symptoms might have been encountered. Nonetheless, we used CSC-treated EAE samples and cell culture to explore how CSC affects inflammation. Our results indicate that CSC both activates microglia, and eventually becomes cytotoxic to the cells. Other studies have shown that low concentrations of CSC induce inflammatory cytokine release from pulmonary macrophages, while higher concentrations cause cell death [54]. These reports support our findings that CSC enhances inflammation in EAE mice. We and others have previously shown that inhibition of microglia/macrophage function protects from EAE (e.g., Bhasin et al., 2007), further suggesting that CSC adversely affects EAE scores. Further, we have shown that inhibition of acrolein in CSC by hydralazine significantly reduces cell death in treated primary microglia. However, this effect does not fully rescue this phenotype, as there is still significantly more

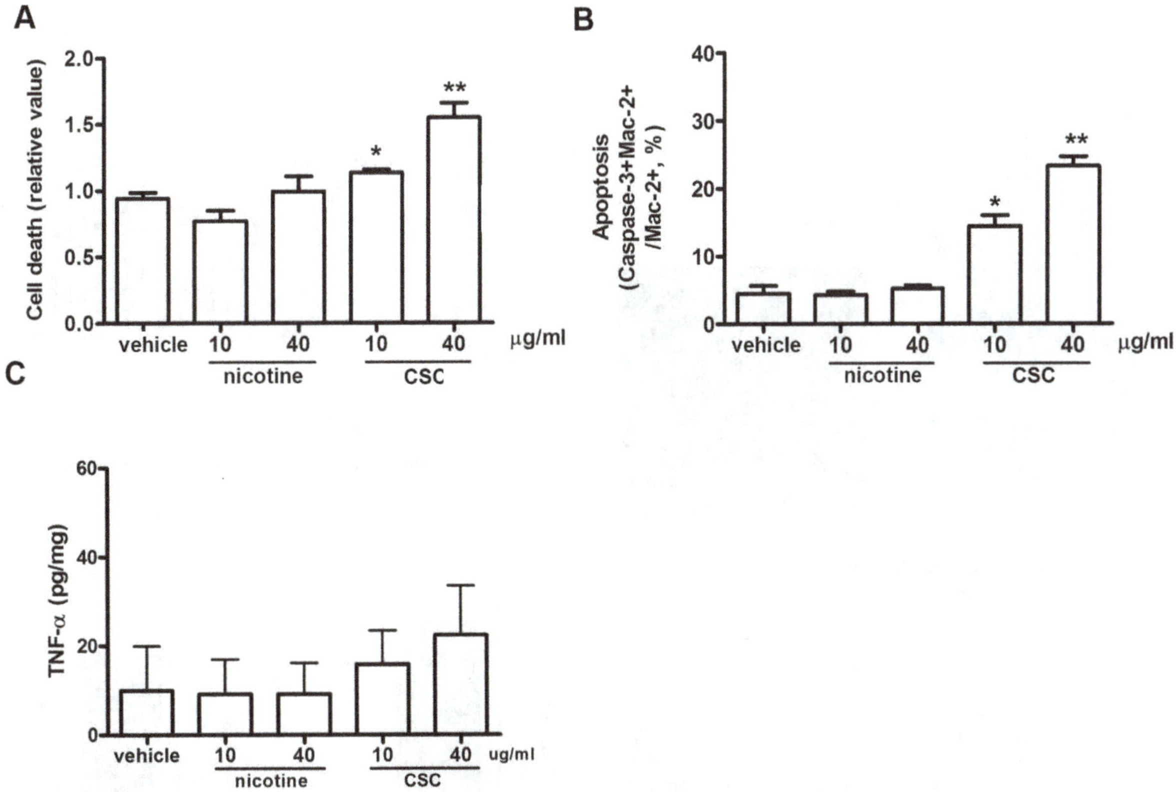

Figure 8. CSC exposure induces microglia apoptosis. Primary microglia were treated with the indicated concentrations of CSC or nicotine for 24 hours. **(A)** Media were collected and cell death was measured with a live/dead assay kit according to the manufacturer's instruction; (n = 4–7). Vehicle used was DMSO/saline. **(B)** apoptosis quantified through double staining with anti-Mac2 and anti-caspase-3. **(C)** TNF-α levels measured by ELISA as described in Methods. (n = 3; $^{**}p<0.01$; $^{*}p<0.05$ compared to vehicle).

cell death compared to controls. This suggests that acrolein could mediate part, but not all, of CSC's negative effects *in vitro* and *in vivo*.

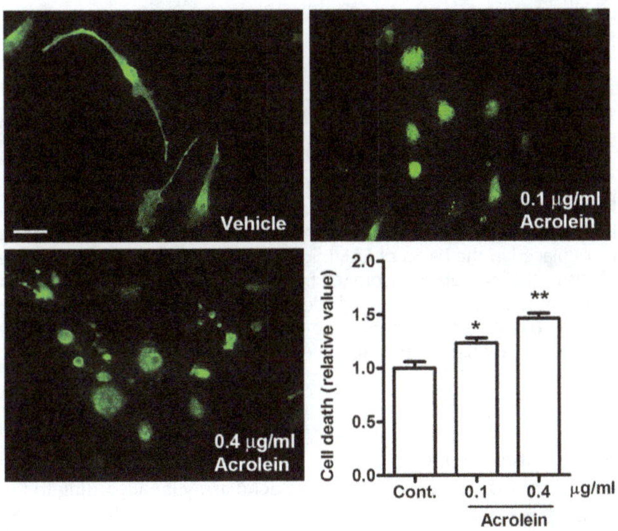

Figure 9. Acrolein induces cell death. Primary microglia were treated with acrolein for 24 hours and stained with Mac2 antibody. Cell death was quantified using a live/dead assay. Bar = 20 µm (n = 3; $^{**}p<0.01$; $^{*}p<0.05$).

As discussed previously, M1 microglia have detrimental effects during MS/EAE. However, it does not mean that pro-inflammatory mediators like M1 microglia and Th1 cells only contribute adversely to MS/EAE. Controlled microglial activation and T cell infiltration promote optic nerve recovery from injury [55]. Appropriate amounts of M1 differentiation have been shown to promote neurogenesis and oligogenesis, whereas excessive activation is inhibitory [48,49]. Rebalancing the pro-inflammatory and anti-inflammatory factors is critical for disease progression and recovery, which is supported by our results showing the opposite courses of disease development of CSC- and nicotine-treated EAE animals. Results from our lab and others suggest that nicotine could be a good candidate as an inflammatory regulator since it suppresses pro-inflammatory differentiation of microglia and T cells [45] without affecting cell viability. We also demonstrated that nicotine administration significantly limits exacerbation and disease severity in established EAE. This is the first study that provides evidence to support the proposal that nicotine could be used as a therapy for on-going MS. The therapeutic effect of nicotine transdermal patches on MS/EAE is currently under investigation. However, some considerations may apply to the proposal to use nicotine. Although nicotine ameliorated symptoms of EAE in our study here, it has been associated with inflammation in the respiratory system and cancer [56–58]. The potential side effects of nicotine patches will need to be evaluated carefully.

Recent studies by Odoardi *et al.* have demonstrated that the lung contributes to the T cell activation and migration that are required for MS/EAE initiation [59]. This may explain why lung infections are associated with MS progression. Importantly, there

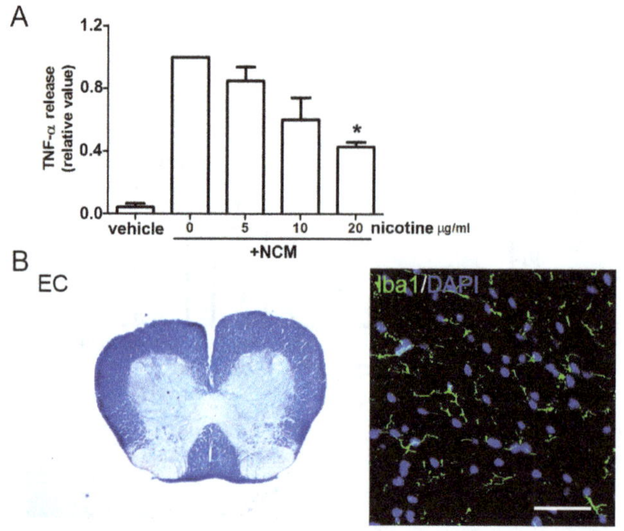

Figure 10. Nicotine has an anti-inflammatory function under MS/EAE relevant conditions in culture. (A) Primary microglia were exposed to nicotine for 30 minutes and then treated with conditioned medium from glutamate-stimulated neurons (NCM) for 24 hours. The media from the treated microglia were collected and TNF-α levels measured by ELISA as described in Methods (n = 4). **(B)** Frozen sections of spinal cords were isolated from mice treated with nicotine (28 days, 200 mg/ml nicotine ditartrate). EC staining was applied to visualize myelination in spinal cord sections. Inflammation was evaluated by staining of Iba1, CD45, Arg1 and iNOS. Staining of caspase-3 was used to visualize cell death. The results were compared with those from vehicle-injected mice. Bar = 50 μm (n = 3–4; *p<0.05).

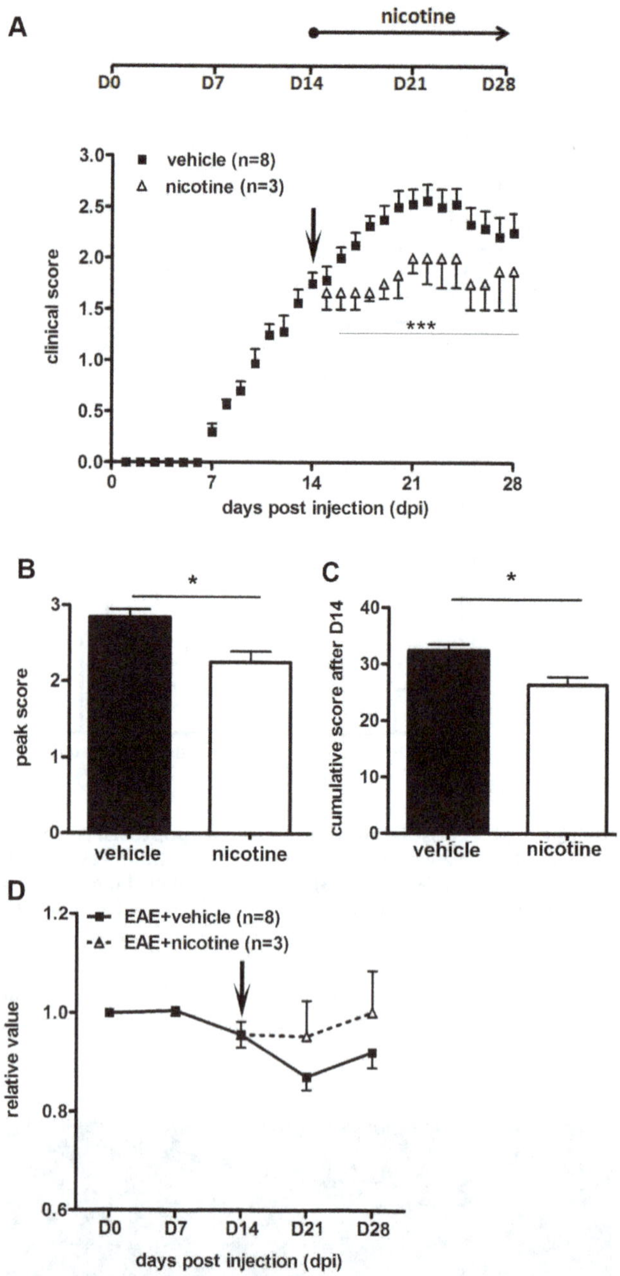

Figure 11. Therapeutic administration of nicotine attenuates EAE symptoms. (A) 14-day pumps filled with 200 mg/ml nicotine were placed in the backs of EAE mice at day 14 (***<0.001). Peak score **(B)** as well as cumulative score **(C)** from day 14 to day 28 were recorded and compared between the vehicle (n = 8) and nicotine-treated (n = 3) groups. **(D)** Weekly weights were plotted as a percentage of day 0 weights. (***p<0.001; *p<0.05)

are many components in cigarette smoke that can modify the physiology of the lung but have not yet been shown to have direct effects on the CNS. It is possible that one of the pathways through which CSC affects EAE is through changing the inflammatory environment in the lungs and thus altering T cell differentiation. However, the respiratory system was not included in our study because we used osmotic pumps to deliver the CSC systemically into mice and thus the CSC components did not directly interact with the respiratory system. As this method is not an accurate representation of the delivery of cigarette smoke in human MS patients, to better model the effects of CSC on MS/EAE, a method that subjects mice directly exposed to cigarette smoke, such as an inhalation chamber [60], may need to be employed.

Supporting Information

Figure S1 EAE scores using saline or saline/DMSO vehicles. EAE was induced by injection of MOG_{35-55} in CFA and pertussis toxin. Saline or DMSO in saline (50%) was infused into EAE mice starting at day 0 of EAE for 28 days. Peak score and cumulative score were compared.

Figure S2 Lower concentrations of nicotine do not have significant effects on EAE. EAE was induced by injection of MOG_{35-55} in CFA and pertussis toxin. Nicotine (10 mg/ml) was infused into the mice starting at Day 0, with saline as vehicle (n = 3 for each treatment).

Figure S3 Nicotine exposure does not affect microglial death. Primary microglia were treated with the indicated concentrations of nicotine for 24 hours. Media were collected and cell death was measured with a live/dead assay kit according to the manufacturer's instruction (n = 4).

Figure S4 Hydralazine reverses CSC-mediated cell death. Primary microglia were treated with 450 nM hydralazine, 40 μg/ml CSC, or both for 24 hours, with DMSO for control. Media were collected and cell death was measured with a live/

dead assay kit according to the manufacturer's instruction (n = 3, **p<0.01; *p<0.05).

Figure S5 CSC induces oxidative stress in mouse spinal cords during EAE. Spinal cord sections from D0 control and DMSO or CSC-infused animals on D14 and D28 post EAE induction were stained for nitrotyrosine (green), a marker for oxidative stress, or DAPI (blue). Bar = 50 μm.

Acknowledgments

We would like to thank members of the Tsirka lab and Drs. David Talmage and Michael Frohman for discussions and editing of the manuscript.

Author Contributions

Conceived and designed the experiments: ZG JN ST. Performed the experiments: ZG JN. Analyzed the data: ZG JN ST. Contributed reagents/materials/analysis tools: ZG JN KJ. Wrote the paper: ZG JN ST.

References

1. Handel AE, Williamson AJ, Disanto G, Dobson R, Giovannoni G, et al. (2011) Smoking and multiple sclerosis: an updated meta-analysis. PLoS One 6: e16149.
2. Hernan MA, Olek MJ, Ascherio A (2001) Cigarette smoking and incidence of multiple sclerosis. Am J Epidemiol 154: 69–74.
3. Pittas F, Ponsonby A, van der Mei I, Taylor B, Blizzard L, et al. (2009) Smoking is associated with progressive disease course and increased progression in clinical disability in a prospective cohort of people with multiple sclerosis. J Neurol 256: 577–585.
4. Sundstrom P, Nystrom L (2008) Smoking worsens the prognosis in multiple sclerosis. Mult Scler 14: 1031–1035.
5. Rowland LM, Beason-Held L, Tamminga CA, Holcomb HH (2010) The interactive effects of ketamine and nicotine on human cerebral blood flow. Psychopharmacology (Berl) 208: 575–584.
6. Hawkins BT, Abbruscato TJ, Egleton RD, Brown RC, Huber JD, et al. (2004) Nicotine increases in vivo blood-brain barrier permeability and alters cerebral microvascular tight junction protein distribution. Brain Res 1027: 48–58.
7. de Vries HE, Kooij G, Frenkel D, Georgopoulos S, Monsonego A, et al. (2012) Inflammatory events at blood-brain barrier in neuroinflammatory and neurodegenerative disorders: implications for clinical disease. Epilepsia 53 Suppl 6: 45–52.
8. Razani-Boroujerdi S, Boyd R, Davila-Garcia M, Nandi J, Mishra N, et al. (2007) T cells express alpha7-nicotinic acetylcholine receptor subunits that require a functional TCR and leukocyte-specific protein tyrosine kinase for nicotine-induced Ca2+ response. J Immunol 179: 2889–2898.
9. Wang H, Yu M, Ochani M, Amella C, Tanovic M, et al. (2003) Nicotinic acetylcholine receptor alpha7 subunit is an essential regulator of inflammation. Nature 421: 384–388.
10. Jin H, Li H, Sui H, Xue M, Wang Y, et al. (2012) Nicotine stimulated bone marrow-derived dendritic cells could augment HBV specific CTL priming by activating PI3K-Akt pathway. Immunol Lett 146: 40–49.
11. Shi FD, Piao WH, Kuo YP, Campagnolo DI, Vollmer TL, et al. (2009) Nicotinic attenuation of central nervous system inflammation and autoimmunity. J Immunol 182: 1730–1739.
12. Carlens C, Hergens MP, Grunewald J, Ekbom A, Eklund A, et al. (2010) Smoking, use of moist snuff, and risk of chronic inflammatory diseases. Am J Respir Crit Care Med 181: 1217–1222.
13. Hedstrom AK, Baarnhielm M, Olsson T, Alfredsson L (2009) Tobacco smoking, but not Swedish snuff use, increases the risk of multiple sclerosis. Neurology 73: 696–701.
14. van Noort J, van den Elsen P, van Horssen J, Geurts J, van der Valk P, et al. (2011) Preactive multiple sclerosis lesions offer novel clues for neuroprotective therapeutic strategies. CNS Neurol Disord Drug Targets 10: 68–81.
15. Zhang Z, Zhang ZY, Schittenhelm J, Wu Y, Meyermann R, et al. (2011) Parenchymal accumulation of CD163(+) macrophages/microglia in multiple sclerosis brains. J Neuroimmunol 237: 73–79.
16. Mikita J, Dubourdieu-Cassagno N, Deloire MS, Vekris A, Biran M, et al. (2011) Altered M1/M2 activation patterns of monocytes in severe relapsing experimental rat model of Multiple Sclerosis. Amelioration of clinical status by M2 activated monocyte administration. Mult Scler 17: 2–15.
17. Bhasin M, Wu M, Tsirka SE (2007) Modulation of microglial/macrophage activation by macrophage inhibitory factor (TKP) or tuftsin (TKPR) attenuates the disease course of experimental autoimmune encephalomyelitis. BMC Immunol 8: 10.
18. Defaux A, Zurich MG, Honegger P, Monnet-Tschudi F (2011) Minocycline promotes remyelination in aggregating rat brain cell cultures after interferon-gamma plus lipopolysaccharide-induced demyelination. Neuroscience.
19. Rasmussen S, Imitola J, Ayuso-Sacido A, Wang Y, Starossom SC, et al. (2011) Reversible neural stem cell niche dysfunction in a model of multiple sclerosis. Ann Neurol 69: 878–891.
20. Wu M, Nissen JC, Chen EI, Tsirka SE (2012) Tuftsin promotes an anti-inflammatory switch and attenuates symptoms in experimental autoimmune encephalomyelitis. PLoS One 7: e34933.
21. Matta SG, Balfour DJ, Benowitz NL, Boyd RT, Buccafusco JJ, et al. (2007) Guidelines on nicotine dose selection for in vivo research. Psychopharmacology (Berl) 190: 269–319.
22. Wu M, Tsirka S (2009) Endothelial NOS-deficient mice reveal dual roles for nitric oxide during experimental autoimmune encephalomyelitis. Glia 57: 1204–1215.
23. Benowitz NL (1996) Biomarkers of Cigarette Smoking. In: National Cancer Institute (U.S.). The FTC cigarette test method for determining tar n, and carbon monoxide yields of US cigarettes: report of the NCI Expert Committee., editor. Smoking and tobacco control monograph. Bethesda, MD: NIH (NIH Publication No 96-4028). pp. 93–111.
24. Paulson JR, Yang T, Selvaraj PK, Mdzinarishvili A, Van der Schyf CJ, et al. (2010) Nicotine exacerbates brain edema during in vitro and in vivo focal ischemic conditions. J Pharmacol Exp Ther 332: 371–379.
25. Matsuda R, Kezuka T, Nishiyama C, Usui Y, Matsunaga Y, et al. (2012) Suppression of murine experimental autoimmune optic neuritis by mature dendritic cells transfected with calcitonin gene-related Peptide gene. Invest Ophthalmol Vis Sci 53: 5475–5485.
26. Rogove A, Tsirka S (1998) Neurotoxic responses by microglia elicited by excitotoxic injury in the mouse hippocampus. Curr Biol 8: 19–25.
27. Zhai H, Heppner F, Tsirka S (2011) Microglia/macrophages promote glioma progression. Glia 59: 472–485.
28. Zhang W, Fang M, Song F, Windsor LJ (2011) Effects of cigarette smoke condensate and nicotine on human gingival fibroblast-mediated collagen degradation. J Periodontol 82: 1071–1079.
29. Hao J, Simard AR, Turner GH, Wu J, Whiteaker P, et al. (2011) Attenuation of CNS inflammatory responses by nicotine involves alpha7 and non-alpha7 nicotinic receptors. Exp Neurol 227: 110–119.
30. Murphy AC, Lalor SJ, Lynch MA, Mills KH (2010) Infiltration of Th1 and Th17 cells and activation of microglia in the CNS during the course of experimental autoimmune encephalomyelitis. Brain Behav Immun 24: 641–651.
31. Leung G, Sun W, Zheng L, Brookes S, Tully M, et al. (2011) Anti-acrolein treatment improves behavioral outcome and alleviates myelin damage in experimental autoimmune encephalomyelitis mouse. Neuroscience 173: 150–155.
32. Chen J, Higby R, Tian D, Tan D, Johnson MD, et al. (2008) Toxicological analysis of low-nicotine and nicotine-free cigarettes. Toxicology 249: 194–203.
33. Caito S, Rajendrasozhan S, Cook S, Chung S, Yao H, et al. (2010) SIRT1 is a redox-sensitive deacetylase that is post-translationally modified by oxidants and carbonyl stress. FASEB J 24: 3145–3159.
34. Roemer E, Schramke H, Weiler H, Buettner A, Kausche S, et al. (2012) Mainstream Smoke Chemistry and In Vitro and In Vivo Toxicity of the Reference Cigarettes 3R4F and 2R4F. Beitr Tabakforsch Int 25: 316–335.
35. Intorp M, Purkis S, Wagstaff W (2012) Determination of Carbonyl compounds in cigarette mainstream smoke. The CORESTA 2010 collaborative study and recommended method. Beitr Tabakforsch Int 25: 361–374.
36. Liu-Snyder P, Borgens RB, Shi R (2006) Hydralazine rescues PC12 cells from acrolein-mediated death. J Neurosci Res 84: 219–227.
37. Burcham P, Pyke S (2006) Hydralazine Inhibits Rapid Acrolein-Induced Protein Oligomerization: Role of Aldehyde Scavenging and Adduct Trapping in Cross-Link Blocking and Cytoprotection. Mol Pharmacol 69: 1056–1065.
38. Centonze D, Muzio L, Rossi S, Cavasinni F, De Chiara V, et al. (2009) Inflammation triggers synaptic alteration and degeneration in experimental autoimmune encephalomyelitis. J Neurosci 29: 3442–3452.
39. Pitt D, Werner P, Raine C (2000) Glutamate excitotoxicity in a model of multiple sclerosis. Nature Med 6: 67–70.
40. Salzer J, Hallmans G, Nystrom M, Stenlund H, Wadell G, et al. (2012) Smoking as a risk factor for multiple sclerosis. Mult Scler.
41. Cloez-Tayarani I, Changeux JP (2007) Nicotine and serotonin in immune regulation and inflammatory processes: a perspective. J Leukoc Biol 81: 599–606.
42. Rogers SW, Gregori NZ, Carlson N, Gahring LC, Noble M (2001) Neuronal nicotinic acetylcholine receptor expression by O2A/oligodendrocyte progenitor cells. Glia 33: 306–313.
43. Pillai S, Chellappan S (2012) alpha7 nicotinic acetylcholine receptor subunit in angiogenesis and epithelial to mesenchymal transition. Curr Drug Targets 13: 671–679.
44. Fletcher JM, Lalor SJ, Sweeney CM, Tubridy N, Mills KH (2010) T cells in multiple sclerosis and experimental autoimmune encephalomyelitis. Clin Exp Immunol 162: 1–11.
45. Nizri E, Irony-Tur-Sinai M, Lory O, Orr-Urtreger A, Lavi E, et al. (2009) Activation of the cholinergic anti-inflammatory system by nicotine attenuates neuroinflammation via suppression of Th1 and Th17 responses. J Immunol 183: 6681–6688.

46. Becher B, Bechmann I, Greter M (2006) Antigen presentation in autoimmunity and CNS inflammation: how T lymphocytes recognize the brain. J Mol Med 84: 532–543.
47. Li WW, Setzu A, Zhao C, Franklin RJ (2005) Minocycline-mediated inhibition of microglia activation impairs oligodendrocyte progenitor cell responses and remyelination in a non-immune model of demyelination. J Neuroimmunol 158: 58–66.
48. Butovsky O, Landa G, Kunis G, Ziv Y, Avidan H, et al. (2006) Induction and blockage of oligodendrogenesis by differently activated microglia in an animal model of multiple sclerosis. J Clin Invest 116: 905–915.
49. Butovsky O, Ziv Y, Schwartz A, Landa G, Talpalar A, et al. (2006) Microglia activated by IL-4 or IFN-gamma differentially induce neurogenesis and oligodendrogenesis from adult stem/progenitor cells. Mol Cell Neurosci 31: 149–160.
50. Moon JH, Kim SY, Lee HG, Kim SU, Lee YB (2008) Activation of nicotinic acetylcholine receptor prevents the production of reactive oxygen species in fibrillar beta amyloid peptide (1-42)-stimulated microglia. Exp Mol Med 40: 11–18.
51. Suzuki T, Hide I, Matsubara A, Hama C, Harada K, et al. (2006) Microglial alpha7 nicotinic acetylcholine receptors drive a phospholipase C/IP3 pathway and modulate the cell activation toward a neuroprotective role. J Neurosci Res 83: 1461–1470.
52. Ohnishi M, Katsuki H, Takagi M, Kume T, Akaike A (2009) Long-term treatment with nicotine suppresses neurotoxicity of, and microglial activation by, thrombin in cortico-striatal slice cultures. Eur J Pharmacol 602: 288–293.
53. Orr-Urtreger A, Kedmi M, Rosner S, Karmeli F, Rachmilewitz D (2005) Increased severity of experimental colitis in alpha 5 nicotinic acetylcholine receptor subunit-deficient mice. Neuroreport 16: 1123–1127.
54. Wickenden JA, Clarke MC, Rossi AG, Rahman I, Faux SP, et al. (2003) Cigarette smoke prevents apoptosis through inhibition of caspase activation and induces necrosis. Am J Respir Cell Mol Biol 29: 562–570.
55. Shaked I, Porat Z, Gersner R, Kipnis J, Schwartz M (2004) Early activation of microglia as antigen-presenting cells correlates with T cell-mediated protection and repair of the injured central nervous system. J Neuroimmunol 146: 84.
56. Liu J, Liang Q, Frost-Pineda K, Muhammad-Kah R, Rimmer L, et al. (2011) Relationship between biomarkers of cigarette smoke exposure and biomarkers of inflammation, oxidative stress, and platelet activation in adult cigarette smokers. Cancer Epidemiol Biomarkers Prev 20: 1760–1769.
57. Momi N, Ponnusamy M, Kaur S, Rachagani S, Kunigal S, et al. (2013) Nicotine/cigarette smoke promotes metastasis of pancreatic cancer through alpha7nAChR-mediated MUC4 upregulation. Oncogene 32: 1384–1395.
58. Warren G, Singh A (2013) Nicotine and lung cancer. J Carcinog 12: 1.
59. Odoardi F, Sie C, Streyl K, Ulaganathan VK, Schlager C, et al. (2012) T cells become licensed in the lung to enter the central nervous system. Nature 488: 675–679.
60. Mehra D, Geraghty PM, Hardigan AA, Foronjy R (2012) A comparison of the inflammatory and proteolytic effects of dung biomass and cigarette smoke exposure in the lung. PLoS One 7: e52889.

13

The Support for Smoke Free Policy and How It Is Influenced by Tolerance to Smoking – Experience of a Developing Country

Abdul Rashid[1]*, Azizah Ab Manan[2], Noorlia Yahya[2], Lailanor Ibrahim[2]

1 Department of Public Health Medicine, Penang Medical College, Georgetown, Penang, Malaysia, **2** Penang State Health Department, Georgetown, Penang, Malaysia

Abstract

This cross sectional survey was conducted to determine the support in making Penang UNESCO World Heritage Site (GTWHS) smoke free and to determine the influence of tolerance towards smoking on this support. This is the first phase in making Penang, Malaysia a smoke free state. A multistage sampling process was done to select a sample of respondents to represent the population of GTWHS. Attitude towards smoking was assessed using tolerance as a proxy. A total of 3,268 members of the community participated in the survey. A big majority (n = 2969; 90.9%) of the respondents supported the initiative. Support was lowest among the owners and residents/tenants, higher age groups, the Chinese, men, respondents who had poor knowledge of the places gazetted as smoke free, and respondents with poor knowledge of the health effects on smokers and on passive smokers. The odds (both adjusted and unadjusted) of not supporting the initiative was high among those tolerant to smoking in public areas. Tolerance towards smoking was associated with 80.3% risk of non-support in the respondents who were tolerant to smoking and a 57.2% risk in the population. Health promotion and education concerning the harm of tobacco smoke in Malaysia, which has mainly targeted smokers, must change. Health education concerning the risks of second hand smoke must also be given to non-smokers and efforts should be made to denormalize smoking.

Editor: Qinghua Sun, The Ohio State University, United States of America

Funding: The funding for this study was provided by the Malaysian health promotion board (MySihat), Grant number LPKM/04/061/01/321. The funder had no role in the study design, data collection and analysis, decision to publish or preparation of the manuscript.

Competing Interests: The authors have declared that no competing interests exist.

* Email: drrashid10@gmail.com

Introduction

Although smoking prevalence has reduced worldwide, both in men and women, the number of smokers has increased significantly and cigarette smoking is still the chief preventable killer in most countries [1–3]. In Malaysia, according to the Global Adult Tobacco Survey (GATS) 2011, 31% of adults aged 15 years and older were current tobacco smokers, more men (43.9%) than women (1.0%) and highest in the 25 to 44 age group. On the average an adult Malaysian smoked 14 cigarettes a day and among those who had ever smoked on daily basis only 9.5% had quit [4]. The World Health Organization (WHO) recommends a 30% relative reduction in current tobacco use in persons age 15 years and above [5].

Burning of tobacco produces a complex mixture of more than 7000 compounds which are risks for a wide range of diseases and premature deaths [2]. Cigarette smokers have an average 10 years reduced life span and the mortality among cigarette smokers is two to three times the mortality among persons who had never smoked [6]. At present most tobacco related deaths are reported in the developed countries but due to the change in smoking trends it is expected that more tobacco related deaths will occur in underdeveloped and developing countries [2],[6]. In Malaysia, tobacco related diseases accounted for the main causes of deaths in the hospitals operated by the Ministry of Health. Heart and pulmonary circulation diseases ranked first due to tobacco related illnesses followed by malignant neoplasms and cerebrovascular diseases [7]. Smoking not only effects morbidity and mortality but also quality of life, participation in workplace and increased health care costs [2].

Second hand smoke is equally if not more injurious to health [8]. In the United States (US) almost 2.5 million non-smoking Americans died from heart diseases and lung cancer due to exposure to second hand smoke. The loss of productivity due to exposure to second hand smoke is estimated to be about USD5.6 billion per year [2]. In Malaysia, it is estimated that 39.8% of adults who worked indoors have been exposed to second hand smoke and 38.4% adults exposed to second hand smoke at home, 84.9% in cafes/coffee shops/bistros, 78.7% in bars/nightclubs, 71% in restaurants, 28.2% in government buildings, 13.6% in indoor shopping complexes and 8.7% in health care facilities [7].

There are several interventions to combat smoking and the hazards of tobacco smoke. One is to target individual's smoking related attitudes or social influence by implementing anti-smoking policies including laws which discourage smoking [2],[9],[10]. Creation of smoke free areas is an effective intervention because it is easier to discourage people from smoking rather than encourage people to quit smoking once they have started [11],[12]. These smoke free areas not only help educate people on the dangers of second hand smoke but also help denormalize smoking by making smoking less socially acceptable and less convenient [2],[13],[14]. According to MPOWER which is a technical package on evidence based tobacco control interventions to reduce tobacco use to protect people from second hand smoke, all public places should be completely smoke free or at least 90% of the population should be covered by complete subnational smoke free legislation. Forty three countries comprising 1.1 billion people have achieved this level [11].

Malaysia became a signatory of the WHO Framework Convention on Tobacco Control (WHO FCTC) on the 23rd September 2003 and ratified it in 2005 and became an official party to the convention in December 2005. In 2011, as part of an initiative to comply with article 8 of the WHO FCTC, a proposal to create a smoke free zone in Penang, Malaysia was submitted to the Penang State Government with the objective to protect people from second hand smoke. The Ministry of Health had earlier gazetted 21 areas to be smoke free and as a start the Penang State Government had gazetted 6 recreational areas as smoke free zones. The current proposal was to include areas which had commercial and residential units. It was decided that George Town World Heritage Site (GTWHS) would be the first phase in making Penang a smoke free state. Studies conducted elsewhere had shown high level of support towards smoke free policies but different social and cultural values affect smoking habits and attitudes towards second hand smoke differently [15]. Thus before implementing the smoke free policy, a preliminary survey was conducted in this area to assess the level of support of the public to the proposal. The objective of this paper is to show the level of support towards the smoke free policy and the influence of tolerance to smoking on it.

Materials and Methods

Study design and Location

This cross sectional survey was conducted in Penang UNESCO World Heritage Site. The survey was commissioned by the Malaysian Health Promotion Board and the Penang State Government to determine the public and the stakeholders' support towards making Penang a smoke free state. The survey commenced from the middle of 2012 and ended in April 2013. Penang is one of the 14 states in Malaysia with a multi-ethnic population. It is one of the most densely populated states in the country with a population of 1,561,853. George Town, the capital of Penang, was inscribed as a UNESCO World Heritage Site on 7th July 2008 under Cultural Heritage Site category. This site features residential, commercial buildings, tourist sites and public open areas.

Sample

Multistage sampling process was done to select a sample of respondents to represent the population of GTWHS. Samples were taken from eating outlets, accommodation & hotels, places of worship, private and government offices, residences, retail & businesses, hawkers, education facilities, places of tourist attraction and public open spaces. Stata was used to calculate the sample size. Because each premise had a different population size, the sample from each premise was taken with a 5% margin of error. Within each premise/location, the type of respondent ranged from owner or senior management, employee, clients and the general public. This allowed the investigators to capture a wide range of respondents from the different levels. However because of the dynamic population, the study unit from each premise was taken based on the willingness to participate in the study.

Tool

Data were collected using face to face interviews by trained interviewers. The interviewers were trained comprehensively on accurate methods of data collection to avoid variations and to ensure uniformity. A uniform protocol covering the questionnaire, inclusion and exclusion criteria for each question was set up to minimize error and bias. Besides the baseline demographic information, the questionnaire was used to gather information on the support for making GTWHS a smoke free zone. Other independent variables related to the support including knowledge, attitudes and practices were also included in the questionnaire. Attitude towards smoking was assessed using tolerance as a proxy [16]. There were 16 items in the tolerance scale, the respondents were asked if they would tolerate smoking in 16 different public locations. Respondents were considered not tolerant to smoking if they answered they would not tolerate smoking in all the public places. The smoking tolerance items were examined using Mokken scaling to assess for fit to a single underlying dimension of tolerance. All items on the tolerance scale were selected by the Mokken scaling procedure, and the final scale had an H coefficient of 0·77, indicating that the items met the criteria for a unidimensional scale. The scale had high consistency level (Cronbach alpha reliability 0.97). The scale used to assess the tolerance towards smoking is in Appendix S1.

Analysis

Data were tabulated and cross tabulated. SPSS version 18 was used to analyse the relationship between the variables using Chi square test. Odds ratio was used to quantify the odds of not supporting the proposal and regression analysis to estimate support for smoke free zone using tolerance as predictor. Stata was used to measure the attributable risk in the exposed and in the population. A probability value of $P<0.05$ was considered to be statistically significant.

Ethics

The research had received the approval of the Joint Penang independent ethics committee (JPEC 01-13-0014). All respondents were asked to give a written informed consent before starting the interview. The anonymity of the respondents was assured.

Results

A total of 3,268 members of the community participated in the survey. Most of the participants were interviewed in business premises (n = 771, 23.6%) followed by offices (both government and private) (n = 455, 13.9%) and education premises (n = 404, 12.4%). The majority of the participants were clients/customers/ patrons/tourists/general public (44.6%) followed by owners (26.0%), employees (19.9%) and residents/tenants (11.4%). The majority were men (58.8%), age group 25 to 44 (37.6%), Chinese (60.3%), married (61.4%), income group of between RM1001 to 3000 (66.0%) and the highest level of education up to secondary school (51.7%). Most had never smoked (79.4%) and were aware of the national laws prohibiting smoking in certain areas (86.6%)

Table 1. Factors associated with non-support to making GTWHS a smoke free zone.

Variable	N	No support	Support	Chi square/P value
Respondent Type				24.76/<0.001
Owner	851	92 (10.8)	759 (89.2)	
Employee	584	38 (6.5)	546 (93.5)	
Clients/customers/patrons/tourists/general public	1459	114 (7.8)	1345 (92.2)	
Residents/tenants	374	55 (14.7)	319 (85.3)	
Age				9.99/0.01
≤24	688	61 (8.9)	627 (91.1)	
25–44	1229	91 (7.5)	1125 (92.5)	
45–64	1052	110 (10.5)	942 (89.5)	
≥65	299	37 (12.4)	262 (87.6)	
Gender				16.61/<0.001
Men	1923	209 (10.9)	1714 (89.1)	
Women	1345	90 (6.7)	1255 (93.3)	
Marital Status				0.38/0.95
Married	2008	186 (9.3)	1822 (90.7)	
Divorce	28	3 (10.7)	25 (89.3)	
Widow/widower	17	1 (5.9)	16 (94.1)	
Single	1215	109 (9.0)	1106 (91.0)	
Race				18.74/<0.001
Malay	634	43 (6.8)	591 (93.2)	
Chinese	1970	215 (10.9)	1755 (89.1)	
Indian	462	28 (6.1)	434 (93.9)	
Others	202	13 (6.4)	189 (93.6)	
Highest Level of Education				45.29/<0.001
Illiterate	61	12 (19.7)	49 (80.3)	
Non formal	29	24 (18.6)	105 (81.4)	
Primary	296	46 (15.5)	250 (84.5)	
Secondary	1691	144 (8.5)	1547 (91.5)	
Tertiary	1091	73 (6.7)	1018 (93.3)	
Income				9.71/0.01
≤RM1000	592	72 (12.2)	520 (87.8)	
RM1001 to 3000	2158	191 (8.9)	1967 (91.1)	
≥RM3001	518	36 (6.9)	482 (93.1)	
Smoking status				219.89/<0.001
Never smokers	2596	146 (5.6)	2450 (94.4)	
Past smokers	167	20 (12.0)	147 (88.0)	
Current smokers	505	133 (26.3)	372 (73.7)	
Awareness on the existence of national laws prohibiting smoking in certain areas				20.72/<0.001
Yes	2827	236 (8.3)	2591 (91.7)	
No	129	24 (18.6)	105 (81.4)	
Unsure	312	39 (12.5)	273 (87.5)	
Knowledge of places which are smoke free according to law				30.16/<0.001
Poor knowledge	998	133 (13.3)	865 (86.7)	
Good knowledge	2270	166 (7.3)	2104 (92.7)	
Health effects on smokers				122.59/<0.001
Poor knowledge	2825	103 (23.3)	340 (76.7)	
Good knowledge	443	196 (6.9)	2629 (93.1)	
Health effects on passive smokers				83.48/<0.001
Poor knowledge	1070	115 (18.7)	499 (81.3)	

Table 1. Cont.

Variable	N	No support	Support	Chi square/P value
Good knowledge	2198	184 (6.9)	2479 (75.6)	

and had good knowledge of places which were smoke free (69.5%). Most had good knowledge of the health effects of tobacco smoke on smokers (86.4%) as well as on passive smokers (81.2%). Although the majority were not tolerant to tobacco smoke (67.3%), a substantial proportion of the participants were tolerant (32.7%).

A big majority of the respondents supported (n = 2969; 90.9%) the smoke free initiative. As shown in Table 1, more than 10% of the owners and residents/tenants did not support the smoke free zone initiative ($\chi 2 = 24.76$; $P<0.001$). The support for the initiative decreased as the age group increased ($\chi 2 = 9.99$; $P = 0.01$). Among the races, Chinese had the highest non-support proportion ($\chi 2 = 18.74$; $P<0.001$). The support for the initiative increased with increasing education levels ($\chi 2 = 45.29$; $P<0.001$), similarly the support increased as the income bracket increased ($\chi 2 = 9.71$; $P = 0.01$). Support was highest among those who never smoked followed by past smokers and lowest among current smokers ($\chi 2 = 219.89$; $P<0.001$). The support for the initiative was lower among the men ($\chi 2 = 16.16$; $P<0.001$), respondents who had poor knowledge of places gazetted as smoke free ($\chi 2 = 30.16$; $P<0.001$), poor knowledge of health effects on smokers ($\chi 2 = 122.59$; $P<0.001$) and among passive smokers ($\chi 2 = 83.48$; $P<0.001$).

The tolerance to smoking among the respondents was 32.7%. As shown in Table 2, there is a six fold odds of not-supporting the smoke free initiative among those tolerant to smoking in public areas. Regression analysis showed that there was a fourfold odds of not supporting the initiative among those tolerant to smoking in public areas. Tolerance towards smoking was associated with 80.3% risk of non-support in the respondents who were tolerant to smoking and a 57.2% risk in the population.

Discussion

Tobacco control measures have avoided an estimated 8 million premature deaths and extended the mean life span by 19 to 20 years [17]. Although Malaysia is relatively new in actively adopting tobacco control policies, the ministry of health and several Non-Governmental Organizations (NGO) have been actively and consistently disseminating information pertaining to the risks associated with smoking to the public. This could explain the high level of support for the proposed smoke free policy which is comparable with that of developed countries [18–21] and other developing countries like Thailand [22]. The implementation of smoke free legislation has been shown to be effective even in low and middle income countries like Malaysia. In Uruguay the exposure to second hand smoke decreased greatly in indoor public places and workplaces after the implementation of the smoke free legislation [23].

In the present study, a higher proportion of owners and residents/tenants and the Chinese compared to others were non-supportive of the smoke free zone initiative probably because most owners of the premises/businesses in the area are Chinese and they fear that this proposal may affect their businesses. The support for the initiative was higher among women which is similar to the findings of studies conducted elsewhere [10],[16],[19],[24]. This could be because the prevalence of smoking among women is much lower compared to men. The correlation between education and level of support is because of the ability to understand the information on health and the increased self-awareness leading to the decision not to support unhealthy choices [10],[21]. Similarly poor knowledge is associated with lower support of smoke free policies [10],[20],[25],[26]. Better knowledge is associated with improved understanding of the risks associated with smoking and second hand smoke. Hence it is important to create awareness of the smoke free policies which has been shown to be associated with higher intolerance to smoking [27]. Education could also be a reason for the decrease in the support among the older age groups in this study. This finding contradicts the findings of studies conducted elsewhere which showed higher support among older respondents [10],[16],[18–20],[24]. In a relatively young country like Malaysia the younger age groups are more aware of the dangers of smoking and second hand smoke compared to the elderly whose level of education is lower and the knowledge on the adverse effect of smoking on health is limited [25]. The support from adolescents is important because they influence each other's habits though peer influence and social norms [27]. In general, support is high among those who never smoked and lowest among current smokers [18],[21],[26–28]. Although smokers and non-smokers generally believe that there is a harmful effect in passive smoking and both groups support tobacco control measures, non-smokers are usually more in favour of smoking bans than smokers [29]. Furthermore smokers whose social environments condone smoking are even less likely to support tobacco control policies [10].

The authors used tolerance to smoking as an indicator for attitudes towards smoking. Gilpin [16] indicated that a population's belief where smoking should not be allowed can be considered as an indicator of its attitude towards smoking. This study found about one in every third respondents was tolerant

Table 2. Tolerance to smoking and its associated risks of non-support to making GTWHS a smoke free zone.

Variable	Prevalence	Unadjusted Odds ratio	Adjusted odds ratio	Attributable risk exposed	Attributable risk population
Tolerance to smoking	32.7%	6.1 (4.7;7.9)	4.0 (3.0;5.4)	80.3%	57.2%

towards cigarette smoke and the attributable risk of tolerance to non-support was high. The tolerance to tobacco smoke is also high among European Union (EU) citizens where only about half of its citizens (57%) are bothered by the exposure to second hand smoke while 30% are rarely and 27% never bothered and most were concerned about the smell rather than the health consequences [19]. People living in countries with weak smoke free policies are more likely to be exposed to second hand smoke compared with people living in countries with comprehensive smoke free policies [30]. In Thailand where the tobacco control policies are better compared to Malaysia, Thai smokers are more likely to be concerned about harm to others than Malaysian smokers are and they are also more likely to support smoke free policies [22]. In Malaysia, health education and promotion has always mainly targeted smokers in an attempt to get them to quit smoking by primarily educating them on the hazards of smoking. Very little health promotional effort is made to educate the public concerning the harmful effects of second hand smoke. This has resulted in a lower proportion of people believing that breathing other peoples smoke causes serious illness in non-smokers [4]. One of the strategies to change the attitudes towards smoking is by adopting comprehensive smoke free policies which make smoking socially unacceptable. Strong smoke free policies are associated with favourable attitudes [31]. Even with minimal initial support, the adoption of smoke free policy has been shown to increase support over time and the resistance towards such policies diminish once implemented [24],[31–33]. Smoke free policies which are markers for denormalization and social unacceptability of smoking [25],[34] help protect non-smokers from exposure to second hand smoke and reduce tobacco use. Such policies also encourage cessation by providing a supportive environment to quit smoking and these policies reduce tobacco initiation among young people because of the lower visibility of role models, fewer opportunities and diminished social acceptability and social advantages for smoking. These policies eventually result in improved health [2],[12],[16],[29,35–44]. In the US, smoking was acceptable and considered normal prior to the 1964 surgeon general's report on the health effects of smoking. This changed after the report was published, non-smokers rights movement emerged and public policies were introduced to change the attitudes of the public to denormalize smoking by making it socially unacceptable to smoke everywhere. This resulted in reduced smoking rates and the protection of more than half of Americans from second hand smoke [2],[11],[13],[36],[45]. In California the tobacco programme aimed at changing social norms related to smoking by educating the public regarding the dangers of second hand smoke and the setting up of smoke free venues has been shown to be effective in changing population attitudes. Such was its success that smokers have been shown to be more considerate about not smoking in the presence of non-smokers. Furthermore because positive attitudes to smoke free public places stimulate adoption of smoke free homes,[46] more than half of all California smokers' homes were reported smoke free [47]. In most developed countries, as a result of the denormalisation and unacceptance of smoking in public areas, smoking habits now carry a connotation of being a filthy habit [48] and is associated with unemployment, low socioeconomic status and low education [49]. Smokers are ostracised and are obliged to smoke in unpleasant surroundings and in extreme weather conditions and are not eligible for insurance premium reductions as non-smokers [48]. These have helped reduce the prevalence of smoking and reduce the morbidity and mortality related to smoking [50].

Conclusions

Malaysian health promotion and education on tobacco control has mainly targeted smokers. This must change; education concerning the risks of second hand smoke should also be targeted towards non-smokers. The education provided can increase the knowledge on the adverse effects of tobacco smoke which will help reduce social acceptability of smoking. This will result in the acceptance of policies restricting second hand smoke and the reduction in smoking rates [35–37],[51–54] leading to reduced adverse health consequence [2],[55],[56]. Educating the public on the dangers of second hand smoke using mass media campaigns have been shown to be effective even on people with low levels of education [16],[53]. This would be an effective tool especially among the elderly Malaysians who have lower levels of education compared with the younger population. The information given can empower non-smokers to speak out against smoking habits [34] and win the support of smokers who will better understand the risks associated with second hand smoke which can trigger acceptance of society wide anti-smoking policies [9]. Mass media campaigns aimed at restructuring perception rather than sending pure anti-use messages [57] can also be used to assure hospitality industries that there is no negative economic impact on their businesses and that sales do not decline as a result of smoke free laws [44],[58].

Limitations

There are several limitations to the study. The main one concerns sampling. Due to the dynamic population in this study the investigators were unable to do probability sampling. However every effort was made to collect data from different levels of the sample units which included the owners or senior management, employees, clients and the general public.

What This Paper Adds

Denormalization of smoking has been shown to be an effective method of tobacco consumption control in most developed countries. In a developing country like Malaysia the focus of health education and promotion has been towards smokers in an effort to get them to quit smoking. Although this has been shown to be successful to some extent, the high tolerance to smoking is a cause of concern. There is a need to change the tobacco control strategies by focussing the health educational efforts towards non-smokers. The denormalization of smoking will not only help reduce uptake but also increase quit rates.

Acknowledgments

The authors would like to thank the Malaysian Health Promotion Board (MySihat), Ministry of Health Malaysia and the Penang State Government in making this survey a success. The authors would also like to thank Prof Ronan Conroy from the Royal College of Surgeons in Ireland for helping in the data analysis.

Author Contributions

Conceived and designed the experiments: AR AM NY LI. Performed the experiments: AR AM. Analyzed the data: AR. Wrote the paper: AR AM NY LI.

References

1. Communication D-Gf (2012) Attitudes of Europeans towards Tobacco. European Union: European Commission. 1–101 p.
2. Department of Health and Human Services US (2014) The Health Consequences of Smoking—50 Years of Progress. A Report of the Surgeon General. Atlanta, GA: Department of Health and Human Services, Centers for Disease Control and Prevention, National Center for Chronic Disease Prevention and Health Promotion, Office on Smoking and Health.
3. Ng M, Freeman MK, Fleming TD, Robinson M, Dwyer-Lindgren L, et al. (2014) Smoking prevalence and cigarette consumption in 187 countries, 1980–2012. JAMA 311: 183–192.
4. Health IfP (2012) Report of the Global Adult Tobacco Survey (GATS) Malaysia, 2011; Health NIo, editor: Ministry of Health Malaysia.
5. Organization WH (2013) Draft action plan for the prevention and control of non-communicable diseases 2013–2020. Geneva: World Health Assembly, World Health Organization.
6. Jha P, Peto R (2014) Global Effects of Smoking, of Quitting, and of Taxing Tobacco. New England Journal of Medicine 370: 60–68.
7. Malaysia MoH (2006) Annual report; System IaD, editor. Kuala Lumpur, Malaysia Ministry of Health Malaysia.
8. Diethelm PA, Rielle JC, McKee M (2005) The whole truth and nothing but the truth? The research that Philip Morris did not want you to see. Lancet 366: 86–92.
9. Zlatev M, Pahl S, White M (2008) Perceived risk and benefit for self and others as predictors of smokers' attitudes towards smoking restrictions. Psychology & Health 25: 167–182.
10. Doucet JM, Velicer WF, Laforge RG (2007) Demographic differences in support for smoking policy interventions. Addict Behav 32: 148–157.
11. Frieden TR (2014) Tobacco control progress and potential. JAMA 311: 133–134.
12. Chapman S, Borland R, Scollo M, Brownson RC, Dominello A, et al. (1999) The impact of smoke-free workplaces on declining cigarette consumption in Australia and the United States. Am J Public Health 89: 1018–1023.
13. Gutman M (2011) Social Norms and Attitudes About Smoking, 1991–2010. Princeton, New Jersey: Robert Wood Johnson Foundation.
14. Malone RE, Grundy Q, Bero LA (2012) Tobacco industry denormalisation as a tobacco control intervention: a review. Tob Control 21: 162–170.
15. Markham WA, Lopez ML, Aveyard P, Herrero P, Bridle C, et al. (2009) Mediated, moderated and direct effects of country of residence, age, and gender on the cognitive and social determinants of adolescent smoking in Spain and the UK: a cross-sectional study. BMC Public Health 9: 1471–2458.
16. Gilpin EA, Lee L, Pierce JP (2004) Changes in population attitudes about where smoking should not be allowed: California versus the rest of the USA. Tob Control 13: 38–44.
17. Holford TR, Meza R, Warner KE, Meernik C, Jeon J, et al. (2014) Tobacco control and the reduction in smoking-related premature deaths in the United States, 1964–2012. JAMA 311: 164–171.
18. Bakhturidze GD, Mittelmark MB, Aaro LE, Peikrishvili NT (2013) Attitudes towards smoking restrictions and tobacco advertisement bans in Georgia. BMJ Open 3: 2013–003461.
19. European Commission (2009) Attitudes of Europeans towards tobacco.
20. Danishevski K, Gilmore A, McKee M (2008) Public attitudes towards smoking and tobacco control policy in Russia. Tob Control 17: 276–283.
21. Maguire RL, Brinkley J, Mansfield C (2010) Custom Attitudes Toward Smoking Restrictions in Work Sites, Restaurants, and Bars Among North Carolinians. N C Med J 71: 511–518.
22. Yong HH, Foong K, Borland R, Omar M, Hamann S, et al. (2010) Support for and reported compliance among smokers with smoke-free policies in air-conditioned hospitality venues in Malaysia and Thailand: findings from the International Tobacco Control Southeast Asia Survey. Asia Pac J Public Health 22: 98–109.
23. Blanco-Marquizo A, Goja B, Peruga A, Jones MR, Yuan J, et al. (2010) Reduction of secondhand tobacco smoke in public places following national smoke-free legislation in Uruguay. Tob Control 19: 231–234.
24. Rosenberg M, Pettigrew S, Wood L, Ferguson R, Houghton S (2012) Public support for tobacco control policy extensions in Western Australia: a cross-sectional study. BMJ Open 2: 2011–000784.
25. Koh HK, Alpert HR, Judge CM, Caughey RW, Elqura LJ, et al. (2011) Understanding worldwide youth attitudes towards smoke-free policies: an analysis of the Global Youth Tobacco Survey. Tob Control 20: 219–225.
26. Ashley MJ, Cohen JE (2003) What the public thinks about the tobacco industry and its products. Tob Control 12: 396–400.
27. Unger JB, Rohrbach LA, Howard KA, Boley Cruz T, Johnson CA, et al. (1999) Attitudes toward anti-tobacco policy among California youth: associations with smoking status, psychosocial variables and advocacy actions. Health Educ Res 14: 751–763.
28. Poland BD, Cohen JE, Ashley MJ, Adlaf E, Ferrence R, et al. (2000) Heterogeneity among smokers and non-smokers in attitudes and behaviour regarding smoking and smoking restrictions. Tob Control 9: 364–371.
29. Thyrian JR, Panagiotakos DB, Polychronopulos E, Willemsen MC, Zatonski W, et al. (2010) The exposure to environmental tobacco smoke and attitudes towards tobacco control measures–a comparison of 5 European countries. Cent Eur J Public Health 18: 87–92.
30. Thrasher JF, Nayeli Abad-Vivero E, Sebrie EM, Barrientos-Gutierrez T, Boado M, et al. (2013) Tobacco smoke exposure in public places and workplaces after smoke-free policy implementation: a longitudinal analysis of smoker cohorts in Mexico and Uruguay. Health Policy Plan 28: 789–798.
31. Hyland A, Higbee C, Borland R, Travers M, Hastings G, et al. (2009) Attitudes and beliefs about secondhand smoke and smoke-free policies in four countries: findings from the International Tobacco Control Four Country Survey. Nicotine Tob Res 11: 642–649.
32. Thrasher JF, Boado M, Sebrie EM, Bianco E (2009) Smoke-free policies and the social acceptability of smoking in Uruguay and Mexico: findings from the International Tobacco Control Policy Evaluation Project. Nicotine Tob Res 11: 591–599.
33. Walsh RA, Paul CL, Tzelepis F, Stojanovski E, Tang A (2008) Is government action out-of-step with public opinion on tobacco control? Results of a New South Wales population survey. Australian and New Zealand Journal of Public Health 32: 482–488.
34. Glantz SA, Jamieson P (2000) Attitudes toward secondhand smoke, smoking, and quitting among young people. Pediatrics 106.
35. Callinan JE, Clarke A, Doherty K, Kelleher C (2010) Legislative smoking bans for reducing secondhand smoke exposure, smoking prevalence and tobacco consumption. Cochrane Database Syst Rev: CD005992.
36. Cummings KM (2002) Programs and policies to discourage the use of tobacco products. Oncogene 21: 7349–7364.
37. Fichtenberg CM, Glantz SA (2002) Effect of smoke-free workplaces on smoking behaviour: systematic review. Bmj 325: 188.
38. Fong GT, Hyland A, Borland R, Hammond D, Hastings G, et al. (2006) Reductions in tobacco smoke pollution and increases in support for smoke-free public places following the implementation of comprehensive smoke-free workplace legislation in the Republic of Ireland: findings from the ITC Ireland/UK Survey. Tob Control 15: iii51–58.
39. Hammond D, Fong GT, Zanna MP, Thrasher JF, Borland R (2006) Tobacco denormalization and industry beliefs among smokers from four countries. Am J Prev Med 31: 225–232.
40. Hublet A, Schmid H, Clays E, Godeau E, Gabhainn SN, et al. (2009) Association between tobacco control policies and smoking behaviour among adolescents in 29 European countries. Addiction 104: 1918–1926.
41. Hyland A, Li Q, Bauer JE, Giovino GA, Steger C, et al. (2004) Predictors of cessation in a cohort of current and former smokers followed over 13 years. Nicotine Tob Res 6: S363–369.
42. Martinez-Sanchez JM, Fernandez E, Fu M, Gallus S, Martinez C, et al. (2010) Smoking behaviour, involuntary smoking, attitudes towards smoke-free legislations, and tobacco control activities in the European Union. PLoS ONE 5: e13881.
43. Thomson G, Wilson N, Edwards R, Woodward A (2008) Should smoking in outside public spaces be banned? Yes. Bmj 337: a2806.
44. Viswanathan B, Plumettaz C, Gedeon J, Bovet P (2011) Impact of a smoking ban in public places: a rapid assessment in the Seychelles. Tob Control 20: 427–430.
45. Borland R, Yong HH, Siahpush M, Hyland A, Campbell S, et al. (2006) Support for and reported compliance with smoke-free restaurants and bars by smokers in four countries: findings from the International Tobacco Control (ITC) Four Country Survey. Tob Control 15: iii34–41.
46. Borland R, Yong HH, Cummings KM, Hyland A, Anderson S, et al. (2006) Determinants and consequences of smoke-free homes: findings from the International Tobacco Control (ITC) Four Country Survey. Tob Control 15: iii42–50.
47. Gilpin EA, Farkas AJ, Emery SL, Ake CF, Pierce JP (2002) Clean indoor air: advances in California, 1990–1999. Am J Public Health 92: 785–791.
48. Chapman S, Freeman B (2008) Markers of the denormalisation of smoking and the tobacco industry. Tob Control 17: 25–31.
49. Siahpush M, Borland R, Yong HH (2007) Sociodemographic and psychosocial correlates of smoking-induced deprivation and its effect on quitting: findings from the International Tobacco Control Policy Evaluation Survey. Tob Control 16.
50. Bayer R (2008) Stigma and the ethics of public health: not can we but should we. Soc Sci Med 67: 463–472.
51. Ashley MJ, Cohen J, Bull S, Ferrence R, Poland B, et al. (2000) Knowledge about tobacco and attitudes toward tobacco control: how different are smokers and nonsmokers? Can J Public Health 91: 376–380.
52. Cohen JE, de Guia NA, Ashley MJ, Ferrence R, Northrup DA, et al. (2002) Predictors of Canadian legislators' support for tobacco control policies. Soc Sci Med 55: 1069–1076.
53. Pierce JP, Macaskill P, Hill D (1990) Long-term effectiveness of mass media led antismoking campaigns in Australia. Am J Public Health 80: 565–569.
54. Rennen E, Nagelhout GE, van den Putte B, Janssen E, Mons U, et al. (2014) Associations between tobacco control policy awareness, social acceptability of smoking and smoking cessation. Findings from the International Tobacco Control (ITC) Europe Surveys. Health Educ Res 29: 72–82.

14

Hyperbolic Discounting: Value and Time Processes of Substance Abusers and Non-Clinical Individuals in Intertemporal Choice

Jiuqing Cheng*, Claudia González-Vallejo

Department of Psychology, Ohio University, Athens, Ohio, United States of America

Abstract

The single parameter hyperbolic model has been frequently used to describe value discounting as a function of time and to differentiate substance abusers and non-clinical participants with the model's parameter k. However, k says little about the mechanisms underlying the observed differences. The present study evaluates several alternative models with the purpose of identifying whether group differences stem from differences in subjective valuation, and/or time perceptions. Using three two-parameter models, plus secondary data analyses of 14 studies with 471 indifference point curves, results demonstrated that adding a valuation, or a time perception function led to better model fits. However, the gain in fit due to the flexibility granted by a second parameter did not always lead to a better understanding of the data patterns and corresponding psychological processes. The k parameter consistently indexed group and context (magnitude) differences; it is thus a mixed measure of person and task level effects. This was similar for a parameter meant to index payoff devaluation. A time perception parameter, on the other hand, fluctuated with contexts in a non-predicted fashion and the interpretation of its values was inconsistent with prior findings that supported enlarged perceived delays for substance abusers compared to controls. Overall, the results provide mixed support for hyperbolic models of intertemporal choice in terms of the psychological meaning afforded by their parameters.

Editor: Pablo Brañas-Garza, Middlesex University London, United Kingdom

Funding: The authors have no support or funding to report.

Competing Interests: The authors have declared that no competing interests exist.

* Email: jc311609@ohio.edu

These authors contributed equally to this work.

Introduction

Psychological research on behavioral control has widely used the intertemporal choice paradigm with results generally demonstrating a preference for immediate, smaller rewards over delayed, larger ones by animals and humans. This result is termed "temporal discounting" and the degree to which individuals discount has been linked to important life consequences such as creditworthiness [1] and indices of health behaviors such as exercise and smoking [2].

Early studies with pigeons showed that it was possible to find a point of indifference between a standard alternative with a constant reinforcement, and a moving alternative for which the contingencies changed depending on the choices of the subject [3]. The adjustment consisted of increasing or decreasing a delay to reinforcement based on the animal's previous choice. This procedure allows for the empirical derivation of a point of indifference between the two alternatives. The magnitude of this indifference point is conceived as a measure of the degree to which a future value is discounted.

Research on substance abuse has used the basic intertemporal choice paradigm to better understand impulsivity. The paradigm reflects the everyday choice that a substance abuser confronts: the drug offers an immediate euphoria (a sooner smaller reward), whereas not taking the drug offers future happiness and healthiness (a delayed larger reward). To date, studies have shown that substance abusers exhibit excessive preference for the sooner reward when compared to the behavior of healthy individuals [4]; hence, they are more impulsive [5]. The basis for the observed group difference is still not fully understood because temporal discounting may result from time distortions, differential time weighting, or from differential subjective valuation processes. Indeed, there is neural evidence suggesting that the evaluation of delayed rewards involves different psychological processes from those of self-control [6].

The mathematical representation of temporal discounting was first depicted by the exponential model, which assumed that value was discounted at a constant rate (delay-independent), and was amount-independent [7]. The behavioral anomaly of dynamic inconsistency-people reverse their time preference when a constant delay is added to both options-poses challenges to this model resulting in further mathematical refinements. In this study we focus on the hyperbolic model, which is the most widely used mathematical description of the discounting phenomenon [7–9]

$$V = \frac{A}{1 + k * D} \qquad \text{(Equation1)}$$

with V representing the value of the reinforcement delivered after a fixed delay D, A is the amount of the reinforcement, and k is a free parameter with greater values indicating greater discounting [7]. This one-parameter model (we refer to it as the base-model in what follows) is able to describe the diminishing value of A as the delay increases and assumes no devaluation of A at D = 0. This model has been useful in representing differences between substance abusers and the non-clinical population via differences in k. For example, a meta-analysis showed that a great proportion of studies used the parameter k to compare the behavior of substance abusers and healthy individuals [4]. Further, this study showed that on average, the substance abusers exhibited a larger parameter k compared to healthy people. More recently, a field study on social cooperation [10] used k as a measure of individuals' impatience and examined its relationship to the likelihood of inflicting punishments on free riders when playing a one-shot, public good game with punishment. Results showed that punishment by highly cooperative individuals was carried out by the more patient, whereas punishment by low cooperators was carried out by impatient individuals. These results suggest interesting relationships between self-control as measured by k, and the application of sanctions in social domains.

In the present study, we focus on further exploring the differences between discounting by healthy and substance dependent individuals via modeling and parametric analyses of models based on Equation 1. In particular, we seek to examine group differences in terms of valuation versus time processes. We note that we restrict our models to functions that have been widely used to describe the behavior of substance abusers. Hence, models such as Laibson's quasi-hyperbolic model [11,12] or forms based on the exponential model [13] are not included in the current study.

Valuation Processes

A large body of literature contends that payoffs are subjectively represented within each individual (going back to at least to Bernoulli [14]), and most theories, including prospect theory, contend that the subjective value is non-linearly related to the nominal value [15]. Lowestein and Prelec reviewed the economic utility and the discounted utility functions when describing anomalies in intertemporal choice and proposed a more general discounting model based on both the hyperbolic model and a value function similar to prospect theory's [16]. We follow this work and take a non-linear valuation function in accord with Steven's law to represent subjective value. In essence Steven's law captures the relationship between physical intensity and perceived intensity via a power function [17]. The following equation represents the addition of a valuation function to the base-model, where V, k, A, and D are as previously defined.

$$V = \frac{A^a}{1 + k * D} \qquad (a\text{–model})$$

The added parameter a ($0<a$) adjusts the perceived valuation of the amount $A>0$; parameter $a<1$ represents diminishing subjective value, which is commonly assumed in utility models. It is possible that average group differences in discounting between substance abusers and non-clinical participants stem from different valuation functions with substance abusers having smaller a, everything else constant.

An interesting phenomenon in substance abusers is that they are readily willing to give up money in order to get drugs; they are likely to purchase the drugs right after they get their paychecks, and presumably before they are in the craving stage [18]. Thus, money may be conceived as a secondary reinforcer with its value depending on how soon the cash is exchanged for drugs. Because exchanging the money for drugs requires time, money may be further discounted; that is, substance abusers may perceive an additional delay between receiving the secondary reinforcer (money) and the primary reinforcer (drugs). The a-model may be rewritten into a representation that elucidates this property: first multiplying the right side of the equation by A^{1-a}/A^{1-a}, we return to A in the numerator, and the denominator becomes ($c+k$*D). We label this model as the c-model:

$$V = \frac{A}{c + k * D} \qquad (c\text{–model})$$

with $c = A^{1-a}$ and with $a = 1 - \ln(c)/\ln(A)$ for a constant A. Values of $c>1$ imply $a<1$ for a constant $A>1$. In this model the subjective value of A dampens when $c>1$ (for $A>1$), everything else constant, thus representing the property of marginally decreasing subjective value. Re-expression of the denominator in the c-model results in: $(1+k*(d+D))$ with $c = 1+k*d$. Here we take the addition of the quantity d to the delay D to stand for the additional time that takes to exchange the money into drugs (we thank an anonymous reviewer for this expression). This representation makes the secondary nature of money more evident as an additional subjective delay slows down receiving a primary reinforcer. Thus, it is possible that substance abusers experience elongated delays that further reduce the subjective value of money, compared to controls.

Time Processes

The excessive preference of substance abusers towards the sooner, smaller reward may be due to their abnormal time perception [19]. For example, it was found that stimulant-dependent individuals tended to overestimate a period [20]. We take two commonly used models in the literature to explore the time related processes. The first one was derived by Rachlin and contains a power function to represent subjective time [8],

$$V = \frac{A}{1 + k * D^s} \qquad (\text{Rachlin} - \text{model})$$

with parameter s indicating the subjective sensitivity to delay; $0<s<1$ implies subjective values of D that are smaller than D, or a diminished time sensitivity. The finding that subjective time estimation changed less than corresponding changes in objective time [21] provided support for parameter values in this range. In this experiment, participants were given a 180 mm line with end-points labeled "very short" and "very long" to indicate how long they perceived a delay to be. It was found that the subjective times that corresponded to 3 months, 1 year, and 3 years were 105.9 mm, 131.3 mm, and 140.0 m, respectively. Thus, the perception of time was negatively accelerated with objective time. For values of $s>1$, time is enhanced (such as the feeling that time stretches when waiting in a long queue). A smaller V results when $s>1$, all else equal, thus resulting in greater discounting of A; the opposite pattern holds when $s<1$.

The second model in this class is the one advanced by Green and colleagues [22,23]. In this model, the parameter s scales the sensitivity toward delay in a more global manner. Myerson & Green (1995) [24] indicated that the s parameter is to reflect individual differences in scaling amount and time and was defined as the ratio of two exponents that scale time and amount, respectively. The paper [24] further stated that "...the exponent s might be expected to remain constant when the same individual confronts different choice situations." (p. 274).

$$V = \frac{A}{(1 + k * D)^s} \qquad \text{(Green – model)}$$

In the equation above, at a fixed s, greater k results in greater discounting. Similarly, for a constant k, a greater s results in greater discounting.

Function Form Analysis

The models under consideration stem from different psychological assumptions about the process of discounting. Needless to say, they all conserve the parameter k as a means of representing time discounting via a weight on delay; however, because the function forms do vary as the result of the other parameters (namely c and s), the same k will not have the same impact on V across models and this is important from the perspective of interpreting values of k. Thus, to the extent that other parameters vary across groups, they may shed light on psychological differences stemming from valuation or time perception, or both. Note that all models reduce to the base-model when $a = c = s = 1$.

In this section we briefly demonstrate the changes in the discounting curves defined by the two-parameter models reviewed. We show that the models do not always overlap, but model differences may be hard to detect depending on the conditions of testing. In particular, because in the limit the functions go to 0 as D approaches infinity, larger values of D present more challenging testing situations for model discrimination. In addition, the amount A affects the valuation directly not only influencing the intercept but also affecting the slope (i.e., amount of value decrease per unit of time increment). We adopt different magnitudes of the parameter values to show their effect on the subjective value of A (i.e., V). In addition, because the a- and c-models are equivalent, we only present results of the c-model.

Figure 1 plots V for c-, Rachlin-, and Green-models for two levels of k ($k = 0.5$ and $k = 2$), two levels of c ($c = 1$ and $c = 10$), and one level of s ($s = 0.5$). The figure also displays the functions at two levels of A (A = 100 and A = 1000). First, Figure 1 shows the greater discounting with larger values of k in all models. Furthermore, the behavior of the Rachlin- and Green-models are fairly similar for a constant s = 0.5 with greater differentiation when k is greater. The c-model produces greater discounting with a larger c, but the effect of k is important. When k is large, the c parameter produces little change in discounting as a result of a rather large change in c (going from $c = 1$ to $c = 10$). When k is small, on the other hand, the change in c is more pronounced. Both the base-model ($c = 1$) and the c-model with larger c tend to produce greater discounting in all conditions, but the differences are more salient with greater A. Furthermore, the change in value per unit of time is larger at greater A. This is particularly clear when k is large (right hand-side panels). By 100 units of delay D, the subjective value of A = 100 is nearly zero for all models; this is not so for A = 1000.

In order to explore the effects of the s parameter in the Rachlin- and Green-models, Figure 2 shows plots that vary s (0.5 and 1.5), and k (0.5 and 2) and the size of A (100 and 1000). In Figure 2, greater discounting is observed with greater s (dotted lines). The difference between the models is small in most situations but they have less overlap with smaller s (solid lines). When $s<1$ (solid lines) and $k<1$, Green-model produces greater discounting than Rachlin-model and the reverse is true when $k>1$; however, the effect is more easily observed at greater A (bottom panels) and in some range of D. As D increases, nevertheless, all models make similar predictions as they approach 0 in the limit. Figure 2 also shows how the s parameter regulates the effect of k. A relatively small s can counteract the discounting effect of a large k in both the Rachlin- and Green-models (comparing solid to dotted lines in Figure 2). Thus s tends to regulate the inflection and slope of the curves whereas k is more closely related to the general base level of discounting.

As seen in Figures 1 and 2, the ability to distinguish the models depends greatly on the levels of A and D for any given set of parameter values. In particular, the slopes of the functions (measuring the change in value per unit of time) vary with changes in the different conditions. Furthermore, expanding the time horizon diminishes model differences. Interestingly, the models are silent with regards to the actual units of D. If D were days in Figure 2 at A = 100, $k = 2$, the models predict similar subjective values of A beyond 100 days (i.e., approximately 3 months, or ¼ year). If D were weeks, on the other hand, the models predict similar behavior beyond 100 weeks, 24 months, or approximately 2 years.

Overview

The goal of this study is to use the mathematical models presented and examine the factors underlying discounting of substance abusers (SA) and non-clinical (NC) people. More specifically, we use available behavioral data for both SA and NC with the aim of elucidating the different psychological processes underlying discounting with a modeling comparison approach. This approach analyzes both model fit and parameter interpretability. In particular, we set to understand if the basis for group differences resides in value versus time processes. We also examine the behavior of model parameters in terms of describing a well known contextual effect that shows changes in discount tendencies as a function of payoff size-*the magnitude effect.*

Methods

Data Selection

Previous research on intertemporal choice used aggregate (i.e. group) data or individual data to test model fitting (e.g. [8,25]). Because mathematical representations of behavior on the aggregate level may not reflect individual level behavior [26,27], we sought data that would allows us to fit the models at the level of each individual in each condition tested (i.e. indifference curve level). Data were obtained from published and unpublished sources (see Table 1) and the study fitted the models to $N = 471$ indifference curves.

For data selection, we used three inclusion criteria that were pertinent to our goals. 1) The studies had adopted a typical intertemporal choice task that either used staircase procedure or titration procedure. These studies asked participants to make repeated choices between an immediate, smaller reward, versus a delayed larger reward in order to derive a point of indifference that reflects the subjective present value of a future amount. With the staircase procedure, the immediate magnitude was presented in a staircase manner with same increment while the delayed magnitude was fixed. With the titration procedure, the immediate magnitude was adjusted based on participants' previous responses so that the immediate magnitude gradually approached the subjective value of the delay magnitude. With a series of indifference points assessed at different delays, the models could be fitted. 2) The study had fitted a hyperbolic model. This allowed us to begin with data that were feasible for our aim of model comparison. 3) The studies included either substance abusers (SA) or non-clinical participants (NC).

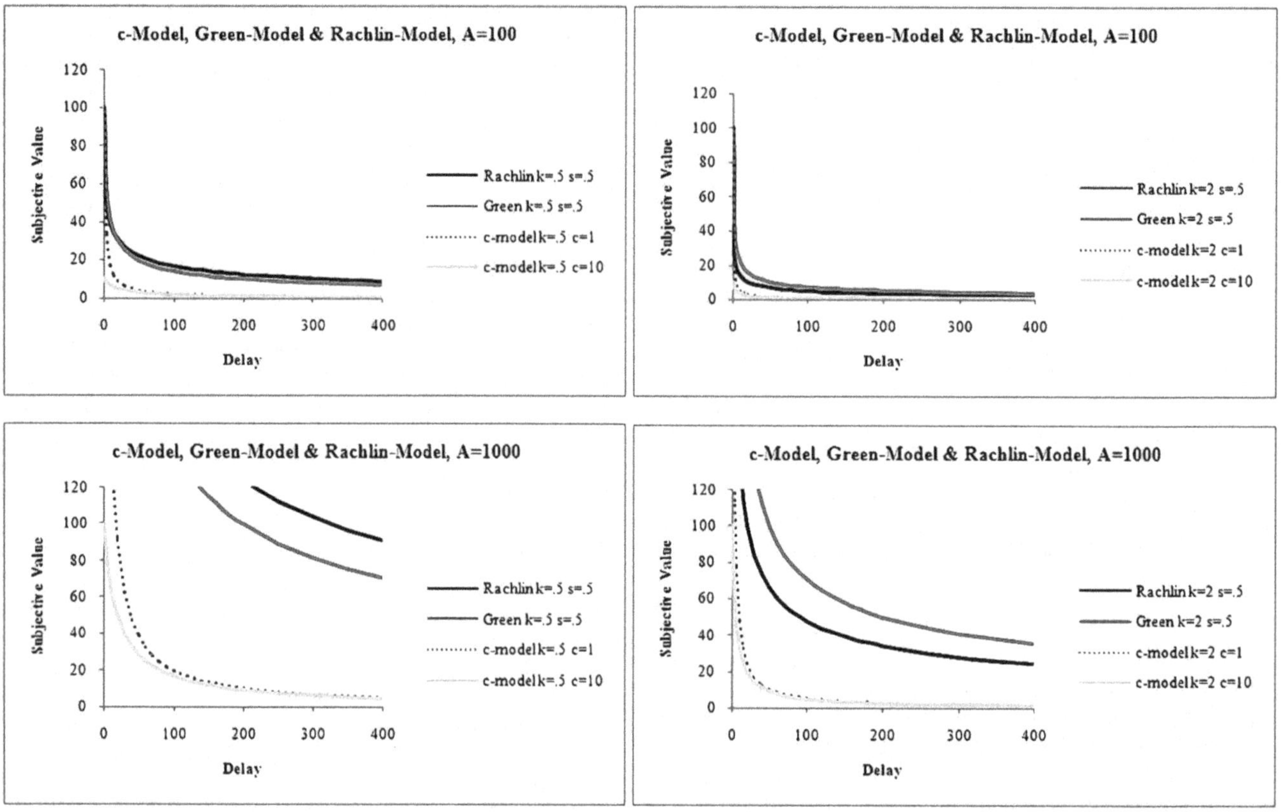

Figure 1. Subjective Value of A from *c*-, Rachlin- with parameters $k=0.5$ and 2; $c=1$ and 10; $s=0.5$. $A=100$ and 1000.

Based on these criteria and a literature search, we contacted seven authors who had several publications and three of them provided us with the data from those publications (the data were chosen by those authors). In addition, we included data from our lab (one published and one unpublished set). We note that our inclusion criteria was not exhaustive of all studies on temporal discounting, because our aim was to both have a uniform set of studies (with similar methodologies) and enough data so that individual model fitting for both SA and NC was possible.

Table 1 details the characteristics of the studies [22,28–30] included in the present manuscript. Each study is described in terms of number of participants, age, gender, education level and drug type (if substance abusers). In describing each experimental design, we included the nature of the rewards (real or hypothetical), the magnitude of the rewards, the delays associated with the rewards and procedure of the task (staircase or titration). It should be noted again that the sample sizes described are not the number of participants. In some studies, one participant completed the temporal discounting tasks in more than one condition (e.g. different magnitudes). Therefore, sample size here indicated the number of actual discounting curves in each condition that was obtained from each of the different individuals. In other words, model fitting was performed at the level of each person's curve. Fitting at discounting curve level allowed us to test if a parameter was able to capture the magnitude effect by comparing this parameter between different magnitude conditions within a same group of participants.

In order to easily identify the different studies in the text of this manuscript we label them using the authors' names as found in Table 1 (from top to bottom): Bickel A, Bickel B, Bickel C, Odum, Cheng Heroin small, Cheng Heroin large, Estle 1 small, Estle 1 large, Estle 3 small, Estle 3 medium, Estle 3 large, Cheng control small, Cheng control large, and OU. The reader can easily find the testing conditions (e.g., whether the study was done with SA or NC; the size of the payoffs, etc.) by referring to Table 1. As seen in Table 1, there are a total of 14 studies.

Model fitting and Parametric Analyses

Indifference points were directly obtained from the studies. We note that in model fitting we maintained the time units used by the authors of the original studies. For example, although in [22] some delays were presented in years to participants the delays were transformed to months when fitting the Green-model by the authors. We followed the same procedure so that the delay units in our study were the same as those in the original studies. All models were fitted via non-linear regression on individual level using SPSS. The estimated parameters and goodness of fit results were checked for consistency, whenever possible, by comparing them to the results of the original studies when provided by the authors (this was the case for Odum [29]; and for Estle 1 and Estle 3 [22]). We compared the models by focusing on R^2, but importantly, estimated parameters were examined with regards to meaningfulness because models may fit data with nonsensical values. Further SA and NC groups were compared in terms of their parametric representations.

Results

Goodness of Fit Analyses

Table 2 and Table 3 list median R^2 for all models in each study separating for studies having SA (Table 2) and for those having NC (Table 3). In each study, but Bickel condition B, the R^2 of

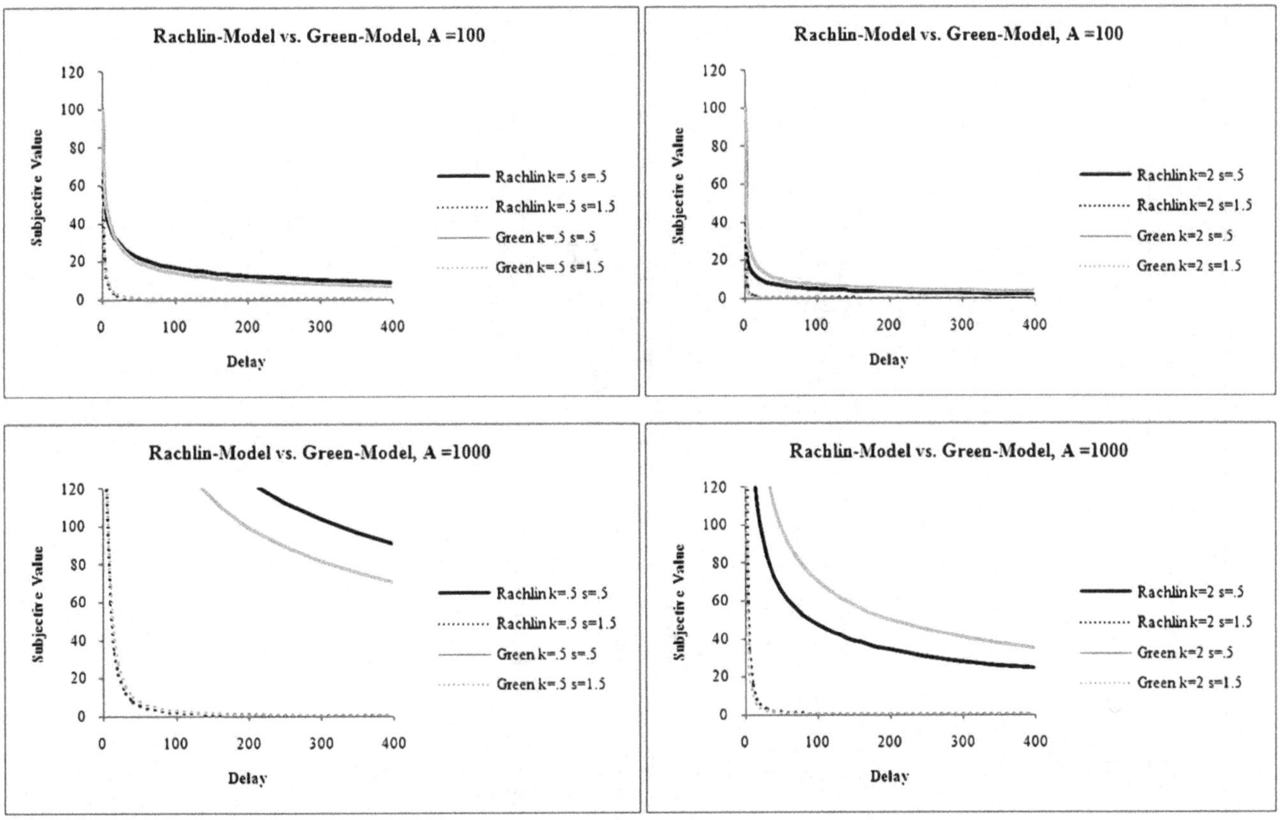

Figure 2. Rachlin- and Green-Models with varying parameters s = 0.5 and 1.5; k = 0.5 and 2. A = 100 and 1000.

base-model was lower than that of the other models, Wilcoxon Signed Rank Z≥3.408, p-values <.01. In Bickel condition B, there was no difference in R^2 between base-model and c-model, p-value>.1. However, base-model fitted more poorly when compared to Rachlin- and Green-models in this study, Wilcoxon Z≥ 3.629, p-values <.01. The R^2 differences between the base (one parameter) and the other models (two parameters) were not surprising, however, as a model with more parameters was expected to fit better and in general the base-model fitted well (median R^2 = .881 across all studies).

To further test whether adding a parameter to the base-model was useful, we compared the models using a statistics that penalizes model for being over-parameterized. Schwarz Bayesian Criteria (*SBC*) is a measure of model selection derived by modifying the Bayesian information criterion [31]. It reflects the posterior probability of a specific model being the true model based on the observed data. SBC makes a trade-off between variance that can be accounted for and the complexity of the models. A model with smaller SBC is favored because it explains sufficient variance (compared to competing models) in a relative concise manner; if models provide equal fit from the perspective of variance accounted for, *SBC* penalizes the model with more parameters. *SBC* was computed for each model in each study by first obtaining the median indifference points across participants, then fitting the models to these values. In each case, $SBC = n * \ln(SSE/n) + p * \ln(n)$, where n was the number of median indifference points corresponding to the number of time delays, SSE was the residual variance, and p was the number of parameters. Results showed that *SBC* from base-model was larger than *SBC* from any two-parameter model in each study. Across all the studies, mean *SBC* for base-model, c-model, Rachlin-model and Green-model were 60.2, 50.9, 46.8, and 49.2, respectively. Thus, the Rachlin-model fitted best from this perspective.

We proceeded to compare the median R^2 values between two-parameter models using the Wilcoxon Signed Rank Z test. First, Rachlin- and Green-models did not show a difference in 10 out of 14 studies, p-values>.1. In four conditions in [30], Rachlin-model fitted better, p-values <.05. Second, Rachlin-model was superior to the c-model in 8 out of 14 studies (Bickel B, Cheng heroin large, Estle 1 large, Estle 3 all three magnitude conditions, Cheng control small, and OU), p-values <.05, and marginally better in two studies (Cheng heroin small and Estel 1 small), p-values <.1. When comparing c- and Green-models, the Green-model was significantly better in 6 out of 14 studies (Bickel B, Cheng heroin large, Estle 1 large, Estle 3 all three magnitude conditions), p-values <.05, and marginally better in one study (OU), p-value < .1. Hence, the Rachlin-model tended to provide better fits than the c-model, but only slightly better fits than the Green-model. This is consistent with the simulation results found in Figures 1 and 2 showing that the Rachlin- and Green-models tend to overlap.

We further compared the median R^2 of the two-parameter models for SA and NC, respectively, across all of the studies. We note that the studies were not combined in this analysis as each person's set of data was fitted individually. To the extent that a model was fitted at this micro-level, all specifics of the study were assumed to be reflected in the estimated parameter values. Table 4 displays the median R^2 for each model in SA and NC.

In both populations, Rachlin-model had the highest median R^2. Green-model took the second place and c-model had the lowest fit

Table 1. Demographic Information of Participants and Experimental Design.

	Basic demographic information of participants					General information of experimental design		
Study	**N***	**Mean age**	**Gender**	**Mean education**	**Substance abusers or non-clinical participants**	**Rewards**	**Delays**	**Staircase or titration**
Bickel, Yi, Landes, Hill & Baxter (2010) condition A [28]	27	38.6	20 males and 7 females	12.2	20 cocaine users, 5 methamphetamine users and 2 mixed users	Real $100	1 day, 1 week, 1 month and 6 months	Staircase
Bickel, Yi, Landes, Hill & Baxter (2010) condition B and C [28]	54	Same as above				Hypothetical $100 and hypothetical $1,000, respectively	1 day, 1 week, 1 month, 6 months, 1 year, 5 years and 25 years	Same as above
Odum, Madden, Badger & Bickel (2000) [29]	17	32.7	11 males and 6 females	12.8	Opium (non-needle sharing)	Hypothetical $1,000	1 week, half a month, 1 month, 6 months, 1 year, 5 years and 25 years	Staircase
Cheng, Lu, Han, Gonzalez-Vallejo & Sui (2012) heroin abusers [30]	112	34.1	41 males and 15 females	10.2	Herion abusers	Hypothetical 200RMB and 50,000RMB (Chinese currency)	1 day, 1 week, 1 month, 6 months, 1 year, 5 years, 10 years and 20 years	Titration
Cheng, Lu, Han, Gonzalez-Vallejo & Sui (2012) controls [30]	112	36.0	Same as above	10.6	non-clinical participants	Same as above		
Estle, Green, Myerson & Holt (2006, Exp 1) [22]	40	19.5	7 males and 13 females	undergraduate	non-clinical participants	Hypothetical $200 and $40,000	1 month, 6 months, 1 year, 3 years, 5 years, 10 years and 20 years	Titration
Estle, Green, Myerson & Holt (2006, Exp 3) [22]	81	19.2	15 males and 12 females	undergraduate	non-clinical participants	Hypothetical $100, $20,000 and $60,000	1 month, 6 months, 1 year, 3 years, 5 years, 8 years, 12 years, and 20 years	Titration
Cheng & Gonzalez-Vallejo (unpublished data)	28	NA	NA	undergraduate	non-clinical participants	Hypothetical $600	1, 10, 30, 50, 100, and 150 days	Staircase

*: The number of actual discounting curves in each condition that was obtained from different individuals.

Table 2. Median R^2 for SA Group in Each Study.

Study	Bickel A	Bickel B	Bickel C	Odum	Cheng Heroin	Cheng Heroin
Magnitude	100	100	1000	1000	200	50000
Base-model	.000 (.88)	.753 (.90)	.471 (.90)	.777 (.81)	.855 (.78)	.829 (.77)
c-model	.817 (.76)	.753 (.90)	.840 (.50)	.921 (.28)	.959 (.05)	.884 (.09)
Rachlin-model	.700 (.66)	.882 (.40)	.853 (.57)	.940 (.11)	.964 (.03)	.967 (.04)
Green-model	.848 (.89)	.855 (.55)	.859 (.68)	.945 (.16)	.941 (.06)	.963 (.08)

Note: Numbers in parentheses are the interquartile range.

among the three, all p-values $<.01$, but again all models demonstrated excellent fit (median $R^2>.93$).

Another way of examining the predictive validity of the models was to perform a linear regression with predicted and observed values as the predictor and the criterion, respectively. A perfect prediction would result in a line with slope equal to one and an intercept equal to zero. This analysis was conducted using each person's observed and predicted values and Figure 3 depicts the scatter plot of predicted and observed indifference points and the linear fits for each model in SA and NC. Table 5 provides R^2s, slopes, and intercepts of the linear fits in Figure 3. In both populations, the linear fit of Rachlin-model was closest to the optimal values; Green and c-models followed (we note that we kept outliers in this analysis so that all models had the same number of observations). Taken together, all analyses indicated that Rachlin-model provided the best fit.

Analyses of Estimated Parameter Values

As is well known in the mathematical psychology literature, models may fit well but with non-interpretable parameters. Therefore, analysis with modeling must be concerned not only with fitting, but also with the meaningfulness of the parameters obtained [32]. We proceeded to examine outliers in the estimated parameters in order to gain a better sense of the performance of the models. We looked for very strange parameter values that could not be interpretable. For example, a participant had estimated parameters of k and s from Green-model equal to 5.6×10^{11} and.0711, respectively. The extremely large value for k in this case implies an indifference curve that drops immediately after the intercept A and remains essentially flat in the range of values of D studied. Instead of adopting conventional mean $\pm$ 3SD to detect outliers, we used this rather conservative approach to select outliers (i.e., selecting extremely large or extremely small estimated values), and found that across all studies, only 11 cases (out of 472, or 2.33%) were found to have outliers for c-model. The Rachlin-model had 4 cases (0.85%); and Green-model had 22 cases (4.66%). The cases identified by this procedure also had very low R^2s ($R^2\leq.201$). Because the outlying cases constitute a very small percentage of the data, we keep them in all of the analyses except when focusing on the interpretation of mean parameter values as will be noted. We performed all previously reported group analyses by taking the outliers out and the conclusions remained unchanged.

The analyses with SBC revealed that the two-parameter models improved model fitting beyond simply increasing model complexity. We proceeded to test the specific values of the estimated parameters c and s in order to better understand the contribution they make to the base-model because when c $(a)=s=1$ the models reduce to the base-model. Table 6 shows the median and mean values of the parameters for each model in each study. We note that values in Table 6 were calculated without the outliers. Doing so had little impact on medians, but was important in interpreting the mean values.

As shown in Table 6, in all studies the median and mean c were greater than 1. In terms of the c-model's alternative representations, this implies that $a<1$ (or $d>0$; see c-model descriptions). The median and mean s were smaller than 1 with two exceptions for mean Rachlin-s and four exceptions for mean Green-s. Table 7 further displays the percentage of the parameter values that were above (for c) or below (for s) the default value of 1 in each study.

As shown in Table 7, for c- and Rachlin-models, 11 out of 14 (78.6%) studies showed that the new parameters were different from 1. For Green-model, 10 out of 14 (71.4%) displayed such a pattern. Binomial test showed that a significant proportion of the values were above or below the target value of 1.

Relationship Between Estimated Parameters and Discount Tendency

Previous studies using the Rachlin-model and/or Green-model [8,22–24] did not examine a possible association between the parameters, but it may be useful to do so in order to understand their behavior in representing discount tendency. Given the non-normal distributions and the few outliers, and in order to keep the number of data points constant for all models, we adopted Spearman rank correlation for these analyses without deleting observations. Table 8 shows the Spearman rank correlations between the two parameters in each model in each study.

As seen in Table 8, there is a general negative relationship between parameters k and s in Rachlin- and Green-models. A larger k in both models led to a greater devaluation whereas a smaller s reduced this trend. Theoretical analyses of the function forms (Figure 2) show that s regulates the inflection and slope of the curves whereas k is more closely related to the general base level of discounting. Thus, the negative correlations between k and s indicated that these parameters tended to counteract their impact on discounting, allowing the functions to have greater flexibility. In contrast, parameters c and k in the c-model behaved more independently; with c determining the base level of discounting and k further adjusting the curvature of the subjective value function over time as shown in Figure 1.

In order to further explore the relationship of the observed discounting and the estimated parameters, we used the area under the curve (AUC) as a parameter-free measure of the discounting tendency. AUC is a non-parametric measure adopted by [33], which is based on adding the segments enclosed by the empirically obtained indifference curve. AUC is standardized and thus ranges from 0 to 1. A larger AUC indicates that the participants discount future outcome to a lesser extent, whereas a smaller AUC represents higher discounting. We note that theoretically, the area under a curve is the integral of the function used to represent

Table 3. Median R^2 for NC Group in Each Study.

Study	Estle 1	Estle 1	Estle 3	Estle 3	Estle 3	Cheng Control	Cheng Control	OU
Magnitude	**200**	**40000**	**100**	**20000**	**60000**	**200**	**50000**	**600**
Base-model	.922 (.26)	.898 (.11)	.884 (.11)	.844 (.28)	.881 (.31)	.923 (.23)	.930 (.09)	.921 (.15)
c-model	.956 (.17)	.922 (.11)	.930 (.23)	.895 (.16)	.912 (.43)	.980 (.03)	.979 (.03)	.952 (.05)
Rachlin-model	.962 (.08)	.939 (.09)	.946 (.18)	.921 (.18)	.947 (.30)	.989 (.02)	.981 (.03)	.978 (.04)
Green-model	.949 (.07)	.949 (.07)	.938 (.17)	.901 (.20)	.948 (.23)	.981 (.04)	.975 (.04)	.964 (.05)

Note: Numbers in parentheses are the interquartile range.

discounting. This integral depends on the model parameters and in some cases, for Rachlin-model for example, the close form is quite complex. It is beyond of the scope of this paper to present a detailed analysis of such definite integrals, but suffice it to say that in general for these models the integral is inversely proportional to k. Thus, to the extent that the models are close approximations to the data, we expect that the relationship between k and AUC to be negative.

Table 9 shows Spearman rank correlations between AUC and parameters in each study. Table 9 shows that the k parameters in base-model and c-model were highly negatively related with AUC. The pattern was more varied for Rachlin- and Green-models. The k in Rachlin-model was significantly and negatively related with AUC in 9 out of 14 studies (64.3%). In contrast, k was related with AUC in only three studies in the Green-model (21.0%). The parameter s was significantly correlated with AUC in 9 studies (64.3%) in each of Rachlin and Green-models. In all, but the heroin and control participants in [30], the significant relationships between s and AUC were also negative.

In order to better understand the independent contribution of the parameters in predicting the discounting behavior as measured by AUC, partial Spearman rank correlations between AUC and a single parameter when controlling for the other were obtained. Table 10 displays these partial correlations.

Results in Table 10 show that in the c-model, the parameter k was negatively associated with AUC after controlling for c. In contrast, c did not reveal a consistent relationship with AUC in the presence of k. This is consistent with model analyses (Figures 1) as c sets the base level of subjective value independently of delay, whereas k affects subjective value via the weighting of delay. In Rachlin- and Green-models k and s were significantly negatively related with AUC after controlling for the other parameter, which further demonstrated their more complex relationship in determining subjective value as exhibited in Figures 1 and 2. In addition, the net relationship between AUC and k, or s was also negative in [30]. Hence, in the c-model, k uniquely described the AUC. Whereas in Rachlin- and Green-models, both k and s related to AUC with a greater k (or s) being associated with a smaller AUC (i.e., greater discounting).

Analysis of the Magnitude Effect

The magnitude effect refers to the phenomenon that greater discounting is observed for smaller than for larger gains [22]. This effect is due to changes in the conditions (payoff level) and provides additional tests of models' parameters. In particular, the parameter s has been described as a person measure [24] and hence would not be expected to change with conditions. The k parameter of Green- and the base-model has often been used to describe individual differences as earlier described, but it has also been used to describe changes due to situations (e.g., to account for sign and magnitude effects [25,30]); hence, the meaning of k may be broader to account for both person and situation based variability. The c parameter is directly indexing a valuation process and hence it is expected to vary with payoff level. We examine these possibilities in tests of the magnitude effect.

We tested the effect in studies that contained a within-subjects manipulation of payoff size: Bickel B (A = 100) vs. Bickel C (A = 1000); Cheng heroin small (A = 200) vs. Cheng heroin large (A = 50000); Cheng control small (A = 200) vs. Cheng control large (A = 50000); Estle 1 small (200) vs. Estle 1 large (A = 40000); Estle 3 small (A = 100) vs. Estle 3 medium (A = 20000); Estle 3 small (A = 100) vs. Estle 3 large (A = 60000); and Estle 3 medium (A = 20000) vs. Estle 3 large (A = 60000). In [28], the magnitude effect was not reported and we found that there was no difference

Table 4. Median R^2 Within SA and NC.

	SA	NC
c-model	.906 (.192)	.960 (.070)
Rachlin-model	.953 (.119)	.971 (.058)
Green-model	.937 (.133)	.964 (.073)

in AUC between condition B (mean AUC = .431) and condition C (mean AUC = .398), paired $t(26) = .91, p = .37$. In [30], the authors reported that there was a magnitude effect in both heroin participants and controls. In [22], it was found that the magnitude effect existed in all comparisons listed above except when comparing medium and large magnitudes in Experiment 3.

For studies in which the magnitude effect was not revealed by mean AUC changes, no changes of parameters were observed in any of the tests conducted. For the studies with magnitude effects, Wilcoxon Signed Ranked on parameter values within each study showed that k from all models was able to reflect this effect with smaller values in the large than in the small magnitude conditions, all p-values $\leq .05$. In terms of parameter c, it reflected the magnitude effect in all studies (p-values $\leq .01$), but in Cheng control participants and Estle 1. Similar to k, c was smaller in the large than in the small magnitude conditions. Note that c can be expressed in terms of a in the a-model and thus it is of particular interest to analyze whether the a parameter is constant, or whether it changes with magnitude depicting intrinsic changes in subjective valuation due to payoff size. We proceeded to analyze the magnitude effect in terms of the parameter a by first estimating it at each curve level and confirming its relationship with c. Wilcoxon Signed Ranked test on parameter a for each study showed that a indexed the magnitude effect in all studies with a smaller a in the small magnitude conditions, all p-values $< .05$. Parametric tests (paired samples t-test) on mean parameter values replicated these results with the following exceptions: k parameter of Green-model did not show an effect in [30]; a parameter did not show an effect in the Estle 1 study.

In terms of s, using Rachlin-model the changes were sometimes in the direction of the magnitude effect (i.e., smaller s in the large than the small payoff condition) but other times the change was in the opposite direction. In Estle 3 (small vs. large; small vs. medium), the parameter s showed an opposite magnitude effect: s was greater in the large than in the small magnitude conditions, p-values $< .05$. There was no change of s in Estle 1 between the two magnitude conditions, p-value$> .1$. In Cheng control and heroin groups the direction of the magnitude effect was not consistently shown by parameter s, and the parameter values did not change significantly.

Parameter s in Green-model showed that it changed significantly with magnitude in both Cheng heroin participants and control participants in the direction of the effect, p-values $< .01$. The change was in the opposite direction in Estle 3 when comparing the small and large magnitude conditions, $p < .05$, but no effect when comparing the small and medium conditions. Similarly, there was no effect of s in Estle 1 when comparing small and large conditions.

Taken together, k, c and a, varied consistently in the direction of the magnitude effect with smaller values in conditions with larger A. In contrast, s did not show a consistent pattern and this may be in agreement with the expectation that s must remain constant because it was to reflect an individual level tendency [24]. In order to further clarify the extent to which each parameter moved in the predicted direction, we computed the effect size (Cohen's d) in each study. Following the methods provided by [34], weighted average d across the studies were obtained along with its 95% confidence interval. The results appear in Table 11.

Table 11 shows that the 95% CIs include the value of zero only for the effect of the s parameter in both Rachlin- and Green-models. Although the sample size made the conclusions from this meta-analysis tentative (we have five studies demonstrating the magnitude effect), it was safe to say that there was no evidence of a consistent magnitude effect with parameter s. This lends support to the assumption that s should remain constant with changes in contexts, but further studies are needed to clarify its role in describing context effects.

Parameter Comparison between SA and NC in an Experimental-Control Design

The groups of SA and NC participants come from different studies and conditions; therefore direct comparisons of parameter values is limited. Among these studies, however, [30] has both heroin-dependent patients and controls, and the groups were globally matched on age, gender, education, and income (for more details refer to [30]). Focusing on participants in this study, we

Table 5. Linear Regression of Predictive Validity of Models in SA and NC.

	slope	intercept	R^2 of linear fit
c-model SA	.883	592.50	.873
Rachlin-model SA	.979	−48.846	.942
Green-model SA	.978	−99.155	.883
c-model NC	.969	533.763	.940
Rachlin-model NC	.979	27.628	.969
Green-model NC	.972	54.236	.957

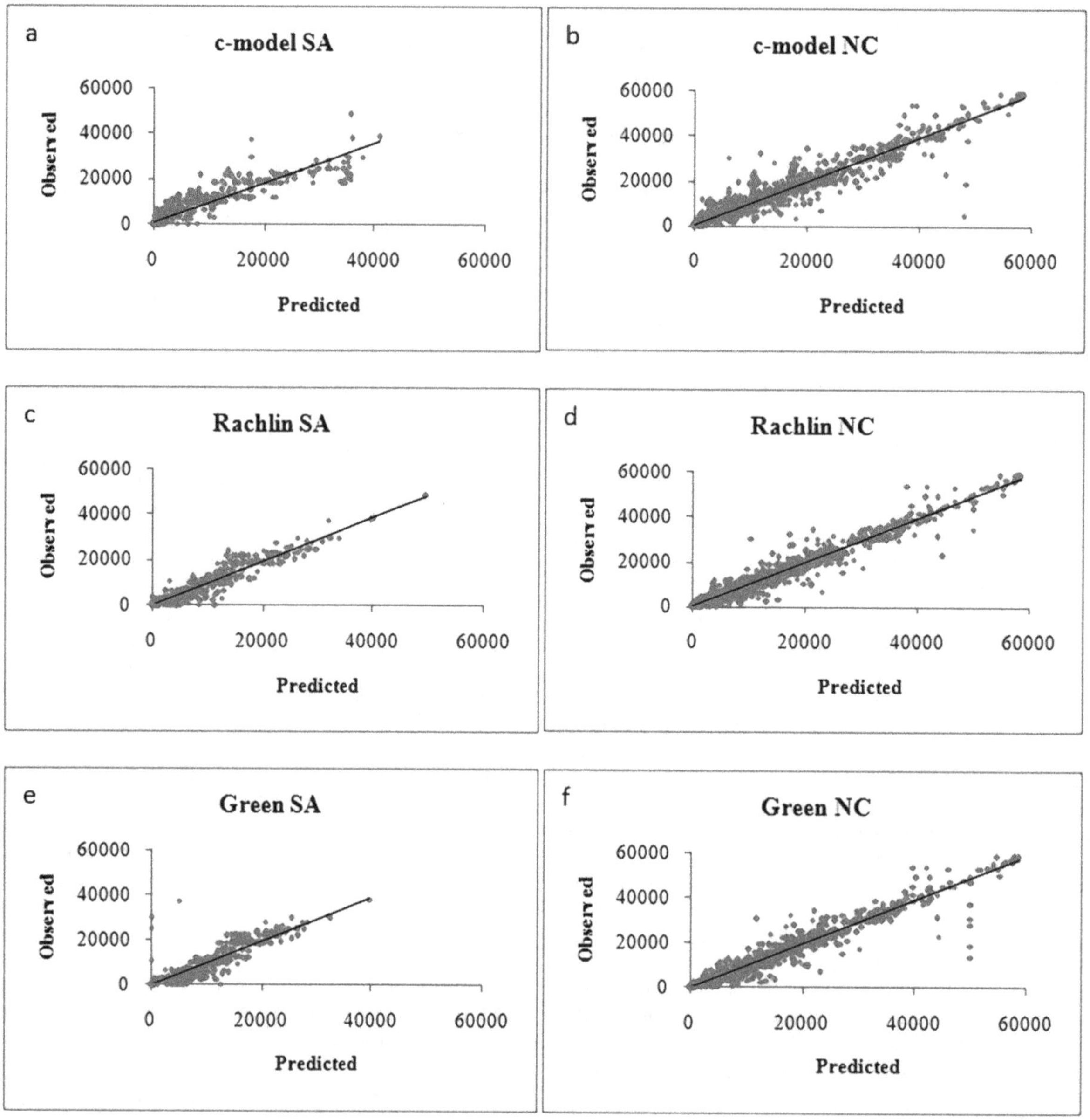

Figure 3. Scatter Plots of Predicted and Observed Indifference Points for Each Model in each SA and NC Groups.

compared the parameter values keeping study conditions separate (i.e., small and large magnitude conditions). The mean and median parameter values are found in Table 6, but to facilitate reading of the results, we present them in Table 12.

In terms of median c and k, they were larger in SA than in NC in both small and large magnitude conditions, both Mann-Whitney test p-values $<.01$. In Rachlin- and Green-models k was larger in SA than in NC, and the reverse was true for s in all conditions, all Mann-Whitney test p-values $<.01$. Therefore, the parameter k in all models indexed the difference between SA and NC in both magnitude conditions; so did the c parameter and both parameters moved in the expected direction, i.e., they were smaller in NC participants. Parameter a from a-model performed similar to parameter c: a was significantly smaller in SA than in NC. The s parameter, on the other hand, moved in the opposite direction with smaller values for the SA individuals. As seen in Figure 2, greater s implies greater discounting which would be expected for the SA participants instead.

There are limitations to using non-parametric tests when making comparisons because the magnitude of the quantities being compared is lost. Hence we performed tests of mean differences between the SA and NC groups. In order to conduct these tests, we identified the outliers by the procedure earlier described. We also assessed departures from symmetry of the distributions and transformed them using the natural log function when needed.

Independent t-tests were performed for each parameter between heroin-dependent and the non-clinical groups. For c-model, parameter k was larger in SA than in NC in the small magnitude condition, $t(110) = 5.24$, $p<.001$, and in the large magnitude condition, $t(109) = 5.17$, $p<.001$. Parameter c was also larger in SA in both small and large magnitude conditions, $t(110) = 5.11$, $p<.001$ and $t(109) = 5.0$, $p<.001$, respectively.

Table 6. Median and Mean Values of Parameters in Each Study.

		c-model		Rachlin-model		Green-model	
		k	*c*	*k*	*s*	*k*	*s*
Bickel A[SA]	Median	.004 (.03)	1.133 (.50)	.096 (.43)	.257 (.60)	1.251 (6.9)	.273 (.43)
	Mean	.020 (.03)	1.589 (1.3)	.456 (1.0)	.474 (.63)	15.14 (29.4)	1.651 (4.68)
Bickel B[SA]	Median	.002 (.009)	1.092 (.20)	.041(.13)	.486 (.55)	.040 (.613)	.252 (.44)
	Mean	.058 (.009)	2.839 (8.46)	1.468 (7.2)	.603 (.51)	4.564 (10.9)	.307 (.27)
Bickel C[SA]	Median	.002 (.009)	1.092 (.38)	.066 (.24)	.423 (.49)	.178 (1.6)	.288 (.59)
	Mean	.030 (.08)	1.330 (.83)	.269 (.67)	.604 (.91)	5.112 (16.1)	.399 (.36)
Odum[SA]	Median	.013 (.641)	1.067 (.32)	.259 (2.4)	.980 (1.6)	3.97(10.7)	.175 (85)
	Mean	2.41 (6.81)	1.511 (1.53)	3.089 (7.8)	1.438 (1.5)	10.27 (16.2)	.483 (.50)
Cheng Heroin small[SA]	Median	.008 (.007)	1.276 (.35)	.117 (.24)	.512 (.27)	.122 (.72)	.333 (.17)
	Mean	.010 (.01)	1.527 (.91)	.270 (.43)	.556 (.19)	1.965 (5.25)	.382 (.20)
Cheng Heroin large[SA]	Median	.002 (.002)	1.151 (.23)	.051 (.11)	.520 (.23)	.047 (.23)	.286 (.13)
	Mean	.002 (.001)	1.292 (.39)	.153 (2.7)	.539 (.32)	.754 (3.25)	.260 (.12)
Estle 1 small[NC]	Median	.054 (.10)	1.058 (.39)	.193 (.42)	.867 (.56)	.268 (1.30)	.767 (.71)
	Mean	.109 (.19)	1.202 (.40)	.265 (.42)	.878 (.47)	1.122 (2.5)	.694 (.41)
Estle 1 large[NC]	Median	.009 (.02)	1.032 (.07)	.024 (.07)	.774 (.37)	.035 (.15)	.419 (.76)
	Mean	.040 (.09)	1.046 (.13)	.070 (.11)	.864 (.38)	.150 (.266)	.920 (1.7)
Estle 3 small[NC]	Median	.051 (.17)	1.192 (.38)	.205 (.20)	.641 (.43)	.549 (1.15)	.439 (.52)
	Mean	.114 (.16)	1.270 (.37)	.316 (.32)	.705 (.27)	1.106 (.25)	.694 (.63)
Estle 3 medium[NC]	Median	.007 (.02)	1.026 (.08)	.020 (.03)	.871 (.45)	.027 (.12)	.550 (.87)
	Mean	.013 (.02)	1.056 (.10)	.037 (.06)	.834 (.38)	.508 (1.84)	3.76 (13.3)
Estle 3 large[NC]	Median	.006 (.02)	1.019 (.13)	.012 (.05)	.846 (1.04)	.019 (.27)	.732 (37.4)
	Mean	.013 (.01)	1.072 (.16)	.066 (.10)	1.004 (.61)	.344 (1.2)	17.40 (26.1)
Cheng Control small[NC]	Median	.004 (.002)	1.040 (.07)	.012 (.02)	.808 (.20)	.009 (.01)	.653 (.22)
	Mean	.005 (.004)	1.088 (.16)	.043 (.01)	.789 (.17)	.187 (.95)	.586 (.23)
Cheng Control large[NC]	Median	.001 (.0004)	1.061 (.06)	.008 (.01)	.663 (.20)	.005 (.005)	.381 (.19)
	Mean	.0009 (.0005)	1.067 (.06)	.014 (.02)	.753 (.27)	.008 (.06)	.535 (1.2)
OU[NC]	Median	.008 (.01)	1.036 (.09)	.014 (.04)	.844 (.44)	.008 (.02)	.525 (1.61)
	Mean	.011 (.01)	1.056 (.08)	.041 (.06)	.832 (.30)	.079 (.23)	3.045 (7.2)
SA	Median	.003 (.009)	1.157 (.34)	.086 (.26)	.503 (.38)	.120 (4.07)	.282 (.31)
	Mean	.346 (2.74)	1.645 (3.06)	3.078 (9.8)	.419 (1.36)	.754 (3.9)	.958 (4.7)
NC	Median	.004 (.015)	1.043 (.95)	.016 (.05)	.771 (.34)	.012 (.09)	.465 (.54)
	Mean	.041 (.23)	1.099 (.21)	.355 (1.35)	1.742 (6.2)	.086 (.19)	.827 (.35)

Table 6. Cont.

		c-model		Rachlin-model		Green-model	
		k	*c*	*k*	*s*	*k*	*s*
Total	Median	.004 (.01)	1.071 (.21)	.032 (.14)	.646 (.40)	.024 (.16)	.347 (.44)
	Mean	.173 (1.82)	1.278 (1.99)	.382 (2.61)	.725 (.52)	.468 (1.37)	.865 (3.24)

Note: Numbers in parentheses are IQR and standard deviation for median and mean values, respectively. SA: median and mean of parameter values computed across all cases in studies having substance abusers; NC: median and mean of parameter values computed across all cases in studies having non-clinical participants. The Total has the median and mean computed across all cases and studies. When SA and NC are superscripts, they indicate whether the study contains substance abusers or non-clinical people.

For Rachlin-model, parameter k demonstrated the group difference in both magnitude conditions, $t(110) = 7.20$, $p < .001$, and $t(104) = 7.38$, $p < .001$, respectively. Parameter s, however, was smaller in SA than in NC in small and large magnitude conditions, with $t(110) = -7.20$, $p < .001$ and $t(110) = -5.28$, $p < .001$, respectively.

Similar to the other models, in Green-model, SA displayed a larger k when compared to NC, $t(107) = 3.42$, $p = .001$ in the small magnitude condition; $t(105) = 2.38$, $p < .05$ in the large magnitude condition. Parameter s moved in the opposite direction of parameter k. In each case, s was smaller in SA: $t(104) = -6.024$, $p < .001$ in the small condition; $t(110) = -4.013$, $p < .001$ in the large condition. Thus, in agreement with the non-parametric tests the parameters k and c consistently represented the group differences whereas the parameter s did not.

Discussion

The present study aimed to better understand the basis of the observed discounting behavior of both substance abusers and non-clinical individuals. Traditionally the single parameter model of Equation 1 has been used to describe group differences with parameter k being on average greater for the substance abusers than for the non-clinical individuals. Our results replicate these findings. However, the k parameter is too general and differences in discounting tendency may be due to valuation process differences, or to time perception distortions that in turn affects the subjective value of a future amount. The present study sought to clarify the psychological basis for discounting in intertemporal choice and the observed group differences using a modeling approach. The models tested represent valuation, time perception, and general time/amount scaling functions: c-, Rachlin-, and Green-models, respectively. Rachlin- and Green-models have been widely used with substance abusers and hence served as benchmarks for investigating individual differences. The c-model, as it derives from the a-model, has been theoretically considered but not tested. This study advances our understanding of the manner in which models of discounting behavior represent different psychological process for different individual and conditions.

The analyses first elucidated the similarities and differences of the function forms and how model parameters produce varying discounting tendencies for different A and D levels. Through such simulations, it was shown that Rachlin- and Green-models predicted very similar discounting for a wide array of delays. In contrast, the base-model, and c-model with greater $c > 1$, can produce deeper discounting patterns than the Rachlin- and Green-models at a fixed k. Furthermore, the analyses demonstrated the different roles of k in the different models. In c-model, k had a greater influence in regulating the shape of the discounting curve, whereas c set the overall base-level of discounting. In contrast, in Rachlin- and Green-models, parameter s appeared to regulate the changes of subjective value over time with k serving to set the base level of discounting. However, the relationship between k and s was very interactive; a large s could counteract a small k and vice versa. Results of the simulation also demonstrated that A affected the rate of discounting (change in subjective value per unit of time).

Moreover, discounting rate is not constant throughout the delay periods and this implies that individuals are more sensitive to delay differences closer to the present moment than later. Tests of such implications are needed to further study the models' validity. For example, assume a participant has estimated $k = 0.08$ and $s = 0.5$ and let us use the Rachlin-model without loss of generality. The

Table 7. Percentage of Deviation of Parameters From The Value of 1 in Each Study.

	c>1 (%)	Rachlin-*s* <1 (%)	Green-*s* <1 (%)
Bickel A^{SA}	85***	93***	85**
Bickel B^{SA}	85***	89***	81**
Bickel C^{SA}	81***	93***	89**
Odum^{SA}	65	53	65
Cheng Heroin small^{SA}	96***	98**	100***
Cheng Heroin large^{SA}	80*	75*	75*
Estle 1 small^{NC}	70	60	70
Estle 1 large^{NC}	80*	75*	75*
Estle 3 small^{NC}	81**	85**	85**
Estle 3 medium^{NC}	78**	74*	67
Estle 3 large^{NC}	63	59	56
Cheng Control small^{NC}	88***	91***	100***
Cheng Control large^{NC}	84***	89***	93***
OU^{NC}	82**	71*	71*
SA	89***	92***	90***
NC	80***	82***	79***
Total	84***	84***	86***

Note: **p*<.05; ***p*<.01; ****p*<.001. SA: percentage computed across all cases in studies with substance abuse individuals; NC: percentage computed across all cases in studies with non-clinical individuals. Total: percentage computed across all cases in all studies. When SA and NC are superscripts, they indicate whether the study contains substance abusers or non-clinical people.

model predicts a subjective value of 798.09 for the option (A = 1000, D = 10) and a value of 736.5 for (A = 1000, D = 20); this is a 61.59 drop in subjective value of A in a period difference of 10 D units. In later periods (between D = 20 and D = 30) the drop in subjective value of A is of 41.17. This implies that the preference for the sooner option would be stronger in the first than in the second comparison. However, it is likely that by dominance a decision maker confronted with such pairs of options would select

Table 8. Spearman Rank Correlations Between the Model Parameters.

	c-model (*k,c*)	Rachlin-(*k,s*)	Green-(*k,s*)
Bickel A^{SA}	.181	−.239	−.505**
Bickel B^{SA}	−.161	−.363	−.733***
Bickel C^{SA}	.204	−.243	−.541**
Odum^{SA}	−.397	−.162	−.834***
Cheng Heroin small^{SA}	.266*	−.845***	−.845***
Cheng Heroin large^{SA}	−.273*	−.977***	−.640***
Estle 1 small^{NC}	−.429	−.442	−.829***
Estle 1 large^{NC}	−.053	−.439	−.433
Estle 3 small^{NC}	−.266	−.447*	−.584**
Estle 3 medium^{NC}	−.041	−.597**	−.814***
Estle 3 large^{NC}	−.410*	−.808***	−.925***
Cheng Control small^{NC}	.140	−.903***	−.353**
Cheng Control large^{NC}	.492***	−.963***	−.374**
OU^{NC}	0.0	−.822***	−.455*
SA	.078	−.621***	−.494***
NC	−.018	−.408***	−.583***
Total	−.012	−.620***	−.555***

Note: **p*<.05; ***p*<.01; ****p*<.001. SA: correlation computed across cases in studies with substance abusers. NC: correlation computed across all cases in studies with non-clinical individuals. Total: correlation computed across all cases in all studies. When SA and NC are superscripts, they indicate whether the study contains substance abusers or non-clinical people.

Table 9. Spearman Correlations Between AUC and Estimated Parameters.

	Base k	c model k	c	Rachlin-k	Rachlin-s	Green-k	Green-s
Bickel A[SA]	$-.971^{***}$	$-.718^{***}$	$-.063$	$-.692^{**}$	$-.410^{*}$	$-.199$	$-.479^{*}$
Bickel B[SA]	$-.955^{***}$	$-.903^{***}$	$-.075$	$-.269$	$-.676^{***}$	$.162$	$-.662^{***}$
Bickel C[SA]	$-.957^{***}$	$-.958^{***}$	$-.284$	$-.467^{*}$	$-.665^{***}$	$.087$	$-.731^{***}$
Odum[SA]	$-.912^{***}$	$-.765^{***}$	$-.044$	$-.873^{***}$	$-.044$	$-.345$	$-.010$
Cheng Heroin small[SA]	$-.793^{***}$	$-.788^{***}$	$-.485^{***}$	$-.608^{***}$	$.305^{***}$	$-.615^{***}$	$.274^{*}$
Cheng Heroin large[SA]	$-.687^{***}$	$-.736^{***}$	$-.116$	$-.224$	$.068$	$-.209$	$-.182$
Estle 1 small[NC]	$-.937^{***}$	$-.973^{***}$	$.355$	$-.532^{*}$	$-.380$	$-.098$	$-.329$
Estle 1 large[NC]	$-.985^{***}$	$-.983^{***}$	$.015$	$-.580^{**}$	$-.347$	$-.302$	$-.671^{**}$
Estle 3 small[NC]	$-.990^{***}$	$-.940^{***}$	$.081$	$-.501^{**}$	$-.405^{*}$	$-.194$	$-.548^{**}$
Estle 3 medium[NC]	$-.992^{***}$	$-.993^{***}$	$-.015$	$-.299$	$-.531^{**}$	$.161$	$-.634^{***}$
Estle 3 large[NC]	$-.979^{***}$	$-.968^{***}$	$.263$	$-.064$	$-.466^{*}$	$.244$	$-.526^{**}$
Cheng Control small[NC]	$-.510^{***}$	$-.807^{***}$	$-.179$	$-.524^{***}$	$.300^{*}$	$-.563^{***}$	$-.106$
Cheng Control large[NC]	$-.968^{***}$	$-.789^{***}$	$-.500^{***}$	$-.586^{***}$	$.412^{**}$	$-.600^{***}$	$-.196$
OU[NC]	$-.993^{***}$	$-.980^{***}$	$-.071$	$-.207$	$-.310$	$.137$	$-.414^{*}$
SA	$-.779^{***}$	$-.792^{***}$	$-.243^{***}$	$-.405^{***}$	$-.363^{***}$	$-.075$	$-.462^{***}$
NC	$-.131^{*}$	$-.241^{***}$	$-.121$	$-.190^{**}$	$-.069$	$-.047$	$-.279^{***}$
Total	$-.471^{***}$	$-.442^{***}$	$-.274^{***}$	$-.371^{***}$	$-.059$	$-.185^{***}$	$-.226^{***}$

Note: $^{*}p<.05$; $^{**}p<.01$; $^{***}p<.001$. SA: correlation computed across cases in studies with substance abusers. NC: correlation computed across all cases in studies with non-clinical individuals. Total: correlation computed across all cases in all studies. When SA and NC are superscripts, they indicate whether the study contains substance abusers or non-clinical people.

Table 10. Partial Spearman Rank Correlations Between Model Parameters and AUC.

	c-model *k*	*c*	Rachlin-*k*	Rachlin-*s*	Green-*k*	Green-*s*
Bickel A^{SA}	−.776***	−.690***	−.892***	−.820***	−.477*	−.630**
Bickel B^{SA}	−.930***	−.520**	−.750***	−.862***	−.635***	−.810***
Bickel C^{SA}	−.959***	−.317	−.868***	−.908***	−.537**	−.816***
Odum^{SA}	−.853***	−.588*	−.892***	−.384*	−.639**	−.573*
Cheng Heroin small^{SA}	−.770***	−.460***	−.688***	−.492***	−.744***	−.580***
Cheng Heroin large^{SA}	−.804***	−.486***	−.749***	−.735***	−.430**	−.420**
Estle 1 small^{NC}	−.972***	−.297	−.845***	−.811***	−.701**	−.736**
Estle 1 large^{NC}	−.984***	−.205	−.870***	−.823***	−.887***	−.933***
Estle 3 small^{NC}	−.955***	−.512**	−.834***	−.812***	−.758***	−.831***
Estle 3 medium^{NC}	−.994***	−.455*	−.906***	−.926***	−.794***	−.879***
Estle 3 large^{NC}	−.978***	−.586**	−.847***	−.882***	−.749***	−.814***
Cheng Control small^{NC}	−.802***	−.112	−.618***	−.474***	−.645***	−.393**
Cheng Control large^{NC}	−.721***	−.209	−.772***	−.700***	−.567***	−.740***
OU^{NC}	−.983***	−.362	−.853***	−.862***	−.063	−.398*
SA	−.799***	−.298***	−.722***	−.708***	−.521***	−.651***
NC	−.245***	−.129*	−.285***	−.227***	−.183**	−.327***
Total	−.463***	−.311***	−.520***	−.396***	−.383***	−.402***

Note: *$p<.05$; **$p<.01$; ***$p<.001$. SA: correlation computed across cases in studies with substance abusers. NC: correlation computed across all cases in studies with non-clinical individuals. Total: correlation computed across all cases in all studies. When SA and NC are superscripts, they indicate whether the study contains substance abusers or non-clinical people. When SA and NC are superscripts, they indicate whether the study contains substance abusers or non-clinical people.

the sooner options with 100 percent certainty in both situations; thus show no reduced time sensitivity in choice. This means that the models' predicted preferences may not agree with participants' behavior once the models are tested with another method. More generally, cross-validation studies are much needed, and by this we mean that a function derived via the indifference point methodology is then used to predict behavior outside of the data employed in model fitting.

In terms of model testing, the analysis inspected not only model fit and the corresponding proportion of variance accounted for, but also examined the meaning of the estimated parameters in different groups and in different magnitude conditions. Ultimately, it is the meaning of such parameters that can provide psychological understanding. First, compared to the base-model, all the two-parameter models improved fit non-trivially as demonstrated with the SBC measure and with the tests of mean and median parameter values against the default value of 1. Among the two-parameter models, Rachlin-model displayed the best fit at the individual level in both SA and NC. This result contrasts with that of [8,23] finding that no difference was found between Rachlin- and Green-models. A possible reason for this difference was that a greater number of studies were included, with a wider range of D. We note, however, that all of the models performed extremely well when considering R^2, and that the function forms tend to overlap in many situations as shown in the function form analysis. Thus, not finding differences may be more the rule than the exception.

In terms of estimated parameters, previous research found that the parameter *s* in Green- and Rachlin-models was smaller than 1 [23]. We replicated this finding in fourteen studies. Additionally, we found that a significant proportion of cases had a *c* larger than 1 in *c*-model. Therefore, from the perspective of whether the two-parameter models may be easily reduced to the one-parameter

Table 11. Meta-Analysis of Effect Size (Cohen's d) When Testing Magnitude Effect.

Parameters	Avg(*d*)	SD(δ^a)	95% CI
c-model *k*	0.851	0.472	[.415–1.29]
c	0.312	0.141	[.132–.492]
a-model *k*	0.861	0.53	[.377–1.35]
a	0.616	0.273	[.343–.899]
Rachlin -*k*	0.39	0.0	[.283–.497]
Rachlin-*s*	−0.087	0.529	[−.569–.395]
Green-*k*	0.317	0.035	[.184–.450]
Green-*s*	−0.008	0.674	[−.613–.597]

Note. a: According to Hunter & Schmidt (2004), the population variance of effect size (δ^2) is obtained by subtracting variance due to sampling error from observed variance adjusted by sample size.

Table 12. Median and Mean Values of the Parameters of Heroin and Control Participants in [30].

		c-model		Rachlin-model		Green-model	
		k	*c*	*k*	*s*	*k*	*s*
Heroin^S	Median	.008 (.007)	1.276 (.35)	.117 (.24)	.512 (.27)	.122 (.72)	.333 (.17)
	Mean	.010 (.01)	1.527 (.91)	.270 (.43)	.556 (.19)	1.965 (5.25)	.382 (.20)
Heroin^L	Median	.002 (.002)	1.151 (.23)	.051 (.11)	.520 (.23)	.047 (.23)	.286 (.13)
	Mean	.002 (.001)	1.292 (.39)	.153 (2.7)	.539 (.32)	.754 (3.25)	.260 (.12)
Control^S	Median	.004 (.002)	1.040 (.07)	.012 (.02)	.808 (.20)	.009 (.01)	.653 (.22)
	Mean	.005 (.004)	1.088 (.16)	.043 (.01)	.789 (.17)	.187 (.95)	.586 (.23)
Control^L	Median	.001 (.0004)	1.061 (.06)	.008 (.01)	.663 (.20)	.005 (.005)	.381 (.19)
	Mean	.0009(.0005)	1.067 (.06)	.014 (.02)	.753 (.27)	.008 (.06)	.535 (1.2)

Note: Superscripts ^{S} and ^{L} index small and large payoffs. Numbers in parentheses are IQR for median, and standard deviation for means; means computed without outliers.

base model, our results indicated that this was not the case. Psychologically, in terms of the valuation process, c being larger than 1 implies a power function for subjective value that is concave (i.e., $a<1$ in a-model). This is consistent with the general value function of prospect theory and other utility functions that assume diminishing returns [15]. That the parameter s was also not equal to 1 echoed the notion that subjective time was different from objective time [19–21]. However, we note that having $s<1$ meant that time was not enhanced, but rather shrunk, and the fact that s was smaller in SA than in NC implied that the subjective delays were smaller for SA than NC. This contradicts the expectation that SA's would overestimate the duration of time as reported in [20]. Indeed, more generally $s<1$ reduces discounting as observed in Figures 1 and 2, everything else constant. This means that the greater discounting observed in SA cannot be attributed to time perception processes in the manner represented by s in Rachlin- and Green-models. It is the compensation of a smaller s by a greater k that accounts for greater discounting in the SA individuals.

Another finding was that Rachlin- and Green-models produced estimated parameters that were statistically and negatively related to each other. This suggests that the models improved fitting in part by having parameters compensated for each other. As the function form analyses showed, the parameter s could counteract the effects of k and vice versa. This was not so for the parameter c in the c-model. Furthermore, the models' parameters showed that the parameters k and s were negatively related to AUC when controlling for the other, whereas this was not the case for c. In combination, this shows that c is a less redundant parameter.

Additional analyses on contextual differences showed that the parameter k in all models was consistently greater in the small versus the large magnitude conditions, thus being able to describe the *magnitude effect*. The same was true in almost all cases for the c parameter and in all cases for the corresponding a parameter. In contrast, parameter s in either the Rachlin- or the Green-model did not show a consistent pattern in relationship to the magnitude effect. These results reestablish that the k parameter may be conceived as a situation specific, or context effect index, but not s.

In a similar vein, when testing models with data from heroin patients and control participants within a single study, k was larger in the heroin group than in controls. This was also true for the c parameter. In contrast s was smaller for the substance abuse individuals than the non-clinical group. Hence, parameters k and c systematically measured the average individual tendencies, whereas s allowed for better model fit but its values did not advance additional meaning that could describe, or explain these person level effects.

Overall, we found that Rachlin-model provided the best description of the data across studies from the perspective of variance accounted for, followed by Green-model. This indicated that a time perception function (Rachlin-model), or a general amount-to-time scaling function (Green-model) was beneficial to the base model in explaining additional variance. However, both models have challenges with regards to the interpretation of their parameters. In particular, the finding that the SA individuals had s values that would result in less rather than greater discounting is problematic; model fitting was significantly improved with s, but psychological understanding was not. Furthermore the s parameter negatively correlated with k which resulted in small changes in s that counteracted the movements of k across the many studies reviewed. Thus, s adds flexibility to the models, but it does not add explanatory power to them. Further studies are needed to establish s as a person level index. In terms of k, it described both context and person level effects well, but this success is also its weakness as it does not uniquely represent either factor.

In terms of *c*-model, it also performed better than the base-model. Its parameter *c* varied with magnitude and revealed group differences in the expected direction (i.e., greater *c* for the SA than the NC groups), and it tended to do so independently of *k* as correlation analysis showed. Hence, *c*-model may be a viable descriptive and explanatory model of the general discounting tendencies observed between SA and NC. Nonetheless, this model is not free of issues altogether. $c>1$ implied that individuals had a marginally decreasing utility function, and this was confirmed upon estimation of the parameter *a*. Analyses of the magnitude effect revealed that *a* varied as a function of magnitude, which positioned *a* as a weight on outcome. It is not entirely clear why such weighting would change with levels of payoffs; one possibility may be that individuals pay greater attention to larger quantities. If so, *a* is not an index of a person level trait.

An alternative interpretation of $c>1$ is that the delay D is enlarged by a subjective additional delay as shown in the equivalent form, $c = 1+kd$, with *d* representing additional time units added to the denominator of the base-model, denominator $= 1+k(d+\text{D})$. In this re-expression, the greater discounting by substance abusers can be attributed to an increased subjective delay that stems from money not changing fast enough to their most preferred reinforcer-drugs. The secondary nature of money as a reinforcer may not always depend on internal individual proclivities. For example, people suffering from hyperinflation in Zimbabwe were shown to purchase things as soon as they received their salary [35]. In late 1980s in China, inflation was extremely high due to the economic structural reform (21.3 percent in 1988 and 16.0 percent in 1989) and a survey conducted on 150,000 urban households during that period reported that consumers had strong motives to transfer savings to products [36]. Irrespective of whether the additional discounting is internally or externally determined, the *c*-model allows for a positive shift in delay that reduces subjective value. This conclusion demands further empirical studies and highlights the inability of the current data to provide a clear meaning of the parameter *c* (or *a*). As is true for *k*, the *c* parameter did not reveal itself as a pure person or task level measure.

In sum, the present study replicated the finding that known models (base-, Rachlin-, and Green-models) could describe indifference curves derived from standard intertemporal choice staircase or titration procedures extremely well. In particular, Rachlin-model appeared as the most successful one in terms of model fitting. The *k* parameter across all models was able to consistently describe both situation and person dependent variability in discounting. In addition, we showed that a value based model, *c*-model (or *a*-model), also provided excellent fit and its parameters also tracked group and task differences. But the descriptive ability of a model does not guarantee its explanatory power. Because the *k* parameter was so essential to representing both group and context differences across the models, it remains unclear whether value or time perception processes lead to greater discounting. In addition, the ambiguity of *k* as both a person and situation based index demands further research to unpack its meaning. The same is true for the *c*-model which advances interpretations of *c* as a weight on the nominal amount A, via the *a*-model, or as an additional subjective delay that reflects the secondary reinforcing nature of money. These interpretations are quite different, thus necessitating further research. Additionally, the results showed that the *s* parameter was perhaps too volatile to render a clear meaning. It is also not known if *s* is time-unit dependent. For example, many studies present delays in one unit to the participants (e.g., months) but then transform them to another unit for hyperbolic model fitting (e.g., days). It is unclear whether such transformations improve model fitting but at the expense of understanding time perception via the power function with *s*.

Additional considerations pertain to the methodology used to derive hyperbolic models. The indifference point methodology typically presents participants with an immediate smaller option versus a delayed larger one to derive the function. However, participants are typically not asked to compare binary options defined by payoffs and delays at other combinations of delays to further assess the predictive validity of the derived function. A vast literature in preferential choice has demonstrated that individuals vary their preferences among options depending on the method and conditions that are used to assess them [37–39]. Thus, it stands to test whether the implied changes in subjective value per unit of time derived from the indifference point methodology can predict choices that require the decision maker to directly compare binary choice options with varying monetary and delay differences. Indeed, using a general choice paradigm researchers [40–42] have begun to show limitations of the base- hyperbolic model. In addition, we point that the hyperbolic functions tested are silent to the units of delay making the models incomplete from the perspective of being full psychological accounts of how individuals contrast monetary versus delay differences. As earlier stated, for any given model, the prediction would be the same if D were days or D were years, but clearly these units would have great effect on individuals' discounting.

Author Contributions

Analyzed the data: JC CG. Wrote the paper: JC CG.

References

1. Meier S, Sprenger C (2011) Time discounting predicts creditworthiness. Psychological Science, 23(1): 56–58.
2. Chabris CF, Laibson DL, Morris CL, Schuldt JP, Taubinsky D (2008) Individual laboratory-measured discount rates predict field behaviour. Journal of Risk Uncertainty, 37: 237–269.
3. Rodriguez ML, Logue AW (1988) Adjusting delay to reinforcement: Comparing choice in pigeons and humans. Journal of Experimental Psychology: Animal Behavior Processes, 14: 105–117.
4. MacKillop J, Amlung MT, Few LR, Ray LA, Sweet LH (2011) Delayed reward discounting and addictive behavior: a meta-analysis. Psychopharmacology, 216(3): 305–321.
5. de Wit H (2008) Impulsivity as a determinant and consequence of drug use: a review of underlying processes. Addiction Biology, 14: 22–31.
6. Figner B, Knoch D, Johnson EJ, Krosch AR, Lisanby SH, et al. (2010) Lateral prefrontal cortex and self-control in inter-temporal choice. Nature Neuroscience, 13: 538–539.
7. Mazur JE (1987) An adjusting procedure for studying delayed reinforcement. In: Commons ML, Mazur JE, Nevin JA, Rachlin H (Eds.) Quantitative Analyses of Behavior: The Effect of Delay and of Intervening Events on Reinforcement Value, Erlbaum, Hillsdale, NJ, pp 55–73.
8. Rachlin H (2006) Notes on discounting. Journal of Experimental Analysis of Behavior, 85(3): 425–435.
9. Green L, Myerson J (2004) A discounting framework for choice with delayed and probabilistic rewards. Psychological Bulletin, 130(5): 769–792.
10. Espín AM, Brañas-Garza P, Herrmann B, Gamella JF (2012) Patient and Impatient Punishers of Free-riders. Proceedings of the Royal Society B: Biological Sciences, 279(1749): 4923–8.
11. Laibson D (1997) Golden Eggs and Hyperbolic Discounting. Quarterly Journal of Economics, CXII(2), 443–477.
12. Burks SV, Carpenter JP, Goette L, Rustichini A (2009) Cognitive skills affect economic preferences, strategic behavior, and job attachment. Proceedings of the National Academy of Sciences 106 (19): 7745–7750.
13. Andersen S, Harrison GW, Lau MI, Rutström EE (2008) Eliciting Risk and Time Preferences. Econometrica, 76: 583–618.
14. Bernoulli D (1954) Exposition of A New Theory On The Measurement Of Risk. Econometrica, 22: 23–36.

15. Kahneman D, Tversky A (1979) Prospect theory: An analysis of decision under risk. Econometrica, 47: 263–291.
16. Loewenstein G, Prelec D (1992) Anomalies in inter-temporal choice-evidence and an interpretation. Quarterly journal of economics, 107(2): 573–597.
17. Stevens SS (1957) On the psychophysical law. Psychological Review 64(3): 153–181.
18. Mercer D, Woody G (1999) An Individual Drug Counseling Approach to Treat Cocaine Addiction: The Collaborative Cocaine Treatment Study Model (Therapy Manuals for Drug Abuse: Manual (3). National Institute of Drug Abuse.
19. Takahashi T (2011) A neuroeconomic theory of rational addiction and nonlinear time-perception. Neuro Endocrinology Letters, 32(3): 221–225.
20. Wittmann M, Leland D, Churan J, Paulus MP (2007) Impaired time perception and motor timing in stimulant-dependent subjects. Drug Alcohol Depend, 90: 183–192.
21. Zauberman G, Kim K, Malkoc A, Bettman J (2009) Discounting Time and Time Discounting: Subjective Time Perception and Intertemporal Preferences. Journal of Marketing Research, 46(4): 543–556.
22. Estle SJ, Green L, Myerson J, Holt DD (2006) Differential effects of amount on temporal and probability discounting of gains and losses. Memory & Cognition, 34(4): 914–28.
23. McKerchar T, Green L, Myerson J, Pickford T, Hill J, et al. (2009) A comparison of four models of delay discounting in humans. Behavioral Processes, 81: 256–259.
24. Myerson J, Green L (1995) Discounting of delayed rewards: Models of individual choice. Journal of Experimental Analysis of Behavior, 64: 263–276.
25. Johnson MW, Bickel WK (2002) Within-subject comparison of real and hypothetical money rewards in delay discounting. Journal of Experimental Analysis Behavior, 77(2): 129–46.
26. Estes WK (1956) The problem of inference from curves based on group data. Psychological Bulletin, 53: 134–140.
27. Sidman M (1952) A note on the functional relations obtained from group data. Psychological Bulletin, 49(3): 263–269.
28. Bickel WK, Yi R, Landes RD, Hill PF, Baxter C (2011) Remember the future: working memory training decreases delay discounting among stimulant addicts. Biological psychiatry, 69: 260–265.
29. Odum AL, Madden GJ, Badger GJ, Bickel WK (2000) Needle sharing in opioid-dependent outpatients: psychological processes underlying risk. Drug and alcohol dependence, 60: 259–266.
30. Cheng J, Lu Y, Han X, González-Vallejo C, Sui N (2012) Temporal discounting in heroin-dependent patients: no sign effect, weaker magnitude effect, and the relationship with inhibitory control. Experimental & Clinical Psychopharmacology, 20 (5): 400–409.
31. Schwarz G (1978) Estimating the Dimension of a Model. Annals of Statistics, 6: 461–464.
32. French S (1986) Decision Theory: an Introduction to the Mathematics of Rationality. Ellis Horwood, Chichester.
33. Myerson J, Green L, Warusawitharana M (2001) Area under the curve as a measure of discounting. Journal of Experimental Analysis Behavior, 76(2): 235–243.
34. Hunter JE, Schmidt FL (2004) Methods of meta-analysis: Correcting error and bias in research findings (Second edition). Thousand Oaks, CA: Sage.
35. Hadiati W (2011) Long Queues in Zimbabwe. Available: http://www.help-ev.de/blog/allgemein/long-queues-in-zimbabwe/.
36. Aaberge R, Zhu Y (2001) The pattern of household savings during a hyperinflation: the case of urban China in the late 1980s. Review of Income and Wealth, 47 (2): 181–202.
37. González-Vallejo C, Wallsten TS (1992) Effects of probability mode on preference reversal. Journal of Experimental Psychology: Learning, Memory, and Cognition, 18 (4): 855–64.
38. González-Vallejo C, Erev I, Wallsten TS (1994) Do decision quality and preference order depend on whether probabilities are verbal or numerical? The American journal of psychology, 157–172.
39. González-Vallejo C, Moran E (2001) The evaluability hypothesis revisited: Joint and separate evaluation preference reversal as a function of attribute importance. Organizational Behavior and Human Decision Processes, 86 (2): 216–233.
40. Scholten M, Read D (2006) Discounting by intervals: A generalized model of intertemporal choice. Management Science, 52: 1426–1438.
41. Scholten M, Read D (2010) The Psychology of Intertemporal Tradeoffs. Psychological Review, 117(3): 925–44.
42. Roelofsma P, Read D (2000) Intransitive intertemporal choice. Journal of Behavioral Decision Making, 13(2): 161–177.

15

IL-17A and Serum Amyloid A Are Elevated in a Cigarette Smoke Cessation Model Associated with the Persistence of Pigmented Macrophages, Neutrophils and Activated NK Cells

Michelle J. Hansen*, Sheau Pyng J. Chan, Shenna Y. Langenbach, Lovisa F. Dousha, Jessica E. Jones, Selcuk Yatmaz, Huei Jiunn Seow, Ross Vlahos, Gary P. Anderson, Steven Bozinovski

Lung Health Research Centre, Department of Pharmacology and Therapeutics, The University of Melbourne, Victoria, Australia

Abstract

While global success in cessation advocacy has seen smoking rates fall in many developed countries, persistent lung inflammation in ex-smokers is an increasingly important clinical problem whose mechanistic basis remains poorly understood. In this study, candidate effector mechanisms were assessed in mice exposed to cigarette smoke (CS) for 4 months following cessation from long term CS exposure. BALF neutrophils, $CD4^+$ and $CD8^+$ T cells and lung innate NK cells remained significantly elevated following smoking cessation. Analysis of neutrophil mobilization markers showed a transition from acute mediators (MIP-2α, KC and G-CSF) to sustained drivers of neutrophil and macrophage recruitment and activation (IL-17A and Serum Amyoid A (SAA)). Follicle-like lymphoid aggregates formed with CS exposure and persisted with cessation, where they were in close anatomical proximity to pigmented macrophages, whose number actually increased 3-fold following CS cessation. This was associated with the elastolytic protease, MMP-12 (macrophage metallo-elastase) which remained significantly elevated post-cessation. Both GM-CSF and CSF-1 were significantly increased in the CS cessation group relative to the control group. In conclusion, we show that smoking cessation mediates a transition to accumulation of pigmented macrophages, which may contribute to the expanded macrophage population observed in COPD. These macrophages together with IL-17A, SAA and innate NK cells are identified here as candidate persistence determinants and, we suggest, may represent specific targets for therapies directed towards the amelioration of chronic airway inflammation.

Editor: Thomas H. Thatcher, University of Rochester Medical Center, United States of America

Funding: This work was supported by NHMRC (National Health and Medical Research Council) Australia (www.NHMRC.gov.au), project grant number 628492. The funders had no role in study design, data collection and analysis, decision to publish, or preparation of the manuscript.

Competing Interests: The authors have declared that no competing interests exist.

* Email: mjhansen@unimelb.edu.au

Introduction

Chronic Obstructive Pulmonary Disease (COPD) is a debilitating lung condition that is characterized by chronic airway inflammation. COPD is now the third cause of death worldwide and kills more than 3.5 million people per year. About 85% of all COPD is caused by inhalation of irritants mostly cigarette smoke (active and passive), ambient air pollutants and poor indoor air quality caused by biomass cooking and heating fumes. Inflammation induced by these irritants contributes to key pathological processes in COPD including small airway narrowing, destruction of alveolar walls (emphysema) and mucous hypersecretion (reviewed in [1]). Innate immune cells including macrophages and neutrophils accumulate and are considered essential for disease progression [2], as are immune cells of the adaptive response including $CD8^+$ T cells [3]. $CD4^+$ T cells and B cells also aggregate and can organize into lymphoid follicles, the percentage of which increases with progression of COPD [2]. The close association of de novo lymphoid follicles with persistence and severity of COPD strongly suggests their contribution to deleterious autoimmunity in the airways although beneficial effects in terms of mounting a rapid immune response to respiratory pathogens have not been formally excluded. The combined activity of the these inflammatory cells is thought to drive the accelerated decline in lung function that is a hallmark of the disease.

Cigarette smoke (CS) cessation currently remains the single most effective strategy to reduce the accelerated decline in lung function attributable to COPD. At least in developed countries there is clear evidence that smoking rates have fallen, in part due to effective cessation strategies. However, cross-sectional and longitudinal studies have shown that in individuals with established disease, airway inflammation does not fully resolve with CS cessation [4,5] and post cessation persistent lung disease is an increasingly important clinical problem. In particular, airway and sputum neutrophils persist and in some cases, increase with cessation [4–6]. Neutrophilic inflammation is particularly damaging in COPD due to a deficiency in efferocytosis (clearance of moribund cells) mediated by excessive oxidative stress [7,8], which can lead to excessive degranulation of necrotic neutrophils. Activated neutrophils release neutrophil elastase and other serine proteases, which increases with the severity of COPD and these processes are intrinsically insensitive to inhaled glucocorticosteroids [9]. Neutrophil elastase degrades extracellular matrix components including elastin, collagens I–IV and fibrinogen and the degree of elastase localized to lung elastic fibers correlates with the degree of emphysema [10]. Neutrophil elastase can also promote mucin production [11] and activate TLR4-dependent production of IL-8 via epidermal growth factor receptor (EGFR) transactivation mechanisms [12].

Macrophages also accumulate in COPD airways and are positively associated with disease severity [2]. Importantly, depletion of macrophages protected against the development of emphysema in a chronic smoke exposure model; demonstrating a pathogenic role for this immune cell [13]. Furthermore, it is now recognized that macrophages acquire a distinct phenotype associated with the progressive induction of M2-related programs as a consequence of smoke exposure and COPD [14]. Macrophages can initiate neutrophilic inflammation as they are a major source of neutrophil chemokines. Several neutrophil chemokines such as IL-8 (CXCL8), KC (CXCL1) and MIP-2α (CXCL2) are implicated in COPD as they are elevated in CS exposure models [15] and during exacerbations [16]. In addition, Interleukin-17A (IL-17A) can promote neutrophil mobilization through its regulation of leukocyte growth factors and cytokines. Immunoreactive IL-17A$^+$ cells increase in frequency in the submucosa of COPD patients [17] and IL-17A expression is elevated in CS exposure models, where mice lacking IL-17RA were protected from developing emphysema [18]. Serum Amyloid A (SAA) can also mobilize neutrophils into the airways, and SAA is elevated in COPD lung tissue [19] and is related to neutrophilic lung infiltration [20]. In this study, a CS cessation model was used to identify which molecular markers most closely relate to the persistence of innate immune responses. We identify IL-17A and SAA inflammatory cytokine networks in the persistence of inflammation following CS cessation and suggest that targeting these networks may be of therapeutic benefit in augmenting the benefit of smoking cessation in this disease group.

Materials and Methods

Animals

Specific pathogen-free male BALB/c mice obtained from the Animal Resource Centre (Perth, Australia) arrived at 6 weeks of age were housed at in sterile micro-isolator cages, and maintained on a 12:12 h light/dark cycle. This study was carried out in strict accordance with the National Health and Medical Research Council (NHMRC) of Australia. All procedures were approved by the Animal Experimentation Ethics Committee of the University of Melbourne.

Treatment

After a one week acclimatization period, mice were randomly divided into 4 groups (n = 14–18 per group) that were matched for body weight. Two groups of animals were exposed to cigarette smoke (CS) and two groups were sham exposed according to our published protocol [21,22]. Briefly, animals underwent whole body exposure to the smoke of 1 filtered cigarette inside an 18 liter plastic chamber (Winfield Red, 16 mg or less of tar, 1.2 mg or less of nicotine and 15 mg or less of CO, Philip Morris) over 15 min with a 5 minute recovery interval and this was then repeated such that mice received 2 cigarettes over a 30 min period. Smoke was generated in 50-ml tidal volumes over 10 seconds by use of timed draw-back. The mean total suspended particulate (TSP) mass concentration in the chamber containing cigarette smoke generated from one cigarette, measured from 3 min 13 s to 15 min, was 419 mg/m^3 as previously published [22]. This exposure protocol was repeated three times a day (8 am, 12 pm and 4 pm exposures) for 6 days a week and generates carboxyhemoglobin levels within the range observed in human smokers [22]. Sham animals were handled identically without cigarette smoke exposure. After 16 weeks of CS one group of mice was sacrificed, as described below. The remaining groups were then sacrificed after a period without CS of 4 and 12 weeks. Body weight was measured twice per week.

Tissue Collection

The study protocol included 4 groups (n = 11–14 per group). Mice were weighed and given an anesthetic overdose (ketamine and xylazine, 180 and 32 mg/kg i.p., respectively) and allocated to the following experimental protocols. Cohort 1 (n = 8) were subjected to bronchoalveolar lavage (BAL). Briefly, lungs from each mouse were lavaged in situ with 0.4 ml PBS, followed by three 0.3 mL of PBS, with 1 ml of BAL fluid (BALF) recovered from each animal. Smoke exposure had no effect on the recovered volume as previously shown [22]. Whole lungs were perfused free of blood via right ventricular perfusion with 10 ml of saline, rapidly excised en bloc, blotted. The large left lobe was snap frozen in liquid nitrogen and stored at −80°C for QPCR analysis. The remaining lung tissue was retained and subjected to flow cytometry analysis as detailed in the flow cytometry methods section. Cohort 2 (n = 5–6) were subjected to histology as detailed in the histology methods section.

Cellular Inflammatory Response

Bronchoalveolar lavage fluid (BALF) was collected as previously described [22]. Cytospins were prepared at 400 rpm for 10 min on a Cytospin 3 (Shandon, UK). Cytospin slides were stained with DiffQuik (Dade Baxter, Australia) and 500 cells per slide were by standard morphological criteria.

Flow Cytometry

BALF cells were resuspended in FACS buffer (PBS 1% FCS). Lungs were perfused with ice-cold PBS to remove excess blood before single cell suspensions were obtained using collagenase. Briefly, whole lungs were digested with RPMI containing collagenase D (1 mg/mL) and DNase I (Roche, Mannheim, Germany) and cells were washed and recovered by centrifugation. Erythrocytes were lysed by incubation with RBC lysis buffer. To avoid non-specific binding of Abs to FcRγ, FACS Buffer containing anti-mouse CD16/32 mAb (Mouse BD Fc Block) (2.4G2, BD) was added to all primary stains. Cells were labeled with fluorophore-conjugated antibodies at pre-optimized dilutions to CD3-FITC, CD4-PE, CD8-PE, CD49b-PE (NK/NK T marker) and CD69-FITC (all from Becton Dickinson) for 1 h at 4°C and then washed twice in FACS buffer and resuspended in a final volume of 0.5 ml of FACS buffer. Data was acquired on a BD FACSCalibur flow cytometer (Becton Dickinson) and typically up to 10^5 viable cell events were collected for analysis. A strict gating strategy was used to determine different immune cell populations as follows: single cell gate (FSC-H vs FSC-A), live cells (propidium iodide exclusion), granularity/size cell gate (FSC-A vs SSC-A) and specific surface marker gates. Flowjo software (version 7.2.4, Tree Star, OR) was used to generate plots for data analysis.

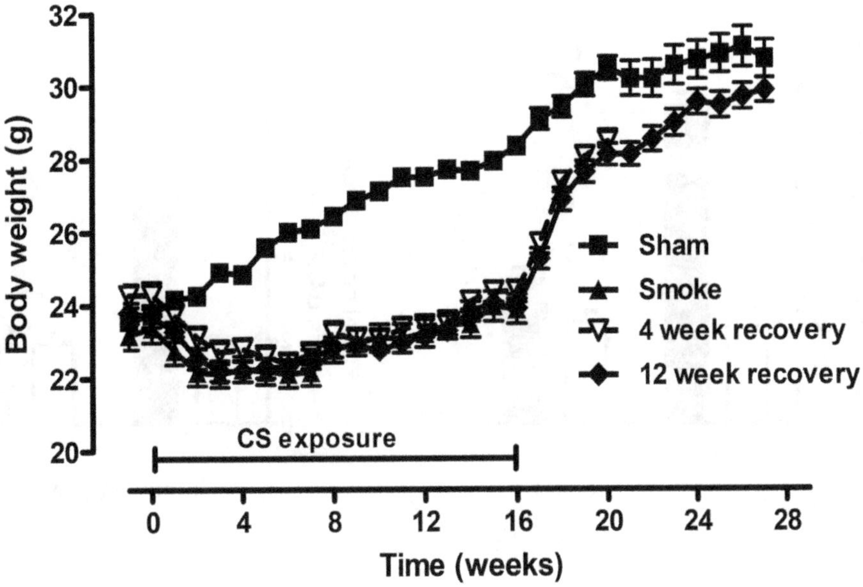

Figure 1. Smoke-induced weight loss was reversed 12 weeks after CS cessation. Male BALB/c mice were either exposed to 6 cigarettes/day, 6 days/week (■) or sham handled (▲) for 16 weeks. After smoke exposure, groups of mice were then exposed to room air without cigarette smoke for either 4 weeks (∇) or 12 weeks (◆). For all groups body weight was determined weekly. Data are shown as mean ± SE for n = 14–18 per treatment group.

Histology

Mouse lungs (n = 5–6 per group) were perfusion fixed *in situ* via a tracheal cannula with 10% neutral buffered formalin (NBF) at 25 cm H_2O pressure. After 10 min, the trachea was ligated and the lungs were left *in situ* for 1 hr, then removed and immersed in 10% NBF for at least 24 hr and then embedded in paraffin. After paraffin embedding, 4 µm sections were prepared and stained with hematoxylin and eosin. The number of pigmented macrophages was counted by a treatment-blind observer at x200 magnification, with at least 8 fields captured per sample for analysis using ImageJ software. Assessment of the number of lymphoid follicles per mm^2 of lung tissue was determined as previously published [23].

Quantitative RT-PCR

Total RNA was isolated from lung tissue using an RNeasy kit (Qiagen, MD, USA) and was used as a template to generate first-strand cDNA synthesis using SuperScript III (Invitrogen, CA, USA). TaqMan low density arrays (Applied Biosystem, CA, USA) were used for determining gene expression of individual samples using an ABI 7900 HT Sequence Detection System (Applied Biosystems). Gene expression was quantified using 18S rRNA as an internal control as previously described [22].

Statistical Analyses

Results are expressed as mean ± SE. All data were analyzed using two-way ANOVA and when statistical significance was achieved a *post hoc* Bonferroni test for multiple comparisons was used to compare between treatment groups. All statistical analyses were performed with GraphPad Prism for Windows (version 6.02). In all cases, probability values less than 0.05 ($P<0.05$) were considered statistically significant.

Results

Cessation of CS exposure restored body weight

As previously reported [24,25] mice exposed to CS failed to gain as much body weight as the Sham handled mice and were 15% lighter at the conclusion of the 16 week exposure period ($P<0.05$; Figure 1). After smoking cessation mice rapidly gained weight but remained significantly lighter by 6% after 4 weeks of recovery ($P<0.05$). By 12 weeks of recovery the body weight of mice previously exposed to CS was no different to the sham handled mice. Since the systemic effects of cigarette smoke resolve by 12 weeks, the cellular and molecular markers were characterized at this time point. In addition, following 16 weeks of smoke exposure, no significant increase in airspace enlargement was observed in BALB/c mice, which is consistent with previous studies that show an increase in mean linear intercept and destructive index in longer term chronic exposure models (i.e. 6 months) [26].

Neutrophil and lymphocyte cell number remained elevated after 12 weeks of CS cessation

Mice exposed to CS for 16 weeks (6 cigarettes/day, 6 days/week) had a significant increase in total, macrophage and neutrophil number in BALF compared to sham mice ($P<0.05$, Figure 2A–C). Following 12 weeks of CS cessation BALF macrophage and total cell number decreased to sham levels. Peak neutrophil numbers in CS exposed mice declined by approximately 10-fold in the 12 weeks CS cessation group, however remained significantly elevated by 5-fold compared to Sham mice ($P<0.05$, Figure 2C). FACS analysis was used to determine the number of Ly6G+ neutrophils in the lung tissue, which showed that tissue neutrophils accumulated with CS exposure, resulting in a 1.6-fold increase above sham exposed mice (Figure 2D). Unlike neutrophil numbers in the BALF, tissue associated neutrophil numbers in the CS cessation group normalized to sham levels (Figure 2D).

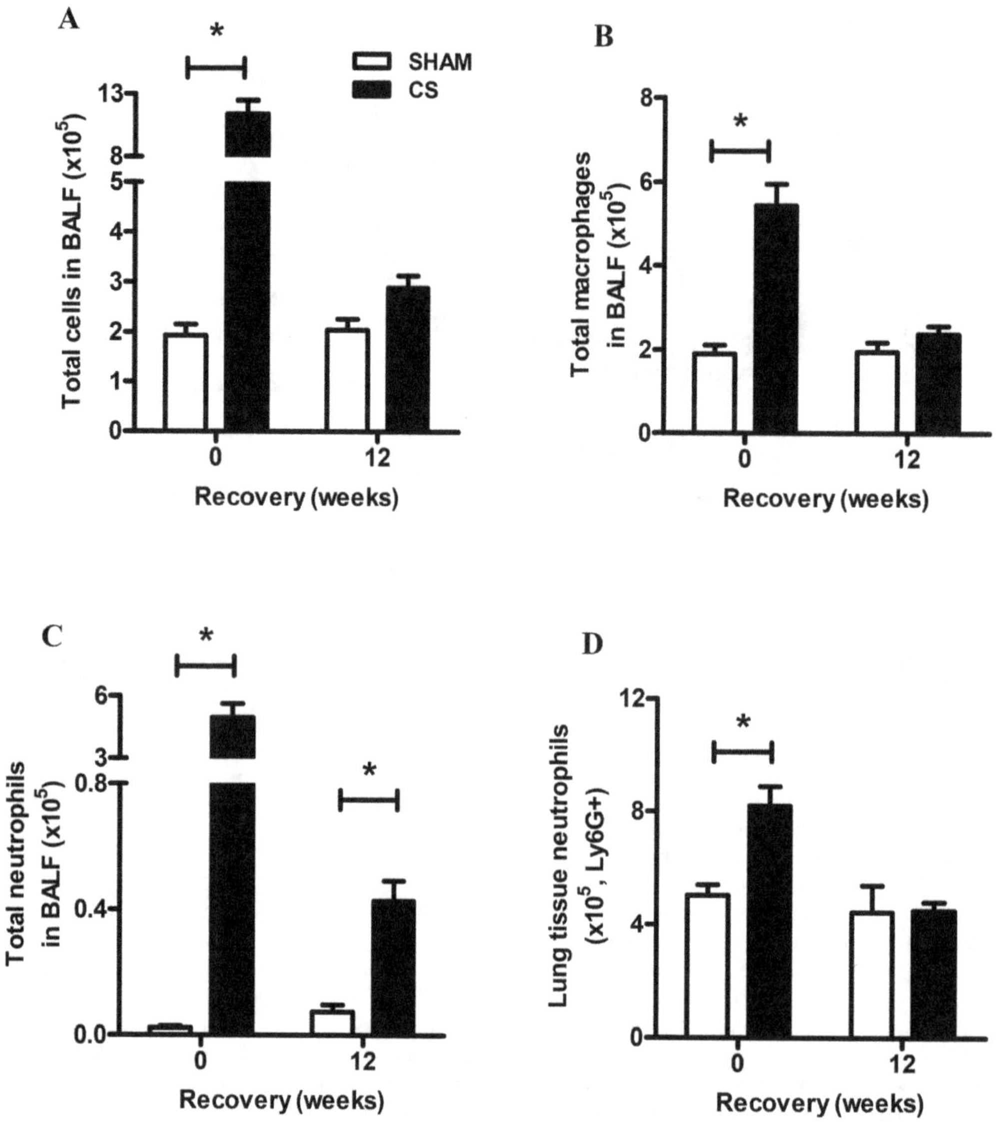

Figure 2. Effect of sub-chronic smoke exposure and 12 weeks of CS cessation on BALF cellularity and lung neutrophilia. Male BALB/c mice were either exposed to 6 cigarettes/day, 6 days/week (■) or sham handled (□) for 16 weeks. After smoke exposure a group of mice was then exposed to room air without cigarette smoke for 12 weeks. Total cells (A), macrophages (B) and neutrophils (C) were determined in BALF. Data are shown as mean ± SE for n = 8–11 per treatment group. (D) Single cell suspension of the lungs was used to determine neutrophil numbers in the lung tissue by flow cytometry. Data were analysed by two-way ANOVA and when significance was achieved a *post hoc* Bonferroni test was performed. #$P<0.05$ significant *post hoc* effect of CS compared to sham animals at the same recovery time-point.

FACS analysis was used to determine $CD3^+$ $CD4^+$ and activated $CD69^+CD8^+$ T cell number in BALF and lung tissue (Figure 3A–F). In lung tissue, CS had no effect on $CD4^+$ T cell numbers and no change in frequency was observed in the cessation groups (Figure 3A). $CD4^+$ T cells were also analyzed in the BALF compartment following 12 weeks CS recovery, demonstrating a 1.6-fold increase above Sham exposed mice (Figure 3B). Activated $CD8^+$ T cells were also quantified by flow cytometry in the lung tissue, demonstrating a significant 2.3-fold increase in CS-exposed mice above Sham controls (Figure 3C). There was also a trend towards increased $CD8^+$ T cell numbers in the CS cessation group (1.5-fold); however this failed to reach statistical significance. Analysis of BALF $CD8^+$ T cells numbers demonstrated a 2.4-fold increase in the recovery group compared to the Sham controls (Figure 3D). In addition, activated NK cells were quantified in the lung and BAL compartment demonstrating a 2-fold increase in the lung tissue that was maintained in the CS cessation group (Figure 3E). In contrast there was no increase in activated NK cells in the BAL compartment (Figure 3F).

Cigarette smoke exposure induced lymphoid aggregates and the prolonged elevation in pigmented macrophages

Hematoxylin and eosin staining of lung sections revealed the presence of structures consistent with the formation of lymphoid aggregates, a hallmark of chronic inflammation in CS exposed mice, which persisted following 12 weeks of cessation (Figure 4A). Quantification of the number of tertiary lymphoid aggregates demonstrated that these structures appeared with 16 weeks of CS exposure and consistent with a recent study [23], persisted in the cessation group where numbers appeared to slightly increase over time (Figure 4B). The lymphoid aggregates were anatomically located in close proximity to pigmented macrophages. The

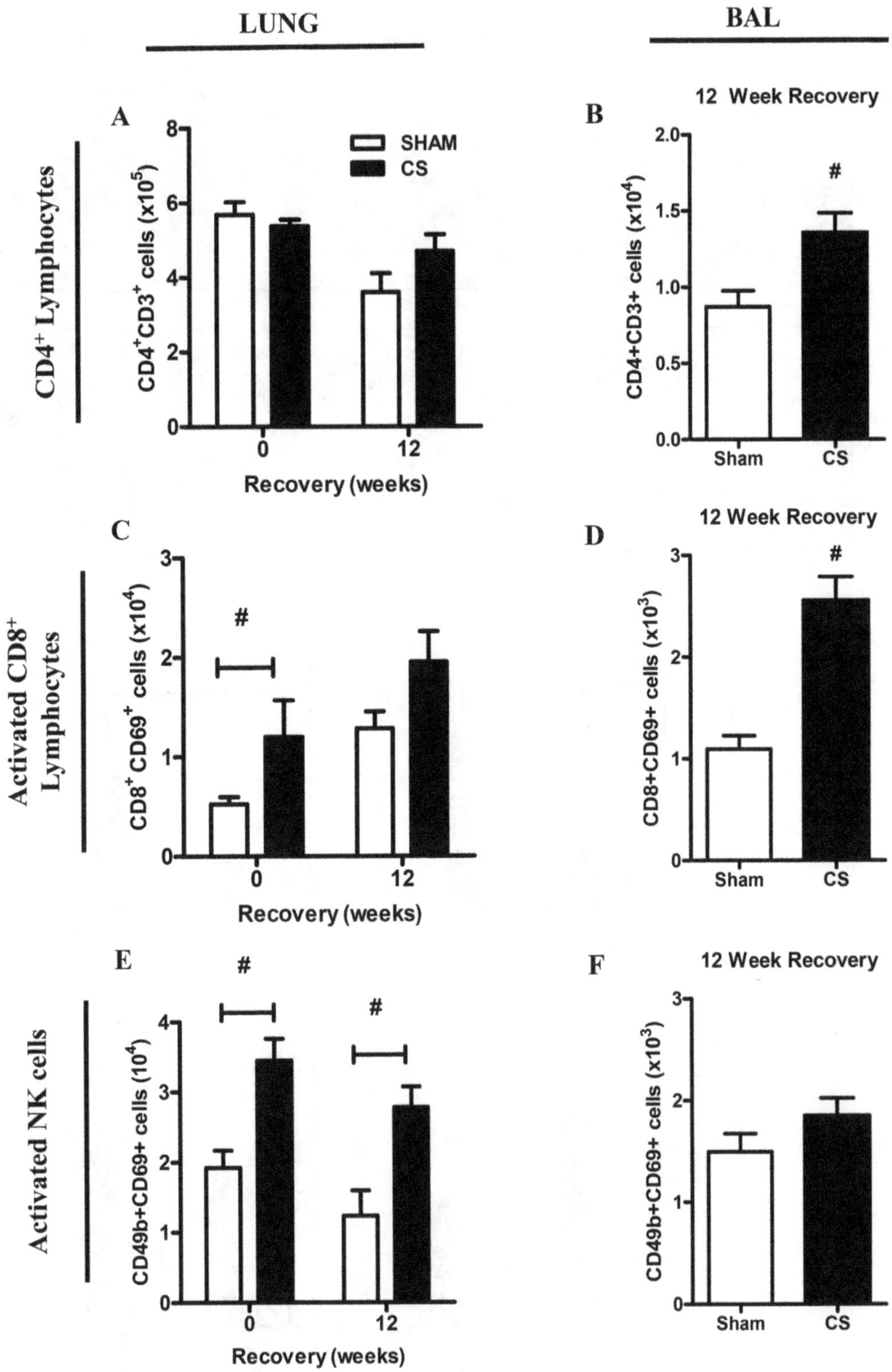

Figure 3. Effect of sub-chronic smoke exposure and 12 weeks of CS cessation on BALF and lung CD4$^+$ and activated CD8$^+$ lymphocytes. Male BALB/c mice were either exposed to 6 cigarettes/day, 6 days/week (■) or sham handled (□) for 16 weeks. After smoke exposure a group of mice was then exposed to room air without cigarette smoke for 12 weeks. CD4$^+$CD3$^+$ lymphocyte number was determined in individual lung single cell suspensions (A) and BALF cells (B) using FACS analysis. Activated CD8$^+$CD69$^+$ lymphocyte number was determined in individual lung single cell suspensions (C) and BALF cells (D) using FACS analysis. In addition, activated NK cell numbers were quantified in individual lung single cell suspensions (E) and BALF cells (F). Data are shown as mean ± SE for n = 7–8 per treatment group. Data were analysed by two-way ANOVA and when significance was achieved a *post hoc* Bonferroni test was performed. #P<0.05 significant *post hoc* effect of CS compared to sham animals at the same recovery time-point.

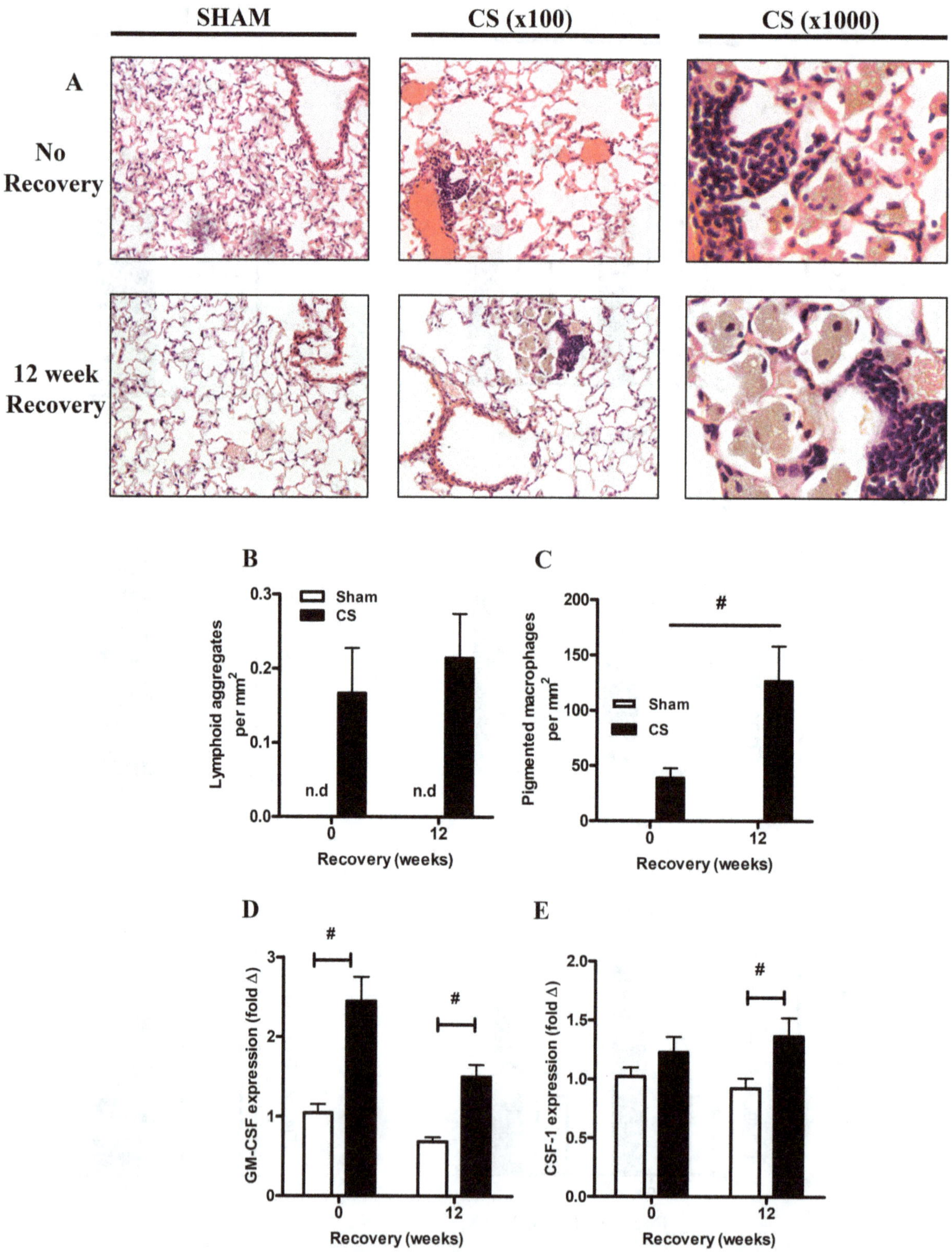

Figure 4. Sub-chronic smoke exposure resulted in the prolonged presence of pigmented macrophages. Representative histological staining of hematoxylin and eosin sections from sham and CS exposed mice and after 12 weeks of recovery (A). Magnification, x100 and x1000. The histological sections were scored for the number of lymphoid aggregates (B). The histological sections were scored for the presence of pigmented macrophages (C). Gene expression of the macrophage survival cytokines GM-CSF (D) and CSF-1 (E) was determined by Q-PCR, normalized to 18S rRNA and expressed as a fold change relative to the Sham no recovery group. Data are shown as mean ± SE for n = 7–8 per treatment group for QPCR and n = 4–6 for immunhistochemistry. Data were analysed by two-way ANOVA and when significance was achieved a *post hoc* Bonferroni test was performed. #P<0.05 significant *post hoc* effect.

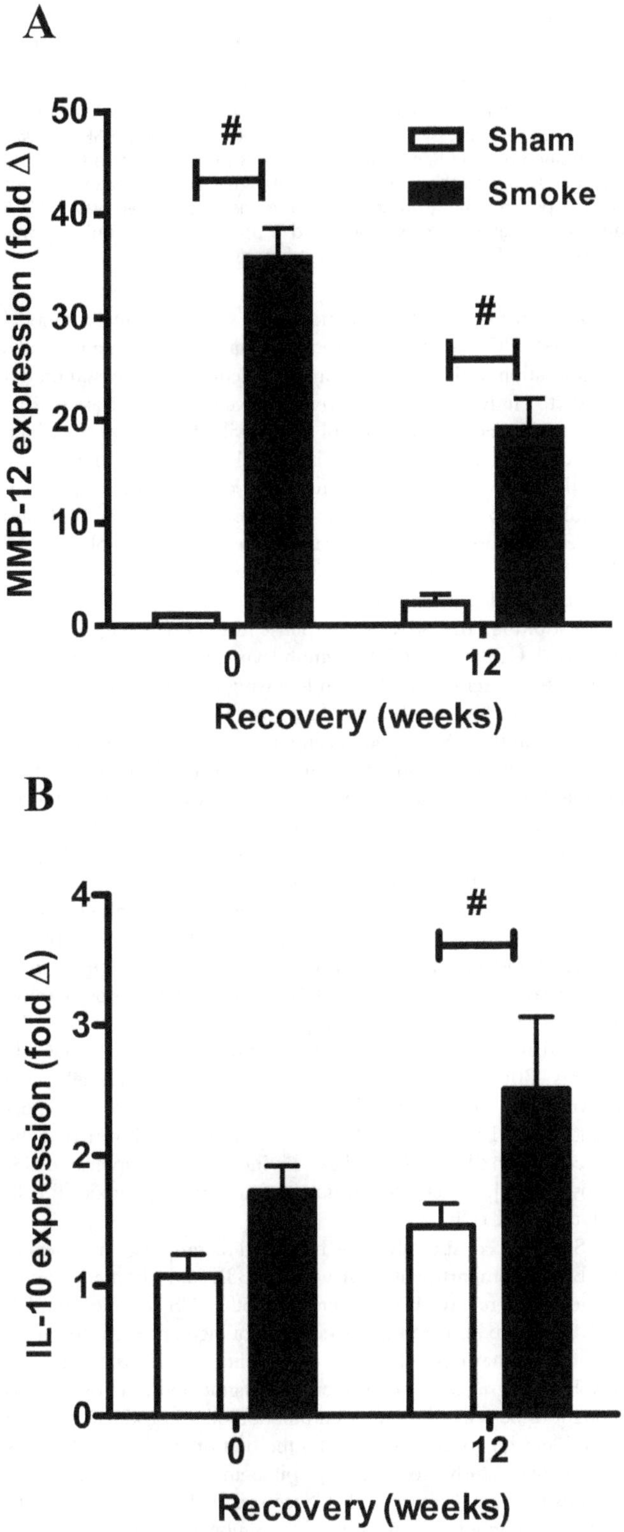

Figure 5. Effect of sub-chronic smoke exposure and 12 weeks of CS cessation on alternative macrophage marker mRNA expression in lung tissue. Male BALB/c mice were either exposed to 6 cigarettes/day, 6 days/week (■) or sham handled (□) for 16 weeks. After smoke exposure a group of mice was then exposed to room air without cigarette smoke for 12 weeks. Gene expression of the alternative macrophage markers, MMP-12 (A) and IL-10 (B) was determined by Q-PCR, normalized to 18S rRNA and expressed as a fold change relative to the Sham 0 weeks recovery group. Data are shown as mean ± SE for n = 7–8 per treatment group. Data were analysed by two-way ANOVA and when significance was achieved a *post hoc* Bonferroni test was performed. #P<0.05 significant *post hoc* effect.

accumulation of brown pigmented macrophages in the CS mice was quantified by a blind observer. CS exposure induced a significant increase in pigmented macrophages compared to sham mice (P<0.05, Figure 4C). Cessation resulted in a further 3-fold increase in the numbers of pigmented macrophages when compared to mice analyzed immediately after the 16 weeks of CS exposure (P<0.05, Figure 4C). Gene expression analysis of macrophage colony stimulating factors known to promote the survival and proliferation of leukocytes demonstrated that CS exposure caused a significant induction of GM-CSF mRNA compared to sham animals and this increase persisted following 12 weeks of cessation (P<0.05, Figure 4D). The mRNA expression of CSF-1 was also significantly induced after 12 weeks of CS cessation (P<0.05, Figure 4E).

Differential effects of CS cessation on markers of alternative macrophage activation and neutrophil mobilization

Expression of markers of alternative macrophage activation, MMP-12 and IL-10, was examined by QPCR of the lung tissue. CS caused a marked induction of MMP-12 gene expression (36-fold) and this remained significantly elevated by 19-fold after 12 weeks of cessation compared to sham animals (P<0.05, Figure 5A). IL-10 mRNA expression was also significantly elevated in the CS group after 12 weeks of smoking cessation compared to sham mice (P<0.05, Figure 5B).

The mRNA expression of neutrophil mobilization mediators was also examined. CS exposure significantly increased the mRNA expression of MIP-2α, KC and G-CSF compared to sham mice (P<0.05, Figure 6). 12 weeks of CS cessation resulted in a significant reduction in the mRNA expression of MIP-2α (2.3-fold), KC (2.3-fold) and G-CSF (2.1-fold) when compared to mice that were analyzed immediately following CS (P<0.05). Expression of the alternative neutrophil mobilizing mediators, IL17A and SAA, significantly increased by 9-fold and 33-fold above sham exposed mice respectively (P<0.05, Figure 7). IL-17A transcript levels did not decrease with CS cessation, where there was a 13-fold increase in the CS cessation group (Figure 7A). Although there was a trend towards reduced expression of SAA transcript in the CS cessation group (17-fold above sham), this was not significantly different to levels in CS exposed mice (Figure 7B). In addition, the well characterized T_H17 polarising cytokines IL-6 (Figure 7C) and IL23 (Figure 7D) were measured by QPCR in the lung tissue. IL-6 levels were increased by 16 weeks of CS exposure; however there was no difference in IL-6 expression in the CS cessation arm. IL23 levels did not significantly increase with 16 weeks CS exposure.

Discussion

COPD is a disease that displays a complex immunological profile associated with the engagement of innate and adaptive cellular processes in response to chronic CS exposure. Immune cells of both the innate and adaptive response persisted in our CS cessation model and this was previously associated with a modest reduction of alveolar enlargement and increased pulmonary compliance [27]. The innate response is particularly active in COPD, where macrophages and neutrophils accumulate in COPD airways [28], and neutrophilic inflammation fails to fully

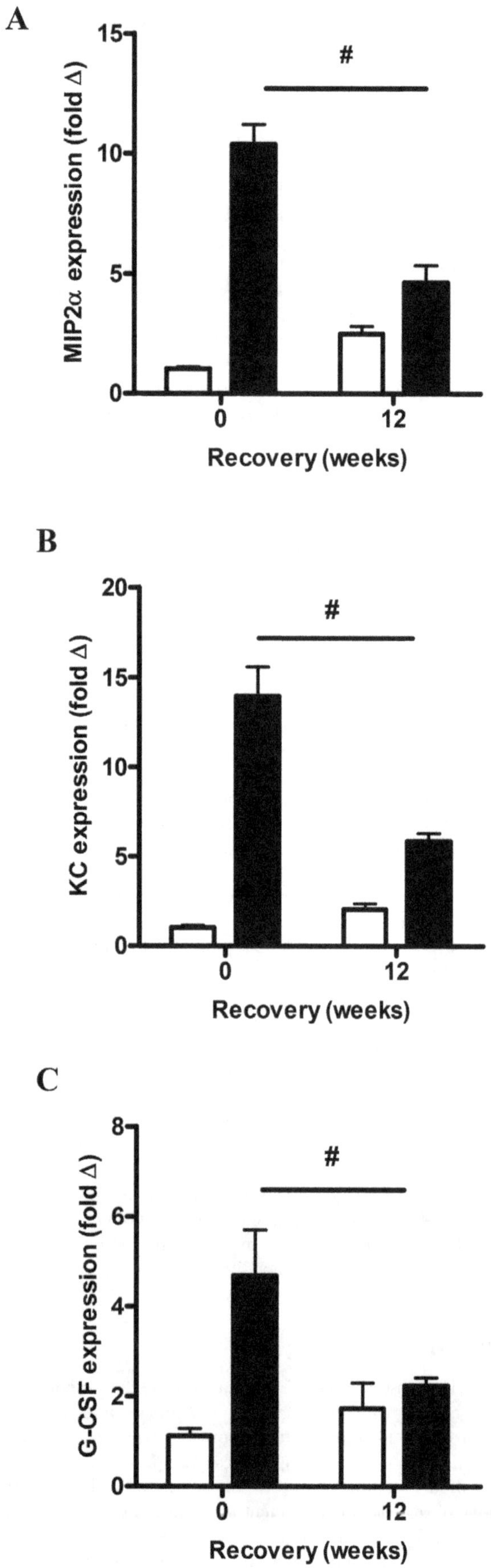

Figure 6. Effect of sub-chronic smoke exposure and 12 weeks of CS cessation on classic neutrophil mobilization mediators. Male BALB/c mice were either exposed to 6 cigarettes/day, 6 days/week (■) or sham handled (□) for 16 weeks. After smoke exposure a group of mice was then exposed to room air without cigarette smoke for 12 weeks. Gene expression of MIP-2α (A), KC (B) and G-CSF (C) was determined by Q-PCR, normalized to 18S rRNA and expressed as a fold change relative to the Sham group. Data are shown as mean ± SE for n = 7–8 per treatment group. Data were analysed by two-way ANOVA and when significance was achieved a *post hoc* Bonferroni test was performed. #P<0.05 significant *post hoc* effect.

resolve in response to CS cessation [4,5]. Our experimental model displayed a similar response to CS cessation where neutrophilic inflammation in the BAL compartment reduced with cessation but failed to fully resolve to control levels. In contrast, tissue neutrophils declined to control levels with CS cessation, which was consistent with the decline in G-CSF, a major hematopoietic growth factor required for mobilization and maturation of granulocyte precursors. Given the short-lived nature of blood derived neutrophils, the low level persistence of neutrophils in the BAL compartment is characteristic of an inflammatory response that has failed to fully resolve.

In addition, the adaptive response was also engaged, where increased $CD4^+$ and $CD8^+$ lymphocyte numbers in the BALF compartment remained elevated following CS cessation. Although total lymphocyte numbers in lung tissue were not significantly increased in the CS cessation group, there was an accumulation of lymphoid follicle-like structures in response to CS exposure that persisted in the cessation group. This is consistent with a recent report, where the persistence of lymphoid aggregates was associated with increased anti-nuclear autoantibody (ANA) production [23]. The role of these organized structures remain to be fully resolved, however therapeutic targeting of lymphoid follicle formation in mice chronically exposed to CS failed to suppress airway remodeling and alveolar enlargement [29]. There was also an increase in innate lymphoid NK cells in CS exposed mice, which persisted in the cessation group. This is consistent with the observed increase in NK cells in the induced sputum of COPD patients [30]. In a chronic CS challenge model, NK cells were shown to be more primed to release inflammatory mediators including IL-12 and IL-18 [31]. It has also been shown that the NK cell group 2D (NKG2D) ligand is increased in response to CS-exposure [32], which can sustain activation of cytotoxic T cells including NK cells.

CS models consistently show increased macrophage numbers in the BALF compartment (reviewed in [33]) and elevated macrophage numbers have been observed in other CS cessation models [27]. Here, we observed the persistence of pigmented macrophage populations that typically clustered together in regions adjacent to lymphoid aggregates. The presence of pigmented macrophages is thought to be related to the accumulation of CS products ingested by resident lung macrophages. To the best of our knowledge, this is the first study to quantify pigmented macrophages and demonstrate an increase with CS cessation. In conjunction with increased pigmented macrophage numbers, leukocyte colony stimulating factors, GM-CSF and CSF-1 transcript were significantly increased in the CS cessation group. Both CSFs are known to promote survival, proliferation and differentiation of myeloid lineages, and the findings presented here suggest that pigmented macrophages may proliferate in response to increased CSF expression. Whether these pigmented macrophages represent a distinct phenotype in COPD that contribute to disease pathobiology remains to be determined. There is however, growing evidence that macrophages do not conform to the classic M1/M2

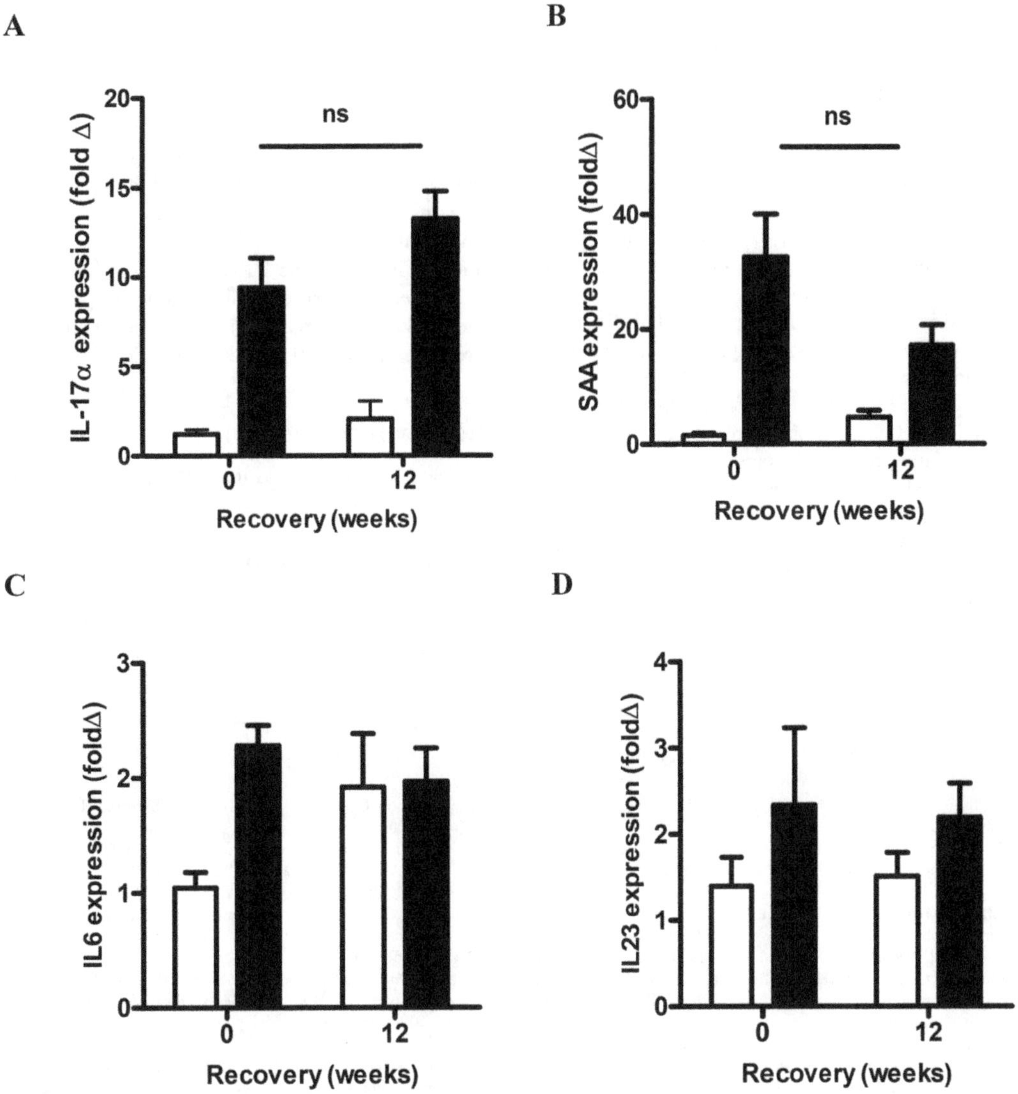

Figure 7. Effect of sub-chronic smoke exposure and 12 weeks of CS cessation on IL-17A and SAA expression. Male BALB/c mice were either exposed to 6 cigarettes/day, 6 days/week (■) or sham handled (□) for 16 weeks. After smoke exposure a group of mice was then exposed to room air without cigarette smoke for 12 weeks. Gene expression of IL-17A (A), SAA (B), IL-6 (C) and IL23 (D) was determined by Q-PCR, normalized to 18S rRNA and expressed as a fold change relative to the Sham group. Data are shown as mean ± SE for n = 6–8 per treatment group. Data were analyzed by two-way ANOVA and when significance was achieved a *post hoc* Bonferroni test was performed.

dichotomy in COPD [14,34]. In this study, IL-10 and MMP-12 expression were used as markers for differential macrophage polarization as previously reported [34], and increased expression suggest that alternative macrophage populations persist and contribute to chronic inflammation.

Previous global expression studies have shown that the majority of CS-inducible genes decline with cessation [35]. In our study, there was a focus on genes involved in neutrophil mobilization that are known to be upregulated in COPD. We have shown that IL-17A and SAA were not significantly reduced in the CS cessation group, in contrast to MIP-2α, KC and G-CSF that significantly declined with recovery. Our previous studies have demonstrated intense SAA immunoreactivity [19] and a positive correlation with neutrophilic airway inflammation [20] in the lungs of COPD patients. SAA is also a ligand for the GPCR termed ALX/FPR2, where SAA is a potent chemotactic factor that mediates phagocyte migration via this receptor [36]. SAA also promotes airway neutrophilic inflammation in a manner that is opposed by the eicosanoid, LipoxinA_4 [19]. Lipoxins and resolvins are alternative lipid-based ALX/FPR2 ligands that can oppose the actions of SAA and actively promote the resolution of inflammation (reviewed in [37,38]). Hence, the relative abundance of alternative ALX/FPR2 ligands may contribute to the impairment of resolution, where increased SAA may skew the balance towards a pro-inflammatory state.

SAA has also been shown to promote airway neutrophil recruitment via IL-17A dependent mechanisms [20]. There is also emerging evidence for an important role for IL-17A in COPD. IL-17A$^+$ cells have been shown to be increased in the bronchial submucosa of chronic smokers and stable COPD subjects [17,39]. Furthermore, genetic ablation of the IL-17R in experimental CS models protected the mice against the development of emphysema [18], hence identifying IL-17A as a major inflammatory cytokine that can drive pathological inflammation. Recent studies also demonstrate that neutrophilic inflammation induced by CS exposure is potently suppressed in mice deficient in IL-17A [40] and in response to neutralisation with a blocking antibody [41]. Furthermore, inhibition of IL-17A signaling in an experimental COPD model also suppressed accumulation of macrophages in response to CS exposure [18]. Our finding of persistent IL-17A expression in the CS cessation group is consistent with a recent study that identified an increase in the frequency of IL-17A expressing $CD4^+$ (T_H17) and $CD8^+$ (T_C17) T cells in CS exposed mice [42]. In our study, known T_H17 cytokines were also quantified by QPCR and showed that IL-6, but not IL23 was significantly increased in response to CS exposure. This finding is consistent with our previous study that investigated T_H17 cytokine expression in response to SAA stimulation, where IL-6 was predominately induced [20]. Although SAA levels were not significantly reduced with CS cessation, there was a trend towards reduced expression relative to the non-cessation group and IL-6 levels were not increased in the CS cessation group. This data suggests that SAA and IL-6 can be sufficient to initiate polarization and maturation of IL-17A expressing cellular populations in CS exposed lungs, however once established, IL-$17A^+$ cells may be maintained in the mucosa independently of T_H17 cytokines.

In addition to classic T_H17 pathways, there is also emerging evidence for alternative innate cellular sources of IL-17A in inflammatory lung models. This may be particularly relevant to COPD as NOD. SCID mice deficient in B and T cells still develop airspace enlargement in response to chronic CS exposure, to suggest a more prominent role for innate immune responses [43]. Indeed, innate sources of IL-17A have been identified in inflammatory lung models including macrophages, neutrophils, NK cells and $\gamma\delta$ T cells [20,44] and the predominant source of IL-17A in COPD is yet to be defined. In conclusion, this study has investigated innate and adaptive responses following CS cessation and has identified the IL-17A and SAA innate cytokine networks as markers of persistent inflammatory responses. The targeting of the IL-17A axis may represent a novel therapeutic strategy to promote the resolution of inflammation following CS cessation.

Acknowledgments

The authors would like to thank Debbie Allen, Oliver Ferdinando and Lindsay Kosack for their technical assistance.

Author Contributions

Conceived and designed the experiments: MH SB GA RV. Performed the experiments: SC SL LD JJ HS SY. Analyzed the data: MH SB GA RV SC SL JJ HS. Contributed to the writing of the manuscript: MH SB GA RV.

References

1. Barnes PJ (2008) Immunology of asthma and chronic obstructive pulmonary disease. Nat Rev Immunol 8: 183–192.
2. Hogg JC, Chu F, Utokaparch S, Woods R, Elliott WM, et al. (2004) The nature of small-airway obstruction in chronic obstructive pulmonary disease. N Engl J Med 350: 2645–2653.
3. Saetta M, Di Stefano A, Turato G, Facchini FM, Corbino L, et al. (1998) CD8+ T-lymphocytes in peripheral airways of smokers with chronic obstructive pulmonary disease. Am J Respir Crit Care Med 157: 822–826.
4. Rutgers SR, Postma DS, ten Hacken NH, Kauffman HF, van Der Mark TW, et al. (2000) Ongoing airway inflammation in patients with COPD who Do not currently smoke. Chest 117: 262S.
5. Willemse BW, ten Hacken NH, Rutgers B, Lesman-Leegte IG, Postma DS, et al. (2005) Effect of 1-year smoking cessation on airway inflammation in COPD and asymptomatic smokers. Eur Respir J 26: 835–845.
6. Stanescu D, Sanna A, Veriter C, Kostianev S, Calcagni PG, et al. (1996) Airways obstruction, chronic expectoration, and rapid decline of FEV1 in smokers are associated with increased levels of sputum neutrophils. Thorax 51: 267–271.
7. Bozinovski S, Vlahos R, Zhang Y, Lah LC, Seow HJ, et al. (2011) Carbonylation caused by cigarette smoke extract is associated with defective macrophage immunity. Am J Respir Cell Mol Biol 45: 229–236.
8. Hodge S, Hodge G, Ahern J, Jersmann H, Holmes M, et al. (2007) Smoking alters alveolar macrophage recognition and phagocytic ability: implications in chronic obstructive pulmonary disease. Am J Respir Cell Mol Biol 37: 748–755.
9. Vlahos R, Wark PA, Anderson GP, Bozinovski S (2012) Glucocorticosteroids differentially regulate MMP-9 and neutrophil elastase in COPD. PLoS One 7: e33277.
10. Damiano VV, Tsang A, Kucich U, Abrams WR, Rosenbloom J, et al. (1986) Immunolocalization of elastase in human emphysematous lungs. J Clin Invest 78: 482–493.
11. Shao MX, Nadel JA (2005) Neutrophil elastase induces MUC5AC mucin production in human airway epithelial cells via a cascade involving protein kinase C, reactive oxygen species, and TNF-alpha-converting enzyme. J Immunol 175: 4009–4016.
12. Walsh DE, Greene CM, Carroll TP, Taggart CC, Gallagher PM, et al. (2001) Interleukin-8 up-regulation by neutrophil elastase is mediated by MyD88/IRAK/TRAF-6 in human bronchial epithelium. J Biol Chem 276: 35494–35499.
13. Beckett EL, Stevens RL, Jarnicki AG, Kim RY, Hanish I, et al. (2013) A new short-term mouse model of chronic obstructive pulmonary disease identifies a role for mast cell tryptase in pathogenesis. J Allergy Clin Immunol 131: 752–762.
14. Shaykhiev R, Krause A, Salit J, Strulovici-Barel Y, Harvey BG, et al. (2009) Smoking-dependent reprogramming of alveolar macrophage polarization: implication for pathogenesis of chronic obstructive pulmonary disease. J Immunol 183: 2867–2883.
15. Stevenson CS, Coote K, Webster R, Johnston H, Atherton HC, et al. (2005) Characterization of cigarette smoke-induced inflammatory and mucus hypersecretory changes in rat lung and the role of CXCR2 ligands in mediating this effect. Am J Physiol Lung Cell Mol Physiol 288: L514–522.
16. Qiu Y, Zhu J, Bandi V, Atmar RL, Hattotuwa K, et al. (2003) Biopsy neutrophilia, neutrophil chemokine and receptor gene expression in severe exacerbations of chronic obstructive pulmonary disease. Am J Respir Crit Care Med 168: 968–975.
17. Di Stefano A, Caramori G, Gnemmi I, Contoli M, Vicari C, et al. (2009) T helper type 17-related cytokine expression is increased in the bronchial mucosa of stable chronic obstructive pulmonary disease patients. Clin Exp Immunol 157: 316–324.
18. Chen K, Pociask DA, McAleer JP, Chan YR, Alcorn JF, et al. (2011) IL-17RA is required for CCL2 expression, macrophage recruitment, and emphysema in response to cigarette smoke. PLoS One 6: e20333.
19. Bozinovski S, Uddin M, Vlahos R, Thompson M, McQualter JL, et al. (2012) Serum amyloid A opposes lipoxin A(4) to mediate glucocorticoid refractory lung inflammation in chronic obstructive pulmonary disease. Proc Natl Acad Sci U S A 109: 935–940.
20. Anthony D, Seow HJ, Uddin M, Thompson M, Dousha L, et al. (2013) Serum amyloid A promotes lung neutrophilia by increasing IL-17A levels in the mucosa and gammadelta T cells. Am J Respir Crit Care Med 188: 179–186.
21. Hansen MJ, Chen H, Jones JE, Langenbach SY, Vlahos R, et al. (2013) The lung inflammation and skeletal muscle wasting induced by subchronic cigarette smoke exposure are not altered by a high-fat diet in mice. PLoS One 8: e80471.
22. Vlahos R, Bozinovski S, Jones JE, Powell J, Gras J, et al. (2006) Differential protease, innate immunity, and NF-kappaB induction profiles during lung inflammation induced by subchronic cigarette smoke exposure in mice. Am J Physiol Lung Cell Mol Physiol 290: L931–945.
23. Morissette MC, Jobse BN, Thayaparan D, Nikota JK, Shen P, et al. (2014) Persistence of pulmonary tertiary lymphoid tissues and anti-nuclear antibodies following cessation of cigarette smoke exposure. Respir Res 15: 49.
24. Chen H, Hansen MJ, Jones JE, Vlahos R, Bozinovski S, et al. (2007) Regulation of hypothalamic NPY by diet and smoking. Peptides 28: 384–389.
25. Chen H, Vlahos R, Bozinovski S, Jones J, Anderson GP, et al. (2005) Effect of short-term cigarette smoke exposure on body weight, appetite and brain neuropeptide Y in mice. Neuropsychopharmacology 30: 713–719.
26. Motz GT, Eppert BL, Sun G, Wesselkamper SC, Linke MJ, et al. (2008) Persistence of lung CD8 T cell oligoclonal expansions upon smoking cessation in a mouse model of cigarette smoke-induced emphysema. J Immunol 181: 8036–8043.
27. Braber S, Henricks PA, Nijkamp FP, Kraneveld AD, Folkerts G (2010) Inflammatory changes in the airways of mice caused by cigarette smoke exposure are only partially reversed after smoking cessation. Respir Res 11: 99.
28. Hogg JC (2004) Pathophysiology of airflow limitation in chronic obstructive pulmonary disease. Lancet 364: 709–721.

29. Bracke KR, Verhamme FM, Seys LJ, Bantsimba-Malanda C, Cunoosamy DM, et al. (2013) Role of CXCL13 in cigarette smoke-induced lymphoid follicle formation and chronic obstructive pulmonary disease. Am J Respir Crit Care Med 188: 343–355.
30. Urbanowicz RA, Lamb JR, Todd I, Corne JM, Fairclough LC (2010) Enhanced effector function of cytotoxic cells in the induced sputum of COPD patients. Respir Res 11: 76.
31. Motz GT, Eppert BL, Wortham BW, Amos-Kroohs RM, Flury JL, et al. (2010) Chronic cigarette smoke exposure primes NK cell activation in a mouse model of chronic obstructive pulmonary disease. J Immunol 184: 4460–4469.
32. Borchers MT, Wesselkamper SC, Curull V, Ramirez-Sarmiento A, Sanchez-Font A, et al. (2009) Sustained CTL activation by murine pulmonary epithelial cells promotes the development of COPD-like disease. J Clin Invest 119: 636–649.
33. Vlahos R, Bozinovski S (2014) Recent advances in pre-clinical mouse models of COPD. Clin Sci (Lond) 126: 253–265.
34. Woodruff PG, Koth LL, Yang YH, Rodriguez MW, Favoreto S, et al. (2005) A distinctive alveolar macrophage activation state induced by cigarette smoking. Am J Respir Crit Care Med 172: 1383–1392.
35. Halappanavar S, Russell M, Stampfli MR, Williams A, Yauk CL (2009) Induction of the interleukin 6/signal transducer and activator of transcription pathway in the lungs of mice sub-chronically exposed to mainstream tobacco smoke. BMC Med Genomics 2: 56.
36. Su SB, Gong W, Gao JL, Shen W, Murphy PM, et al. (1999) A seven-transmembrane, G protein-coupled receptor, FPRL1, mediates the chemotactic activity of serum amyloid A for human phagocytic cells. J Exp Med 189: 395–402.
37. Levy BD, Vachier I, Serhan CN (2012) Resolution of inflammation in asthma. Clin Chest Med 33: 559–570.
38. Serhan CN, Chiang N, Van Dyke TE (2008) Resolving inflammation: dual anti-inflammatory and pro-resolution lipid mediators. Nat Rev Immunol 8: 349–361.
39. Doe C, Bafadhel M, Siddiqui S, Desai D, Mistry V, et al. (2010) Expression of the T helper 17-associated cytokines IL-17A and IL-17F in asthma and COPD. Chest 138: 1140–1147.
40. Chang Y, Al-Alwan L, Audusseau S, Chouiali F, Carlevaro-Fita J, et al. (2014) Genetic deletion of IL-17A reduces cigarette smoke-induced inflammation and alveolar type II cell apoptosis. Am J Physiol Lung Cell Mol Physiol 306: L132–143.
41. Shen N, Wang J, Zhao M, Pei F, He B (2011) Anti-interleukin-17 antibodies attenuate airway inflammation in tobacco-smoke-exposed mice. Inhal Toxicol 23: 212–218.
42. Duan M-C, Tang H-J, Zhong X-N, Huang Y (2013) Persistence of Th17/Tc17 Cell Expression upon Smoking Cessation in Mice with Cigarette Smoke-Induced Emphysema. Clinical and Developmental Immunology 2013: 11.
43. D'Hulst A I, Maes T, Bracke KR, Demedts IK, Tournoy KG, et al. (2005) Cigarette smoke-induced pulmonary emphysema in scid-mice. Is the acquired immune system required? Respir Res 6: 147.
44. Essilfie AT, Simpson JL, Horvat JC, Preston JA, Dunkley ML, et al. (2011) Haemophilus influenzae infection drives IL-17-mediated neutrophilic allergic airways disease. PLoS Pathog 7: e1002244.

16

Prevalence of Depression, Suicidal Ideation, Alcohol Intake and Nicotine Consumption in Rural Central India. The Central India Eye and Medical Study

Jost B. Jonas[1,2◑¶]*, **Vinay Nangia**[1◑¶]*, **Marcella Rietschel**[3◑¶], **Torsten Paul**[3], **Prakash Behere**[1,4], **Songhomitra Panda-Jonas**[1,2]

1 Suraj Eye Institute, Nagpur, Maharashtra, India, **2** Department of Ophthalmology, Medical Faculty Mannheim of the Ruprecht-Karls-University Heidelberg, Mannheim, Germany, **3** Department of Genetic Epidemiology in Psychiatry, Central Institute of Mental Health, Medical Faculty Mannheim of the Ruprecht-Karls-University Heidelberg, Mannheim, Germany, **4** Department of Psychiatry, Datta Meghe Institute of Medical Sciences, Wardha, Maharashtra, India

Abstract

Background: To investigate the prevalence of depression, suicidal ideations, alcohol and nicotine consumption in adults in an agrarian society mostly unchanged by the effects of urbanization.

Methods: The Central India Eye and Medical Study is a population-based study in rural Central India close to the tribal belt and included 4711 subjects (aged 30+ years). Depression was assessed by the Center for Epidemiologic Studies Depression Scale (CESD), suicidal ideation by six standardized questions, nicotine use by the Fagerstroem Nicotine Tolerance Questionnaire (FTNQ), and alcohol consumption by the Alcohol Use Disorders Identification Test (AUDIT).

Results: Mild to moderate depression (CESD sum score: 15–21) was detected in 1862 (39.6%) individuals (33.5% of men, 44.8 of women), and major depression (CESD sum score >21) in 613 (13.0%) individuals (8.1 of men, 17.3% of women). Suicide attempt was reported by 199 (4.2%) participants and suicidal thoughts during the last 6 months by 238 (5.1%) individuals. There were 887 (18.9%) smokers and smokeless tobacco was consumed by 1968 (41.8%) subjects. Alcohol consumption was reported by 1081 (23.0%) participants; 283 (6.0%) subjects had an AUDIT score ≥8 (hazardous drinking), and 108 (4.63%) subjects a score ≥13 (women) or ≥15 (men) (alcohol dependence).

Conclusions: In rural Central India, prevalence of major depression was comparable to figures reported from other developing countries. Prevalence of smoking and hazardous alcohol consumption was higher than as reported from urban regions. Measures should be taken to address the relatively high prevalence of suicide attempts and thoughts on suicide in rural Central India.

Editor: Osama Ali Abulseoud, Mayo Clinic, United States of America

Funding: Support was provided by an unrestricted grant from Om Drishti Trust Nagpur; Heidelberg Engineering Co. Heidelberg, Germany; Rotary Sight Saver Netherlands; Orbis India; and Carl Zeiss Meditec Co., Jena, Germany. The funders had no role in study design, data collection and analysis, decision to publish, or preparation of the manuscript.

Competing Interests: The authors advise of the following: The authors received unrestricted grants from Heidelberg Engineering Co. Heidelberg, Germany and Carl Zeiss Meditec Co., Jena, Germany. Co-author Jost B. Jonas is an Editor of PLOS ONE. This does not alter the authors' adherence to PLOS ONE policies on sharing data and materials.

* Email: nagpursuraj@gmail.com (VN); jost.jonas@medma.uni-heidelberg.de (JBJ)

◑ These authors contributed equally to this work.

¶ These authors share first authorship on this work.

Introduction

Depression with a lifetime prevalence of 2% to 15% is one of the most important risk factors for substantial disability and is one of the major leading causes of disease burden in 2010 [1–5]. Smoking has become the leading cause of preventable death with yearly about 5 million premature deaths worldwide [1,2,6–8]. Alcohol consumption, among other risk factors such as dietary risks, tobacco smoking, high blood pressure, high fasting plasma glucose and physical inactivity, belongs to the leading risk factors related to DALYs [1,2,9–13]. Results from the Global Burden of Disease study showed that especially mental health disorders constitute an enormous and growing problem in developed and developing regions [14]. Despite the worldwide importance of depression, suicide, smoking and alcohol consumption, and although India is the second largest nation by the number of inhabitants, relatively little has been known about the prevalence of depression, suicide ideation, alcohol and nicotine consumption in India. It holds true in particular for the rural population in the under-developed regions of the Indian subcontinent. The present study was therefore conducted to assess the prevalence of depression, nicotine and alcohol abuse and possibly associated health issues in adults living in rural Central India in villages bordering the so-called tribal belt. Since the living conditions in these communities have not markedly changed within the last 100 years, the study additionally offered the possibility of assessing the prevalence of depression, smoking and alcohol consumption in an environment which has remained mostly untouched by factors associated with a developed technical and medical infrastructure.

Methods

The Central India Eye and Medical Study (CIEMS) is a population-based cross-sectional study in Central India [15]. The Medical Ethics Committee of the Medical Faculty Mannheim of the Ruprecht-Karls-University Heidelberg and the ethical committee of Suraj Eye Institute/Nagpur approved the study and all participants gave informed written consent, according to the Declaration of Helsinki. The study was carried out in 8 villages in the rural region of Central Maharashtra at a distance of about 40 km from Nagpur. The villages were at the border of tribal regions. All villagers aged 30+ were invited to participate in the study which included a bus ride to the hospital, a one-day long examination, meals, and a return bus ride to the village in the evening all free of charge. All examinations were carried out on site in the hospital. Trained social workers interviewed the participants with the help of a standardized questionnaire including 200 questions on the socioeconomic background, living conditions, daily food, smoking or other types of tobacco consumption, alcohol consumption, amount and type of daily physical activity, known diagnosis of major diseases, and intake of medication. Addressing the questionnaire usually took about 30 to 40 minutes with the help of an experienced interviewer. If the study participants appeared to be fatigued, a break was made to make the study participant refresh.

The psychiatric status was assessed by the use of several questionnaires. Current depressive mood disorders were recorded by the Center for Epidemiologic Studies Depression Scale (CES-D) with a 20-item self-report depression scale [16]. A clinical episode of major depression was defined as a score of >21 in the CES-D. Six standardized questions concerning suicidal thoughts, suicidal behavior and suicidal attempts during the last 6 months and lifetime were asked. Individuals identified with suicidal thoughts were visited during the repeated visits to the villages as well as after the end of the study since the Suray Eye Institute continued serving visually handicapped villagers with cataract surgery. We used the Fagerstrom Test for Nicotine Dependence (FTND) to assess the smoking behavior [17]. In addition to the FTND, the history of former nicotine consumption (age of onset of tobacco consumption, cessation age, estimated pack years) and consumption of different tobacco products like hookah, bidis and smokeless tobacco products like snuff, chewing tobacco and bethel was recorded by 9 additional standardized questions. To determine alcohol consumption, the Alcohol Use Disorders Identification Test (AUDIT) was utilized [18]. The Audit is a 10-item self-report questionnaire with a sum score of 8 or more being associated with harmful or hazardous drinking, and a score of 13 or more in women and 15 or more in men, being likely to indicate alcohol dependence. In addition to the AUDIT, the history of former alcohol consumption (starting age of alcohol consumption, cessation age) and the current drinking behavior (e.g. type of drink) was assessed by a further 4 standardized questions.

Statistical analysis was performed using a commercially available statistical software package (SPSS for Windows, version 21.0, SPSS, Chicago, IL). We examined the mean values (presented as mean ± standard error for frequency parameters; presented as mean ± standard deviation for other parameters). All P-values were 2-sided and were considered statistically significant when the values were less than 0.05.

Results

Out of total population of 13,606 villagers, 5885 subjects fulfilled the inclusion criterion of an age of 30+ years. Out of these 5885 subjects, 4711 people participated, resulting in a response rate of 80.1% (Table 1). The representativeness of the study population compared to the total population of India had been examined in previous investigations with no major difference detected between the population structure of the study and the general Indian population (Table 1) [15].

There were 2520 (53.5%) women. Mean age of the study participants was 49.5±13.4 years (Table 2). Among the 1174 non-participants were 685 (58.3%) men; mean age was 48.6±14.1 years (median: 45 years; range: 30–95 years). The group of study participants and the group of non-participants did not differ significantly in age ($P = 0.06$), while the proportion of men was significantly ($P<0.001$) higher in the group of non-participants. Further details about the sub items of the non-psychiatric questionnaire, the socioeconomic background and the medical records were presented previously [15].

The mean body mass index was 19.7±3.4 kg/m^2. Mean duration of daily work was 7.4±2.2 hours. The subjects went to work by foot or by bike in 6.6±1.2 days per week. 2394 (50.8%) subjects were purely vegetarians, 35 (0.7%) subjects reported to eat fish and eggs in addition to vegetables, but no meat, and 2275 (48.3%) subjects had a mixed diet. Mean reported monthly income was 1584±1233 Rupee (1 US$ was roughly the equivalent of 50 Rupee). The reported monthly family income was less than 1500 Rupee for 2377 subjects (50.4%). Hinduism was the predominant religion (97.2% of the study population). Out of the total 4711 subjects, 1623 (34.5%) subjects reported to be illiterate, 1310 (27.8%) subjects to have visited school up the 5th standard, 533 (11.3%) subjects to have visited school between the 6th to 8th standard, 1070 (22.7%) subjects to have attended school between the 9th and 12th standard, and 165 (3.5%) subjects reported to have received a higher level of education such as graduation. Out of the 4711 subjects, 139 (3.0%) participants had a mobile. The majority of the study population lived in houses made out of mud without bricks and mortar ("kacha"; 1109 (23.5%) subjects) or made partially out of mud ("semi pucca2330 (49.5%) subjects). Out of the total 4711 subjects, 2206 (46.9%) subjects indicated that they did not have a toilet facility in their houses. Water source was a public tap, hand pump or well for 1719 (36.5%) subjects.

Depression

Data on depression were available on 4698 (99.7%) subjects with a mean age of 49.5±13.4 years. The group of subjects with data on depression and the group of subjects without assessment of depression (mean age: 55.2±13.9 years) did not differ significantly in age ($P = 0.67$).

The mean of the valid CESD sum scores was 14.1±7.5 points (median: 15; range: 0–58) (Fig. 1, 2). Men had a mean CESD sum score of 12.3±6.9 points (median: 13; range: 0–51), while female participants had a mean CESD sum score of 15.7±7.6 points (median: 16; range: 0–58). 1862 individuals (39.57%) showed a CESD sum score between 15 and 21 points indicating a mild to moderate depression within the last week, while 613 individuals (13.03%) scored >21 points in the CESD, indicating the possibility of a major depression. With respect to gender 734

Table 1. Demographic data of the Central India Eye and Medical Study (Part I) and the whole of India according to the National Census - India (2001).

	Central India Eye and Medical Study			India (Total; in Millions)			India (Rural; in Millions)		
Age	Total	Males	Females	Total	Males	Females	Total	Males	Females
30–34 Years	405 (17%)	173 (16%)	232 (18%)	74.3 (19%)	37.4 (19%)	36.9 (19%)	51.8 (19%)	25.7 (18%)	26.1 (19%)
35–39 Years	381 (16%)	154 (14%)	227 (18%)	70.6 (18%)	36.0 (18%)	34.5 (18%)	49.0 (18%)	24.9 (18%)	24.1 (18%)
40–44 Years	336 (14%)	161 (15%)	175 (14%)	55.7 (14%)	29.9 (15%)	25.9 (14%)	38.6 (14%)	20.4 (15%)	18.1 (13%)
45–49 Years	256 (11%)	118 (11%)	138 (11%)	47.4 (12%)	24.9 (12%)	22.5 (12%)	33.0 (12%)	17.0 (12%)	15.9 (12%)
50–54 Years	248 (10%)	123 (11%)	125 (10%)	36.6 (9%)	19.9 (10%)	16.7 (9%)	25.8 (9%)	13.8 (10%)	12.0 (9%)
55–59 Years	141 (6%)	66 (6%)	75 (6%)	27.7 (7%)	13.6 (7%)	14.1 (7%)	20.0 (7%)	9.6 (7%)	10.3 (8%)
60–64 Years	214 (9%)	91 (8%)	123 (10%)	27.5 (7%)	13.6 (7%)	13.9 (7%)	20.7 (7%)	10.1 (7%)	10.5 (8%)
65–69 Years	172 (7%)	66 (6%)	106 (8%)	19.8 (5%)	9.5 (5%)	10.3 (5%)	14.8 (5%)	7.1 (5%)	7.7 (6%)
70–74 Years	176 (7%)	95 (9%)	81 (6%)	14.7 (4%)	7.5 (4%)	7.2 (4%)	11.1 (4%)	5.7 (4%)	5.4 (4%)
75–79 Years	48 (2%)	40 (4%)	8 (1%)	6.6 (2%)	3.3 (2%)	3.3 (2%)	4.8 (2%)	2.4 (2%)	2.4 (2%)
80+ Years	37 (2%)	27 (2%)	10 (1%)	8.0 (2%)	3.9 (2%)	4.1 (2%)	6.0 (2%)	3.0 (2%)	3.0 (2%)
Total	2414 (100%)	1114 (100%)	1300 (100%	388.9 (100%)	199.4 (100%)	189.5 (100%)	275.5 (100%)	139.8 (100%)	135.7 (100%)

men (33.52%) and 1128 (44.83) women scored between 15 and 21 points, while 178 men (8.13%) and 435 females (17.29%) scored more than 21 points in the CESD.

For 4702 (99.8%) of the 4711 participants three standardized questions concerning suicidal behavior and suicidal attempts during their lifetime could be assessed. 199 participants (4.2%) admitted to have made an attempt at suicide. Out of these, 79 (39.7%) were men. For 3890 of the 4711 participants, three standardized questions concerning suicidal thoughts during the last 6 months or earlier were recorded. Out of these, 238 (5.1% total; 83 men (34.9%)) reported to have thought of committing suicide in the last 6 months. The most often reported reason for attempts at suicide were family related (68.4%), financial problems (22.4%) and long illness (7.9%) for men, and family related (91.7%), financial problems (5.8%) and long illness (0.8%) for women. Reasons for thoughts of committing suicide were similar: family related (79.0%), financial problems (8.6%) and long illness (9.9%) for men, and family related (93.5%), financial problems (2.6%) and long illness (3.9%) for men.

Smoking

With respect to smoking, 887 (18.84%) subjects reported to be or to have been smokers, with 184 (20.74%) being former smokers, and with 398 (44.87%) subjects who had tried to quit smoking previously without success. The mean package year number was 26.6±20.6 (median: 20.0). The mean starting age for smoking was 22.4±9.2. Stratified by gender, 883 men (40.3%) and 4 (0.02%) women reported current or former smoking. Of the 883 male smokers, 701 (79.3%) were current smokers, while of the 4 female smokers 3 still smoked on the examination date. Smokeless tobacco was consumed by 1968 (41.8%) subjects, with 1792 (91.1%) subjects being current users and 176 (8.9%) subjects being former users. Out of the 1968 users of smokeless tobacco, 275 (14.0%) subjects additionally smoked cigarettes/bidis. Gender distribution of the smokeless tobacco users was 1066 men (48.7%) and 902 women (35.8%). A complete Fagerstrom Test for Nicotine Dependence (FTND) could be calculated for 855 smokers (96.4%). The mean of the 855 valid FTND sum scores was 3.87±2.5 points (median: 4). A FTND sum score between 0 and 3 points (low level of addiction) was reported by 424 smokers (49.59%), a score between 4 and 6 points (moderate level of nicotine addiction) was reported by 281 smokers (32.87%), and 150 smokers (17.5%) scored between 7 and 10 FTND points (high level of addiction). Concerning smokeless tobacco no valid sum score was available. For 1957 smokeless tobacco users (99.44%), the mean number of daily consumptions was 4.23±2.2 times (median: 4).

Alcohol consumption

3628 (77.0%) participants reported to have never drunken alcohol; 287 (6.1%) participants reported on a consumption of alcohol once per month or less often, 264 (5.6%) participants an alcohol consumption of 2–4 times/month, 310 (6.6%) subjects an alcohol consumption of 2–3 times/week; 166 (3.5%) subjects an alcohol consumption of 4 times/week; and 54 (1.1%) subjects declared a daily alcohol consumption. Mean AUDIT sum scores was 1.4±3.8 points (median: 0). For the 1081 individuals reporting to drink alcohol the AUDIT sum score was 6.0±5.8 points (median: 4). An AUDIT sum score of 8 or more (harmful or hazardous drinking) was scored by 283 subjects (6.0% of the study population/26.2% of the individuals consuming alcohol). An AUDIT sum score of ≥13 in women or ≥15 or more in men (alcohol dependence) was achieved by 108 subjects (4.6% of the

Table 2. Demographic Parameters and Data on Daily Activities, Smoking and Alcohol Consumption, and Depression in the Central India Eye and Medical Study.

Parameter	Mean ± Standard Deviation	Median	Range
Age (Years)	49.5±13.4	47.0	30, 100
Body Mass Index (kg/m^2)	19.7±3.4	19.1	11.0, 46.3
Duration of Daily Work (Hours)	7.4±2.2	8	0.8, 18
Walking or Biking to Work (Days per Week)	6.6±1.2	7	1, 7
Diet	Purely vegetarians: 2394 (50.8%) subjects; Eating fish and eggs in addition to vegetables, but no meat: 35 (0.7%) subjects, Mixed diet: 2275 (48.3%) subjects		
Reported Monthly Income (Rupee)	1584±1233	1350	200, 15000
Family Income	<1500 Rupee: 2372 (50.5%); 1500–5000 Rupee: 2153 (45.8%); >5000 Rupee: 166 (3.5%)		
Family Type	Joint: 1968 (41.8%); Nuclear: 2607 (55.4%); Single: 133 (2.8%)		
Religion	Hindu: 4562 (96.9%); Muslim: 121 (2.6%); Others: 6 (0.6%)		
Level of Education	Illiterate: 1623 (34.5%); School up 5th standard: 1310 (27.8%); School between 6th to 8th standard: 533 (11.3%); School between 9th and 12th standard: 1070 (22.7%); Higher level of education: 165 (3.5%)		
Possession of Mobile Telephone	139 (3.0%) participants		
Housing	Houses made out of mud ("kacha"): 1109 (23.5%); Houses made partially out of mud ("semi pucca"): 2330 (49.5%)		
House Ownership	Own house: 4486 (95.6%); Rented house: 194 (4.1%); Mortgaged: 13 (0.1%)		
Light Source	Electricity: 4315 (92.0%); Kerosene, gas or oil: 333 (3.5%);		
Room for Cooking in the House	Yes: 4209 (89.7%); No: 485 (10.3%)		
Toilet Facility	No toilet facility in the houses: 2206 (46.9%) subjects		
Water Source	Public tap, hand pump or well: 1719 (36.5%); Pipe, Hand pump or well in the residency/compound: 2904 (62.6%); Other: 18 (0.4%)		
Agricultural Land Ownership	No land; 2062 (44.0%); <2 acres: 482 (10.3%); 2.0–4.9 acres: 833 (17.8%); 5+ acres: 1313 (28.0%)		
Durable Goods Ownership	Mattress, pressure cooker, chair cot/bed, table or clock: 569 (14.3%); Bicycle, electric fan, radio/Transistor, sewing machine: 2941 (63.8%); Moped/scooter, motorcycle, fixed telephone or mobile telephone: 965 (20.9%); Car, tractor: 41 (0.9%); None: 92 (2.0%)		
Livestock Ownership	Yes: 1920 (41.0%); No: 2762 (59.0%)		
Irrigated Land Ownership	No: 2049 (58.8%); Owns at least some irrigated land: 1433 (41.2%);		
Depression Score CESD	14.1±7.5	15	0, 58
Smoking	Current and/or former smokers: 887 (18.9%) (883 men; 4 women); Former smokers: 184 (20.7%); Current smokers with unsuccessful try to quit: 398 (44.9%)		
Package Years	26.6±20.6	20.0	
Fagerstrom Test for Nicotine Dependence	3.87±2.5 points	4	
Fagerstrom Test for Nicotine Dependence	0–3: 424 smokers (49.6%); 4–6: 281 smokers (32.9%); 7–10: 150 smokers (17.5%)		
Smokeless Tobacco	1957 (mean daily consumptions: 4.23±2.2 times (median: 4)		
Alcohol Consumption			
No Alcohol	3628 (77.0%) participants		
consumption of alcohol once per month or less often,	287 (6.1%) participants		
alcohol consumption of 2–4 times/month,	264 (5.6%) participants		
alcohol consumption of 2–3 times/week	310 (6.6%) subjects.		
alcohol consumption of 4 times/week	166 (3.5%) subjects		
daily alcohol consumption	54 (1.1%) subjects		
AUDIT sum score (1081 individuals)	6.0±5.8 points (median: 4)		
AUDIT sum score of 8 or more (harmful or hazardous drinking)	283 subjects (6.0% of the study population/26.2% of the individuals consuming alcohol).		
AUDIT sum score of ≥13 in women or ≥15 or more in men (alcohol dependence)	108 subjects (4.6% of the study population; 51 women (8.9% of women consuming alcohol), 57 men (11.2% of men consuming alcohol).		

study population; 51 women (8.9% of women consuming alcohol), 57 men (11.2% of men consuming alcohol).

Discussion

In our rural Central Indian study, 13.0% of the participants fulfilled the criteria for a major depression and an additional 39.6% of the study population showed mild to moderate depression. Suicide attempt was reported by 199 (4.2%) participants and suicidal thoughts during the last 6 months by 238 (5.1%) participants. Alcohol consumption was reported by 1081 (23.0%) participants; 283 (6.0%) subjects had an AUDIT sum score of ≥8 (harmful or hazardous drinking), and 108 (4.63%) subjects scored an AUDIT sum of ≥13 in women and ≥15 in men indicating alcohol dependence.

The figure of 13.0% for the prevalence of major depression is in agreement with results reported for developing countries by the WHO and the GBD [1,2]. Previous studies from India estimated the prevalence of depression in Indian community samples [19–24]. The most recent and largest population-based study reported by Poongothai and colleagues in 2009 screened more than 24,000 subjects in the city of Chennai (South India) and reported an overall prevalence of depression of 15.1% [19]. Earlier studies which mostly used screening instruments with poorer sensitivity, reported lower frequencies: Nandi and colleagues who performed their studies in the same region in 1972 reported prevalence rates for depression of 5.0% which by 1992 had increased to 7.4% [20]. A review by Math and Chandrashekar in 2006 suggested that the data reported on prevalence rates for psychiatric disorders from epidemiological studies was inconclusive with a high discrepancy in the prevalence rates, ranging from 9.5 to 370/1000 populations in India [23]. They concluded that the prevalence of mental disorders reported in epidemiological surveys could be considered lower estimates rather than accurate reflections of the true prevalence in the population.

The WHO estimated that 170 000 people die of suicide in India out of nearly 900 000 people worldwide, with about another 200 000 subjects in China and 140 000 in high-income countries [25]. In a recent survey on suicide mortality in India, Patel and colleagues found that about 3% of surveyed deaths in individuals aged 15 years or older were due to suicide [26]. A 15-year-old subject in India had a cumulative risk of about 1.3% of dying before the age of 80 years by suicide, with men having a higher risk (1.7%) than had women (1.0%). According to the recent global Burden of Disease Study GBD 2010, suicide was the most common cause of death among Indian women aged between 15 and 49 years, followed by maternal disorders, fire, tuberculosis, and diarrhea [27,28]. Beside these and other studies on the death rate by suicide in India [29–31], none of the major investigations have addressed the prevalence of suicide thoughts and unsuccessful suicide attempts in the Indian population, in particular not in the rural population. A WHO publication based on data collected by India's National Crime Records Bureau, Ministry of Home Affairs showed a rising suicide rate from 1980–2009 [32]. In 1980, there was a total rate of 6.3 suicides per 100.000 people, in 2009 the total rate was 10.5 per 100.000. In this publication the suicide

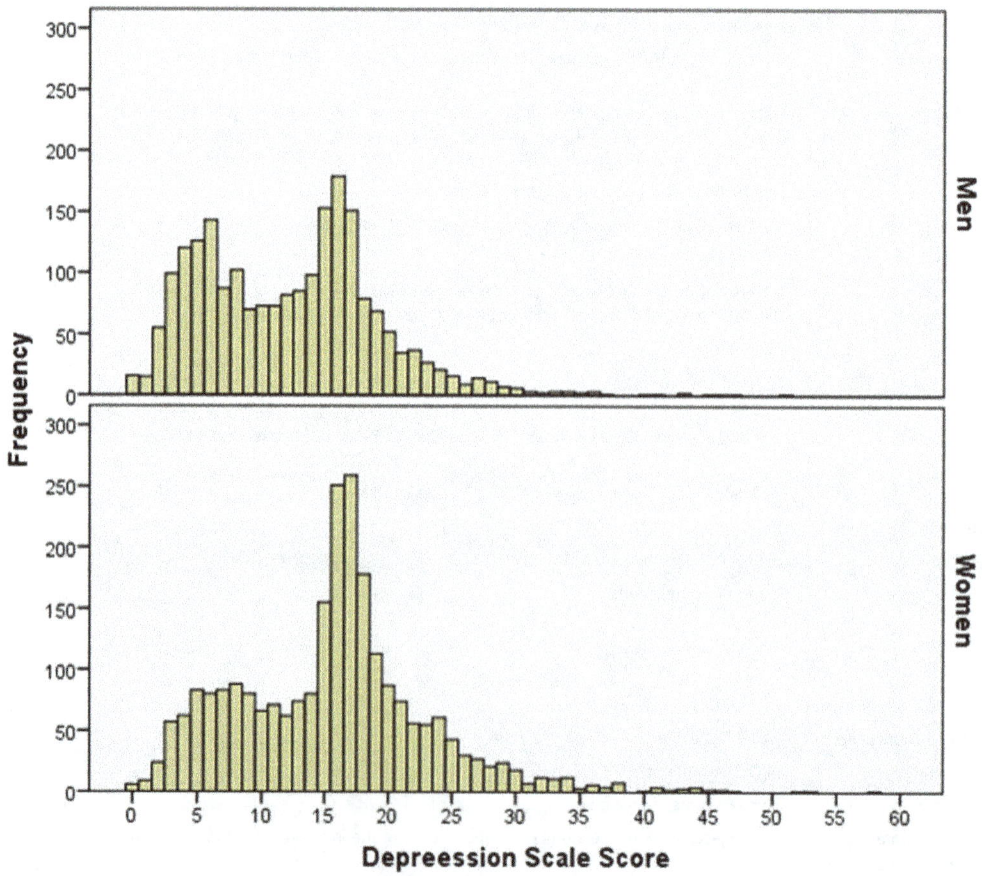

Figure 1. Histograms Showing the Distribution of the Depression Scale Score Stratified by Gender in the Central India Eye and Medical Study.

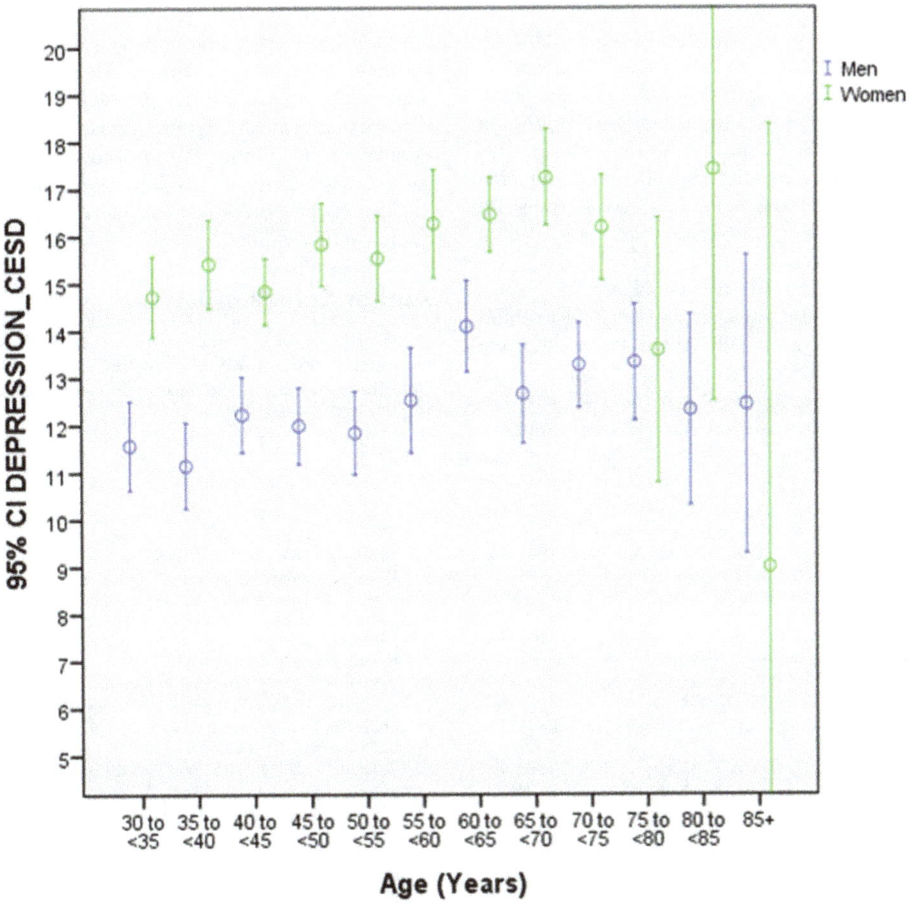

Figure 2. Graph Showing the Distribution of the Depression Score Stratified by Age and Gender in the Central India Eye and Medical Study.

rate for women only showed a slight increase from 1980 to 2009 with a peak in the year 2000, while the rate of suicides among the male population nearly doubled (7.3 in 1980 to 13.0 in 2009).

In the study population, 19% of the individuals reported to be or to have been smokers, with the majority of smokers being men (40.3% of men versus 0.02% of women). Smokeless tobacco was consumed by 1968 (41.8%) subjects. These figures were higher than those reported in the Indian National Family Health Survey-2 from 1998–99 [33]. That survey on 315,598 individuals 15 years or older revealed that 30% of the population (47% men and 14% of women) either smoked or chewed tobacco. It also showed that individuals with no education were 2.7 times more likely to smoke and chew tobacco than those with postgraduate education, and that scheduled tribes had a 23% higher probability to consume tobacco than other social groups [34]. Compared with the figures from a survey focused on 14 low-income and middle-income countries including India, 48.6% of men and 11.3% of women were tobacco users [35]. Again these figures were lower than those for our rural study population. It indicates that our study population had a relatively high prevalence of using tobacco corresponding to the association between lower socio-economic background or lower educational level and tobacco use [34,36].

Out of our study population, 77.0% of the participants reported to have never drunken alcohol, while an AUDIT sum score of 8 or more (harmful or hazardous drinking) was scored by 6.0% of the study population or 26.2% of the individuals consuming alcohol. In the Indian National Sample Survey as a representative survey of 471,143 people over the age of 10 years in 1995–96 revealed a national prevalence of regular use of smoking tobacco is estimated to be 16.2%, chewing tobacco 14.0%, and alcohol 4.5%. Men were 9.7 times more likely to regularly use alcohol [36]. Respondents belonging to scheduled castes and tribes (recognized disadvantaged groups), people from rural areas and those without formal education were significantly more likely to report regular use of alcohol [37,38].

Potential limitations of our study should be discussed. First, a major concern in any prevalence study is nonparticipation. The Central India Eye and Medical Study had a reasonable response rate of 80.1%, however, differences between participants and non-participants can lead to a selection artifact. Second, our study included only those who resided in a purely rural region, a region that can be considered to be markedly rural based on responses to the questionnaire regarding socioeconomic background and lifestyle. The study did not include subjects from an urban region, so we can provide no information on any differences between rural and urban regions with respect to the examined parameters. Third, our study as cross-section investigation does not allow firm statements on a longitudinal association, i.e. temporal causation cannot be established with the current cross-sectional design. Fourth, our study only included participants over the age of 30 years and therefore the frequency we report only refer to this age-group. This is important as cohort effects exist for major depression and generally age at onset is declining. Fifth, epidemiological studies using questionnaires such as the CES-D, usually assessed "depressive symptoms" rather than "depression", so the findings of our study can give information only about depressive symptoms. To make a definitive diagnosis of depression would need additional tests. Sixth, due to the study design, our investigation could not assess relationships between outcome parameters, such as a potential association between smoking and prevalence of depression, or an association between alcohol consumption and depression.

In conclusion, the rural Central Indian population living in a purely agrarian society showed a prevalence of major depression of 13.0% (8.1 of men, 17.3% of women). About 4% of the study population reported about suicide attempt, and 5% indicated to have had suicidal thoughts during the last 6 months. Approximately 20% of the population was present or former smokers. Harmful or hazardous drinking or alcohol dependence was reported by 12% and 5% of the study population, respectively. As in other population and societies, depression was a very common psychiatric disorder. Measures should be taken to address the relatively high prevalence of suicide attempts and thoughts on suicide. Future research focused on the general population, longitudinal (prospective), multi-center, co-morbid studies, assessment of disability, functioning, family burden and quality of life studies involving a clinical service providing approach, is required.

Author Contributions

Conceived and designed the experiments: JBJ VN MR PB SPJ. Performed the experiments: JBJ VN MR PB SPJ. Analyzed the data: JBJ MR TP. Contributed reagents/materials/analysis tools: JBJ VN. Wrote the paper: JBJ VN MR TP PB SPJ.

References

1. Murray CJ, Vos T, Lozano R, Naghavi M, Flaxman AD, et al. (2012) Disability-adjusted life years (DALYs) for 291 diseases and injuries in 21 regions, 1990–2010: a systematic analysis for the Global Burden of Disease Study 2010. Lancet 380: 2197–2223.
2. Lim SS, Vos T, Flaxman AD, Danaei G, Shibuya K, et al. (2012) A comparative risk assessment of burden of disease and injury attributable to 67 risk factors and risk factor clusters in 21 regions, 1990–2010: a systematic analysis for the Global Burden of Disease Study 2010. Lancet 380: 2224–2260.
3. Lieb K, Zanarini MC, Schmahl C, Linehan MM, Bohus M (2004) Borderline personality disorder. Lancet 364: 453–461.
4. Moussavi S, Chatterji S, Verdes E, Tandon A, Patel V, et al. (2007) Depression, chronic diseases, and decrements in health: results from the World Health Surveys. Lancet 370: 851–858.
5. Patton GC, Coffey C, Romaniuk H, Mackinnon A, Carlin JB, et al. (2014) The prognosis of common mental disorders in adolescents: a 14-year prospective cohort study. Lancet 383: 1404–1411.
6. Peto R, Lopez AD, Boreham J, Thun M, Heath C Jr (1992) Mortality from tobacco in developed countries: indirect estimation from national vital statistics. Lancet 339: 1268–1278.
7. Glassman AH, Covey LS, Stetner F, Rivelli S (2001) Smoking cessation and the course of major depression: a follow-up study. Lancet 357: 1929–1932.
8. Williamson DF, Madans J, Anda RF, Kleinman JC, Giovino GA, et al. (1991) Smoking cessation and severity of weight gain in a national cohort. N Engl J Med 324: 739–745.
9. Renaud S, de Lorgeril M (1992) Wine, alcohol, platelets, and the French paradox for coronary heart disease. Lancet 339: 1523–1526.
10. Biederman J, Faraone SV (2005) Attention-deficit hyperactivity disorder. Lancet 366: 237–248.
11. Room R, Babor T, Rehm J (2005) Alcohol and public health. Lancet 365: 519–530.
12. Hawton K, van Heeringen K (2009) Suicide. Lancet 373: 1372–1381.
13. Moran P, Coffey C, Romaniuk H, Olsson C, Borschmann R, et al. (2012) The natural history of self-harm from adolescence to young adulthood: a population-based cohort study. Lancet 379: 236–243.
14. Lim SS, Vos T, Flaxman AD, Danaei G, Shibuya K, et al. (2012) A comparative risk assessment of burden of disease and injury attributable to 67 risk factors and risk factor clusters in 21 regions, 1990–2010: a systematic analysis for the Global Burden of Disease Study 2010. Lancet 380: 2224–2260.
15. Jonas JB, Nangia V, Joshi PP, Matin A, Panda-Jonas S (2010) Diabetes mellitus in rural India. Epidemiology 21: 754–755.
16. Radloff LS (1977) 'The CES-D scale: A self report depression scale for research in the general population'. Applied Psychological Measurement 1: 385–401.
17. Heatherton TF, Kozlowski LT, Frecker RC, Fagerstrom KO (1991) The Fagerstrom Test for Nicotine Dependence: A revision of the Fagerstrom Tolerance Questionnaire. Br J Addict 86: 1119–1127.
18. Saunders JB, Aasland OG, Babor TF, de la Fuente JR, Grant M (1993) Development of the alcohol use disorders identification test (AUDIT): WHO collaborative project on early detection of persons with harmful alcohol consumption —II. Addiction 88: 791–803.
19. Poongothai S, Pradeepa R, Ganesan A, Mohan V (2009) Prevalence of depression in a large urban South Indian population - The Chennai Urban Rural Epidemiology Study (CURES-70). PloS One 4: E7185.
20. Nandi DN, Banerjee G, Mukherjee SP, Ghosh A, Nandi PS, et al. (2000) Psychiatric morbidity of a rural Indian community changes over a 20 year interval. Br J Psych 176: 351–356.
21. Nandi PS, Banerjee G, Mukherjee SP, Nandi S, Nandi DN (1997) A study of psychiatric morbidity of the elderly population of a rural community in West Bengal. Indian J Psych 39: 122–129.
22. Tiwari SC (2000) Geriatric Psychiatric morbidity in rural Northern India: Implications for the future. Int Psychogeriatrics 12: 35–48.
23. Math SB, Chandrashekar CR, Bhugra D (2007) Psychiatric epidemiology in India. Indian J Med Res 126: 183–192.
24. Ganguli HC (2000) Epidemiological findings on prevalence of mental disorders in India. Indian J Psychiatry 42: 14–20.
25. WHO (2008) The global burden of disease: 2004 update. Geneva: World Health Organization, 2008.
26. Patel V, Ramasundarahettige C, Vijayakumar L, Thakur JS, Gajalakshmi V, et al. (2012) Suicide mortality in India: a nationally representative survey. Lancet 379: 2343–2351.
27. Salomon JA, Wang H, Freeman MK, Vos T, Flaxman AD, et al. (2010) Healthy life expectancy for 187 countries, 1990–2010: a systematic analysis for the Global Burden Disease Study 2010. Lancet 380: 2144–2162.
28. Lozano R, Naghavi M, Foreman K, Lim S, Shibuya K, et al. (2012) Global and regional mortality from 235 causes of death for 20 age groups in 1990 and 2010: a systematic analysis for the Global Burden of Disease Study 2010. Lancet 380: 2095–2128.
29. Lester D, Natarajan M, Agarwal K (1999) Suicide in India. Arch Suicide Res 5: 91–96.
30. Aaron R, Joseph A, Abraham S, Muliyil J, George K, et al. (2004) Suicides in young people in rural southern India. Lancet 363: 111–118.
31. Borges G, Nock MK, Haro Abad JM, Hwang I, Sampson NA, et al. (2010) Twelve-month prevalence of and risk factors for suicide attempts in the world health organization world mental health surveys. J Clin Psychiatry 71: 1617–1628.
32. World Health Organization website. Available: http://www.who.int/entity/mental_health/media/indi.pdf. Accessed 2014 Mar 3.
33. Rani M, Bonu S, Jha P, Nguyen SN, Jamjoum L (2003) Tobacco use in India: prevalence and predictors of smoking and chewing in a national cross sectional household survey. Tob Control 12:e4.
34. Subramanian SV, Nandy S, Kelly M, Gordon D, Davey Smith G (2004) Patterns and distribution of tobacco consumption in India: cross sectional multilevel evidence from the 1998–9 national family health survey. BMJ 328: 801–806.
35. Giovino GA, Mirza SA, Samet JM, Gupta PC, Jarvis MJ, et al. (2012) Tobacco use in 3 billion individuals from 16 countries: an analysis of nationally representative cross-sectional household surveys. Lancet 380: 668–679.
36. Neufeld KJ, Peters DH, Rani M, Bonu S, Brooner RK (2005) Regular use of alcohol and tobacco in India and its association with age, gender, and poverty. Drug Alcohol Depend 77: 283–291.
37. Ghosh S, Samanta A, Mukherjee S (2012) Patterns of alcohol consumption among male adults at a slum in Kolkata, India. J Health Popul Nutr 30: 73–81.
38. Srinath Reddy K, Perry CL, Stigler MH, Arora M (2006) Differences in tobacco use among young people in urban India by sex, socioeconomic status, age, and school grade: Assessment of baseline survey data. Lancet 367: 589–594.

17

A Simple and Rapid Method for Standard Preparation of Gas Phase Extract of Cigarette Smoke

Tsunehito Higashi[1], Yosuke Mai[1], Yoichi Noya[2], Takahiro Horinouchi[1], Koji Terada[1], Akimasa Hoshi[1], Prabha Nepal[1], Takuya Harada[1], Mika Horiguchi[1], Chizuru Hatate[1], Yuji Kuge[2], Soichi Miwa[1]*

1 Department of Cellular Pharmacology, Graduate School of Medicine, Hokkaido University, Sapporo, Hokkaido, Japan, **2** Central Institute of Isotope Science, Hokkaido University, Sapporo, Hokkaido, Japan

Abstract

Cigarette smoke consists of tar and gas phase: the latter is toxicologically important because it can pass through lung alveolar epithelium to enter the circulation. Here we attempt to establish a standard method for preparation of gas phase extract of cigarette smoke (CSE). CSE was prepared by continuously sucking cigarette smoke through a Cambridge filter to remove tar, followed by bubbling it into phosphate-buffered saline (PBS). An increase in dry weight of the filter was defined as tar weight. Characteristically, concentrations of CSEs were represented as virtual tar concentrations, assuming that tar on the filter was dissolved in PBS. CSEs prepared from smaller numbers of cigarettes (original tar concentrations ≤15 mg/ml) showed similar concentration-response curves for cytotoxicity versus virtual tar concentrations, but with CSEs from larger numbers (tar ≥20 mg/ml), the curves were shifted rightward. Accordingly, the cytotoxic activity was detected in PBS of the second reservoir downstream of the first one with larger numbers of cigarettes. CSEs prepared from various cigarette brands showed comparable concentration-response curves for cytotoxicity. Two types of CSEs prepared by continuous and puff smoking protocols were similar regarding concentration-response curves for cytotoxicity, pharmacology of their cytotoxicity, and concentrations of cytotoxic compounds. These data show that concentrations of CSEs expressed by virtual tar concentrations can be a reference value to normalize their cytotoxicity, irrespective of numbers of combusted cigarettes, cigarette brands and smoking protocols, if original tar concentrations are ≤15 mg/ml.

Editor: Thomas H. Thatcher, University of Rochester Medical Center, United States of America

Funding: This work was supported by Grant-in-Aids for Scientific Research (B) 24390059 (SM), Scientific Research (C) 25460326 (KT) and Challenging Exploratory Research 25670123 (SM) from Japan Society for the Promotion of Science (http://www.jsps.go.jp/english/index.html), by a grant from the SRFJ (SM), and by a grant from the Akiyama Life Science Foundation (THi). The funders had no role in study design, data collection and analysis, decision to publish, or preparation of the manuscript.

Competing Interests: The authors have declared that no competing interests exist.

* Email: smiwa@med.hokudai.ac.jp

Introduction

Cigarette smoking is a major risk factor for cardiovascular diseases such as stroke and coronary artery disease [1,2], for chronic pulmonary obstructive diseases [3,4] and for several forms of cancer [5–7]. Cigarette smoke is reported to contain more than 4,000 chemical compounds [8,9]. Among these are reactive oxygen species (ROS) such as peroxynitrate and free radicals of organic compounds [1,10]. Although the free radicals are highly reactive to induce cell injury, their lifetime is too short to reach lung of smokers [10]. Recent studies indicate that cigarette smoke contain stable components which have the potential to stimulate cellular ROS production not only in the lung but also in tissues remote from the lung [11–13].

Cigarette smoke consists of two phases; the tar (particle) phase containing nicotine and the gas phase. In view of human health, the gas phase is important, because it can pass through the lung alveolar epithelium to reach the circulating blood and to induce damage in tissues remote from the lung [14,15]. In fact, the gas phase extract contains stable toxic compounds which exert various cytotoxic effects in a wide range of cells [16–18]. In this context, we have recently shown that the gas phase extract of cigarette smoke induces cell death and plasma membrane damage through ROS generation, which is in turn induced by protein kinase C (PKC)-mediated activation of NADPH oxidase (NOX) [19,20]. In addition, the gas phase extract of cigarette smoke can oxidize LDL in vitro, while it can promote atherosclerotic changes in aortas in vivo [14,21,22]. Recently, using LC/MS and GC/MS in combination with functional assays in cultured cells, we have identified several stable cytotoxic compounds responsible for cytotoxicity in the gas phase extract of cigarette smoke: among these compounds are acrolein (ACR), methyl vinyl ketone (MVK), and 2-cyclopentene-1-one (CPO) [23]. We have also shown that like the gas phase extract, these stable cytotoxic compounds induce cell damage in a PKC- and NOX-dependent manner [20,23].

In spite of its importance for human health, no standard method for preparation of the gas phase extract of the cigarette smoke has been established, although the protocols for standard smoking protocols are established by the International Organization for Standardization (ISO) [24] and Health Canada (HC) [25]. Therefore, researchers have performed experiments using the gas phase extracts prepared by their own methods. The gas phase extracts are generally made by passing cigarette smoke through the

Cambridge filter and subsequently bubbling the smoke in aqueous solution. The methods for preparation of the gas phase extracts differ mainly in terms of smoking protocols (puff smoking vs continuous smoking), bubbling conditions (pore sizes of glass ball filters for generating bubbles and temperatures of the aqueous solution) and the number of combusted cigarettes. The most serious problem is the absence of the definition for concentration of the gas phase extracts of cigarette smoke, which makes it difficult to compare the experimental data on the cigarette smoke extract from different laboratories.

In the present study, we attempt to establish a standard method for preparation of gas phase extracts of cigarette smoke, which is simple and rapid. For this purpose, we use continuous smoking protocol, because it does not require an expensive smoking machine and it is rapid. Using that smoking protocol, we optimize methods for extraction of cytotoxic activities from cigarette smoke into aqueous solution. As a measure of concentrations of the gas phase extracts of cigarette smoke, we introduce the virtual tar concentration (w/v), which is calculated on the assumption that the tar phase trapped on the Cambridge filter is dissolved in the aqueous solution used for extraction of cigarette smoke. We show that the virtual tar concentration can be used as a reference value to normalize the cytotoxic activities of gas phase extracts of cigarette smoke, irrespective of smoking conditions (continuous smoking or puff smoking), cigarette brands and the number of combusted cigarettes, as long as the original tar concentrations in the gas phase extracts are ≤15 mg/ml.

Materials and Methods

Materials

The cigarette used was, unless otherwise specified, the Hi-Lite (JT, Tokyo, Japan) containing 17 mg of tar and 1.4 mg of nicotine per cigarette. In some experiments, other brands such as Peace (JT, 28 mg of tar and 2.3 mg of nicotine), Seven Stars (JT, 14 mg of tar and 1.2 mg of nicotine), Mevius (JT, 10 mg of tar and 0.8 mg of nicotine), Mevius Super Light (JT, 6 mg of tar and 0.5 mg of nicotine), Marlboro (Phillip Morris, 12 mg of tar and 1.0 mg of nicotine), Lucky Strike (British American Tobacco, 11 mg of tar and 1.0 mg of nicotine), Kent 9 mg (British American Tobacco, 9 mg of tar and 0.8 mg of nicotine) were used. The materials and reagents were purchased from the following sources: Cambridge filters from Heinr Borgwaldt GmbH (Hamburg, Germany); CellTiter96 Aqueous One Solution Proliferation Assay Kit and CytoTox-One™ Homogenous Membrane Integrity Assay Kit from Promega Corporation (Madison, WI, USA); acetone, CPO and propionaldehyde from WAKO Pure Chemical Industries (Osaka, Japan); Hoechst 33342, O-(2,3,4,5,6-pentafluorobenzyl) hydroxylamine hydrochloride (PFBOA) and diphenyleneiodonium chloride (DPI) from Sigma Aldrich (St Louis, MO, USA); propidium iodide (PI) from Dojindo Laboratories (Kumamoto, Japan); ACR and MVK from Tokyo Chemical Industry (Tokyo, Japan); bisindolylmaleimide I (BIS I) from Calbiochem (San Diego, CA, USA).

Preparation of the gas phase extract of cigarette smoke

The gas phase extract of cigarette smoke (from now on, we refer to this extract as the cigarette smoke extract [CSE]) was prepared using continuous smoking protocol, unless specified otherwise: this CSE was designated cCSE. The preparation of the cCSE was performed as previously described [19,23] with slight modifications. As shown in Fig. 1, one cigarette per trial was combusted, and the main stream of the cigarette smoke was continuously sucked through a standard glass-fiber Cambridge filter with a constant flow rate of 1.050 l/min by an aspiration pump to remove the tar phase and nicotine. According to the rules of ISO4387, cigarettes with and without filters were combusted up to 3 mm from the tipping paper and 23 mm from the end of cigarette, respectively, while the aspiration rate was set at the average flow rate of the 2-seconds puff duration of the puff smoking defined by ISO3308. The remaining gas phase of cigarette smoke was bubbled into 15 ml of phosphate buffered saline (PBS) in a 100 ml graduated cylinder (the diameter is 28 mm) at 25°C (Fig. 1). To increase the bubbling efficiency, bubbling was performed through a Kinoshita-type glass ball filter with the pore size of 20–30 μm (Kinoshita Industry, Tokyo, Japan). After combustion of cigarettes, the Cambridge filter was dried in air at 25°C for 12 h and an increase in the dry weight of the filter was regarded as the amount of the tar phase. The combustion of cigarette (usually Hi-Lite brand) was repeated, unless otherwise specified, until the dry weight of the tar phase trapped on the Cambridge filter reached 150 mg. The concentration of cCSE was expressed in terms of the virtual tar concentration which was calculated on the assumption that the tar trapped on the Cambridge filter is dissolved in the PBS used for cCSE preparation. The cCSE preparations were aliquoted and stored at −80°C until use.

For preparation of the other type of the gas phase extract of cigarette smoke by puff smoking condition (designated pCSE), smoking was performed using conditions as recommended by ISO (ISO3308). In this case, smoke was generated with a mechanical smoking machine (RM200, Heinr Borgwaldt GmbH) according to ISO3308 rules (2 s puff duration, 35 ml puff volume, bell-shaped puff profile, 60 s puff cycle). The procedures after generation of smoke were the same as those for the cCSE. To avoid the inhalation of cigarette smoke, the devices for CSE preparation were put in the fume hood.

Cell culture

Human embryonic kidney HEK293T cells, human cervical carcinoma HeLa cells, C6 rat glioma cells, A7r5 rat aorta smooth muscle cells, EA.hy926 immortalized human umbilical vein endothelial cells (HUVEC), human lung small cell carcinoma SBC-3 cells, human lung squamous cell carcinoma H1299 cells, and human lung adenocarcinoma A549 cells were maintained in Dulbecco's modified Eagle medium (DMEM) supplemented with 10% (v/v) heat-inactivated fetal bovine serum (FBS), 100 units/ml penicillin G, and 100 μg/ml streptomycin sulfate at 37°C in humidified air with 5% CO_2. U937 human monocytes and RAW264.7 mouse macrophages were maintained in RPMI1640 supplemented with 10% (v/v) FBS, 10 μM 2-mercaptoethanol, 100 units/ml penicillin G, and 100 μg/ml streptomycin sulfate at 37°C in humidified air with 5% CO_2. Chinese hamster ovary (CHO) cells were maintained in F-12 Ham medium supplemented with 10% (v/v) FBS, 100 units/ml penicillin G, and 100 μg/ml streptomycin sulfate at 37°C in humidified air with 5% CO_2.

HEK293T cells, HeLa cells, and CHO cells were purchased from RIKEN CELL BANK (Wako, Japan). C6 cells, A7r5 cells, U937 cells, RAW264.7 cells, and H1299 cells were purchased from American Type Culture Collection (Manassas, VA, USA). SBC-3 cells were purchased from Japanese Collection of Research Bioresources (Ibaraki, Japan). HUVEC were provided from Dr. Cora Jean S. Edgell, University of North Carolina at Chapel Hill [26].

Evaluation of cytotoxicity

We used 3-(4,5-dimethylthiazol-2-yl)-5-(3-carboxymethyl)-2-(4-sulfophenyl)-2H-tetrazolium (MTS) reduction assay for evaluation

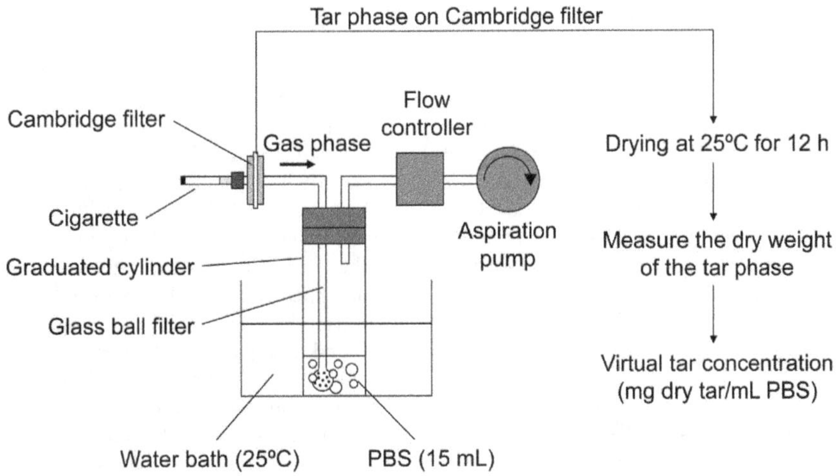

Figure 1. Schematic diagram of an apparatus for preparation of gas phase extracts of cigarette smoke. A standard method for preparation of the gas phase extract of cigarette smoke is as follows. Four cigarettes of Hi-Lite brand, unless otherwise specified, were sequentially combusted and the main-stream smoke was continuously sucked through a Cambridge filter at a constant flow rate of 1.050 l/min by an aspirator, to remove the tar phase. The remaining gas phase was bubbled through a glass ball filter (pore size: 20–30 μm) into phosphate buffered saline (PBS, 15 ml) in a graduated cylinder kept at 25°C. After combustion of cigarette, the filter was dried in air for 12 h at 25°C, and the dry weight of the tar phase trapped on the Cambridge filter was obtained by subtracting the weight of filter before use from that after use. The concentration of the gas phase extract was expressed as the virtual tar concentration (mg tar/ml PBS), assuming that the tar phase trapped on the Cambridge filter is dissolved in the PBS. Four cigarettes of Hi-Lite brand gave the dry tar weight of approximately 150 mg. Notably, cytotoxicity of the gas phase extracts depends not on cigarette brands but on the virtual tar concentration.

of cell viability, PI uptake assay and lactate dehydrogenase (LDH) leakage assay for evaluation of cell membrane damage, and DNA fragmentation assay for evaluation of cell apoptosis.

MTS reduction assay was performed using CellTiter96 Aqueous One Solution Cell Proliferation Assay Kit, as described recently [19,23]. Briefly, the cells were inoculated onto a 96-well plate at a density of 1×10^4 cells per well. After incubation with CSE for 4 h, 20 μl of kit reagent was added to the culture medium (100 μl), and incubated for a further 1 h. The amount of reduced form of MTS was measured by absorbance at 490 nm using a microplate reader (SPECTRA MAX 250, Molecular Devices Corp., Sunnyvale, CA, USA). MTS reduction activity of the CSE-treated cells was represented as a percentage of the absorbance obtained from non-treated cells. MTS reduction activity in culture medium without cells was regarded as zero.

PI uptake assay was performed as recently described [19,20,23]. The cells were incubated with CSE for 4 h in culture medium containing 1 μg/ml PI and 1 μg/ml Hoechst 33342. The fluorescent images of PI and Hoechst 33342 were captured by IX-71 inverted fluorescent microscope (Olympus, Tokyo, Japan) equipped with ×40 objective lens (LUCPlanFL N, NA = 0.60, Olympus).

LDH leakage assay was performed using CytoTox-One™ Homogenous Membrane Integrity Assay Kit according to the manufacture's protocols as recently described [19,20]. The cells were inoculated onto a 96-well plate at a density of 1×10^4 cells per well. After incubation with CSE for 4 h, culture media (100 μl) were transferred to a new 96-well plate (Black Cliniplate; Thermo Fisher Scientific Inc., Rockford, IL, USA) for measurement LDH activity leaked into media. For measurement of total LDH activity, the cells cultured in parallel were disrupted by adding 2 μl of Lysis Buffer to the culture media, and the whole lysates were transferred to the 96-well plate. The enzyme reaction was started by adding 100 μl of CytoTox-ONE™ reagent. After 10-min incubation, at room temperature, the reaction was terminated by adding 50 μl of Stop Solution. The amount of the reaction product (rezorufin) was measured using a microplate spectrofluorometer (Varioscan, Thermo Fisher Scientific Inc.). LDH leakage was represented as a percentage of the total LDH activity. LDH activity in culture media without cells was regarded as zero.

For DNA fragmentation assay, the cells were inoculated onto 6-cm dish at the density of 1×10^6 cells per dish. After 24-h incubation with CSE, the cells were lysed by incubation with lysis buffer (10 mM Tris-HCl [pH 7.4], 5 mM EDTA, 0.5% Triton X-100) for 30 min at 4°C, and centrifuged at 15,000× g for 30 min at 4°C to remove cell debris. The supernatants were transferred to new tubes, and incubated with 40 μg/ml proteinase K for 1 h at 37°C. After purification by phenol/chloroform extraction and ethanol precipitation, the DNA was reconstituted in Tris-EDTA buffer (10 mM Tris-HCl [pH 8.0], 1 mM EDTA) containing 40 μg/ml RNaseA, and incubated for 30 min at 37°C. The purified DNA was subjected to 1.8% agarose gel electrophoresis.

Analysis of CSE by HPLC and GC/MS

Identification of cytotoxic compounds in the CSE was performed using HPLC and GC/MS as described recently [23]. Briefly, the CSE was fractionated by HPLC equipped with a reverse-phase column, each fraction was analyzed for cytotoxic activity using PI uptake assay, and two active fractions inducing PI uptake into cultured C6 glioma cells were analyzed for identification of cytotoxic compounds using GC/MS. Before analysis by GC/MS, the active fractions from HPLC were derivatized with a carbonyl reagent PFBOA to stabilize carbonyl compounds as described [23].

Data analysis

For evaluation of cytotoxic activities of CSEs (cCSE or pCSE) using MTS reduction assay and LDH leakage assay, concentration-response curves were constructed by plotting the activities against virtual tar concentrations of CSEs. MTS reduction activity in the presence of CSEs was represented as a percentage of control value in the absence of CSEs, while LDH activity leaked into culture medium was represented as a percentage of control value in culture medium of cells lysed by 0.2% Triton X-100 in the absence of CSEs. From the concentration-response curves, the values for EC_{50} and maximum inhibition were obtained. The data for experiments performed with or without cultured cells were presented as means ± SE or means ± SD., respectively. The significance of the differences between mean values was evaluated with GraphPad PRISM™ (version 4.0, GraphPad Software Inc., San Diego, CA, USA) by student's unpaired *t*-test or one-way ANOVA, followed by Tukey's multiple comparison test. A *P* value less than 0.05 was considered to indicate statistically significant differences.

Results

Validation of quantification of tar amount

In the present study, we attempted to represent the concentration of the cCSE in terms of the virtual tar concentration which was calculated on the assumption that the tar phase (dry weight [mg]) trapped on the Cambridge filter is dissolved in the PBS (15 ml). Since the tar phase was reported to contain water [27], we first investigated conditions for vaporizing the water in the tar phase on Cambridge filters to estimate the dry weight of the tar phase. To minimize vaporization of volatile chemical components in the tar phase, we tested relatively low temperatures such as 25°C and 55°C for vaporization of water.

For evaluation of vaporizing conditions, smoke from 4 cigarettes of Hi-Lite brand was passed through a Cambridge filter, and the filter was dried at 25°C or 55°C for various lengths of time, and the weight of the filter was measured. The increase in the weight of the filter following smoking was regarded as the weight of the tar phase. As shown in Fig. 2A, the weight of the tar phase on the filter decreased up to 2 h following drying at 25°C, and thereafter, it reached a plateau up to 12 h. Following drying at 55°C, the weight of the tar phase on the filter also decreased in a similar time course, and thereafter, it reached a plateau up to 12 h. Notably, the weight of the tar phase on the filter following drying at 55°C for 12 h is significantly lower than that following drying at 25°C for 12 h, indicating that part of volatile components in the tar phase might have been vaporized. Therefore, in the following experiments, Cambridge filters were dried at 25°C for 12 h.

As shown in Fig. 2B, the weight of the tar phase trapped on the Cambridge filter increased linearly with an increase in the number of combusted cigarettes up to 6 cigarettes (of Hi-Lite brand), which gave approximately 225 mg of tar on the filter. During combustion of cigarettes, the aspiration speed was continuously monitored by a Kofloc flowmeter, and it was found to be constant (1.050 l/min) up to 6 cigarettes. These results indicate that the Cambridge filter functions normally without being saturated with the tar phase at least up to 225 mg. In the following experiments, we usually used 4 cigarettes for preparation of the cCSE. When more than 4 cigarettes were combusted for cCSE preparation, a new Cambridge filter was used every 4 cigarettes to avoid saturation of the filter with tar phase.

Effects of the temperature of PBS and the pore size of the glass ball filter on the cytotoxicity of the gas phase extract of cigarette smoke

Since the water-solubility of chemical compounds is generally affected by temperature, we examined the effect of the temperature of PBS in the graduated cylinder on the cytotoxicity of cCSE preparation. cCSE was prepared by continuous smoking of four cigarettes of Hi-Lite brand which gave 150 mg of tar on the Cambridge filter. The concentrations of the cCSE were expressed in terms of the virtual tar concentration, assuming that the tar trapped on the Cambridge filter was dissolved in cCSE. The tar concentration of the original cCSE was calculated to be 10 mg/ml. The cCSEs prepared with PBS (15 ml) kept at 0°C and 25°C showed similar concentration-response curves for inhibition of MTS reduction activity (Fig. 3A), indicating that the temperature of the PBS has little effect on the recovery of cytotoxic compounds.

The pore size of the glass ball filter used for bubbling smoke might affect the cytotoxicity of cCSE by changing the size of bubbles and hence the efficiency of transfer of cytotoxic compounds from bubbles to PBS. To optimize the pore size of the glass ball filter, we compared the cytotoxicity of cCSEs prepared using glass ball filters with different pore sizes. The cCSEs prepared with glass ball filters of normal pore size (20–30 μm) or large pore size (100–120 μm) showed similar concentration-response curves for inhibition of MTS reduction activity (Fig. 3B), indicating that the pore size of glass ball filters has little effect on the recovery of cytotoxic compounds. Therefore, in the following experiments, we used PBS kept at 25°C and a glass ball filter of normal pore size for preparation of the cCSE.

Effects of the original tar concentrations of cCSEs on their cytotoxic potency

To examine how much cigarette smoke will saturate the PBS (15 ml), we constructed the concentration-response curves for cytotoxicity of cCSEs prepared from varying numbers of cigarettes (Fig. 4A and Table 1). In this experiment, 2–40 cigarettes of Hi-Lite brand were combusted by continuous smoking protocol, and a new Cambridge filter was used every 4 cigarettes, to avoid the saturation of the filter with tar. Again, the concentrations of the cCSE were expressed in terms of the virtual tar concentration, based on the dry weight of tar trapped on the Cambridge filter.

The concentration-response curves for inhibition of MTS reduction activity were similar among cCSEs which were made from 2–6 cigarettes (equivalent to the original tar concentration of 5–15 mg/ml), as demonstrated by comparable values for the EC_{50} and maximal inhibition (Fig. 4A and Table 1). However, the concentration-response curves began to be shifted to the right, when more than 8 cigarettes (equivalent to the original tar concentration ≥20 mg/ml) were used (Fig. 4A and Table 1). The rightward shift of the curves was more marked with an increase in the number of cigarettes, indicating that the cytotoxic activities of cCSEs prepared from larger numbers of cigarettes were lower than expected at a given tar concentration. These results taken together strongly demonstrate that cytotoxic activity in the smoke is efficiently extracted into PBS up to 6 cigarettes of Hi-Lite brand (equivalent to the original tar concentration of ≤15 mg/ml), whereas some part of the cytotoxic activity is leaked with more than 8 cigarettes (equivalent to the original tar concentration of ≥ 20 mg/ml).

To confirm the leakage of the cytotoxic activity, another reservoir containing 15 ml of PBS was incorporated downstream of the first reservoir, and the cytotoxic activity of the PBS in the second reservoir was analyzed using MTS reduction assay. As shown in Fig. 4B, the PBS in the second reservoir showed no cytotoxic activity, when four cigarettes of Hi-Lite brand (equivalent to the original tar concentration of 10 mg/ml) were used for cCSE preparation, but it showed significant cytotoxic activity, when 14 cigarettes (equivalent to the original tar concentration of 35 mg/ml) were used, demonstrating that some part of cytotoxic activity has actually leaked.

These findings taken together show that as long as ≤6 cigarettes of Hi-Lite brand (equivalent to the original tar concentration of ≤ 15 mg/ml) are used for preparation of the original cCSE, nearly

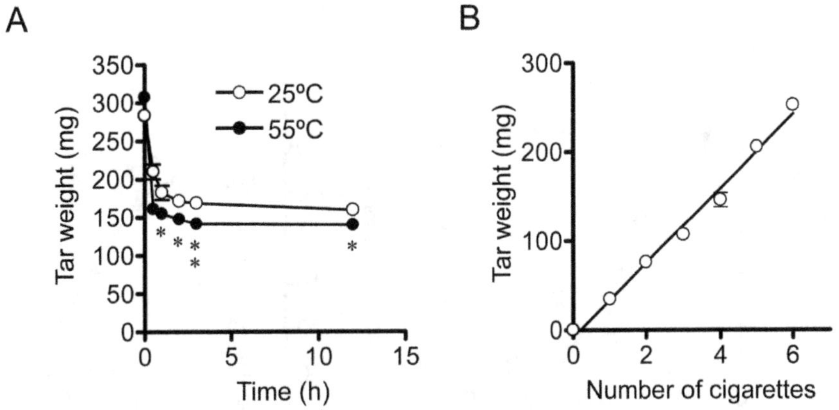

Figure 2. Quantification of the weight of the tar of cigarette smoke trapped on the Cambridge filter. (A) Time-course of a decrease in the weight of the tar phase of cigarette smoke trapped on the Cambridge filter after drying at 25°C (open circle) or 55°C (closed circle). Four cigarettes of Hi-Lite brand were sequentially combusted and the main-stream smoke was sucked through a Cambridge filter at a constant flow rate of 1.050 l/min by an aspiration pump. After combustion of cigarette, the filter was dried for various lengths of time at 25°C (open circle) or 55°C (closed circle), and the weight of the tar phase of cigarette smoke trapped on the Cambridge filter was obtained by subtracting the filter weight before combustion of cigarette from the weight after combustion. (B) The relationship between the number of combusted cigarettes and the dry weight of the tar phase trapped on the Cambridge filter. Various numbers of Hi-Lite brand cigarettes were sequentially combusted as described in A. After combustion, the filter was dried for 12 h at 25°C, and the dry weight of the tar phase on the Cambridge filter was determined as described in A. Values represent means ± SD of three experiments. *, $P<0.05$; **, $P<0.01$ versus 25°C.

100% of the cytotoxic activity is extracted into the PBS, but that with ≥8 cigarettes of Hi-Lite brand (equivalent to the original tar concentration of ≥20 mg/ml), part of cytotoxic activity leaks probably because of saturation of PBS. This means that when cCSEs are prepared at the original tar concentrations of ≤15 mg/ml, the tar concentrations are linearly related with the cytotoxic potency of cCSEs, and hence, that the tar concentrations can be used as a universal measure of cytotoxic potency of cCSE.

To exclude the possibility that the cytotoxicity is caused by a pH change in culture medium (DMEM) following addition of cCSE, we measured the pH values of the medium containing varying concentrations of cCSE. The pH values of DMEM containing cCSE at final tar concentrations of 0, 0.5 and 1.0 mg/ml were 7.48±0.02, 7.45±0.03 and 7.46±0.04, respectively (n = 3 for each group), which were not significantly different from each other. These results suggest that addition of cCSE to culture medium at least up to the virtual tar concentration of 1.0 mg/ml had no effect on the pH of culture medium.

Effects of cigarette brands on the cytotoxicity of cCSE

To clarify whether the potency of cytotoxic activities of cCSE varies depending on cigarette brands, we examined the cytotoxicity of 8 representative cigarette brands (5 brands from JT, Japan, 3 brands from other countries) with different tar contents (Table 2). To prepare the original cCSEs at comparable tar concentrations from various brands of cigarettes, we first determined the dry weight of tar per cigarette which was trapped on the Cambridge filter after combustion of one cigarette by

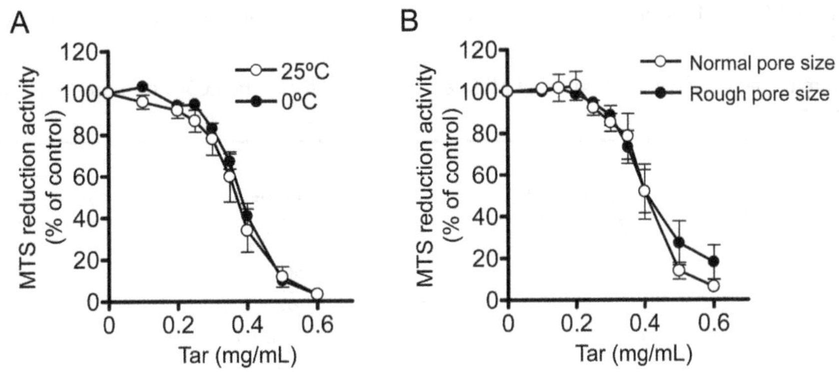

Figure 3. Effects of the bubbling condition on gas phase extracts of cigarette smoke. Effects of the temperature of phosphate-buffered saline (PBS) (A) and pore size of a glass ball filter for bubbling the gas phase of cigarette smoke into PBS (B) on the cytotoxic activities of the gas phase extract were examined. The gas phase extract of cigarette smoke (designated cCSE) was prepared as described in the legend for Fig. 1, by continuous smoking of four cigarettes of Hi-Lite brand which gave the virtual tar concentration of approximately 10 mg/ml PBS. In panel A, the temperature of PBS for extraction of cigarette smoke was kept at either 25°C (open circle) or 0°C (closed circle), and in panel B, the pore size of the glass ball filter was either normal (pore size, 20–30 μm; open circle) or rough (pore size, 100–120 μm; closed circle). For evaluation of the cytotoxicity of cCSE, C6 glioma cells were incubated for 4 h with various concentrations of cCSE and MTS reduction activity was determined as described in Materials and methods. MTS reduction activity in the absence of cCSE was represented as 100%. Values represent means ± SE of three experiments, each in triplicate.

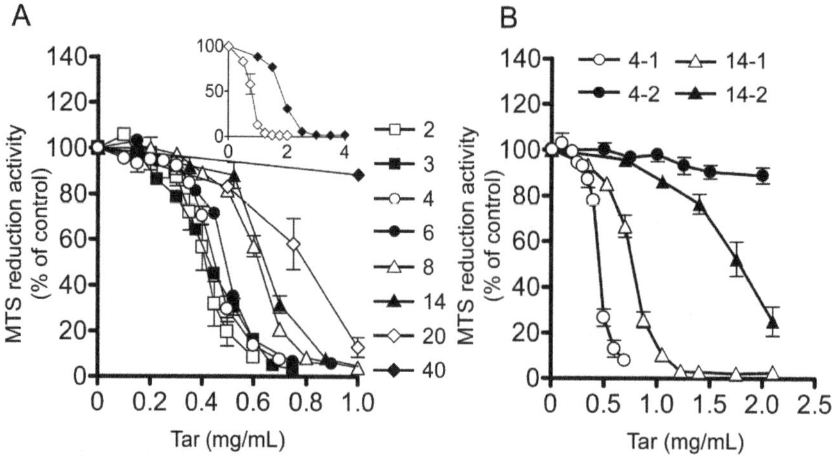

Figure 4. Cytotoxic activities of gas phase extracts of cigarette smoke and the number of cigarette. Concentration-response curves of the gas phase extracts of cigarette smoke prepared from varying numbers of cigarettes (Hi-Lite brand) (A) and of the phosphate buffered saline (PBS) in the second graduated cylinder (B) for inhibition of MTS reduction activity. (A) The gas phase extract of cigarette smoke (designated cCSE) was prepared from varying numbers (2–40) of cigarettes (Hi-Lite brand) based on continuous smoking protocol, while a new Cambridge filter was used every 4 cigarettes. Inset: Concentration-response curves of the cCSE prepared from 20 or 40 cigarettes with a change in scale of concentrations on x axis. (B) In the apparatus for preparation of cCSE, the second graduated cylinder with 15 ml of PBS was incorporated downstream of the first one, and cCSE was prepared from either 4 or 14 cigarettes (Hi-Lite brand). The cytotoxicity of PBS in the original and second graduated cylinders was evaluated using MTS reduction assay. MTS reduction activity in the absence of the gas phase extract was represented as 100%. Values represent means ± SE of three experiments, each in triplicate. 4-1 (14-1) and 4-2 (14-2) represent the cytotoxic activities of the PBS in the first (original) and second graduated cylinders prepared from 4 (14) cigarettes, respectively.

continuous smoking protocol (Table 2). The dry weight of tar per cigarette varied from 18.8 mg to 53.1 mg, which were two to three times larger than the tar content provided by the tobacco company: the difference is mainly due to that the tar content is determined by puff smoking according to the regulation of ISO3308, which discards cigarette smoke during the time interval except puff.

From these cigarettes, we prepared cCSEs, whose original tar concentration was 10 mg/mL (equivalent to the tar concentration of cCSE prepared from four cigarettes of Hi-Lite brand). The concentration-response relationships for inhibition of MTS reduction activity were not significantly different among the cCSEs prepared from different cigarette brands, as demonstrated by comparable values for the EC_{50} and maximal inhibition (Fig. 5 and Table 2). These results demonstrate that the cytotoxic activities of cCSEs depend on the tar concentration but not on either cigarette brands or nominal tar contents of cigarettes. Furthermore, the present results suggest that although cigarettes are highly engineered products containing differing tobacco leave composition and chemical additives [28,29], those factors have little effect on the cytotoxic activities from the toxicological viewpoint.

Comparison of cytotoxic potency of cCSE and pCSE

We compared the cytotoxic potency of two types of CSE, i.e. cCSE and pCSE, which were prepared by continuous or puff smoking protocols, respectively. For both CSEs, the original solutions were prepared at the virtual tar concentration of 10 mg/

Table 1. The EC_{50} and maximal values for inhibition of MTS reduction activity of the cCSEs prepared from varying numbers (2–40) of cigarettes (Hi-Lite brand).

Number of cigarette	EC_{50} (mg/ml)[a]	Maximum inhibition (%)[a]
2	0.411±0.022	91.45±0.70
3	0.431±0.083	96.66±0.54
4	0.451±0.011	92.57±0.66
6	0.494±0.001	94.30±0.46
8	0.618±0.012**	96.95±0.61
14	0.643±0.013**	97.72±0.03
20	0.784±0.059**	97.76±0.53
40	1.797±0.024**	98.17±0.06

[a]The cCSEs at the original tar concentration of 10 mg/ml were subjected to MTS reduction assay in C6 glioma cells. The concentration-response curves for inhibition of MTS reduction activity were constructed, and the EC_{50} values and maximal inhibition were determined. The concentrations of cCSEs were represented by the virtual tar concentrations. MTS reduction activity in the absence of the cCSEs was represented as 100%. Values represent means ± SE of three experiments, each in triplicate.
**$P<0.01$ vs the value for 2 cigarettes.

Table 2. Tar content per cigarette of various brands, the dry weight of tar trapped on the Cambridge filter after combustion of one cigarette and the EC_{50} values of cCSEs for inhibition of MTS reduction activity.

Cigarette brand	Nicotine content per cigarette (mg)[a]	Tar content per cigarette (mg)[a]	Dry tar weight per cigarette (mg)[b]	EC_{50} (mg/ml) for MTS reduction activity[c]
Peace	2.3	28	53.1±2.6	0.521±0.025
Hi-Lite	1.4	17	35.5±1.8	0.463±0.014
Seven Stars	1.2	14	35.6±0.4	0.502±0.023
Mevius	0.8	10	25.9±3.1	0.520±0.019
Mevius Super Light	0.5	6	18.8±2.5	0.534±0.006
Marlboro	1.0	12	26.1±1.1	0.496±0.028
Lucky Strike	1.0	11	22.7±2.4	0.495±0.029
Kent 9 mg	0.8	9	26.4±2.4	0.521±0.025

[a]Nicotine and tar content per cigarette is the value reported by its manufacturer and determined by puff smoking based on ISO regulation.
[b]For determination of dry tar weight per cigarette, smoke of one cigarette from either brand was continuously sucked through the Cambridge filter, and the increase in the dry weight of the filter was determined (represented as means ± SD of three experiments).
[c]For determination of the EC_{50} values, cCSEs at the original tar concentration of 10 mg/ml were prepared from cigarettes of various brands by continuous smoking, and subjected to MTS reduction assay in C6 glioma cells for construction of concentration-response curves from which the EC_{50} values (means ± SE of three experiments, each in triplicate) were determined.

ml and their cytotoxic activities were examined using MTS reduction assay and DNA fragmentation assay for cell death, and LDH leakage assay and PI uptake assay for plasma membrane damage. For preparation of 15 mL of cCSE at that tar concentration, four cigarettes of Hi-Lite brand were required, while nine cigarettes were required for preparation of the same amount of pCSE.

cCSE and pCSE showed similar concentration-response relationships for inhibition of MTS reduction activity (Fig. 6A), induction of LDH leakage (Fig. 6B), induction of DNA fragmentation (Fig. 6C) and induction of PI uptake (Figs. 6D and 6E):

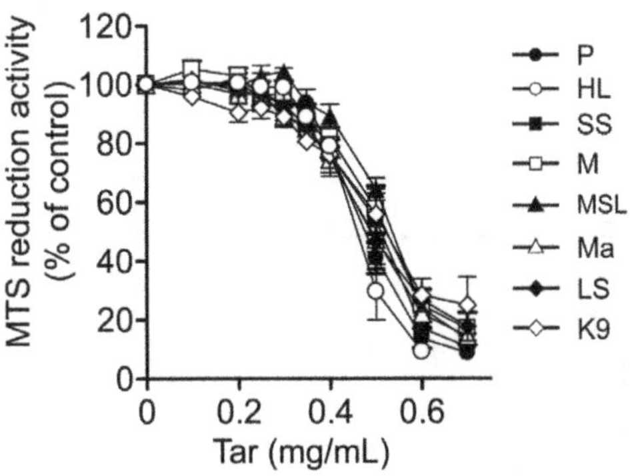

Figure 5. Relationship between cytotoxic activities of gas phase extracts of cigarette smoke and cigarette brand. The gas phase extracts of cigarette smoke (designated cCSE) at the original tar concentration of 10 mg/ml were prepared from cigarettes of various brands by continuous smoking protocol as described in the legend for Fig. 1. The cCSEs were subjected to MTS reduction assay for evaluation of their cytotoxic activities, as described in Fig. 3. MTS reduction activity in the absence of the gas phase extract was represented as 100%. Values represent means ± SE of three experiments, each in triplicate. P, Peace (JT, Japan; 28 mg tar, 2.3 mg nicotine), HL, Hi-Lite (JT, Japan; 17 mg tar, 1.4 mg nicotine), SS, Seven Stars (JT, Japan; 14 mg tar, 1.2 mg nicotine), M, Mevius (JT, Japan; 10 mg tar, 0.8 mg nicotine), MSL, Mevius Super Light (JT, Japan; 6 mg tar, 0.5 mg nicotine), Ma, Marlboro (Phillip Morris, USA; 12 mg tar, 1.0 mg nicotine), LS, Lucky Strike (British American Tobacco, UK; 11 mg tar, 0.9 mg nicotine), K9, Kent 9 mg (British American Tobacco, UK; 9 mg tar, 0.8 mg nicotine).

there was no significant difference between cCSE and pCSE regarding the EC_{50} values for inhibition of MTS reduction activity (0.454±0.004 mg/ml vs 0.469±0.009 mg/ml, respectively) and the EC_{50} values for induction of LDH leakage (0.465±0.035 mg/ml and 0.524±0.025 mg/ml). These results indicate that the cytotoxic potency and property of the gas phase extracts do not depend on smoking protocol.

Comparison of pharmacological properties of cCSE and pCSE

In our recent paper [19,20], we have reported that cCSE induces the plasma membrane damage and cell death in cultured C6 glioma cells, and that total of the plasma membrane damage and part of cell death are induced by ROS which are produced by PKC-dependent activation of NADPH oxidase (NOX), based on the sensitivities to a PKC inhibitor (BIS I) and a NOX inhibitor (DPI). To get insights into the molecular mechanism of action of both types of CSEs, we compared the effects of BIS I and DPI on the cCSE- and pCSE-induced changes in MTS reduction activity (Fig. 7A) and LDH leakage (Fig. 7B).

Following exposure for 4 h to cCSE (final tar concentration, 0.6 mg/ml), MTS reduction activity was decreased to about 10% of the control value without the exposure, and the cCSE-induced decrease in MTS reduction activity was partially recovered (to approximately 70% of the control value) by pretreatment with the maximally effective concentration of BIS I or DPI (Fig. 7A), as reported recently [19,20]. Exposure for 4 h to pCSE (final tar concentration, 0.6 mg/ml) also induced a decrease in MTS reduction activity to the same extent as exposure to cCSE, and the decrease was partially recovered by pretreatment with BIS I or DPI to the extent comparable to that induced by cCSE (Fig. 7A).

LDH leakage was increased to about 100% following exposure for 4 h to cCSE (final tar concentration, 0.6 mg/ml), and the increase was almost totally abrogated by pretreatment with the maximally effective concentration of BIS I or DPI (Fig. 7B), as reported [19,20]. Exposure for 4 h to pCSE (final tar concentration, 0.6 mg/ml) also induced an increase in LDH leakage to the same extent as exposure to cCSE, and the increase induced by pCSE was suppressed by pretreatment with BIS I or DPI to the extent comparable to that induced by cCSE (Fig. 7B). These

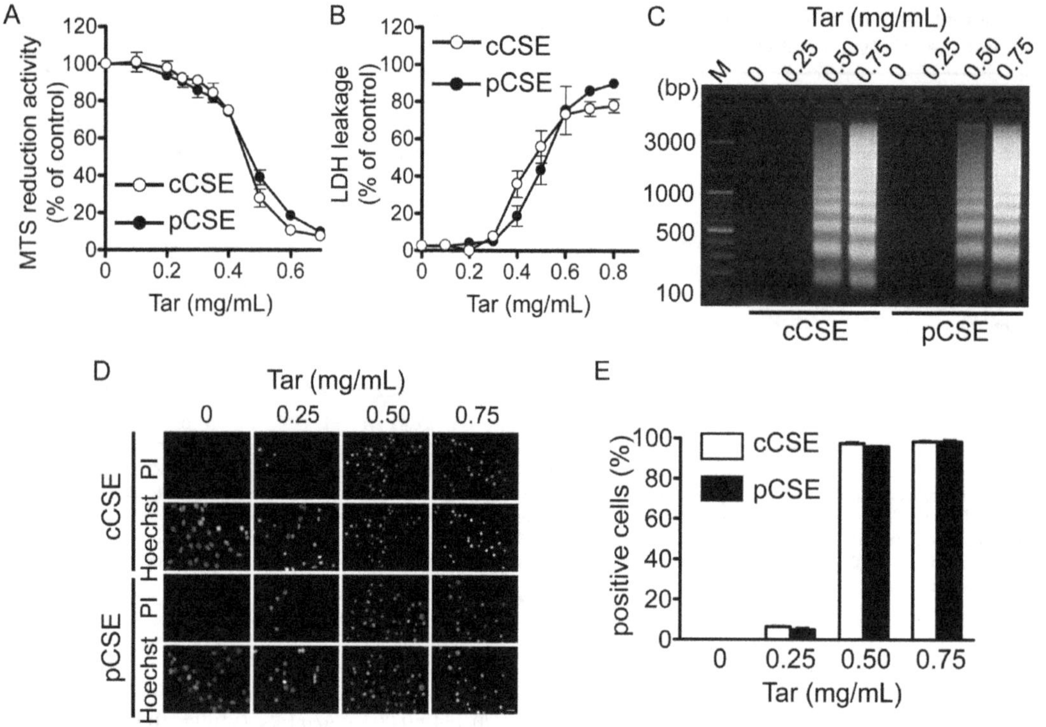

Figure 6. Cytotoxic activities of gas phase extracts of cigarette smoke and smoking methods. The gas phase extracts of cigarette smoke were prepared from Hi-Lite brand cigarettes by either continuous smoking protocol (cCSE) as described in the legend for Fig. 1 or puff smoking (pCSE) as described in Materials and Methods. The original gas phase extracts at the virtual tar concentration of 10 mg/ml PBS were prepared, and they were subjected to MTS reduction assay (A), LDH leakage assay (B), DNA fragmentation assay (C) and PI uptake assay (D, E) in cultured C6 glioma cells for evaluation of their cytotoxic activities. In MTS reduction assay, substrate reduction activity was represented as a percentage of the value in the absence of the gas phase extract; in LDH leakage assay, LDH activity leaked into culture medium was represented as a percentage of total activity in the medium of cells lysed by 0.2% Triton X-100; in PI uptake assay, the number of the cells positive for PI uptake was represented as a percentage of total number of cells identified by Hoechst 33342 for nuclear staining. Values in panels A, B and E represent means ± SE of three experiments, each in triplicate. The results in panels C and D are representative of three separate experiments.

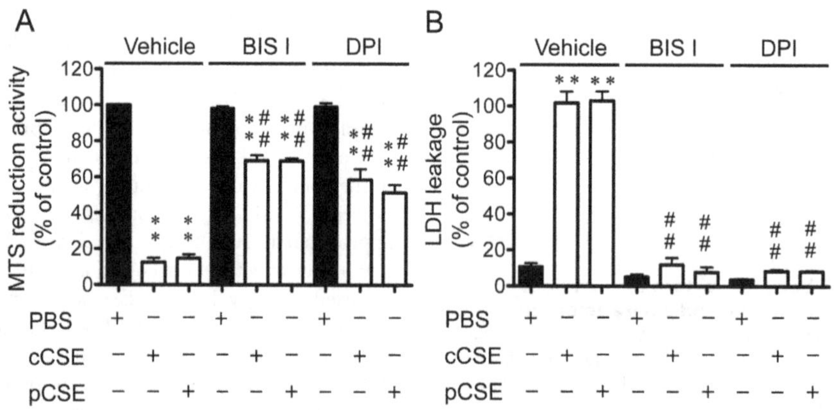

Figure 7. Pharmacological properties of cytotoxic activities of two types of gas phase extracts of cigarette smoke. The gas phase extracts of cigarette smoke at the virtual tar concentration of 10 mg/ml PBS were prepared from Hi-Lite brand cigarettes by either continuous (cCSE) or puff smoking protocol (pCSE), and they were subjected to MTS reduction assay (A) and LDH leakage assay (B). For determination of the effects of inhibitors of protein kinase C or NADPH oxidase, 5 μM BIS I or 1 μM DPI was added to the culture medium of C6 glioma cells, respectively, 30 min before the start of 4-h incubation with cCSE or pCSE. In panel A, MTS reduction activity was represented as a percentage of the control value in the absence of CSEs (PBS) within the vehicle-treated group. In panel B, LDH activity leaked into culture medium was represented as a percentage of total activity in the medium of cells lysed by 0.2% Triton X-100. Values represent means ± SE of three experiments, each in triplicate. $^{**}P<0.01$ vs PBS-treated cells within either of three groups (Vehicle-, BIS I- and DPI-treated groups); $^{\#\#}P<0.01$ vs cCSE- or pCSE-treated cells within the vehicle-treated group.

results taken together indicate that the action mechanisms of two types of CSEs (cCSE and pCSE) for cytotoxicity such as cell death and plasma membrane damage are similar from the pharmacological viewpoint.

Comparison of the concentrations of carbonyl compounds in cCSE and pCSE

In our recent paper [23], we fractionated cCSE into nine fractions with HPLC, found two HPLC fractions to possess cytotoxic activities with functional assays in cultured cells and in those active HPLC fractions, identified ACR, MVK and CPO as stable cytotoxic factors responsible for the cytotoxic activities of cCSE. In addition, in the active HPLC fractions, we identified other carbonyl compounds such as acetone and propionaldehyde which do not possess cytotoxic activities. Therefore, we compared the concentrations of these carbonyl compounds in cCSE with those in pCSE (Table 3). For determination of the concentrations of these carbonyl compounds, both CSEs were first fractionated by reversed-phase HPLC and each fraction was analyzed for cytotoxicity. The fractions showing cytotoxic activities detected by PI uptake assay were subjected to GC/MS after derivatization with a carbonyl reagent PFBOA. As shown in Table 3, there was no significant difference between both types of CSE regarding the concentrations of cytotoxic carbonyls such as ACR and MVK and of noncytotoxic carbonyls such as acetone and propionaldehyde. These results demonstrate that the chemical composition of cCSE and pCSE is equivalent in terms of the concentrations of the major carbonyl compounds.

The sensitivity of various cell lines to cCSE

Finally, we examined the sensitivity to cCSE of various cell lines which are widely used, using MTS reduction assay (Fig. 8). Among these cell lines, CHO cells were the most sensitive to cCSE only in the low tar concentration range (up to 0.2 mg/ml), but they became relatively resistant in the higher tar concentration range. U937 human monocytes, A7r5 rat aorta smooth muscle cells and SBC-3 cells were the second sensitive: the EC_{50} values of cCSE for inhibition of MTS reduction activity were 0.285±0.021 mg/ml, 0.299±0.018 mg/ml and 0.300±0.010 mg/ml (represented by the tar concentration), respectively. C6 rat glioma cells and HEK293T cells were the third in the sensitivity, with the EC_{50} values of 0.423±0.019 mg/ml and 0.446±0.015 mg/ml, respectively. In contrast, HeLa cells, RAW264.7 mouse macrophages, HUVEC, H1299 cells and A549 cells were resistant to CSE up to the tar concentration of 0.6 mg/ml.

Discussion

The gas phase of cigarette smoke is considered to be important from the viewpoint of human health, because it is the gas phase but not the tar phase that can pass through the alveolar epithelium of the lung to enter the circulation, exerting cytotoxic effects in tissues remote from the lung [14,15,30]. However, no standard method for preparation of the gas phase extracts of cigarette smoke has so far been established, and hence, researchers have performed experiments using the gas phase extracts prepared by their own methods. Because of the potential variability in the composition and concentration of those extracts, the comparison of the data from different laboratories has been difficult. In the present study, we have standardized a simple and rapid method for preparation of the gas phase extract of cigarette smoke based on continuous smoking protocol (referred to as cCSE).

The protocol for preparation of cCSE established in the present study is as follows. 1) Cigarette smoke of any brand is continuously sucked through a Cambridge filter with a constant flow rate of 1.050 l/min. 2) The smoke is subsequently bubbled through a glass ball filter of normal pore size into 15 mL of PBS kept at 25°C. 3) The dry weight of the tar phase trapped on the Cambridge filter is determined after drying at 25°C for 12 h, 4) The concentration of cCSE is expressed in terms of the virtual tar concentration which is calculated on the assumption that the tar trapped on the Cambridge filter is dissolved in the PBS used for cCSE preparation, 5) Combustion of cigarette can be repeated as long as the dry weight of tar trapped on the Cambridge filter is ≤ 225 mg.

The most important finding is that the concentration of cCSE expressed in terms of the virtual tar concentration can be used as a reference value to normalize the cytotoxic activities of cCSE, irrespective of the number of combusted cigarettes, cigarette brands and smoking protocols (continuous smoking vs puff smoking), as long as the tar concentrations in the original cCSEs are ≤15 mg/ml of PBS: over this concentration range, part of the cytotoxic activity in the smoke escapes without being extracted into the PBS, causing a lower cytotoxic potency than expected from the tar concentration.

Amongst cigarette brands, the ratio of tar to other gas phase components might vary. Indeed, the ratio of tar to nicotine varies among brands (Table 2). Given this, a given virtual tar concentration may expose cells to differing levels of specific gas phase components despite standardizing by the virtual tar concentration. However, as shown in Figure 5, the concentration-response curves for the cytotoxic activities of the cCSEs prepared from different cigarette brands are not significantly different from each other, when the concentrations of cCSEs are normalized in terms of the virtual tar concentration. This result strongly indicates that the

Table 3. Comparison of concentrations of carbonyl compounds in cCSE and pCSE.

	cCSE[a]	pCSE[a]
Acetone (μM)	287.9±29.2	326.1±20.3
Acrolein (μM)	36.7±1.3	41.7±2.8
Propionaldehyde (μM)	24.4±3.5	28.7±6.9
Methyl vinyl ketone (μM)	17.5±3.0	13.8±0.5

[a]The cCSE and pCSE at the original tar concentration of 10 mg/ml were prepared from Hi-Lite brand cigarettes by either continuous (cCSE) or puff smoking protocol (pCSE). cCSE and pCSE were fractionated by HPLC and each fraction was analyzed for cytotoxic activities using PI uptake assay. The positive fractions were analyzed by GC/MS after derivatization with a carbonyl reagent PFBOA. Values represent means ± SD of three experiments.

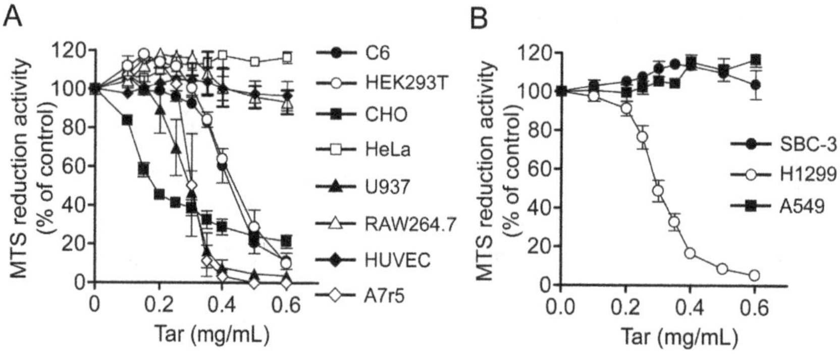

Figure 8. Sensitivities of various cultured cells to the gas phase extracts of cigarette smoke. The gas phase extracts of cigarette smoke (cCSE) at the virtual tar concentration of 10 mg/ml were prepared from Hi-Lite brand cigarettes by continuous smoking protocol, and they were subjected to MTS reduction assay using various cultured cells. MTS reduction activity was represented as a percentage of the control value in the absence of cCSE. Values represent means ± SE of three experiments, each in triplicate. (A) C6, rat glioma cells; HEK293T, human embryonic kidney cells; CHO, Chinese hamster ovary cells; HeLa, human cervical carcinoma cells; U937, human monocytes; RAW264.7, mouse macrophages; HUVEC, immortalized human umbilical vein endothelial cells; A7r5, rat aorta smooth muscle cells. (B) SBC-3, human lung small cell carcinoma; H1299, human lung squamous cell carcinoma; A549, human lung adenocarcinoma.

concentrations of cytotoxic compounds in the CSEs are actually normalized by the virtual tar concentration, and hence that the ratio of cytotoxic compounds to tar is independent of the ratio of nicotine to tar.

Another important finding is that the toxicological properties of cCSE are equivalent to those of pCSE, in terms of potency of cytotoxicity, pharmacology of the cytotoxicity and the concentrations of major cytotoxic compounds such as ACR and MVK. Although there are no experimental data, it has so far been believed that the chemical composition and hence the property of the cytotoxicity of the smoke generated by continuous and puff smoking protocols might be different, mainly based on the consideration that the combustion temperature of cigarette might be different between the two smoking protocols, leading to generation of different spectrum of chemicals [31,32].

The standard method for cCSE preparation established in the present study makes possible the comparison of the experimental data on cCSE from various laboratories, and is expected to accelerate the research on toxicity of smoking and pathophysiology of smoking-related diseases, leading to development of methods for prevention and treatment of smoking-related diseases. However, because cytotoxicity is only one measure of the effects of cigarette smoke, it is noted that other measures such as protease/cytokine expression or mucin production [33,34] might vary among brands despite the virtual tar concentration being controlled.

In the present study, we have proposed a standardized method for preparation of nicotine- and tar-free CSE, i.e. the gas phase extract of cigarette smoke. The other phase (tar phase) containing tar and nicotine is reported to be also important for human health [35–37]. However, a standardized method for preparation of the tar phase extract which is simple and rapid is also absent. Therefore, as a next step, it is important to establish such standardized method and to accelerate the investigation on the cytotoxic effects of nicotine and tar and their molecular mechanisms of action.

In summary, we introduced the virtual tar concentration as a measure of cytotoxic potency of the gas phase extract of cigarette smoke, and established a simple and rapid method for standard preparation of the gas phase extract of cigarette smoke based on continuous smoking protocol. We also demonstrated that from the toxicological viewpoint, the gas phase extract prepared by the present method is equivalent to the extract prepared by a puff smoking machine.

Acknowledgments

We thank Dr. Cora Jean S. Edgell, University of North Carolina at Chapel Hill for providing us with HUVEC.

Author Contributions

Conceived and designed the experiments: T. Higashi SM. Performed the experiments: T. Higashi YM YN AH PN T. Harada MH CH. Analyzed the data: T. Higashi T. Horinouchi KT. Contributed reagents/materials/analysis tools: YK. Contributed to the writing of the manuscript: T. Higashi SM.

References

1. Ambrose JA, Barua RS (2004) The pathophysiology of cigarette smoking and cardiovascular disease: an update. J Am Coll Cardiol 43: 1731–1737.
2. Steenland K, Thun M, Lally C, Heath C, Jr. (1996) Environmental tobacco smoke and coronary heart disease in the American Cancer Society CPS-II cohort. Circulation 94: 622–628.
3. Erhardt L (2009) Cigarette smoking: an undertreated risk factor for cardiovascular disease. Atherosclerosis 205: 23–32.
4. Nussbaumer-Ochsner Y, Rabe KF (2011) Systemic manifestations of COPD. Chest 139: 165–173.
5. D'Agostini F, Balansky R, Steele VE, Ganchev G, Pesce C, et al. (2008) Preneoplastic and neoplastic lesions in the lung, liver and urinary tract of mice exposed to environmental cigarette smoke and UV light since birth. Int J Cancer 123: 2497–2502.
6. Hecht SS, Kassie F, Hatsukami DK (2009) Chemoprevention of lung carcinogenesis in addicted smokers and ex-smokers. Nat Rev Cancer 9: 476–488.
7. Tauler J, Mulshine JL (2009) Lung cancer and inflammation: interaction of chemokines and hnRNPs. Curr Opin Pharmacol 9: 384–388.
8. Burns DM (1991) Cigarettes and cigarette smoking. Clin Chest Med 12: 631–642.
9. Church DF, Pryor WA (1985) Free-radical chemistry of cigarette smoke and its toxicological implications. Environ Health Perspect 64: 111–126.
10. Pryor WA, Stone K (1993) Oxidants in cigarette smoke. Radicals, hydrogen peroxide, peroxynitrate, and peroxynitrite. Ann N Y Acad Sci 686: 12–27; discussion 27–18.
11. Csiszar A, Podlutsky A, Wolin MS, Losonczy G, Pacher P, et al. (2009) Oxidative stress and accelerated vascular aging: implications for cigarette smoking. Front Biosci (Landmark Ed) 14: 3128–3144.

12. Jaimes EA, DeMaster EG, Tian RX, Raij L (2004) Stable compounds of cigarette smoke induce endothelial superoxide anion production via NADPH oxidase activation. Arterioscler Thromb Vasc Biol 24: 1031–1036.
13. Orosz Z, Csiszar A, Labinskyy N, Smith K, Kaminski PM, et al. (2007) Cigarette smoke-induced proinflammatory alterations in the endothelial phenotype: role of NAD(P)H oxidase activation. Am J Physiol Heart Circ Physiol 292: H130–139.
14. Kunitomo M, Yamaguchi Y, Kagota S, Yoshikawa N, Nakamura K, et al. (2009) Biochemical evidence of atherosclerosis progression mediated by increased oxidative stress in apolipoprotein E-deficient spontaneously hyperlipidemic mice exposed to chronic cigarette smoke. J Pharmacol Sci 110: 354–361.
15. Yamaguchi Y, Nasu F, Harada A, Kunitomo M (2007) Oxidants in the gas phase of cigarette smoke pass through the lung alveolar wall and raise systemic oxidative stress. J Pharmacol Sci 103: 275–282.
16. Lambert C, McCue J, Portas M, Ouyang Y, Li J, et al. (2005) Acrolein in cigarette smoke inhibits T-cell responses. J Allergy Clin Immunol 116: 916–922.
17. Su Y, Han W, Giraldo C, De Li Y, Block ER (1998) Effect of cigarette smoke extract on nitric oxide synthase in pulmonary artery endothelial cells. Am J Respir Cell Mol Biol 19: 819–825.
18. Takano S, Matsuoka I, Magami W, Watanabe C, Nakanishi H (1997) Possible existence of platelet aggregation inhibitor(s) in a gas-phase extract of cigarette smoke. Fukushima J Med Sci 43: 1–11.
19. Asano H, Horinouchi T, Mai Y, Sawada O, Fujii S, et al. (2012) Nicotine- and tar-free cigarette smoke induces cell damage through reactive oxygen species newly generated by PKC-dependent activation of NADPH oxidase. J Pharmacol Sci 118: 275–287.
20. Mai Y, Higashi T, Terada K, Hatate C, Nepal P, et al. (2012) Nicotine- and tar-free cigarette smoke extract induces cell injury via intracellular Ca2+-dependent subtype-specific protein kinase C activation. J Pharmacol Sci 120: 310–314.
21. Frei B, Forte TM, Ames BN, Cross CE (1991) Gas phase oxidants of cigarette smoke induce lipid peroxidation and changes in lipoprotein properties in human blood plasma. Protective effects of ascorbic acid. Biochem J 277 (Pt 1): 133–138.
22. Yamaguchi Y, Kagota S, Haginaka J, Kunitomo M (2002) Participation of peroxynitrite in oxidative modification of LDL by aqueous extracts of cigarette smoke. FEBS Lett 512: 218–222.
23. Noya Y, Seki K, Asano H, Mai Y, Horinouchi T, et al. (2013) Identification of stable cytotoxic factors in the gas phase extract of cigarette smoke and pharmacological characterization of their cytotoxicity. Toxicology 314: 1–10.
24. Hammond D, Wiebel F, Kozlowski LT, Borland R, Cummings KM, et al. (2007) Revising the machine smoking regime for cigarette emissions: implications for tobacco control policy. Tob Control 16: 8–14.
25. Stephens WE (2007) Dependence of tar, nicotine and carbon monoxide yields on physical parameters: implications for exposure, emissions control and monitoring. Tob Control 16: 170–176.
26. Edgell CJ, McDonald CC, Graham JB (1983) Permanent cell line expressing human factor VIII-related antigen established by hybridization. Proc Natl Acad Sci U S A 80: 3734–3737.
27. Purkis SW, Cahours X, Rey M, Teillet B, Troude V, et al. (2011) Some consequences of using cigarette machine smoking regimes with different intensities on smoke yields and their variability. Regul Toxicol Pharmacol 59: 293–309.
28. Connolly GN, Wayne GD, Lymperis D, Doherty MC (2000) How cigarette additives are used to mask environmental tobacco smoke. Tob Control 9: 283–291.
29. Rabinoff M, Caskey N, Rissling A, Park C (2007) Pharmacological and chemical effects of cigarette additives. Am J Public Health 97: 1981–1991.
30. Canales L, Chen J, Kelty E, Musah S, Webb C, et al. (2012) Developmental cigarette smoke exposure: liver proteome profile alterations in low birth weight pups. Toxicology 300: 1–11.
31. Kozlowski LT, O'Connor RJ (2002) Cigarette filter ventilation is a defective design because of misleading taste, bigger puffs, and blocked vents. Tob Control 11 Suppl 1: I40–50.
32. Purkis SW, Troude V, Duputie G, Tessier C (2010) Limitations in the characterisation of cigarette products using different machine smoking regimes. Regul Toxicol Pharmacol 58: 501–515.
33. Tamimi A, Serdarevic D, Hanania NA (2012) The effects of cigarette smoke on airway inflammation in asthma and COPD: therapeutic implications. Respir Med 106: 319–328.
34. Yu H, Li Q, Kolosov VP, Perelman JM, Zhou X (2012) Regulation of cigarette smoke-mediated mucin expression by hypoxia-inducible factor-1alpha via epidermal growth factor receptor-mediated signaling pathways. J Appl Toxicol 32: 282–292.
35. Hecht SS (1999) Tobacco smoke carcinogens and lung cancer. J Natl Cancer Inst 91: 1194–1210.
36. Le Houezec J, McNeill A, Britton J (2011) Tobacco, nicotine and harm reduction. Drug Alcohol Rev 30: 119–123.
37. Valavanidis A, Vlachogianni T, Fiotakis K (2009) Tobacco smoke: involvement of reactive oxygen species and stable free radicals in mechanisms of oxidative damage, carcinogenesis and synergistic effects with other respirable particles. Int J Environ Res Public Health 6: 445–462.

18

Luteolin Inhibits Behavioral Sensitization by Blocking Methamphetamine-Induced MAPK Pathway Activation in the Caudate Putamen in Mice

Tinglin Yan[1]ⓒ, Lu Li[1]ⓒ, Baiyu Sun[1], Fei Liu[1], Peng Yang[1], Teng Chen[1,2], Tao Li[1,2]*, Xinshe Liu[1,2]*

1 Department of Forensic Medicine, Xi'an Jiaotong University, School of Medicine, Xi'an, Shaanxi, PR China, **2** The Key Laboratory of Health Ministry for Forensic Science, Xi'an Jiaotong University, Shaanxi, PR China

Abstract

Goal: To investigate the effect of luteolin on methamphetamine (MA)-induced behavioral sensitization and mitogen-activated protein kinase (MAPK) signal transduction pathway activation in mice.

Methods: Mice received a single dose of MA to induce hyperactivity or repeated intermittent intraperitoneal injections of MA to establish an MA-induced behavioral sensitization mouse model. The effect of luteolin on the development and expression of MA-induced hyperactivity and behavioral sensitization was examined. The expression and activity of ΔFosB and the levels of phosphorylated extracellular signal-regulated kinase 1/2 (pERK1/2), phosphorylated c-Jun N-terminal kinase (pJNK), and phosphorylated p38 mitogen-activated protein kinase (pp38) in the caudate putamen (CPu) were measured by western blot.

Results: Luteolin significantly decreased hyperactivity as well as the development and expression of MA-induced behavioral sensitization in mice. ΔFosB, pERK1/2, and pJNK levels in the CPu were higher in MA-treated mice than in control mice, whereas the pp38 level did not change. Injection of luteolin inhibited the MA-induced increase in ΔFosB, pERK1/2, and pJNK levels, but did not affect the pp38 level.

Conclusions: Luteolin inhibits MA-induced hyperactivity and behavioral sensitization in mice through the ERK1/2/ΔFosB pathway. Furthermore, the JNK signaling pathway might be involved in MA-induced neurodegeneration in the CPu, and luteolin inhibits this process.

Editor: Yong-hui Dang, Xi'an Jiaotong University School of Medicine, China

Funding: National Natural Science Foundation of China (No. 81273351), National Natural Science Foundation of China (No. 81373253; http://www.nsfc.gov.cn). 2012 Key Program for International S&T Cooperation Projects of Shaanxi Province (2012kw-36-02; http://www.sninfo.gov.cn). The Fundamental Research Funds for the Central Universities, Shaanxi Key Project on Science and Technology (2013K12-01-09; http://www.xjtu.edu.cn). The funders had no role in study design, data collection and analysis, decision to publish, or preparation of the manuscript.

Competing Interests: The authors have declared that no competing interests exist.

* E-mail: lxins@mail.xjtu.edu.cn (XL); litao@mail.xjtu.edu.cn (TL)

ⓒ These authors contributed equally to this work.

Introduction

Repeated, intermittent administration of addictive drugs (e.g., morphine, amphetamine, cocaine, nicotine, and alcohol) can enhance the locomotor response in experimental animals. The enhancement of behavioral response by repeated drug administration is called behavioral sensitization[1]. Recent studies have demonstrated that behavioral sensitization reflects underlying neuroplastic changes that occur as a result of repeated exposure to drugs of abuse[2–3]. Behavioral sensitization may be involved in relapse and in compulsive drug-seeking and drug-taking behavior[4–6]. Behavioral sensitization represents a robust form of experience-dependent behavioral plasticity and offers a relatively simple model for understanding the neural mechanisms underlying addiction, including relapse[7–10].

The major neuroanatomical substrate of behavioral sensitization appears to be the mesolimbic dopamine system, of which the major components are the ventral tegmental area and its projected regions, including the caudate putamen (CPu)[5,10]. The CPu, which expresses high levels of dopamine receptors (D1R and D2R) and the *N*-methyl-D-aspartate receptor, is a critical site of synaptic plasticity induced by addictive drugs[10–16]. Previous studies have demonstrated that modifications in the CPu are involved in movement initiation, learning of motor patterns, drug-related habit learning, and behavioral sensitization[17,18].

ΔFosB, a truncated product of *fosB*, is a member of the Fos family of transcription factors (others include c-Fos, FosB, Fra1, and Fra2). ΔFosB is induced in the brain's reward regions by chronic exposure to nearly all drugs of abuse[19]. Once induced, the protein persists for long periods because of its unusual stability[19,20]. The inducible expression of ΔFosB increases locomotor activity, reward responses, and incentive motivational effects, which may lead to a propensity for relapse even after prolonged periods of withdrawal from addictive drugs. This provides direct evidence that the induction of ΔFosB is both necessary and sufficient to produce sensitized behavioral responses to drugs of abuse, which would be expected to make an individual more vulnerable to addiction[20–22]. Nestler et al. have shown that the unusual stability of ΔFosB, partly caused by phosphorylation at its N-terminus by casein kinase 2 (CK2), is the basis of its effects on addiction[23].

The mitogen-activated protein kinase (MAPK) pathway is a key signaling pathway involved in the regulation of proliferation, differentiation, and apoptosis in different cells[24–26]. Recent studies suggest that it is composed of the extracellular signal-regulated kinase (ERK), c-Jun N-terminal kinase (JNK), and p38 signaling pathways. The ERK signaling pathway is involved in molecular adaptations and long-term behavioral alterations, including conditioned place preference (CPP) and behavioral sensitization, induced by cocaine or psychostimulants[27,28]. However, the effects of the JNK and p38 signaling pathways on addiction are not yet clear.

In this study, the effects of luteolin, a CK2 inhibitor, on ΔFosB and the MAPK pathway in the CPu were investigated in mice sensitized by methamphetamine (MA). The results suggest that luteolin attenuates the development and expression of MA-induced behavioral sensitization. The results also suggest that the ERK/ΔFosB signaling pathway mediates the beneficial effect of luteolin on behavioral sensitization induced by MA.

Materials and Methods

All experiments were carried out in strict accordance with the Guidelines on the Care and Use of Laboratory Animals issued by the National Institutes of Health, USA, and were approved by the Institutional Animal Care and Use Committee of Xi'an Jiaotong University.

Animals

C57BL/6J mice (male, 18–22 g) were purchased from the Experimental Animal Center of Xi'an Jiaotong University (production license number: SCXK (Shaanxi) 2007-001; license number: SYXK (Shaanxi) 2007-003). Mice were randomly divided into 4 mice/cage and housed under a reverse light cycle (lights on from 7:00 P.M. to 7:00 A.M.) in a climate-controlled colony room (room temperature: 21°C±2°C; humidity: 50%±10%). The animals had access to food and water ad libitum. Two days before the experiments, the mice were adapted to the experimental equipment for 2 h/day. Behavioral testing took place between 8:00 A.M. and 5:00 P.M.

Drugs

Luteolin (Lu) powder (lot number: 62696-5MG; Sigma, USA) was fully dissolved in 100 μl dimethyl sulfoxide and then diluted with saline to the desired concentration. The solution was always freshly prepared before the experiment. Methamphetamine hydrochloride (batch number: 171212200603; China Pharmaceutical and Biological Products, China) was dissolved in saline and was always freshly prepared before the experiment. Animals in the control group were administered vehicle solution (Veh). All drugs were administered via intraperitoneal (i.p.) injection at a dose of 10 ml·kg^{-1}.

Locomotion

All mice were tested in chambers (43 cm×43 cm×43 cm), and their locomotor activities were determined by a SMART Video Tracking System (version 2.5; Panlab Technology for Bioresearch, Spain) after the injections. The "total distance" is the total distance traversed by a mouse as a result of its horizontal locomotor activity during the recording time. This parameter serves as an overall indicator for the increase in locomotor activity induced by the drugs.

The mice (n = 16) were randomly divided into four groups (n = 4/group): control group (Veh+Veh), Lu group (Lu+Veh), Lu and MA combination group (Lu+MA), and MA group (Veh+MA). Lu was administered at 1 mg·kg^{-1}, and MA was administered at 2 mg·kg^{-1}. After the locomotor activity of the mice in all groups was tested for 30 min, the first drug (Lu or Veh) was injected, and testing continued. After 30 min, the animals were administered the second drug (MA or Veh), and the locomotor activity was monitored for a further 60 min with the total distance recorded every 10 min (Fig. 1B). The same procedures were performed for 5 consecutive days (development phase). Administration ceased on day (D)6–D7 (transfer phase). On D8 (expression phase), all animals were administered the corresponding drugs, and their locomotor activities were measured again (Fig. 1A).

Western blot analysis

Within 5 min of the completion of the experiment described above, animals were sacrificed, and the CPu was isolated. Brain tissues were instantly frozen and stored at −80°C. A protein extraction kit (Bio-Rad, USA) was used to extract total tissue proteins, and the concentration was measured using the BCA assay. For protein quantification, 50 μg of protein was added to 5× loading buffer, boiled for 5 min, and then subjected to SDS-PAGE. After electrophoresis, the proteins in the gel were transferred to a nitrocellulose membrane, blocked for 1 h with 5% skim milk at room temperature, and incubated in primary antibody at 4°C overnight. We used primary antibodies against ΔFosB (cat number: 2251S; lot number: 2; Cell Signaling, USA), phosphor-ERK (cat number: 4370S; lot number: 7; Cell Signaling, USA), ERK (cat number: 9102S; lot number: 23; Cell Signaling, USA), phosphor-p38(cat number: 4511S; lot number: 10; Cell Signaling, USA), β-actin (cat number: 4970S; lot number: 5; Cell Signaling, USA) at 1:500 dilutions and phosphor-JNK (cat number: 3893-1; lot number: YH122306C; Epitomics, USA), JNK(cat number: 2037-1; lot number: YJ070405CS; Epitomics, USA), p38(cat number: 1544-1; lot number: YE101902C; Epitomics, USA) at 1:1000 dilutions. The next day, the membrane was washed with TBST for 4 times, 10 min each time, and the HRP-labeled secondary antibody (cat number: 31402; lot number:

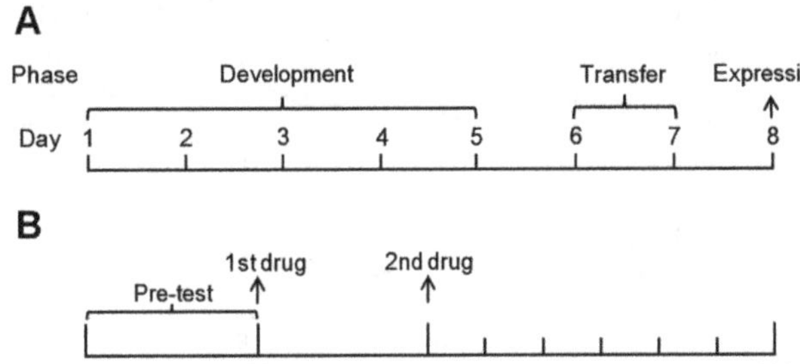

Figure 1. The behavioral sensitization paradigmand dosing schedule. (A) The methamphetamine (MA)induced behavioral sensitization paradigm. On day (D)1-D5,the drugs were injected as schedule. On D6-D7, the drugswere ceased. On D8, the drugs were injected as schedule again. (B)The dosing schedule. Luteolin or vehicle (Veh) wasinjected after pre-testing for 30 min (time point:30 min). MA or Veh was injected after the firstinjections for 30 min (time point: 60 min) andthe test lasts for further 60 min.

31460; Pioneer Biology Company, China) at 1:10000 dilution was added for 1 h at 37°C. The membranes were then washed 4 times with TBST, 10 min each time, and developed using the ECL method (Millipore Corporation, USA). A gel image processing system (Bio-Rad, USA) was used to measure the optical density of each band, and the relative expression levels of the proteins of interest were expressed as the AU ratios of pERK1/2/ERK1/2, pJNK/JNK, and pp38/p38.

Statistical analysis

All data were analyzed using SPSS 17.0 (SPSS, USA). The expression of ΔFosB and the pERK1/2/ERK1/2, pJNK/JNK, and pp38/p38 protein ratios were compared by one-way ANOVA. Locomotor data were analyzed by Student's *t*-test and two-way ANOVA with repeated measures on groups or test sessions. Post hoc multiple comparisons were followed by Student-Newman-Keul tests. "*" and "#" denote P<0.05.

Results

The effect of luteolin on MA-induced behavioral sensitization in mice

The effect of luteolin on hyperactivity induced by a single dose of MA in mice. Two-way repeated-measures ANOVA revealed a significant main effects of time ($F_{(5, 60)} = 22.642$, P< 0.01), group ($F_{(3, 12)} = 37.614$, P<0.01), as well as their interaction ($F_{(15, 60)} = 7.640$, P<0.01) (Fig. 2A). Further multiple comparisons demonstrated, as expected, that a single injection of luteolin (1 mg·kg^{-1}) had no significant effect on the locomotor activity of normal mice. As shown in Figure 2A, MA (2 mg·kg^{-1}) significantly increased locomotor activity in mice, which peaked at the 30–40 min point (P<0.05 vs. the Veh+Veh control group). A single injection of luteolin (1 mg·kg^{-1}) significantly reduced the peak value of locomotor activity acutely induced by MA in mice (P<0.05 at 40 min).

The effect of luteolin on the development and expression of MA-induced behavioral sensitization in mice. Two-way repeated-measures ANOVA revealed a significant main effects of time ($F_{(6, 72)} = 43.319$, P<0.01), group ($F_{(3, 12)} = 28.946$, P<0.01), as well as their interaction ($F_{(18, 72)} = 12.159$, P<0.01) (Fig. 2B). Further multiple comparisons found that multiple injections of luteolin (1 mg·kg^{-1}) had no statistically significant effect on the locomotor activity of normal mice. On D0, no statistically significant difference in the locomotor activities of the mice in any of the experimental groups was detected. The locomotor activity, as reflected by the total distance, increased from D1 to D5 in both the Lu+MA group and the MA group. However, unlike in the Lu+MA group, in the MA group the total distance on D1 was statistically different from that on D8 (P<0.05). In addition, the total distance in the Lu+MA group was significantly lower than that in MA group from D1 to D8 (P<0.05). This suggests that luteolin (1 mg·kg^{-1}) inhibited the development and expression of MA-induced behavioral sensitization in mice.

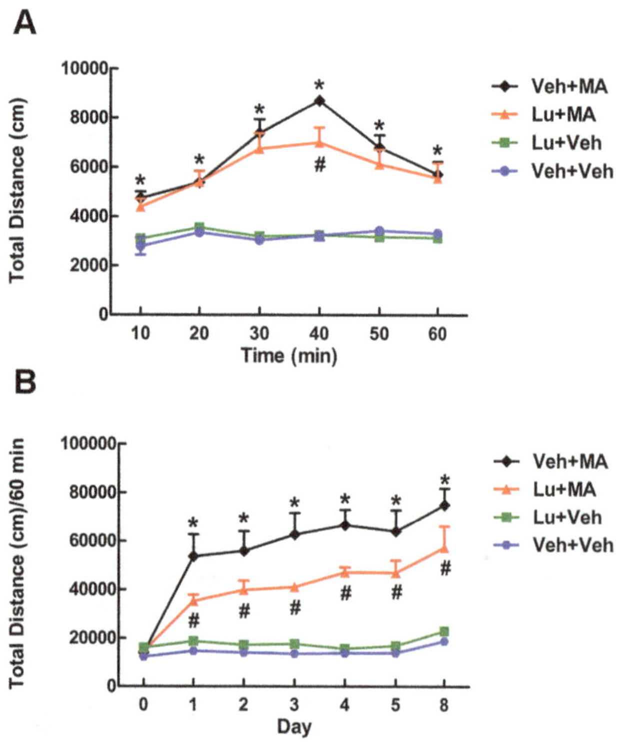

Figure 2. Effect of luteolin on total distance in MA-induced mice. (A) The effect of luteolin (administered 0.5 h before MA injection) on single MA induced mice. (B) The effect of luteolin on the sensitized mice. *P<0.05, compared with the Veh+Veh group. #P<0.05, compared with the Veh+MA group. There was a significant difference between D8 and D1 in the Veh+MA group. Data are presented as the mean ± SEM (n = 4). Data were analyzed using two-way ANOVA and the *t*-test.

The effect of luteolin on MA-induced changes in ΔFosB expression and the MAPK signal transduction pathway in mice

To investigate the mechanisms by which chronic MA administration alters locomotor activity, we examined protein expression in the CPu by western blot.

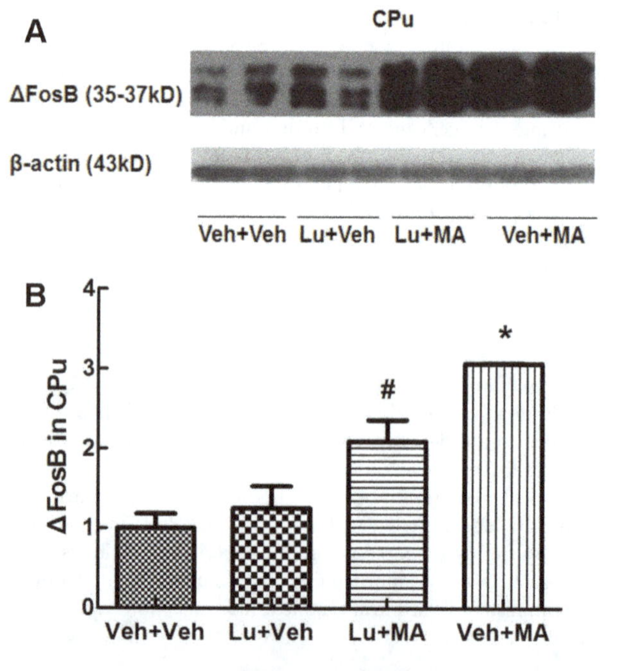

Figure 3. ΔFosB levels in the caudate putamen (CPu) following repeated treatment with methamphetamine. *P<0.05, compared with the Veh+Veh group. #P<0.05, compared with the Veh+MA group. Data are presented as the mean ± SEM (n = 4). Data were analyzed using one-way ANOVA.

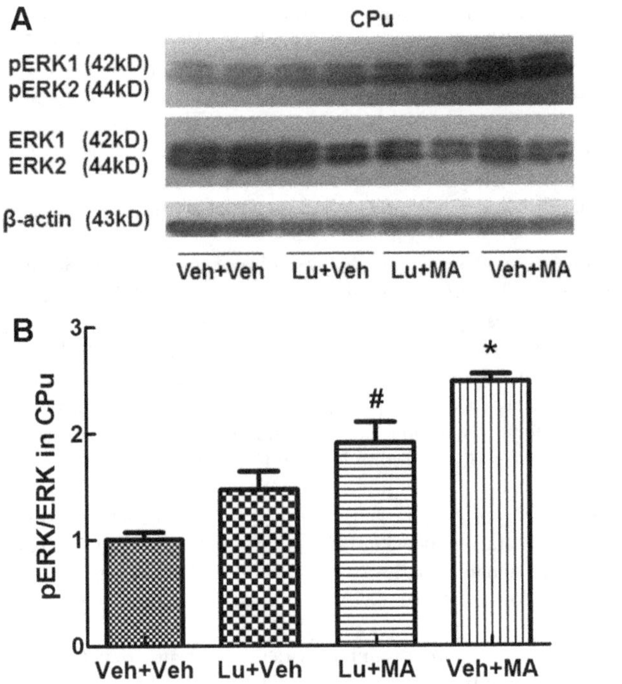

Figure 4. pERK1/2 levels in the CPu following repeated treatment with methamphetamine. (A) Expression of ERK1/2 and pERK1/2 proteins. (B) Ratio of pERK1/2/ERK1/2. *P<0.05, compared with the Veh+Veh group. #P<0.05, compared with the Veh+MA group. Data are presented as the mean ± SEM (n = 4). Data were analyzed using one-way ANOVA.

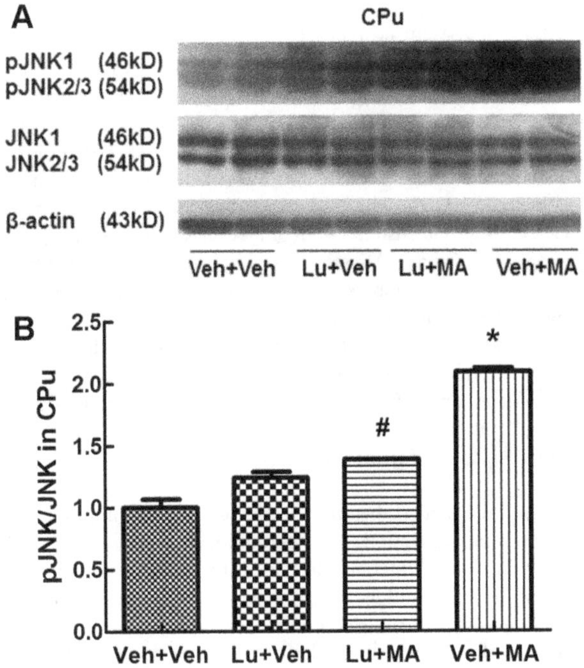

Figure 5. pJNK levels in the CPu following repeated treatment with methamphetamine. (A) Expression of JNK and pJNK proteins. (B) Ratio of pJNK/JNK. *P<0.05, compared with the Veh+Veh group. #P<0.05, compared with the Veh+MA group. Data are presented as the mean ± SEM (n = 4). Data were analyzed using one-way ANOVA.

The effect of luteolin on MA-induced changes in the ΔFosB level in mice. Western blot analysis revealed a significant main effect of group ($F_{(3,\ 12)} = 18.832$, $P<0.01$). Chronic administration of MA significantly increased the ΔFosB level in the CPu ($P<0.05$; Fig. 3). In mice administered Lu+MA, the ΔFosB level was significantly lower than that in mice administered MA alone ($P<0.05$). Luteolin itself had no statistically significant effect on the ΔFosB level in the CPu.

The effect of luteolin on MA-induced changes in the MAPK signal transduction pathway in mice. Western blot analysis revealed different main effects of the groups. Specifically, in the CPu, the main effects on pERK1/2/ERK1/2 ($F_{(3,\ 12)} = 20.565$, $P<0.01$) and pJNK/JNK ($F_{(3,\ 12)} = 117.671$, $P<0.01$) were significant, but the main effects on pp38/p38 ($F_{(3,\ 12)} = 0.027$, NS) were not remarkable. Further multiple comparisons demonstrated that chronic administration of MA increased pERK1/2 (Fig. 4) and pJNK (Fig. 5) levels in the CPu ($P<0.05$). The addition of luteolin attenuated the increases in pERK1/2 and pJNK induced by MA ($P<0.05$). MA did not affect the level of pp38 kinase (Fig. 6). Luteolin itself had no statistically significant effect in any experiment.

Discussion

Many studies have shown that the repeated, intermittent administration of drugs can produce behavioral sensitization. This is manifested by an increase in locomotor activity, rotational behaviors, and stereotyped behaviors[29]. The results of the present study show that multiple, intermittent i.p. administration of MA (2 $mg{\cdot}kg^{-1}$) induces notable behavioral sensitization in mice, consistent with previous reports[30]. Behavioral sensitization is thought to be relevant to animal addiction, and it has been used extensively as a promising animal model to evaluate the key features of addiction, including relapse and drug-seeking and drug-taking behaviors[31]. However, the specific mechanisms underlying the regulation of behavioral sensitization are still unclear.

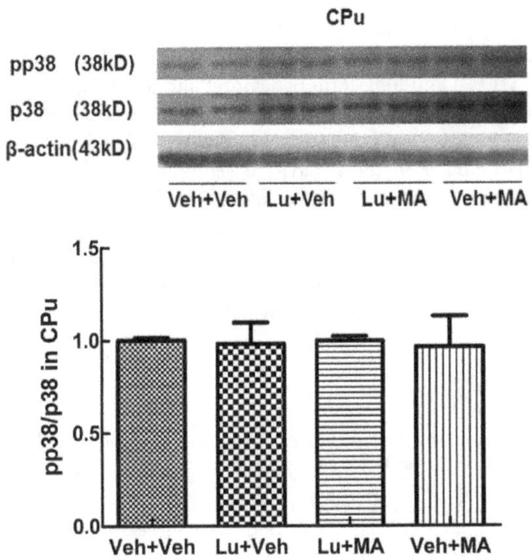

Figure 6. pp38 levels in the CPu following repeated treatment with methamphetamine. (A) Expression of p38 and pp38 proteins. (B) Ratio of pp38/p38. There were no significant differences between the four groups. Data are presented as the mean ± SEM (n = 4). Data were analyzed using one-way ANOVA.

To understand the underlying mechanisms, we measured the expression of ΔFosB protein. The results suggested that MA induced the accumulation of ΔFosB protein. ΔFosB is one of the best-characterized transcription factors known to influence the addiction process. ΔFosB dimerizes with JunD to form activator protein-1 (AP-1) transcription factor complexes. AP-1 complexes then bind to AP-1 sites present in the regulatory regions of many genes, including *Cdk5*, which is responsible for dendritic remodeling[19,32–36]. Consistent with our results, accumulating evidence suggests that ΔFosB increases sensitized behavioral responses, reward responses, and relapse to drugs of abuse[20–22]. These key features of addiction are related to the unusual stability of ΔFosB protein. The stability of ΔFosB is due to two factors: (a) the absence of two degron domains present in the C-terminus of full-length FosB which induce the rapid degradation of other Fos family proteins and (b) the phosphorylation of ΔFosB by CK2 at a serine residue (Ser27) in its N-terminus[19,23].

Because the stability of ΔFosB is regulated by CK2 phosphorylation, we investigated the effect of luteolin, a CK2 inhibitor, on ΔFosB protein expression and locomotor activity. As a CK2 flavonoid inhibitor, luteolin decreases the phosphorylation of serine residues and influences processes such as transcriptional regulation and signal transduction in cells[37,38]. Consistent with previous studies, we found that pre-treatment with luteolin reduced the ΔFosB protein level in the CPu and the locomotor activity of mice sensitized by MA. These finding suggest that ΔFosB mediates the sensitization induced by MA and that luteolin attenuates the expression of ΔFosB and the formation of sensitization.

Increasing evidence indicates that the MAPK signaling pathway is involved in sensitization and the development of neuroplasticity related to the addictive properties of drugs of abuse[27,28,39–41]. Therefore, we assessed the MAPK pathway, including the ERK1/2, JNK, and p38 pathways, and the effect of luteolin on mice sensitized by MA.

Previous studies showed that the ERK1/2 signaling pathway mediates cell metabolism and proliferation, the regulation of cell excitability, synaptic plasticity, and drug-seeking and relapse behavior and plays a key role in the formation of craving during withdrawal[42]. Furthermore, several lines of evidence implicate ERK1/2 in the psychostimulant-induced expression of immediate early genes (IEGs) and long-term behavioral alterations, including CPP, psychomotor sensitization, and craving after late withdrawal[43]. Consistent with previous reports, our results indicate that ERK1/2 participates in the behavioral sensitization induced by chronic exposure to MA. Nestler et al. have shown that ΔFosB mediates neural and behavioral plasticity related to addiction[44]. Furthermore, ERK1/2 activation may be involved in the induction of ΔFosB expression[45]. Taken together, the evidence suggests that MA activates ERK1/2, which induces the expression of the *fosB* gene and the accumulation of ΔFosB. We used luteolin to decrease the stability of ΔFosB and found that luteolin suppressed the increase in the pERK1/2 level induced by MA in the CPu. These results indicate that MA induces behavioral sensitization in part through the ERK1/2/ΔFosB signaling pathway and suggest the presence of a feedback mechanism in this pathway. However, further experiments are needed to determine whether feedback to the upstream ERK signaling pathway is mediated directly by ΔFosB or indirectly by its target genes.

Interestingly, similar results were observed in the JNK signaling pathway. The JNK signaling pathway mediates cell differentiation and regulates apoptosis, depending on the cellular context[46]. Studies suggest that single large doses or multiple small doses of MA produce long-term toxic effects[47–51]. Several studies suggest that reactive oxygen species (ROS) are important players in MA-induced neurodegeneration in the neurites of dopaminergic neurons[52–54]. ROS stimulate the JNK signaling pathway; JNK then phosphorylates c-Jun at Ser63 and Ser73 to activate the transcription of AP-1 target genes[47,52]. This process, consistent with our results, may eventually induce neurodegeneration. Thus, the JNK signaling pathway may mediate neurodegeneration in brain regions related to MA addiction. We found that luteolin suppressed the increase in the pJNK level induced by MA in the CPu. However, circumstantial evidence indicates that CK2 can phosphorylate JNK on Ser407 and Thr404[55]. Therefore, we do not know whether luteolin, as a CK2 inhibitor, suppresses neurodegeneration by inhibiting the phosphorylation of JNK directly or indirectly through ΔFosB. Taken together, our results show that MA might induce neurodegeneration in the CPu through the JNK signaling pathway and that luteolin suppresses this process. Further research is needed to verify that the JNK signaling pathway is involved in regulating the expression of ΔFosB.

Unlike pERK1/2 and pJNK levels, pp38 levels in the CPu did not change when mice were administered MA or Lu+MA. This suggests that the p38 signaling pathway is not involved in behavioral sensitization or the regulation of ΔFosB protein.

Conclusion

In conclusion, our present study shows that luteolin can attenuate MA-induced behavioral sensitization through the ERK1/2/ΔFosB pathway. Furthermore, the JNK signaling pathway might be involved in MA-induced neurodegeneration in the CPu, and luteolin inhibits this process.

Author Contributions

Conceived and designed the experiments: XL TL. Performed the experiments: TY LL BS FL PY. Analyzed the data: TY LL BS FL PY. Contributed reagents/materials/analysis tools: TY LL BS FL PY. Wrote the paper: TY LL BS XL TC.

References

1. Pierce RC, Kalivas PW (1997) A circuitry model of the expression of behavioral sensitization to amphetamine-like psychostimulants. Brain Res Brain Res Rev 25: 192–216.
2. Li J-X, Chen S-Q, Deng Y-P, Liang J-H (2008) Effects of 5-hydroxytryptophan on morphine-induced sensitization in mice. Journal of Chinese Pharmaceutical Sciences 17: 1–5.
3. Robinson TE, Berridge KC (2000) The psychology and neurobiology of addiction: an incentive–sensitization view. Addiction 95: 91–117.
4. Yim DG, Ghosh S, Guy GR, Virshup DM (2014) Casein kinase 1 regulates Sprouty2 in FGF-ERK signaling. Oncogene.
5. Fasano S, D'Antoni A, Orban PC, Valjent E, Putignano E, et al. (2009) Ras-guanine nucleotide-releasing factor 1 (Ras-GRF1) controls activation of extracellular signal-regulated kinase (ERK) signaling in the striatum and long-term behavioral responses to cocaine. Biol Psychiatry 66: 758–768.
6. Scibelli AC, McKinnon CS, Reed C, Burkhart-Kasch S, Li N, et al. (2011) Selective breeding for magnitude of methamphetamine-induced sensitization alters methamphetamine consumption. Psychopharmacology 214: 791–804.
7. Buchanan J, Sparkman N, Johnson R (2010) Methamphetamine sensitization attenuates the febrile and neuroinflammatory response to a subsequent peripheral immune stimulus. Brain, Behavior, and Immunity 24: 502–511.
8. Mitew S, Hay CM, Peckham H, Xiao J, Koenning M, et al. (2013) Mechanisms regulating the development of oligodendrocytes and central nervous system myelin. Neuroscience.
9. Ujike H (2002) Stimulant induced psychosis and schizophrenia: the role of sensitization. Current psychiatry reports 4: 177–184.
10. Rangaswami H, Marathe N, Zhuang S, Chen Y, Yeh JC, et al. (2009) Type II cGMP-dependent protein kinase mediates osteoblast mechanotransduction. The Journal of Biological Chemistry 284: 14796–14808.

11. Do H, Park HJ, Sohn EH, Kim BO, Um SH, et al. (2013) Ethanol induces cell cycle arrest and triggers apoptosis via Sp1-dependent p75NTR expression in human neuroblastoma cells. Cell Biology and Toxicology 29: 365–380.
12. Ryu SY, Kim S (2013) Evaluation of CK2 inhibitor (E)-3-(2,3,4,5-tetrabromophenyl)acrylic acid (TBCA) in regulation of platelet function. European Journal of Pharmacology 720: 391–400.
13. Shrimali D, Shanmugam MK, Kumar AP, Zhang J, Tan BK, et al. (2013) Targeted abrogation of diverse signal transduction cascades by emodin for the treatment of inflammatory disorders and cancer. Cancer Letters 341: 139–149.
14. Stark F, Pfannstiel J, Klaiber I, Raabe T (2011) Protein kinase CK2 links polyamine metabolism to MAPK signalling in Drosophila. Cell Signal 23: 876–882.
15. Han SH, Odathurai Saminathan S, Kim SJ (2010) Insulin stimulates gene expression of ferritin light chain in osteoblast cells. Journal of Cellular Biochemistry 111: 1493–1500.
16. Zhao N, Chen Y, Zhu J, Wang L, Cao G, et al. (2014) Levo-tetrahydropalmatine attenuates the development and expression of methamphetamine-induced locomotor sensitization and the accompanying activation of ERK in the nucleus accumbens and caudate putamen in mice. Neuroscience 258: 101–110.
17. Nikaido T, Akiyama M, Moriya T, Shibata S (2001) Sensitized increase of period gene expression in the mouse caudate/putamen caused by repeated injection of methamphetamine. Mol Pharmacol 59: 894–900.
18. Kaplan GB, Leite-Morris KA, Fan W, Young AJ, Guy MD (2011) Opiate sensitization induces FosB/ΔFosB expression in prefrontal cortical, striatal and amygdala brain regions. PloS One 6: e23574.
19. Nestler EJ (2008) Transcriptional mechanisms of addiction: role of ΔFosB. Philosophical Transactions of the Royal Society B: Biological Sciences 363: 3245–3255.
20. McClung CA, Ulery PG, Perrotti LI, Zachariou V, Berton O, et al. (2004) ΔFosB: a molecular switch for long-term adaptation in the brain. Molecular Brain Research 132: 146–154.
21. Nestler EJ (2001) Molecular basis of long-term plasticity underlying addiction. Nature Reviews Neuroscience 2: 119–128.
22. Kupcova Skalnikova H, Navarro R, Marsala S, Hrabakova R, Vodicka P, et al. (2013) Signaling proteins in spinal parenchyma and dorsal root ganglion in rat with spinal injury-induced spasticity. Journal of Proteomics 91: 41–57.
23. Ulery PG, Rudenko G, Nestler EJ (2006) Regulation of ΔFosB stability by phosphorylation. The Journal of Neuroscience 26: 5131–5142.
24. van der Schaaf ME, Fallon SJ, ter Huurne N, Buitelaar J, Cools R (2013) Working Memory Capacity Predicts Effects of Methylphenidate on Reversal Learning. Neuropsychopharmacology 38: 2011–2018.
25. Huang G, Tang B, Tang K, Dong X, Deng J, et al. (2014) Isoquercitrin inhibits the progression of liver cancer in vivo and in vitro via the MAPK signalling pathway. Oncology Reports 35: 2377–2384.
26. Fan XL, Zhang JS, Zhang XQ, Ma L (2003) Chronic morphine treatment and withdrawal induce up-regulation of c-Jun N-terminal kinase 3 gene expression in rat brain. Neuroscience 122: 997–1002.
27. Valjent E, Corvol J-C, Pagès C, Besson M-J, Maldonado R, et al. (2000) Involvement of the extracellular signal-regulated kinase cascade for cocaine-rewarding properties. The Journal of Neuroscience 20: 8701–8709.
28. Licata SC, Pierce RC (2003) The roles of calcium/calmodulin-dependent and Ras/mitogen-activated protein kinases in the development of psychostimulant-induced behavioral sensitization. Journal of Neurochemistry 85: 14–22.
29. Chinen CC, Faria RR, Frussa-Filho R (2006) Characterization of the rapid-onset type of behavioral sensitization to amphetamine in mice: role of drug-environment conditioning. Neuropsychopharmacology 31: 151–159.
30. Mendez IA, Williams MT, Bhavsar A, Lu AP, Bizon JL, et al. (2009) Long-lasting sensitization of reward-directed behavior by amphetamine. Behavioural Brain Research 201: 74–79.
31. Wise RA, Bozarth MA (1987) A psychomotor stimulant theory of addiction. Psychol Rev 94: 469–492.
32. Borrelli E, Nestler EJ, Allis CD, Sassone-Corsi P (2008) Decoding the epigenetic language of neuronal plasticity. Neuron 60: 961–974.
33. Mierzejewska K, Heo J, Kang JW, Kang H, Ratajczak J, et al. (2013) Genome-wide analysis of murine bone marrowderived very small embryonic-like stem cells reveals that mitogenic growth factor signaling pathways play a crucial role in the quiescence and ageing of these cells. International Journal of Molecular Medicine 32: 281–290.
34. Chen J, Nye HE, Kelz MB, Hiroi N, Nakabeppu Y, et al. (1995) Regulation of delta FosB and FosB-like proteins by electroconvulsive seizure and cocaine treatments. Molecular Pharmacology 48: 880–889.
35. Hiroi N, Marek GJ, Brown JR, Ye H, Saudou F, et al. (1998) Essential role of the fosB gene in molecular, cellular, and behavioral actions of chronic electroconvulsive seizures. The Journal of Neuroscience 18: 6952–6962.
36. Pérez-Otaño I, Mandelzys A, Morgan JI (1998) MPTP-Parkinsonism is accompanied by persistent expression of a ΔFosB-like protein in dopaminergic pathways. Molecular Brain Research 53: 41–52.
37. Jung DH, Park HJ, Byun HE, Park YM, Kim TW, et al. (2010) Diosgenin inhibits macrophage-derived inflammatory mediators through downregulation of CK2, JNK, NF-kappaB and AP-1 activation. International Immunopharmacology 10: 1047–1054.
38. Crozier SJ, Sans MD, Wang JY, Lentz SI, Ernst SA, et al. (2010) CCK-independent mTORC1 activation during dietary protein-induced exocrine pancreas growth. American Journal of Physiology Gastrointestinal and Liver Physiology 299: G1154–1163.
39. Thomas GM, Huganir RL (2004) MAPK cascade signalling and synaptic plasticity. Nature Reviews Neuroscience 5: 173–183.
40. Sweatt JD (2004) Mitogen-activated protein kinases in synaptic plasticity and memory. Current opinion in Neurobiology 14: 311–317.
41. Wang JQ, Tang Q, Parelkar NK, Liu Z, Samdani S, et al. (2004) Glutamate signaling to ras-MAPK in striatal neurons. Molecular Neurobiology 29: 1–14.
42. Cohen-Matsliah SI, Brosh I, Rosenblum K, Barkai E (2007) A novel role for extracellular signal-regulated kinase in maintaining long-term memory-relevant excitability changes. The Journal of Neuroscience 27: 12584–12589.
43. Besnard A, Bouveyron N, Kappes V, Pascoli V, Pages C, et al. (2011) Alterations of molecular and behavioral responses to cocaine by selective inhibition of Elk-1 phosphorylation. The Journal of Neuroscience 31: 14296–14307.
44. Alibhai IN, Green TA, Potashkin JA, Nestler EJ (2007) Regulation of fosB and ΔfosB mRNA expression: In vivo and in vitro studies. Brain Research 1143: 22–33.
45. Pavon N, Martin AB, Mendialdua A, Moratalla R (2006) ERK phosphorylation and FosB expression are associated with L-DOPA-induced dyskinesia in hemiparkinsonian mice. Biol Psychiatry 59: 64–74.
46. Raman M, Chen W, Cobb MH (2007) Differential regulation and properties of MAPKs. Oncogene 26: 3100–3112.
47. Cadet JL, Jayanthi S, Deng X (2005) Methamphetamine-induced neuronal apoptosis involves the activation of multiple death pathways. Review. Neurotoxicity Research 8: 199–206.
48. Chan P, Monte DA, Luo JJ, DeLanney LE, Irwin I, et al. (1994) Rapid ATP loss caused by methamphetamine in the mouse striatum: relationship between energy impairment and dopaminergic neurotoxicity. Journal of Neurochemistry 62: 2484–2487.
49. Chapman DE, Hanson GR, Kesner RP, Keefe KA (2001) Long-term changes in basal ganglia function after a neurotoxic regimen of methamphetamine. Journal of Pharmacology and Experimental Therapeutics 296: 520–527.
50. Hotchkiss AJ, Gibb JW (1980) Long-term effects of multiple doses of methamphetamine on tryptophan hydroxylase and tyrosine hydroxylase activity in rat brain. Journal of Pharmacology and Experimental Therapeutics 214: 257–262.
51. Sonsalla P, Gibb J, Hanson G (1986) Roles of D1 and D2 dopamine receptor subtypes in mediating the methamphetamine-induced changes in monoamine systems. Journal of Pharmacology and Experimental Therapeutics 238: 932–937.
52. Jayanthi S, McCoy MT, Ladenheim B, Cadet JL (2002) Methamphetamine causes coordinate regulation of Src, Cas, Crk, and the Jun N-terminal kinase–Jun pathway. Molecular Pharmacology 61: 1124–1131.
53. Cadet JL, Brannock C (1997) Invited Review Free radicals and the pathobiology of brain dopamine systems. Neurochemistry International 32: 117–131.
54. Sueyoshi N, Nimura T, Ishida A, Taniguchi T, Yoshimura Y, et al. (2009) Ca^{2+}/calmodulin-dependent protein kinase phosphatase (CaMKP) is indispensable for normal embryogenesis in zebrafish, Danio rerio. Archives of Biochemistry and Biophysics 488: 48–59.
55. Kohlstedt K, Brandes RP, Muller-Esterl W, Busse R, Fleming I (2004) Angiotensin-converting enzyme is involved in outside-in signaling in endothelial cells. Circulation Research 94: 60–67.

19

Transient and Persistent Metabolomic Changes in Plasma following Chronic Cigarette Smoke Exposure in a Mouse Model

Charmion I. Cruickshank-Quinn[1], Spencer Mahaffey[1,2], Matthew J. Justice[3], Grant Hughes[4], Michael Armstrong[1], Russell P. Bowler[5], Richard Reisdorph[1,6], Irina Petrache[3,7]*, Nichole Reisdorph[1]*

1 Integrated Department of Immunology, National Jewish Health and University of Colorado School of Medicine, Denver, Colorado, United States of America, 2 Department of Pharmacology, School of Medicine, University of Colorado Denver, Aurora, Colorado, United States of America, 3 Departments of Medicine and of Biochemistry and Molecular Biology, Indiana University, Indianapolis, Indiana, United States of America, 4 Department of Biostatistics and Informatics, University of Colorado Denver, Aurora, Colorado, United States of America, 5 Department of Medicine, National Jewish Health, Denver, Colorado, United States of America, 6 Department of Pediatrics, National Jewish Health, Denver, Colorado, United States of America, 7 Richard L. Roudebush VA Medical Center, Indianapolis, Indiana, United States of America

Abstract

Cigarette smoke exposure is linked to the development of a variety of chronic lung and systemic diseases in susceptible individuals. Metabolomics approaches may aid in defining disease phenotypes, may help predict responses to treatment, and could identify biomarkers of risk for developing disease. Using a mouse model of chronic cigarette smoke exposure sufficient to cause mild emphysema, we investigated whether cigarette smoke induces distinct metabolic profiles and determined their persistence following smoking cessation. Metabolites were extracted from plasma and fractionated based on chemical class using liquid-liquid and solid-phase extraction prior to performing liquid chromatography mass spectrometry-based metabolomics. Metabolites were evaluated for statistically significant differences among group means (p-value$\leq$0.05) and fold change $\geq$1.5). Cigarette smoke exposure was associated with significant differences in amino acid, purine, lipid, fatty acid, and steroid metabolite levels compared to air exposed animals. Whereas 60% of the metabolite changes were reversible, 40% of metabolites remained persistently altered even following 2 months of smoking cessation, including nicotine metabolites. Validation of metabolite species and translation of these findings to human plasma metabolite signatures induced by cigarette smoking may lead to the discovery of biomarkers or pathogenic pathways of smoking-induced disease.

Editor: Ali Önder Yildirim, Institute of Lung Biology and Disease (iLBD), Helmholtz Zentrum München, Germany

Funding: This study was supported by National Heart, Lung and Blood Institute (NHLBI RO1HL 095432, P20 HL-113445-01, U01 HL089856, U01 HL089897); and UL1 RR025780 from NCRR/HIH. The funders had no role in study design, data collection and analysis, decision to publish, or preparation of the manuscript.

Competing Interests: The authors have declared that no competing interests exist.

* Email: ReisdorphN@NJHealth.org (NR); ipetrach@iu.edu (IP)

Introduction

A biological marker (biomarker) is a characteristic that is objectively measured and evaluated as an indicator of normal or pathogenic biological processes, or of pharmacologic responses to a therapeutic intervention [1]. Biomarkers identified in biological fluids such as plasma can be used for early disease diagnoses or to identify those at risk for disease development, which could lead to behavior modification or clinical interventions that may impact disease prognosis. Metabolomics has become a critical tool in clinical research for identifying disease biomarkers associated, for example, with heart disease [2], with cancers of the prostate [3] or lung [4], and with nonalcoholic fatty liver disease [5].

The respiratory tract is the first target of cigarette smoke inhalation and cigarette smoking is a major risk factor for diseases of the airways such as chronic obstructive pulmonary disease (COPD) [6] and head, neck, and lung cancers [7]. It is well established that cigarette smoking is also a risk factor for many systemic diseases, including cardiovascular disease and numerous cancers (e.g. bladder or pancreas), suggesting significant pathogenicity of circulating toxic components or metabolites of absorbed cigarette smoke. However, not all smokers develop disease and progression of diseases such as COPD may persist despite smoking cessation. These observations suggest a critical need for determining pathways through which smoking can lead to disease and for the discovery of useful biomarkers of disease phenotype, severity, and progression.

There are currently few published studies exploring metabolome changes due to smoking. Rather, much of the literature has focused on developing methods to identify compounds in cigarette smoke using techniques such as liquid chromatography tandem mass spectrometry [8,9] and gas chromatography mass spectrometry [10]. Other investigators have looked at specific cigarette smoke metabolites in biological fluids as biomarkers of cigarette smoke exposure [11–13], while other studies have focused on understanding enzyme activities [14] or nicotine biosynthesis [15] of tobacco plants. Xu et al [16] studied the effects of smoking on the human serum metabolome using a targeted metabolomics approach of 140 metabolites with a focus on amino acids and phosphotidylcholines (PC). To our knowledge, no study has yet examined how cigarette smoke affects the entire plasma metabolome. Using state of the art untargeted metabolomics as previously described by Yang et al [17] applied to a cigarette smoking model in mice, we sought to examine changes in the plasma metabolome that are induced by chronic cigarette smoking, and to determine if these changes are stable or transient following smoking cessation.

Materials and Methods

1 Animal studies

Ethics Statement. Animal studies were approved by the Animal Care and Use Committee of Indiana University.

DBA/2J mice (Jackson Labs; male; age 12–14 weeks; n = 2–3 per group) were exposed to ambient air or cigarette smoke as previously described by Schweitzer et al [18]. These mice have been shown to be susceptible to cigarette smoke-induced emphysema-like disease following at least 4 months of exposure [18,19], also demonstrated in this mouse cohort by increased mean linear intercepts (Figure S1). Briefly, mice were exposed 5 hours per day, 5 days a week to 11% mainstream and 89% side-stream smoke from reference cigarettes (3R4F; Tobacco Research Institute, Kentucky) using a Teague 10E whole body exposure apparatus (Teague Enterprise, CA) with monitored suspended particulates (average 90 mg/m^3) and carbon monoxide (average 350 ppm). Five groups of mice were analyzed: 1) ambient air-only exposed at four or six months (controls, n = 3), 2) cigarette smoke-exposed for 4 months (CS-4mo, n = 2), 3) cigarette smoke-exposed for 6 months (CS-6mo, n = 3), and 4) cigarette smoke-exposed for 4 months followed by 2 months in ambient air (CS-cessation, n = 3). At the end of experiments, the mice were euthanized and the plasma was collected by cardiac puncture and then snap-frozen in liquid nitrogen and stored at −80°C.

2 Chemicals and standards

Solvents used for metabolite extraction and LC/MS analysis were of HPLC or LC/MS-grade. Isopropyl alcohol and water were purchased from Honeywell Burdick & Jackson (Muskegon, Michigan). Methyl tert-butyl ether was purchased from J.T. Baker (Central City, Pennsylvania). Acetonitrile, methanol, chloroform, hexane, and acetic acid were purchased from Fisher Scientific (Fair Lawn, New Jersey).

The neutral and phospholipid standards – Triglyceride d5-(20:0/20:1(11Z)/20:0)), C17 ceramide (d18:1/17:0), 1,2-dipentadecanoyl-*sn*-glycero-3-phosphocholine (15:0 PC), and 1,2-diheptadecanoyl-*sn*-glycero-3-phosphoethanolamine (17:0 PE) – were purchased from Avanti Polar lipids Inc. (Alabaster, Alabama). The aqueous standard – creatinine-d3 – was purchased from Sigma Aldrich (St. Louis, MO).

Solid phase extraction (SPE) 12-position vacuum manifold and Strata NH_2 (55 μM, 70 Å) 100 mg/mL SPE cartridges were purchased from Phenomenex (Torrance, California). Glass pipette tips, plastic pipette tips and microcentrifuge tubes were purchased from Fisher Scientific (Fair Lawn, New Jersey). Pyrex glass culture tubes were purchased from Corning Incorporated (Corning, New York).

3 Sample Preparation/Extraction

Standards stored at −20°C and samples stored at −80°C were thawed and kept on ice prior to sample preparation. Samples (n = 2–3/group) were prepared using the liquid-liquid extraction (LLE) and solid-phase extraction (SPE) method previously described by Yang et al [17] with the following changes: subsequent to the extraction steps, the neutral lipid fraction was resuspended in 400 μL 1:1 chloroform: methanol, the phospholipid fraction was resuspended in 400 μL methanol, and the aqueous fraction was resuspended in 100 μL 3% acetonitrile with 0.1% formic acid. Blank samples and a pooled plasma sample were prepared with each batch for sample preparation quality control (QC) purposes. A single pooled plasma sample was prepared at the beginning of the study for use as an instrument QC sample.

4 Liquid chromatography/mass spectrometry

The aqueous fraction samples were analyzed in positive ESI mode at a flow rate of 0.3 mL/min with scan range 50–1050 m/z and scan rate 2.01. 10 μL of sample was injected onto a Zorbax SB-AQ analytical column (1.8 micron, 2.1×50 mm) with a narrow bore SB-AQ guard cartridge (5 micron, 2.1×12.5 mm, 80 Å). Mobile phase A was water with 0.1% formic acid and mobile phase B was 90:10 acetonitrile: water with 0.1% formic acid. Gradient elution was as follows: 0–3 minutes, 2% B, 3–5 minutes 2–40% B, 5–20 minutes 40–100% B, 20–30 minutes 100% B, followed by column re-equilibration. MS source conditions were as follows: gas temperature 300°C, gas flow 10.0 L/min, nebulizer pressure 45 psi, fragmentor 160 V, ESI capillary voltage 4000 V with reference masses 121.05087 and 922.00979 (Agilent reference mix).

The neutral lipid and phospholipid fractions were analyzed in positive ESI mode at a flow rate of 0.5 mL/min with scan range 60–1600 m/z and scan rate 2.01. 10 μL of sample was injected onto an SB-C3 analytical column (5 μM, 2.1×50 mm) with a narrow bore SB-C3 guard cartridge (5 micron, 2.1×1.5 mm, 300 Å). Mobile phase A was water with 5 mM ammonium acetate and mobile phase B was isopropyl alcohol with 5 mM ammonium acetate. Gradient elution was as follows: 0–2 minutes, 30% B, 2–11 minutes 30–100% B, 11–15 minutes 100% B, followed by column re-equilibration. MS source conditions were as follows: gas temperature 300°C, gas flow 7.0 L/min, nebulizer pressure (neutral fraction: 40 psi, phospholipid fraction: 50 psi), fragmentor (neutral fraction: 120 V, phospholipid fraction: 140 V), ESI capillary voltage 2000 V with reference masses 121.05087 and 922.00979 (Agilent reference mix).

Sample analysis was performed on a Time-of-Flight mass spectrometer (6210 TOF-MS, Agilent Technologies) with electrospray source coupled to a high performance liquid chromatography system (Agilent 1200 Series) as described previously [17]. All samples were randomized and injected in triplicate. The analytical quality of the sample preparation, method and instrument were evaluated by injecting the sample prep and instrument QC samples in triplicate during each batch of samples analyzed using TOF, for a total of 7 batches.

The quality control internal standards described in methods section 2 were analyzed to ensure mass accuracy within 3 ppm, retention time reproducibility of less than +/−5% and HPLC pressure curve reproducibility of less than +/−5% at 10 time points. Sample batches that did not meet these criteria were re-analyzed.

5 Data and statistical analysis

Prior to quantitative analysis, data were evaluated for sample preparation reliability and retention time reproducibility by examining the spiked internal standards described in methods sections 3 and 4.

Data was extracted using the following parameters in Mass Hunter software (Agilent Technologies): Find by Molecular

Feature algorithm, single charge, proton and sodium adducts only in positive mode. Data were imported into Mass Profiler Professional software (MPP, Agilent Technologies) for mass (15 ppm) and retention time alignment (0.2 minutes), and data filtered by selecting features which were present in 2 out of 3 technical replicates. Data from sample preparation blanks and instrument blanks were background subtracted to eliminate noise from contaminants. This resulted in 7589 molecular features.

Because LCMS data can result in missing values [20], data was further processed using the 'Find by Formula' algorithm parameters (+H and +Na adducts for positive ionization mode, −H for negative ionization mode, charge states limited to 1, and absolute height >3000 counts). The final data set was then re-imported into MPP for analysis, including normalization ('75% percentile shift' normalization algorithm). The 'Find by Formula' algorithm combined multiple features such as adducts and dimers into a single compound which resulted in 3045 total compounds.

Statistical analysis was performed on the 3045 compounds (1561 in the aqueous fraction, 886 in the neutral fraction and 598 in the phospholipid fraction). ANOVA using Student-Newman-Keuls (SNK) post-hoc test or Student's unpaired t-test were applied. Benjamini-Hochberg false discovery rate (FDR) multiple testing correction using asymptotic p-value computation with a corrected p-value cut-off of 0.05 was used. The list of 3045 compounds was reduced to 656 after FDR<0.05. Fold change cut-off of 1.5 was then applied to this list resulting in 584 compounds following fold change analysis. This final list of significant metabolites were exported into Mass Hunter Quantitative Analysis Software (Agilent) to further reduce the list of potential false positives by removing retention time outliers using a 0.30 minute cut-off window. This final list of 222 metabolites was then re-imported into MPP for annotation, data summary, and visualization purposes.

Finally, annotated compounds and their normalized abundance values were exported to Excel Professional Plus 2010 (Microsoft Corporation, Redmond, WA) for graphing.

6 Identification of plasma metabolites

ID Browser within the Mass Profiler Professional software was used to tentatively identify metabolites (Table S1). This software utilizes an in-house database comprising data from Metlin, Human Metabolome Database (HMDB), Kyoto Encyclopedia of Genes and Genomes (KEGG) and Lipid maps and applies isotope ratios, accurate mass, chemical formulas, and scores to provide preliminary identifications (Table S2). Chosen elements for molecular formula generation were: C, H, N, O, S, and P. A 10 ppm mass error cutoff was used with a neutral mass range up to 2000 Da and positive ions selected as H, Na, K, and NH_4. The database identifications were limited to the top 10 best matches based on score, and charge state was limited to a maximum of 2. Selective solvent extraction implemented during the sample preparation step was applied for additional metabolite information based on lipid chemical class. All identifications are Metabolomics Standards Initiative (MSI) level 2 based on the proposed minimum reporting by Sumner et al [21].

Results and Discussion

1 Quality Control

Quality control (QC) samples were analyzed (n = 31 in the aqueous fraction, n = 31 in the neutral lipid fraction, and n = 32 in the phospholipid fraction) and spike-in standards of known concentration were used to test the LLE and SPE fractionation method efficiency. As expected, only the aqueous spike (creatinine-d3) was detected in the aqueous fraction. Neutral spike-in compounds (TG-d5 and ceramide C17) were detected in the neutral lipid fraction, although the aqueous spike (creatinine-d3) and a phospholipid spike (15:0 PC) were also detected in this fraction, in much lower abundance (29-fold and 2.3-fold lower, respectively). Similarly, the phospholipid spike-in compounds (15:0 PC and 17:0 PE) were detected in the phospholipid fraction, along with small amounts of the aqueous standard creatinine-d3 at 2.5 times lower abundance than in its aqueous fraction. Additionally, the neutral lipid standard ceramide C17 was detected in the phospholipid fraction at 2960-times lower abundance compared to the neutral fraction. The contamination noted was most likely due to minor carryover on the SPE column during the lipid fractionation process. Table 1 shows the reproducibility of the spike-in standards for each QC fraction. These standards were used for quality control purposes rather than for normalization. Although minimal, the few endogenous metabolites which were present in multiple fractions in the sample data were discarded for final quantitative analysis.

2 Mouse plasma metabolomics

2.1 Nicotine metabolites in mouse plasma. We first investigated whether known cigarette smoke components, such as nicotine metabolites, could be detected as indicators of cigarette smoke exposure and to evaluate their persistence in plasma 2 months following cessation of smoking. Water soluble cigarette smoke metabolites were detected in the aqueous fraction of mouse plasma as shown in Figure 1A, adapted from Janne Hukkanen, Peyton Jacob III, and Neal L. Benowitz, Metabolism and Disposition Kinetics of Nicotine, Pharmacol Rev March 2005 57:79–115.

Nicotine itself was not detected in any of the plasma samples. This is likely due to its short half-life in plasma (2–3 hours) compared to urine (11 hours) [22] and the fact that plasma collection was performed 16–24 h following active cigarette smoke exposure. Nicotine metabolites with similarly short half-lives such as anabasine, anatabine, nornicotine, and nicotine isomethonium ion were undetectable or showed minimal elevations in plasma of mice exposed to cigarette smoke. In contrast, the levels of nicotine glucuronide paralleled smoking exposure history and were highly elevated in CS-6mo samples compared to AC-6mo samples ($p = 0.00043$), but were also elevated in CS-cessation compared to AC-6mo ($p = 0.027$). Although levels declined in the CS-cessation group compared to the CS-6mo group, this was not significant ($p = 0.083$). Interestingly, nicotine iminium ion was present in CS-4mo but was absent in the CS-6mo plasma, suggesting that with continued smoking, other routes in the nicotine metabolism pathway, such as conversion to nornicotine, may become more predominant. Nicotyrine also exhibited levels which paralleled smoking exposure with an increase in CS-6mo and CS-cessation compared to AC-6mo (p = 0.013 and p = 0.0037), with a possible decrease in the CS-cessation compared to CS-6mo group (p = 0.57). Additionally, cotinine methonium ion was undetected in AC-4mo and CS-4mo samples, but was present in CS-6mo and CS-cessation indicating that cotinine methonium ion accumulates after chronic cigarette smoke exposure and can still be detected for at least two months following smoking cessation.

Other nicotine metabolites measured were 4-oxo-4-(3-pyridyl)-butanoic acid, which was absent in half of the air controls but present in the smoking samples and 4-hydroxy-4-(3-pyridyl)-butanoic acid, which was detected in low amounts in AC-4mo but was variably elevated in the CS-4mo samples (not reaching statistical significance) and significantly elevated in CS-6mo and CS-cessation plasma (p = 0.0027 and p = 0.00069 respectively,

Table 1. Quality Control using spiked-in standards for each fraction.

Fraction	Standard	n	Average RT (min)	% CV (RT)	Average Area	% CV (area)
Aqueous	Creatinine-d3	31	0.724	0.80%	2217311	3.83%
Neutral lipid	Triglyceride-d5	31	11.299	0.07%	4837032	9.92%
	Ceramide C17	31	7.425	0.19%	12736707	7.86%
Phospholipid	15:0 PC	32	7.013	0.63%	1248929	9.32%
	17:0 PE	32	7.271	0.35%	517234	7.99%

Retention time % CVs are less than 1% and peak area % CVs are less than 10%. Aqueous fraction was analyzed using SB-C3 analytical column and neutral lipid and phospholipid fractions were analyzed using a C18 analytical column on an Agilent 6210 ESI-TOF. Data was analyzed using Agilent Mass Hunter Qualitative and Quantitative Analysis software.

compared to AC-6mo). Similarly, the 4-(3-pyridyl)-butanoic acid metabolite was elevated following prolonged in CS-6mo and CS-cessation samples ($p = 0.0017$ and $p = 0.0012$ respectively, compared to AC-6mo). These metabolites are relevant to human CS exposure, since 4-oxo-4-(3-pyridyl)-butanoic acid has been previously reported in human urine at an average concentration of 228 ng/mL [23] and both the (S) and (R) enantiomers of 4-hydroxy-4-(3-pyridyl)-butanoic acid have been reported in human urine at average concentrations of 14.1 ng/ml and 1120 ng/ml respectively [23].

In addition to nicotine metabolites, additional exogenous compounds representing other tobacco smoke metabolites were identified in mice chronically exposed to cigarette smoke (Figure 1). The identification of these compounds may inform our understanding of tobacco smoke metabolite clearance and persistence. Pyrrolidine, found naturally in the leaves of tobacco and present in cigarette smoke was significantly elevated in the CS-4mo ($p = 0.000025$ vs. AC-4mo) and in the CS-6mo group ($p = 0.022$ vs. AC-6mo). After smoking cessation, pyrrolidine levels declined in plasma compared to those in mice that continued smoking (the CS-6mo group), however this difference was not statistically significant ($p = 0.62$) suggesting a slower clearance from plasma than other metabolites. The low levels of pyrrolidine detected in the plasma of AC-4mo group may be due to its use as a flavoring ingredient, which is present in small quantities in a range of food products including animal food [24]. We also detected 3-methylindole, another component of cigarette smoke [25,26] being elevated in the CS-6mo and CS-cessation groups compared to AC-6mo ($p = 0.0044$ and $p = 0.0073$ respectively), with a non-significant decrease in CS-cessation compared to CS-6mo ($p = 0.77$).

To our knowledge, other than nicotyrine, 4-hydroxy-4-(-pyridyl)-butanoic acid, and 4-oxo-4-(3-pyridyl)-butanoic acid, biological fluid concentrations of the other seven of the cigarette smoke metabolites detected with our methodology (Figure 1) have not yet been reported in the literature. Overall, our data indicate that the majority of cigarette smoke metabolites detected in the plasma of mice exposed to smoking decreased after 2 months following cessation with the exception of 4-(3-pyridyl)-butanoic acid and cotinine methonium ion. In addition to providing insight into the systemic absorption of cigarette smoke components and their long term metabolism, the data presented support the reliability of our methodology used to characterize plasma metabolome changes in response to cigarette smoking.

2.2 Impact of cigarette smoking on endogenous plasma metabolites. When endogenous metabolites found in plasma of mice exposed for 6 months to cigarette smoking, air control, or those recovering for 2 months following 4 months of smoking (smoking cessation group) were compared, 82 significant metabolite differences were identified between at least one pair of groups. From these metabolites, 64 were initially identified (Figures 2 and 3) based on exact mass and isotope ratio, with the other 18 remaining unidentified (Table S4). While 60% of the metabolites exhibited reversible changes following smoking cessation, the remaining 40% were persistently affected, suggesting sustained pathological and/or adaptive effects of chronic smoking.

2.3 Plasma metabolites reversibly changed by chronic cigarette smoking. Upon examination of the differentially regulated metabolites among the six month control chronic smoking and smoking cessation groups, 18 compounds were significantly decreased by cigarette smoking and then had levels restored similar to controls following cessation (Figure 2A). Of these, 11 metabolites were triglycerides (TG) of which 10 belonged to the glycerolipid biochemical class of compounds, and one identified as a fatty acid ester. In addition to these metabolites, 19 additional compounds were significantly increased by smoking but decreased to air control levels following cessation (Figure 2B); 5 of these were TGs of which all were glycerolipids, 4 were glycerophospholipids, and 2 were sphingolipids. Little is known of the glycerolipid involvement in cigarette smoke-induced pathology, but sphingolipids have been linked to COPD (emphysema). Of these, ceramides in particular have been reportedly up-regulated in the lung and lung cells in response to cigarette smoke [27–29]. Their abundance in plasma of smokers or cigarette smoke-exposed animals has not been reported yet. We noted that, of the differentially regulated sphingolipids, ceramide (d18:1/20:0) and galabiosylceramide (d18:1/25:0) increased with smoking. Interestingly, although their levels decreased with smoking cessation, they remained elevated when compared to air control levels. In addition, among the other lipids differentially regulated by smoking in plasma, we detected LysoPC(18:0), which is known to play a role in lipid signaling, smooth muscle contraction, and is associated with atherosclerotic and inflammatory lesions [30]. Also detected was PC(38:3) which was elevated in smokers compared to both air control and CS-cessation groups. Xu et al [16] also reported an elevation of PC(38:3) in current smokers compared to former smokers and never smokers for their targeted analysis of PC's in serum in a human cohort. PC's are involved in cell signaling and are direct substrates of sphingomyelin synthesis which transfer the choline-phosphate head group to a ceramide lipid anchor [31].

2.4 Plasma metabolites persistently changed following smoking cessation. Figure 3 illustrates the metabolites which remained persistently changed following cigarette smoke exposure, despite smoking cessation for 2 months. Five metabolites, including 3 amino acid derivatives and 2 glycerophospholipids,

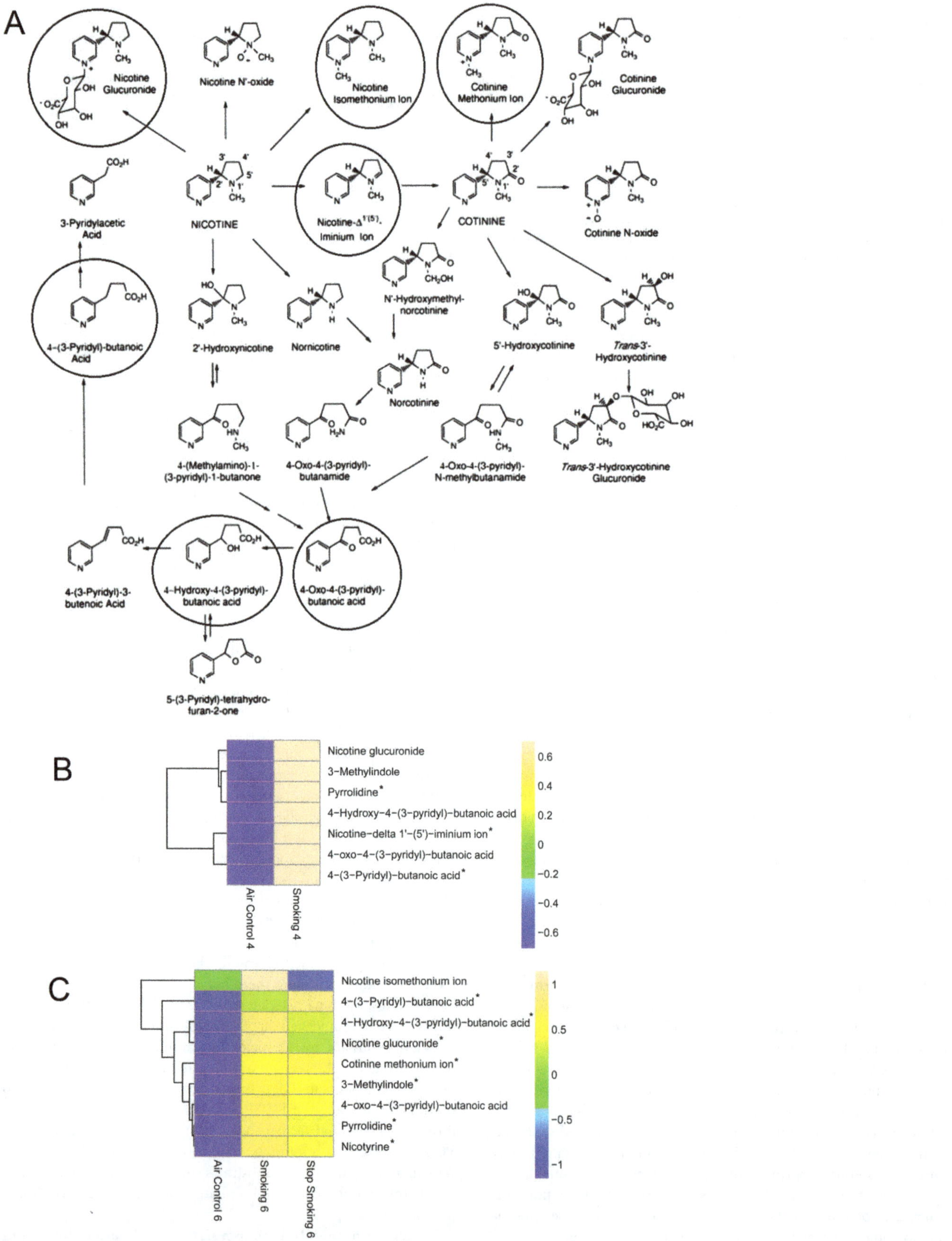

Figure 1. (A) Nicotine pathway and heat maps of CS metabolites in (B) four month and (C) six month comparisons. CS = cigarette smoke. Pathway diagram reprinted with permission from Hukkanen et al. Circled compounds represent the metabolites identified in the plasma of mouse samples in the current study. For each heat map, blue represents a decrease in mean metabolite abundance, and yellow/beige represents an

increase in mean metabolite abundance. For example, nicotine glucuronide is increased in smoking in both the 4- and 6- month smoking mice. Samples were analyzed on an Agilent 6410 ESI-TOF in positive ionization mode, data was processed using Mass Profiler Professional, and quantitative data was obtained using Mass Hunter Quantitative analysis software. Tentative identification was performed using ID Browser within the Mass Profiler Professional software. ID Browser in-house database is comprised of Metlin, Lipid Maps and HMDB. * indicates p-value≤0.05 between the air control and cigarette smoking groups. Differences between other nicotine pathway metabolites are also shown but did not reach statistical significance.

exhibited continued increase in abundance (Figure 3A) despite smoking cessation. Twenty-two metabolites remained decreased despite smoking cessation (Figure 3B), including 3 glycerophospholipids, and 15 glycerolipids. Unlike the majority of TG species listed in Figure 2A which returned to normal levels following smoking cessation, several TG species (detailed in Figure 3B) were found to be persistently decreased in plasma of mice removed from smoking exposure. Six of the ten TGs reversibly decreased were long-chain TGs of 20 carbon chain length while six out of nine TGs persistently decreased were long chain TGs of 18 carbon chain length. It should be noted that the study was limited to 2 months of smoking cessation and that some or all of these compounds may revert to air control levels after longer periods of smoking cessation.

2.5 Unannotated Metabolites. Eighteen additional metabolites were statistically significant and differentially regulated in the 6 month comparison among the air control, smoking and smoking cessation mice. These were present in the aqueous and neutral fractions. Four metabolites were reversibly decreased with smoking, eight were reversibly increased, three were persistently increased, and three were persistently decreased with smoking. These compounds were not identified through database searching. Additional data (m/z, fraction, retention time and regulation) is provided in Table S4.

3 Pathway analysis

Metabolites which showed significant differences and could be tentatively identified at MSI level 2 [21], were grouped based on their distinct chemical classes (Table S3). The recurring classes –

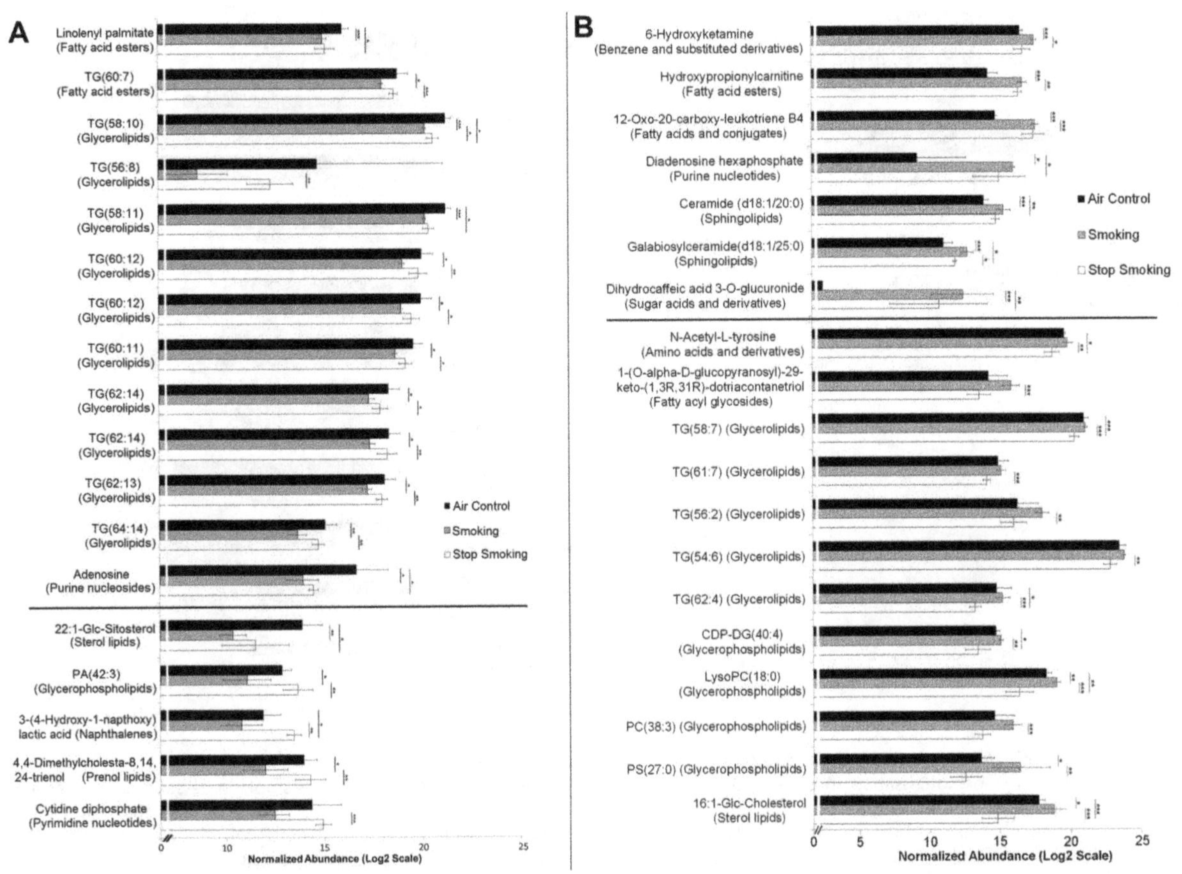

Figure 2. Metabolites which were (A) reversibly decreased and (B) reversibly increased with smoking. In panel A (top), differentially regulated metabolites were higher in air controls, decreased with smoking, and increased toward air control levels following smoking cessation. In panel A (bottom), differentially regulated metabolites were higher in air controls, decreased with smoking, and surpassed air control levels following smoking cessation. In panel B (top) differentially regulated metabolites were lower in air controls, increased with smoking, and decreased following smoking cessation. In panel B (bottom), differentially regulated metabolites were lower in air controls, increased with smoking, and decreased beyond air control levels following smoking cessation. Samples and data were analyzed as described in the methods section. TG = triglyceride, CDP = cytidine-diphosphate, DG = diglyceride, PC = phosphatidylcholine, PS = phosphatidylserine, TG = triglyceride, PA = phosphatidic acid. Fold change ≥1.5; p-value≤0.05, x-axis = Log2 normalized abundance scale; Error bars represent 95% confidence; Significance values *≤0.05, **≤0.01, ***≤0.001.

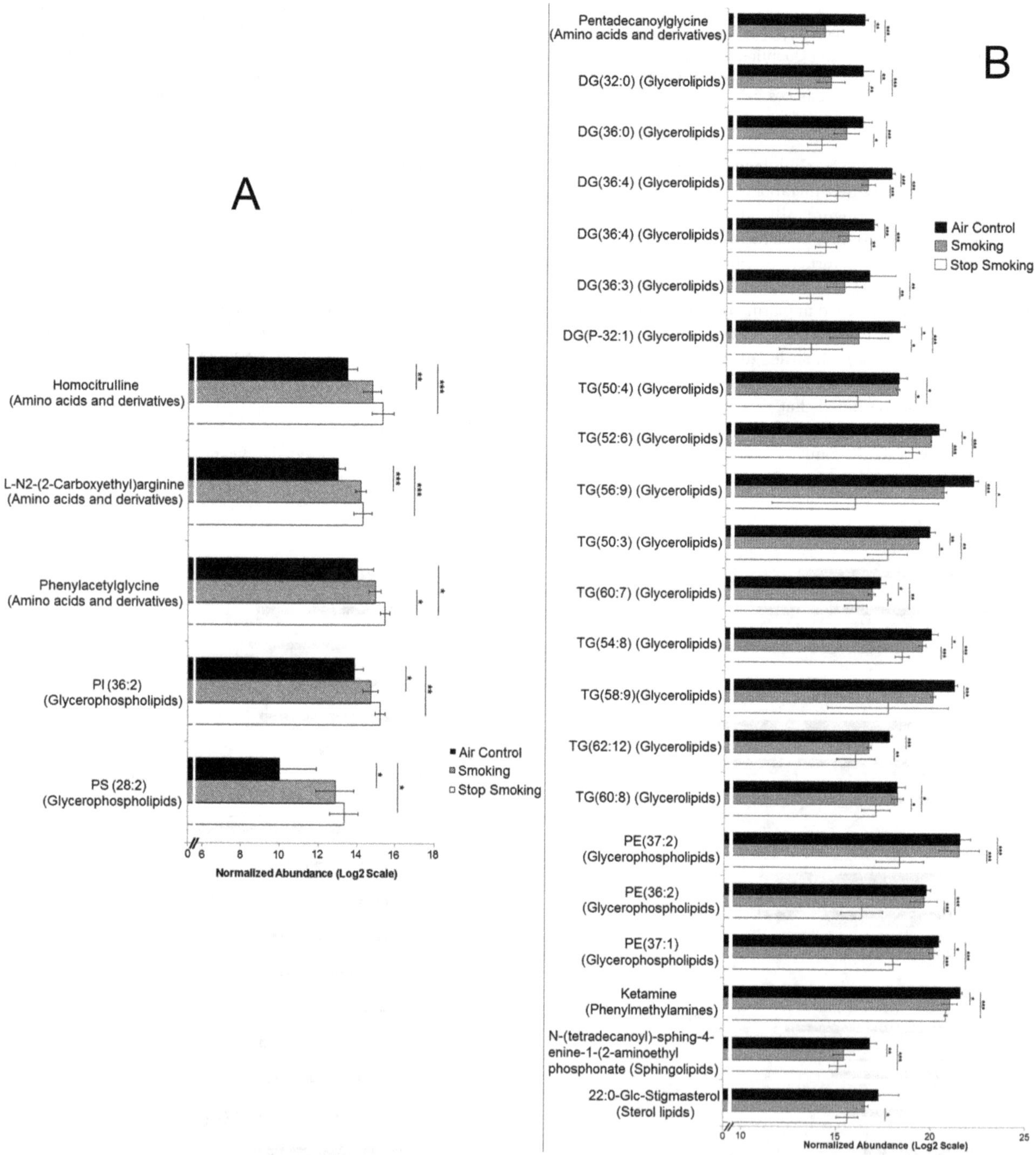

Figure 3. Metabolites which (A) persistently increased and (B) persistently decreased with smoking. In panel A, these metabolites continued increasing even after smoking cessation. In panel B, these metabolites continued decreasing even after smoking cessation. Samples and data were analyzed as described in the methods section. ID Browser in-house database is comprised of Metlin, Lipid Maps and HMDB. PIP = phosphatidylinositol phosphate, PS = phosphatidylserine, TG = triglyceride, DG = diglyceride, PE = phosphatidylethanolamine. Fold change ≥1.5; *p*-value≤0.05, x-axis = Log2 normalized abundance scale; Error bars represent 95% confidence; Significance values *≤0.05, **≤0.01, ***≤0.001.

purines, amino acids, steroids, fatty acid esters, and prenol lipids, and purines - were investigated to determine if distinct metabolic pathway perturbations can be gauged from alterations of plasma metabolites in response to smoking and/or smoking cessation.

3.1 Purine metabolism. Of the nine purine metabolites significantly perturbed by cigarette smoke exposure ($p \leq 0.05$, fold change ≥1.5) in Figure 4A, five were directly embedded within the purine metabolism pathway (Figure 4B).

Compared to air control exposed groups, cigarette smoke exposure led to increased plasma adenosine monophosphate (AMP) after 4 months (p = 0.046 CS-4mo vs. AC-4mo) and decreased adenosine (p = 0.048 CS-cessation vs. AC-6mo; p = 0.019 CS-6mo vs. AC-6mo). CS exposure also elevated

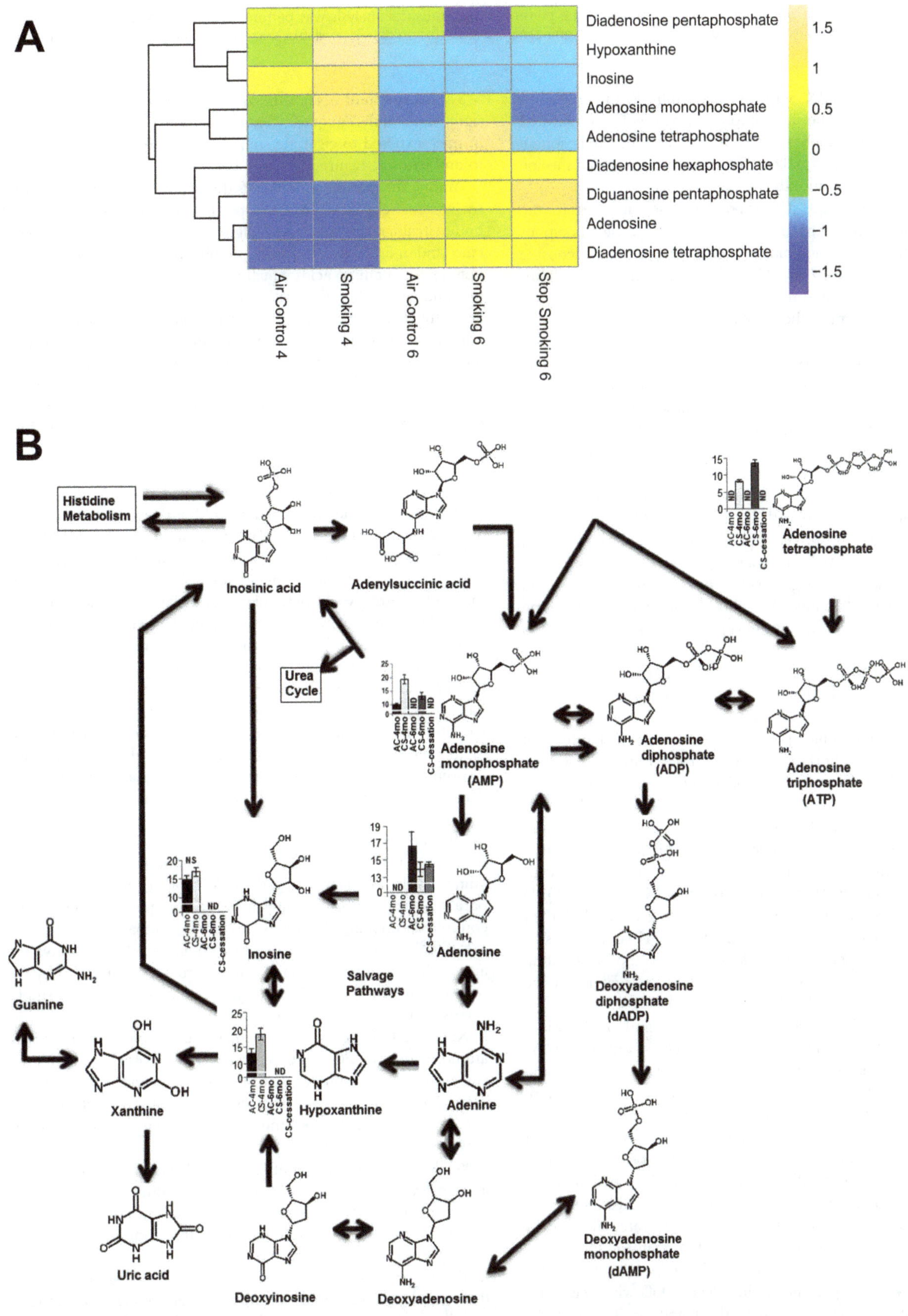

Figure 4. Heat map of (A) purines and (B) purine pathway hits. The mean abundance levels for each of the differentially regulated metabolites detected is shown in the heat map in A. Blue represents a decrease in mean metabolite abundance, and yellow/beige represents an increase in mean metabolite abundance. In panel B, the compounds with indicated abundance levels represent the differentially expressed

metabolites identified in the purine metabolism pathway in the current study. Statistical analysis was performed using Mass Profiler Professional software (Agilent) with *p*-value cutoff ≤0.05, NS indicates not significant, ND indicates no data is available, and error bars represent 95% confidence.

hypoxanthine (p = 0.042 CS-4mo vs. AC-4mo). With continuous smoking (CS-6mo), adenosine tetraphosphate was found elevated (p = 0.0028 CS-6mo vs. CS-4mo) while adenosine monophosphate (AMP) was decreased (p = 0.022 CS-6mo vs. CS4-mo) and inosine was not present after 6 months.

Interestingly, prolonged CS exposure (6mo) also led to the elevations of plasma diguanosine- and diadenosine-polyphosphates, in particular diguanosine pentaphosphate, diadenosine tetraphosphate (p = 0.048 vs. AC-6mo) and diadenosine hexaphosphate (p = 0.050 vs. AC-6mo). Of note, diadenosine pentaphosphate was also present in the plasma of CS-4mo but could not be detected in the CS-6mo group.

The fate and role of purine metabolism in response to cigarette smoking in general, and in COPD in particular remains controversial, perhaps in part because not all studies have followed the same experimental design, but instead covered a range of biological fluids and used multiple detection techniques to study a variety of health conditions. When adenosine was measured in exhaled breath condensate (EBC) its levels, and those of AMP were found to be elevated with increasing COPD severity [32]. Similar to EBC results, Driver et al [33] detected increased levels of adenosine in the BALF of smokers compared to non-smokers, and suggested that their origin may be from plasma extravasation due to epithelial cell injury. In contrast, in sputum, adenosine levels were reportedly lower in smokers with COPD compared to asymptomatic smokers [34], which is a similar trend noted in the murine plasma in our experiments. The short half-life of adenosine (including in plasma) may explain differences in these reports. This underscores the importance of a more global assessment of purine metabolism, which could provide a better understanding of changes induced by short- and long-term exposures to cigarette smoke. Published investigations of other metabolites in this pathway, such as AMP and ATP, detected decreased AMP levels in BALF of COPD smokers compared to control smokers and COPD non-smokers [35] and increased ATP levels in COPD smokers compared to non-smokers [36], whereas no significant differences in ATP levels were measured in EBC among COPD subjects, smokers, and non-smokers [37]. Using a metabolomics approach, we noted significant alterations of AMP and adenosine tetraphosphate in response to smoking, which could be resulting from direct hydrolysis of AMP, ADP, and ATP by cigarette smoke compounds, as suggested by Togna et al [38].

The relevance of changes in diguanosine- and diadenosine-polyphosphates by cigarette smoking is unclear, but it may be important in cardiovascular responses in smokers, since plasma diguanosine pentaphosphate may play a role in blood pressure regulation [39], whereas diadenosine -tetraphosphate, -pentaphosphate, and -hexaphosphate (originally identified in human myocardium [40]) have been associated with eosinophil-related inflammatory and allergic disease and with atherogenesis [24].

While a thorough dissection of the purine metabolism is beyond the scope of our study, our data has to be interpreted in the light that plasma levels of metabolites may reflect a sum of metabolite changes of multiple organs and tissues affected by cigarette smoke. To our knowledge plasma purine levels following cigarette smoking have not been reported in the literature. These results provide novel information linking smoking to perturbed purine metabolism and further studies are being designed to more fully understand their roles in the lung.

3.2 Amino acid metabolism. Several amino acids exhibited significantly different (p≤0.05 and ≥1.5 fold change) plasma levels in mice exposed to cigarette smoking compared to those exposed to ambient air (Figure 5).

Among the plasma amino acids that were significantly increased by chronic cigarette smoke exposure, we putatively identified homocitrulline and phenylacetylglycine, while pentadecanoylglycine and n-acetyltyrosine were significantly decreased. We also noted several amino acids which were found significantly changed in abundance after 6 months when compared to 4 months of cigarette smoke exposure. These were phenylalanine, n-acetylasparagine, n-succinyl-2-amino-6-ketopimelate, tyrosine methylester, ornithine, hexanoylglycine, prenyl-L-cysteine, and sarcosine. In addition histidine and tetracosanoylglycine were present in CS-6mo but were absent or possibly at undetectable concentrations in CS-4mo. N-undecanoylglycine and gamma glutamyl ornithine however were present in CS-4mo but absent in CS-6mo. Tetracosanoylglycine, hexanoylglycine, n-undecanoylglycine, and pentadecanoylglycine are all minor metabolites of fatty acids, while homocitrulline and ornithine are both part of the urea cycle. Therefore, abnormal accumulations of these metabolites during cigarette smoke exposure may indicate marked disruptions not only in the amino acid metabolism, but also in interrelated metabolic pathways, in particular that of fatty acid metabolism.

In a 2012 targeted metabolomics assay, Ubhi et al [41] reported perturbations in amino acid metabolism among patients with COPD, emphysema and cachexia. Serum was analyzed from former smokers, never smokers, COPD Gold stage IV subjects, patients with and without emphysema, and patients with and without cachexia. Interestingly, three of the reported abnormal metabolites reported in this study - sarcosine, phenylalanine, and histidine, overlap with those found in the mouse plasma in our study. The decrease in sarcosine levels in emphysema and cachexia patients compared to controls, was paralleled by a significant decrease in sarcosine levels with continued smoking over time in mouse plasma (p = 0.031). The increased phenylalanine levels in cachexia patients compared to controls, was paralleled by a significant increase in phenylalanine with continued smoking in mouse plasma compared to controls (p = 0.027). Lastly, the increase in histidine levels in emphysema and cachexia subjects compared to controls was paralleled by the presence of histidine in plasma of mice exposed to cigarette smoke versus absence of this amino acid in control mice.

Xu et al [16] performed a targeted metabolomics analysis of amino acids and PC's and reported an increase in ornithine in current smokers compared to former smokers and never smokers. This is consistent with our findings in our mouse model where we detected an increase in ornithine in the CS-6mo compared to the CS-4mo groups (p = 0.010).

While the biological significance of elevation in phenylacetylglycine levels in the CS-cessation plasma compared to AC-6mo group (p = 0.019) remains unclear, it is interesting that elevations of this metabolite was also reported in the urine of heart failure patients compared to healthy controls [42]. In addition to pointing to disruption in these metabolic pathways by cigarette smoking, these results indicate that the mouse model of cigarette smoking may be used to study in more depth the role of relevant metabolic pathways in COPD.

3.3 Steroid Metabolism. We identified six significant steroid metabolites (Figure 6), four of which were upregulated in either the

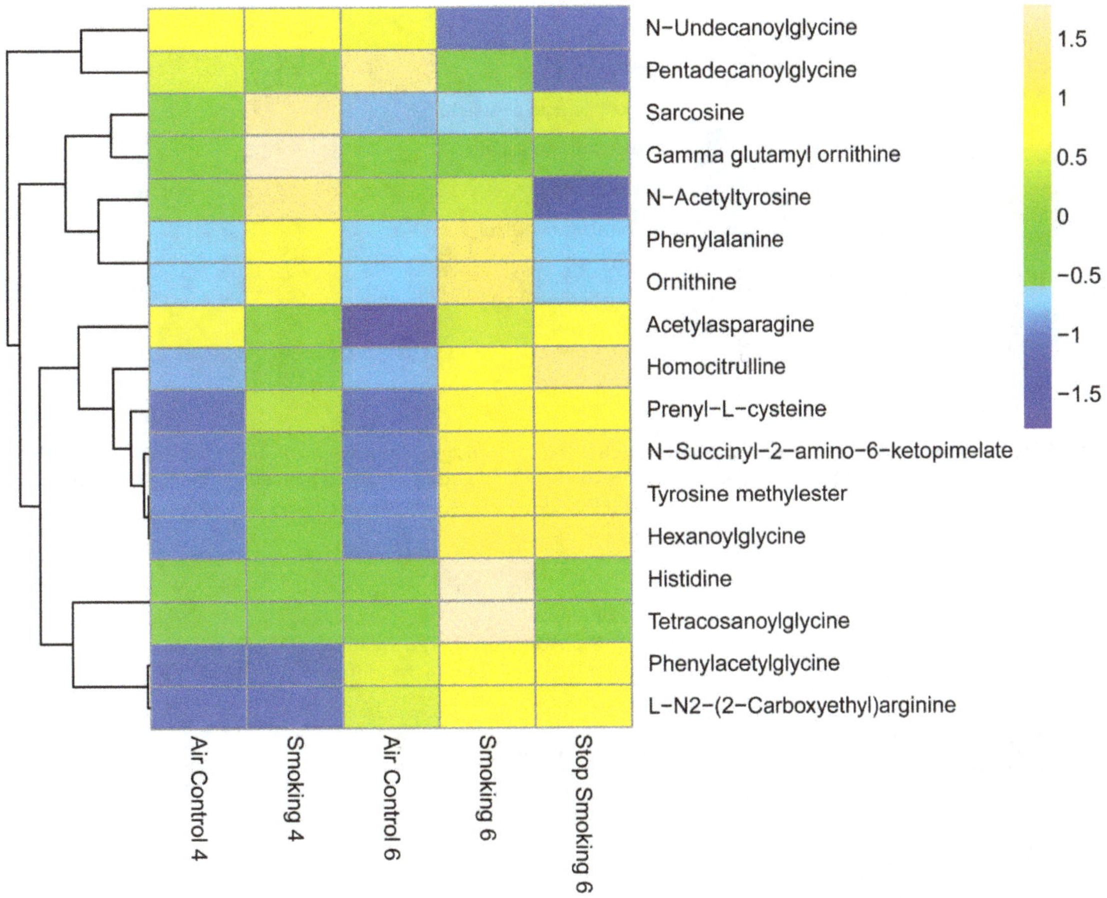

Figure 5. Heat map of differentially regulated amino acids and derivatives. Statistical analysis was performed using Mass Profiler Professional software (Agilent) with p-value cutoff ≤ 0.05. The mean abundance levels for each of the differentially regulated metabolites detected is shown. Blue represents a decrease in mean metabolite abundance, and yellow/beige represents an increase in mean metabolite abundance.

CS-cessation compared to AC-6mo group or higher in CS-6mo compared to CS-4mo. Three of the six steroids (dehydroisoandrosterone 3-glucuronide, CE(22:4), taurocholic acid 3-sulfate) play a role in bile biosynthesis and secretion. One metabolite, pregnanetriol, was decreased following smoking cessation compared to the air controls. To our knowledge, none of the identified steroids have been reported in the literature in association with cigarette smoking; however, targeted studies have been performed to determine the relationship between other steroids and smoking, with an overall increase in steroid levels observed in smokers compared to non-smokers [43,44]. English et al [45] reported increased levels of testosterone in the serum of smokers compared to non-smokers, but found no difference in 17-estradiol between groups. Kapoor and Jones examined the effects of smoking on hormonal levels in humans and reported increased levels of adrenal hormones and parathyroid hormones in smoking groups compared to smoking cessation groups [46]. They also reported that a majority of pituitary hormones were increased in the smoking compared to smoking cessation groups, except for insulin-like growth factor which had decreased levels in smokers. Field et al [43] reported increased serum levels of adrenal steroids in male smokers compared to non-smokers. Our results therefore are in agreement with the published literature and suggest that smoking perturbs steroid hormone levels and significantly alters segments of the steroid metabolism pathway.

3.4 Fatty acid esters and prenol lipids. Six out of the ten fatty acid esters (Figure 7A) identified in the mouse plasma were significantly elevated in the CS-6mo compared to air control group, or elevated in the CS-6mo compared to the CS-4mo. Three of those upregulated in CS-6mo compared to CS-4mo were triglycerides. Two of the fatty acid esters that were up-regulated in the CS-6mo group compared to the AC-6mo group were carnitines. Carnitines are synthesized from the amino acids methionine and lysine [47,48], and are needed for transport of fatty acids during lipid breakdown for energy production [48], demonstrating the interplay among amino acids, fatty acids, and lipids in metabolism. Figure 8 illustrates the complexity of the regulation of fatty acid levels, which depend on other metabolite groups such as acetyl-CoA and lipids, in addition to rates of synthesis and degradation. Our data suggests that a direct link exists between fatty acid esters metabolism and cigarette smoke exposure, with fatty acids and sterol lipids both increased following smoking. However, the role of fatty acid esters accumulation in response to cigarette smoke remains unclear, especially in light of reports of anti-inflammatory protective effects of fatty acids in COPD [49] as opposed to pro-inflammatory effects of fatty acids in asthma [50].

Prenol lipids (Figure 7B) were predominantly down-regulated by cigarette smoke exposure. It is possible that the equilibrium between acetyl-CoA and the mevalonate pathway becomes unstable and a shift occurs either toward sterol lipid and steroid

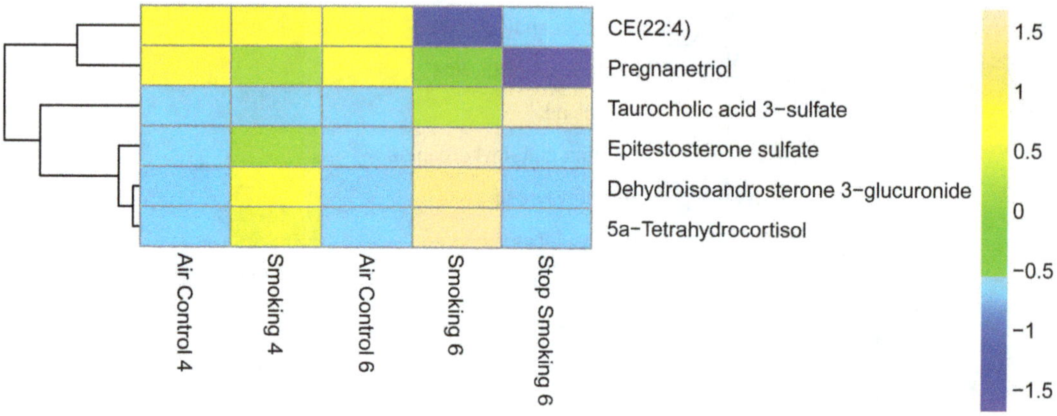

Figure 6. Heat map of differentially regulated steroids and derivatives. Statistical analysis was performed using Mass Profiler Professional software (Agilent) with *p*-value cutoff ≤0.05. The mean abundance levels for each of the differentially regulated metabolites detected is shown. Blue represents a decrease in mean metabolite abundance, and yellow/beige represents an increase in mean metabolite abundance.

metabolism, or fatty acid metabolism where we observed increased levels due to smoking (Figure 8). To our knowledge, alternations of prenol lipid plasma concentrations in response to cigarette smoking have not been reported in the literature and may provide a new target for investigation of analysis of smoking related conditions.

3.5 Additional significant metabolites. Additional metabolites were found to be differentially regulated; however, these

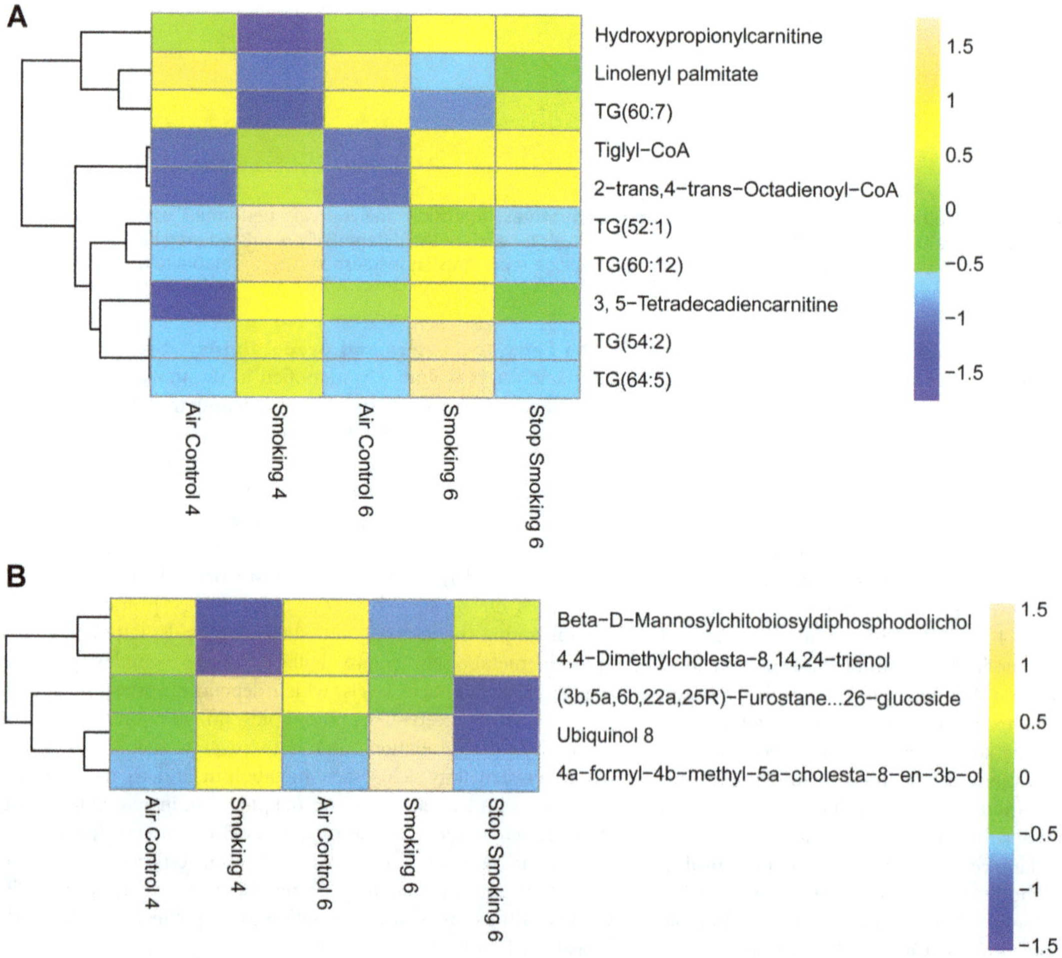

Figure 7. Heat map of differentially regulated (A) fatty acids and (B) prenol lipids. Statistical analysis was performed using Mass Profiler Professional software (Agilent) with *p*-value cutoff ≤0.05. The mean abundance levels for each of the differentially regulated metabolites detected is shown. Blue represents a decrease in mean metabolite abundance, and yellow/beige represents an increase in mean metabolite abundance.

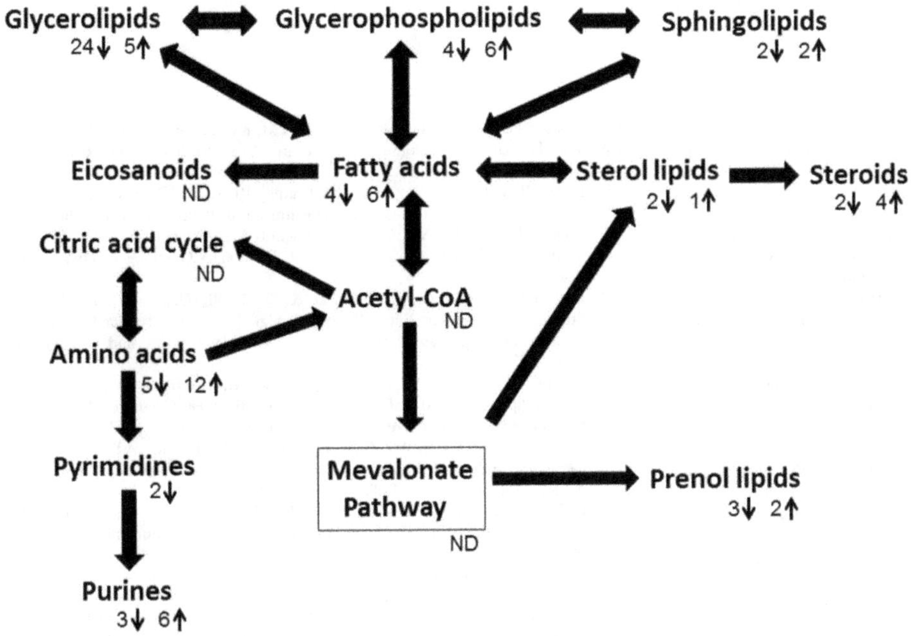

Figure 8. Inter-relation of pathways. Biological relationships among chemical classes of compounds showing the regulation of one group of metabolites and its effects on other biological classes down- or up-stream. Pathway was adapted from KEGG, Lipid Maps, and SMPDB. Metabolites within this pathway passed p-value≤0.05 and fold change ≥1.5 filters. ↓ indicates the number of differentially regulated metabolites which decreased due to smoking, ↑ indicates the number of differentially regulated metabolites which increased due to smoking for a particular chemical class of compounds, [ND]no data was available for these compounds in this dataset.

metabolites are not included in this discussion for several reasons. For example, we did not include compounds that we could not identify through database searching. In addition, some compounds were "orphan" compounds: i.e. the only one present within a specific chemical class. Conversely, the compound may have been annotated as a small peptide and additional analysis was not possible. Finally, because our identifications are tentative, we had increased confidence when multiple compounds mapped to the same pathway. Further information related to these compounds is available at the end of Table S1.

Conclusion

Chronic cigarette smoke exposure increased plasma levels of glycerophospholipids, amino acids, fatty acid esters, purines, and steroids, and decreased prenol lipid, sterol lipid and glycerolipid levels. Sixty percent of the differentially regulated plasma metabolites reversibly changed following smoking cessation while 40% were persistently altered. Our results highlight profound and sustained metabolic changes in plasma, which may reflect systemic changes induced by smoking in various organs. In addition to the 144 annotated metabolites discussed, an additional seventy-eight differentially regulated metabolites were detected, but remain unannotated when matched against MS databases for accurate mass (Table S4). Refinement in the confirmation of metabolite identification following metabolomics detection will provide a new approach to identify unsuspected pathogenetic pathways and biomarkers associated with COPD and its systemic comorbidities. These, in turn can pave the way for identifying molecular targets which can be used to develop novel therapeutics for smoke-induced health conditions.

Supporting Information

Figure S1 Mean linear intercepts (MLI). MLI in DBA2/J mice exposed to ambient air control (AC) or cigarette smoke (CS), as detailed in the methods section, for 4 months (Mean +SEM; $p < 0.05$; Student's t test; n = 5 AC and n = 4 CS).

Table S1 Metabolite Annotations. Annotated metabolites which passed statistical and fold change analyses in the smoking comparisons in mouse plasma.

Table S2 Mass Spectra of Annotated Metabolites. Selected metabolites to demonstrate the experimental vs theoretical isotopic ratios following database searches.

Table S3 Detailed Metabolite Comparisons for Compound Classes.

Table S4 Unannotated Metabolites. Metabolites which passed statistical and fold change analysis but remained unidentified based on MS library searches.

Acknowledgments

We acknowledge Mary Van Demark and Kelly S. Schweitzer, PhD for assistance related to animal experiments and Katerina Kechris, PhD for assistance in statistical analysis.

Author Contributions

Conceived and designed the experiments: IP NR MA RR RB. Performed the experiments: SM RR MA MJJ. Analyzed the data: CICQ. Contributed reagents/materials/analysis tools: IP NR RR. Wrote the paper: CICQ NR IP RB. Provided assistance in statistical analysis: GH.

References

1. Atkinson AJ, Magnuson WG, Colburn WA, DeGruttola VG, DeMets DL, et al. (2001) Biomarkers and Surrogate Endpoints: Preferred Definitions and Conceptual Framework. Clinical Pharmacology & Therapeutics 69: 89–95.
2. Vasan RS (2006) Biomarkers of Cardiovascular Disease: Molecular Basis and Practical Considerations. Circulation 113: 2335–2362.
3. M'Koma AE, Blum DL, Norris JL, Koyama T, Billheimer D, et al. (2007) Detection of pre-neoplastic and neoplastic prostate disease by MALDI profiling of urine. Biochemical and Biophysical Research Communications 353: 829–834.
4. Dong J, Cai X, Zhao L, Xue X, Zou L, et al. (2010) Lysophosphatidylcholine profiling of plasma: discrimination of isomers and discovery of lung cancer biomarkers. Metabolomics 6: 478–488.
5. Barr J, Alonso C, Vázquez-Chantada M, Pérez-Cormenzana M, Mayo R, et al. (2010) Liquid chromatography-mass spectrometry-based parallel metabolic profiling of human and mouse model serum reveals putative biomarkers associated with the progression of nonalcoholic fatty liver disease. Journal of Proteome Research 9: 4501–4512.
6. Barnes PJ (2000) Chronic Obstructive Pulmonary Disease. The New England Journal of Medicine 343: 269–280.
7. Herbst RS, Heymach JV, Lippman SM (2008) Molecular Origins of Cancer: Lung Cancer. New England Journal of Medicine 359: 1367–1380.
8. Xie F, Yu J, Wang S, Zhao G, Xia Q, et al. (2013) Rapid and simultaneous analysis of ten aromatic amines in mainstream cigarette smoke by liquid chromatography/electrospray ionization tandem mass spectrometry under ISO and "Health Canada intensive" machine smoking regimens. Talanta 115: 435–441.
9. Saha S, Mistri R, Ray BC (2013) A rapid and selective method for simultaneous determination of six toxic phenolic compounds in mainstream cigarette smoke using single-drop microextraction followed by liquid chromatography-tandem mass spectrometry. Analytical and Bioanalytical Chemistry 405: 9265–9272.
10. Aragón M, Marcé RM, Borrull F (2013) Determination of N-nitrosamines and nicotine in air particulate matter samples by pressurised liquid extraction and gas chromatography-ion trap tandem mass spectrometry. Talanta 115: 896–901.
11. Murphy SE, Wickham KM, Lindgren BR, Spector LG, Joseph A (2013) Cotinine and trans 3′-hydroxycotinine in dried blood spots as biomarkers of tobacco exposure and nicotine metabolism. Journal of Exposure Science & Environmental Epidemiology 23: 513–518.
12. Jacob P 3rd, Yu L, Duan M, Ramos L, Yturralde O, et al. (2012) Determination of the nicotine metabolites cotinine and trans-3′-hydroxycotinine in biologic fluids of smokers and non-smokers using liquid chromatography–tandem mass spectrometry: Biomarkers for tobacco smoke exposure and for phenotyping cytochrome P450 2A6 activity. Journal of Chromatography B 879: 267–276.
13. Hu CW, Hsu YW, Chen JL, Tam LM, Chao MR (2014) Direct analysis of tobacco-specific nitrosamine NNK and its metabolite NNAL in human urine by LC-MS/MS: evidence of linkage to methylated DNA lesions. Analytical Toxicology 88: 291–299.
14. Wagner R, Feth F, Wagner KG (1986) The regulation of enzyme activities of the nicotine pathway in tobacco. Physiologia Plantarum 68: 667–672.
15. Shoji T, Kajikawa M, Hashimoto T (2010) Clustered transcription factor genes regulate nicotine biosynthesis in tobacco. Plant Cell 22: 3390–3409.
16. Xu T, Holzapfel C, Dong X, Bader E, Yu Z, et al. (2013) Effects of smoking and smoking cessation on human serum metabolite profile: results from the KORA cohort study. BMC Medicine 11: 14 pages.
17. Yang Y, Cruickshank C, Armstrong M, Mahaffey S, Reisdorph R, et al. (2013) New sample preparation approach for mass spectrometry-based profiling of plasma results in improved coverage of metabolome. Journal of Chromatography A 1300: 217–226.
18. Schweitzer KS, Johnstone BH, Garrison J, Rush NI, Cooper S, et al. (2011) Adipose Stem Cell Treatment in Mice Attenuates Lung and Systemic Injury Induced by Cigarette Smoking. American Journal of Respiratory and Critical Care Medicine 183: 215–225.
19. Bartalesi B, Cavarra E, Fineschi S, Lucattelli M, Lunghi B, et al. (2005) Different lung responses to cigarette smoke in two strains of mice sensitive to oxidants. The European respiratory journal 25: 15–22.
20. Hughes G, Cruickshank-Quinn C, Reisdorph R, Lutz S, Petrache I, et al. (2014) MSPrep–Summarization, normalization and diagnostics for processing of mass spectrometry–based metabolomic data. Bioinformatics 30: 133–134.
21. Sumner LW, Amberg A, Barrett D, Beger R, Beale MH, et al. (2007) Proposed Minimum Reporting Standards for Chemical Analysis: Chemical Analysis Working Group (CAWG) Metabolomics Standards Initiative (MSI). Metabolomics Society.
22. Jacob P 3rd, Yu L, Shulgin AT, Benowitz NL (1999) Minor Tobacco Alkaloids as Biomarkers for Tobacco Use: Comparison of Users of Cigarettes, Smokeless Tobacco, Cigars, and Pipes. American Journal of Public Health 89: 731–736.
23. Hecht SS, Hatsukami DK, Bonilla LE, Hochalter JB (1999) Quantitation of 4-Oxo-4-(3-pyridyl) butanoic Acid and Enantiomers of 4-Hydroxy-4-(3-pyridyl) butanoic Acid in Human Urine: A Substantial Pathway of Nicotine Metabolism. Chemical Research in Toxicology 12: 172–179.
24. Wishart DS, Jewison T, Guo AC, Wilson M, Knox C, et al. (2013) HMDB 3.0–The Human Metabolome Database in 2013. Nucleic Acids Research 41 (Database issue): D801–807.
25. Huang TW, Carlson JR, Bray TM, Bradley BJ (1977) 3-Methylindole-Induced Pulmonary Injury in Goats. American Journal of Pathology 87: 647–666.
26. Weems JM, Cutler NS, Moore C, Nichols WK, Martin D, et al. (2009) 3-Methylindole is Mutagenic and a Possible Pulmonary Carcinogen. Toxicological Sciences 112: 59–67.
27. Diab KJ, Adamowicz JJ, Kamocki K, Rush NI, Garrison J, et al. (2010) Stimulation of Sphingosine 1-Phosphate Signaling as an Alveolar Cell Survival Strategy in Emphysema. American Journal of Respiratory and Critical Care Medicine 181: 344–352.
28. Petrusca DN, Gu Y, Adamowicz JJ, Rush NI, Hubbard WC, et al. (2010) Sphingolipid-mediated Inhibition of Apoptotic Cell Clearance by Alveolar Macrophages. Journal of Biological Chemistry 285: 40322–40332.
29. Petrache I, Natarajan V, Zhen L, Medler TR, Richter AT, et al. (2005) Ceramide upregulation causes pulmonary cell apoptosis and emphysema-like disease in mice. Nature Medicine 11: 491–498.
30. Golfman LS, Haughey NJ, Wong JT, Jiang JY, Lee D, et al. (1999) Lysophosphatidylcholine induces arachidonic acid release and calcium overload in cardiac myoblastic H9c2 cells. Journal of Lipid Reseacrch 40: 1818–1826.
31. Gibellini F, Smith TK (2010) The Kennedy Pathway–De Novo Synthesis of Phosphatidylethanolamine and Phosphatidylcholine. IUBMB life 62: 414–428.
32. Esther CR Jr, Lazaar AL, Bordonali E, Qaqish B, Boucher RC (2011) Elevated Airway Purines in COPD. Chest 140: 954–960.
33. Driver AG, Kukoly CA, Ali S, Mustafa J (1993) Adenosine in Bronchoalveolar Lavage Fluid in Asthma. American Review of Respiratory Disease 148: 91–97.
34. Versluis M, Hacken Nt, Postma D, Barroso B, Rutgers B, et al. (2009) Adenosine receptors in COPD and asymptomatic smokers: effects of smoking cessation. Virchows Arch: an international journal of pathology 454: 273–281.
35. Oosterhoff Y, Jong JWD, Jansen MAM, Koëter GH, Postma DS (1993) Airway Responsiveness to Adenosine 5′-Monophosphate in Chronic Obstructive Pulmonary Disease Is Determined by Smoking. American Review of Respiratory Disease 147: 553–558.
36. Lommatzsch M, Cicko S, Müller T, Lucattelli M, Bratke K, et al. (2010) Extracellular Adenosine Triphosphate and Chronic Obstructive Pulmonary Disease. American Journal of Respiratory and Critical Care Medicine 181: 928–934.
37. Lázár Z, Huszár É, Kullmann T, Barta I, Antus B, et al. (2008) Adenosine triphosphate in exhaled breath condensate of healthy subjects and patients with chronic obstructive pulmonary disease. Inflammation Research 57: 367–373.
38. Togna AR, Latina V, Orlando R, Togna GI (2008) Cigarette smoke inhibits adenine nucleotide hydrolysis by human platelets. Platelets 19: 537–542.
39. Tölle M, Giebing G, Tietge UJW, Jankowski J, Jankowski V, et al. (2006) Diguanosine pentaphosphate: an endogenous activator of Rho-kinase possibly involved in blood pressure regulation. Journal of Hypertension 24: 1991–2000.
40. Luo J, Jankowski V, Güngär N, Neumann J, Schmitz W, et al. (2004) Endogenous diadenosine tetraphosphate, diadenosine pentaphosphate, and diadenosine hexaphosphate in human myocardial tissue. Hypertension 43: 1055–1059.
41. Ubhi BK, Cheng KK, Dong J, Janowitz T, Jodrell D, et al. (2012) Targeted metabolomics identifies perturbations in amino acid metabolism that sub-classify patients with COPD. Molecular BioSystems 8: 3125–3133.
42. Kang SM, Park JC, Shin MJ, Lee H, Oh J, et al. (2011) 1H nuclear magnetic resonance based metabolic urinary profiling of patients with ischemic heart failure. Clinical Biochemistry 44: 293–299.
43. Field AE, Colditz GA, Willett WC, Longcope C, McKinlay JB (1994) The relation of smoking, age, relative weight, and dietary intake to serum adrenal steroids, sex hormones, and sex hormone-binding globulin in middle-aged men. Journal of Clinical Endocrinology and Metabolism 79: 1310–1316.
44. Dušková M, Hruškovičová H, Simůnková K, L. Stárka AP (2013) The effects of smoking on steroid metabolism and fetal programming. Journal of Steroid Biochemistry and Molecular Biology.
45. English KM, Pugh PJ, Parry H, Scutt NE, Channer KS, et al. (2001) Effect of cigarette smoking on levels of bioavailable testosterone in healthy men. Clinical Science 100: 661–665.
46. Kapoor D, Jones TH (2005) Smoking and hormones in health and endocrine disorders. European Journal of Endocrinology 152: 491–499.
47. Steiber A, Kerner J, Hoppel CL (2004) Carnitine: a nutritional, biosynthetic, and functional perspective. Molecular Aspects of Medicine 25: 455–473.
48. Virmani A, Binienda Z (2004) Role of carnitine esters in brain neuropathology. Molecular Aspects of Medicine 25: 533–549.
49. Matsuyama W, Mitsuyama H, Watanabe M, Oonakahara K, Higashimoto I, et al. (2005) Effects of Omega-3 Polyunsaturated Fatty Acids on Inflammatory Markers in COPD. Chest 128: 3817–3827.
50. Bolte G, Kompauer I, Fobker M, Cullenz P, Keilk U, et al. (2006) Fatty acids in serum cholesteryl esters in relation to asthma and lung function in children. Clinical and Experimental Allergy 36: 293–302.

20

Patterns and Predictors of Smokeless Tobacco Use among Adults in Bangladesh: Findings from the International Tobacco Control (ITC) Bangladesh Survey

Abu S. Abdullah[1,2*], Pete Driezen[3], Ummul H. Ruthbah[4], Nigar Nargis[4,5], Anne C. K. Quah[6], Geoffrey T. Fong[6,7]

1 Boston University School of Medicine, Boston Medical Center, Boston, Massachusetts, United States of America, **2** School of Public Health, Guangxi Medical University, Nanning, China, **3** Propel Centre for Population Health Impact, University of Waterloo, Waterloo, Ontario, Canada, **4** Department of Economics, University of Dhaka, Dhaka, Bangladesh, **5** World Health Organization, Geneva, Switzerland, **6** Department of Psychology, University of Waterloo, Waterloo, Ontario, Canada, **7** Ontario Institute for Cancer Research, Toronto, Ontario, Canada

Abstract

Background: Although smokeless tobacco (SLT) use is prevalent in South Asian countries including Bangladesh, information about the pattern and correlates of SLT use is scarce. This study described the pattern and predictors of SLT use among Bangladeshi adults.

Methods: The data for this study were derived from the International Tobacco Control Policy Evaluation Bangladesh (ITC BD) Survey, a prospective cohort survey of a nationally representative sample of smokers and non-smokers, conducted during November 2011 and May 2012. The study included 5522 adults aged 15 or above. We used multiple logistic regression models to identify predictors of SLT use.

Results: Of the respondents (N = 5522), 20% were SLT users. In general, SLT use was significantly higher among women, the illiterate and residents of the Dhaka slums or non-tribal/non-border areas outside Dhaka; SLT use increased with age. Several attitudinal factors were also associated with SLT use. Multivariable logistic regression analyses revealed several predictors of SLT use: being female (OR = 1.96, 95% confidence interval, CI: 1.18–3.24), an increasing age, being a resident of a Dhaka slum (OR = 5.86; 95% CI: 3.73–9.21) or non-tribal/non-border areas outside Dhaka (OR = 3.42; 95% CI: 1.94–6.03), being illiterate (OR = 3.37; 95% CI: 1.99–5.71), holding positive opinion towards societal approval of SLT use (OR = 5.84; 95% CI: 3.38–10.09), holding positive opinion towards SLT use by women (OR = 2.63; 95% CI: 1.53–4.54), believing that SLT is addictive (OR = 2.96; 95% CI: 1.51–5.81), and believing SLT is less harmful than bidi (OR = 2.22; 95% CI: 1.36–3.62).

Conclusion: The findings suggest that coordinated efforts of governmental and non-governmental organizations, targeting both smoked tobacco and SLT use reduction and cessation, could be modified to reach each level of population including those who are marginalized, female, less educated and elderly. As most tobacco control programs in Bangladesh target mainly cigarette or bidi smoking, coordinated programs are needed that will also include SLT use within the tobacco control policy and prevention strategies.

Editor: Chris Bullen, The University of Auckland, New Zealand

Funding: The ITC Bangladesh Project was supported by the International Development Research Centre (IDRC Grant 104831-002), Canadian Institutes for Health Research (Operating Grants 79551 and 115016), the US National Cancer Institute (P01 CA138389). Geoffrey T. Fong was supported by a Senior Investigator Award from Ontario Institute for Cancer Research and by a Prevention Scientist Award from the Canadian Cancer Research Institute. Abu S. Abdullah was supported by a Clinical Innovator Award from the Flight Attendant Medical Research Institute, USA through a grant to the American Academy of Pediatrics (AAP) Julius B. Richmond Center. The funders had no role in study design, data collection and analysis, decision to publish, or preparation of the manuscript.

Competing Interests: The authors have declared that no competing interests exist.

* Email: asm.abdullah@graduate.hku.hk

Introduction

Smokeless tobacco (SLT), a general term used in the United States for chewing tobacco and oral snuff products [1] refers to those indigenous smokeless tobacco products that are most frequently used in South Asia, including but not limited to paan, paan masala, zarda, betel quid with tobacco, and gutka [2,3]. SLT can cause oral cancer [4,5] and nicotine addiction [6] and is associated with several other health conditions including oral pain [7], cardiovascular diseases [8], hypertension [9], diabetes [10], loss in bone density [11], and problems during pregnancy and following childbirth [12]. Of the estimated 300 million SLT users globally, 27 million are Bangladeshi adults [13]. The World Health Organization (WHO) estimated that 57,000 people die each year from tobacco-attributable (almost all of it in the form of cigarette smoking) diseases in Bangladesh [14]. In a recent study, Alam et al. reported 25% of all deaths in Bangladeshi men aged 25 to 69 years are attributable to cigarette smoking [15]. These mortality rates underestimate total mortality attributable to tobacco because many Bangladeshi men and women use smokeless tobacco [16]. However, these mortality rates provide an estimate of the bigger public health problem associated with tobacco and smokeless tobacco use in Bangladesh – the world's seventh most populous nation with a population of 150 million. The total cost of SLT-associated diseases in India was US$389 million in 2004 [17], suggesting a high economic burden from SLT use in Bangladesh too. These health and economic consequences underscore the need for urgent public health action to avert the tobacco and SLT-attributable morbidity and mortality in Bangladesh.

Bangladesh has a long history of tobacco use and a variety of ways in which tobacco is smoked and smokeless tobacco is used [18]. The limited data that are available on SLT use in Bangladesh indicate an increasing trend in both male and female adults (aged 15 and above). SLT use has increased from 19.7% (14.8% male and 24.4% female) in 2004 [19] to 27.2% (26.4% male and 27.9% female) in 2009 [16]. By converting these percentages in numbers, we can estimate that the number of SLT users increased by 9 million in five years (from 17.3 million to 25.9 million). Historically, prevalence of smokeless tobacco use is greater among women than among men. However, the growth in SLT use was greater among men during this period.

While these nationally representative prevalence data on SLT use illustrate the magnitude of SLT use in Bangladesh, the socio-demographic, environmental and behavioral level predictors of SLT use are poorly understood. A case-control study of 704 SLT users examined respondents' perceptions and experiences of SLT use and reported associated factors of SLT use: older age, women, widowed, less educated, housewives, and lower socioeconomic status [20]. However, this study was conducted among hospital patients and in an urban setting, limiting it's representativeness at the national level. There has been no comprehensive study on the pattern of SLT use, the determinants of usage or on the correlation between SLT use and smoked tobacco in Bangladesh. Given the paucity of such data on SLT use in Bangladesh, this study examined the patterns and predictors of SLT use among Bangladeshi adults by using data from the Wave 3 International Tobacco Control (ITC) Policy Evaluation Bangladesh Project.

Methods

Data source

Data analysed in this paper came from the Wave 3 ITC Bangladesh (ITC BD) Survey conducted between November 2011 and May 2012. A detailed description of the ITC BD Survey can be found elsewhere [21–23]. Briefly, the ITC BD Survey is a prospective cohort survey of a nationally representative sample of tobacco users and non-users conducted in all six administrative divisions of Bangladesh: Barisal, Chittagong, Dhaka, Khulna, Rajshahi, and Sylhet. The target population of the ITC BD Survey consists of users and non-users of tobacco who are 15 years or older. The Wave 1 survey was conducted in 2009 using a multi-stage probability sampling design. The total sample consisted of two sub-samples: a national sample designed to represent the population of Bangladesh and an urban slum sample, designed to represent the urban poor population of Dhaka. The national sample selected 23 of the 64 districts covering Bangladesh with probability proportional to population size. Another three districts were chosen purposively to include the tribal populations (Garo and Chakma) and a border district between India and Bangladesh. Within randomly selected districts, two upazilas and two villages within upazila were randomly selected, again with probability proportional to population size. A total of 80 villages were selected for the national subsample. Villages contained 300–600 households; a maximum of 450 households per village were enumerated. Households from the enumeration were randomly selected to participate in the Wave 1 survey. The use of a multi-stage probability sampling design guarantees that, in the sense of the theory of probability sampling, the sample is geographically representative of the Bangladesh population.

Household enumeration was conducted to determine basic sociodemographic information of household members as well as tobacco use status of all household members aged 15 or older. Based on the enumeration survey, households were classified into socioeconomic tertiles using a CASHPOR Housing Index. Within each tertile, 10 households having at least one smoker and three households having all non-smokers were randomly chosen to participate in the survey and approached to be interviewed; households that did not respond were replaced. A total of 31,137 households were enumerated in Wave 1, containing 92,853 adults. Of those enumerated, 2000 households were randomly selected for the main survey. One randomly selected adult was interviewed in non-smoking households. In smoker households, all available smokers were selected along with one randomly selected non-smoker.

In the urban slum subsample, 552 households were selected from six urban slums within the city of Dhaka and its surrounding areas. Unlike the national sample, the urban slum sample was designed as a cross-sectional survey due to the insecure nature of housing arrangements in urban slums. In each of the slums, a random starting point was identified and all households in a row were interviewed until the designated number of households for that area had been interviewed. One non-smoker was randomly selected to be interviewed in each household along with all smokers.

Sampling weights were computed for all respondents so that the final sample is broadly representative of the Bangladesh population of adults aged 15 or older. Sampling weights were calibrated to population estimates within predefined geographic and demographic groups (see Wave 1 technical report for more information about the construction of sampling weights).

In Wave 1, 5,771 respondents were interviewed: 1137 were from the urban slums, 256 were from tribal & border areas, 598 were from the city of Dhaka and 3780 were from areas outside the city of Dhaka. Of the 5,771 respondents, 3111 were smokers and 2660 were non-smokers. In Waves 2 and 3, respondents lost to attrition were replaced with newly randomly selected respondents, using the frame of households enumerated in Wave 1. Retention rates were very high from Wave 1 to Wave 2 and from Wave 2 to Wave 3 in the national and purposive samples. Overall, 94% of Wave 1 respondents (not from the urban slums) were re-contacted in Wave 2 while 90% of Wave 2 respondents were re-contacted in Wave 3. None of the Wave 1 slum subsample was followed to Wave 3 so that in Wave 3, 1055 new respondents were recruited to participate in the Wave 3 survey using the same sampling protocol followed in Wave 1 for the slum subsample.

Data were collected using face-to-face interviews. Sampling weights were computed so that results are representative of the Bangladeshi adult population (15 and older).

In all the waves, written consent was obtained from those respondents who can read and write; others gave consent with fingertips. Ethical approval was obtained from the Office of Research Ethics at the University of Waterloo (Waterloo, Canada) (Number. 15019, dated October 03, 2008), and the Ethical Review Committee, Bangladesh Medical Research Council

Table 1. Characteristics of the ITC Bangladesh Wave 3 sample (unweighted), Bangladesh 2011 (N = 5522).

	Frequency[#]	%
Wave of recruitment		
Wave 1	3954	71.6
Wave 2	206	3.7
Wave 3	1362	24.7
Sampling area		
Dhaka non-slum sample	557	10.1
Dhaka slum sample	1055	19.1
Non-tribal, non-border areas outside Dhaka	3666	66.4
Tribal & border areas outside Dhaka	244	4.4
Sex		
Male	3293	59.6
Female	2229	40.4
Age group		
15–24	1190	21.6
25–39	2033	36.8
40–54	1381	25.0
55+	918	16.6
Marital status		
Not married	984	17.9
Married	4519	82.1
Monthly household income		
<5000 taka	497	9.0
5,000 to <10,000 taka	1995	36.1
10,000 taka or more	2314	41.9
not reported	716	13.0
Highest level of education		
Illiterate	1332	24.2
1 to 8 years	2908	52.9
9 years or more	1258	22.9
Muslim		
Non-muslim	919	16.7
Muslim	4570	83.3
Any children in home <= 14		
No children/no children <= 14	1505	27.4
At least one child <= 14	3987	72.6
Any (other) smokers in the home		
No (other) smokers in the home	2175	39.4
At least one (other) smoker in the home	3347	60.6
Anyone (else) uses smokeless tobacco in the home		
No one (else) uses smokeless tobacco	2264	41.0
At least one (other) person uses smokeless tobacco	3258	59.0
Tobacco use status		
Exclusively cigarettes	1723	31.2
Exclusively bidi	267	4.8
Dual user*	207	3.7
Mixed user**	297	5.4
Smokeless	781	14.1
Quitter	242	4.4
Nonsmoker	2005	36.3
Current smokeless user		

Table 1. Cont.

	Frequency#	%
Does not currently use smokeless tobacco	4444	80.5
Current smokeless tobacco user	1078	19.5

*those who use both cigarettes and bidi; **those who use cigarette, bidi and SLT.
#Due to the missing values, the total may not add up to the same in some variables.

(Number: BMRC/ERC/2007–2010/1372; dated February 19, 2009).

Measures

A standardized Bengali questionnaire was used for data collection. Details of the questionnaire are described elsewhere [22]. Briefly, the questionnaire obtained information on the subject's *socio-demographic background* (sex, age, religion, residence (Dhaka non-slum, Dhaka slums, non-tribal/non-border areas outside Dhaka and tribal/border areas), marital status, educational attainment, personal monthly income), whether there are any children (aged 14 or below) at home, *smoking behavior* (non-smoker, exclusively cigarette smokers, exclusively bidi smokers, dual users), *use of any smokeless tobacco (SLT)*, and *any other smokers or SLT users at home*. SLT users were those who answered "yes" to the following question: "Do you currently use any smokeless tobacco products at least once a week?"

Knowledge of the health consequences of SLT use was also assessed, along with *attitudes towards SLT use*. To measure *knowledge of the health consequences of SLT use*, respondents were asked: "Based on what you know or believe, does SLT cause…?" Respondents were then read a list of three diseases or conditions (mouth cancer, gum disease, difficulty to open mouth). To measure *attitudes towards SLT use*, respondents were asked whether they believe SLT is addictive (with response categories of "strongly agree, agree, neutral, disagree, strongly disagree"), whether SLT is less harmful than cigarettes or bidi (with response categories of "less harmful, more harmful and no difference"). Respondents were also asked about societal attitudes (with response categories of "approve, neutral, disapprove"), whether SLT is acceptable for women (with response categories of "strongly agree, agree, neutral, disagree, strongly disagree"), and their overall opinion about SLT use (with response categories of "very good, good, neutral, bad, very bad").

Analyses

The analysis presented here uses descriptive statistics appropriate for complex survey data to estimate the prevalence of current SLT use among Bangladeshi adults. Differences in the prevalence of SLT use across socio-demographic categories and by attitudes toward SLT use were tested using the Rao-Scott chi square test. A logistic regression model then examined predictors of current SLT use. Initial predictors were selected on the basis of the bivariate associations tested with the Rao-Scott chi square test. A backward elimination procedure was conducted within a logistic regression model to select covariates related to current SLT use, using a p-value for inclusion of 0.05 or below. Variables used in construction of the sampling weights (sex, smoking status, and area of residence) were forced into this model to reduce biases in the other coefficients. The final selected model was refit with a weighted logistic regression model that accounts for the stratified multi-stage survey design. The analysis was conducted using the complex survey routines (PROC SURVEYFREQ and PROC SURVEYLOGISTIC) available in SAS Version 9.3 to account for the stratified multi-stage survey design. The only exception to this was the analysis conducted for the selection of predictors of SLT use, which was run using PROC LOGISTIC. Unless otherwise indicated, all results presented in this paper are weighted. In each case, an unweighted analysis was also conducted; since there were no appreciable differences between the two sets of results, only the weighted results are reported here.

Results

Sample characteristics

A total of 5522 respondents were interviewed in the Wave 3 of ITC BD Survey; 72% were recruited in Wave 1 (Table 1). Overall, two-thirds (66.4%) of the sample was from non-tribal, non-border areas outside Dhaka and a greater proportion (59.6%) of the sample was male. Most respondents were married (82.1%), Muslim (83.3%), and had at least one child in their home who was 14 years of age or younger (72.6%). Of the respondents, 36% were non-smokers and 20% were current SLT users (Table 1).

Pattern of SLT use

As shown in Table 2, SLT use was significantly higher in women (23.1%) than men (16.5%) and among those who were illiterate (31.9%) than having 1–8 years (21.5%) or 9 or more years (8.6%) of education. SLT use increased significantly with age: 36% of adults aged 55 and older used smokeless tobacco compared to only 8.5% of adults younger than 25. SLT use was also higher among those who lived in a Dhaka slum (29.9%) and among those living in non-tribal/non-border areas outside of Dhaka (20.3%).

Attitudes toward SLT use

As shown in Table 3, Bangladeshis held differing opinions and attitudes towards SLT use. Bangladeshis who believed smokeless tobacco was less harmful than smoked tobacco (cigarette or bidi) were significantly more likely to be current SLT users. Likewise, Bangladeshis who believed that society approves of smokeless tobacco use were significantly more likely to use SLT (40%) than those who believed society disapproves of SLT use (16%). A significantly higher percentage of respondents (43%) who agree that it is acceptable for women to use SLT currently use SLT themselves compared to only 16% of those who do not agree. A significantly higher proportion of those who believed that SLT use is addictive were current SLT users (20%) than those who did not believe so (9%).

Predictors of current SLT use

Table 4 presents the results of a multivariable logistic regression model estimating the association between socio-demographic factors, attitudes and opinions toward SLT and current SLT use. The multivariable model revealed the following predictors of SLT use: being female (OR = 1.96, 95% CI: 1.18–3.24), being

Table 2. Smokeless tobacco use by demographic characteristics among Bangladeshi residents (weighted), Bangladesh 2011.

				Rao-Scott ChiSq Test		
	Freq.	%	(95% CI)	ChiSq	df	p value
Sampling area						
Dhaka non-slum sample	38/557	10.2	(8.4, 12.2)	42.75	3	<0.001
Dhaka slum sample	304/1055	29.9	(27.1, 32.8)			
Non-tribal, non-border areas outside Dhaka	701/3666	20.3	(16.7, 24.5)			
Tribal & border areas outside Dhaka	35/244	9.1	(4.3, 18.4)			
Sex						
Male	483/3293	16.5	(13.0, 20.6)	8.87	1	0.003
Female	595/2229	23.1	(18.7, 28.1)			
Age group						
15–24	88/1190	8.5	(5.5, 13.1)	66.49	3	<0.001
25–39	335/2033	18.1	(14.0, 23.2)			
40–54	366/1381	23.6	(17.9, 30.4)			
55+	289/918	36.4	(30.3, 42.9)			
Marital status						
Not married	164/984	18.3	(12.3, 26.3)	0.37	1	0.543
Married	907/4519	20.2	(17.0, 23.9)			
Monthly household income						
<5000 taka	95/497	19.5	(14.0, 26.6)	3.46	3	0.326
5,000 to <10,000 taka	400/1995	21.2	(17.2, 25.7)			
10,000 taka or more	441/2314	20.6	(15.1, 27.4)			
not reported	142/716	13.8	(8.4, 21.9)			
Highest level of education						
Illiterate	426/1332	31.9	(27.2, 37.0)	112.58	2	<0.001
1 to 8 years	550/2908	21.5	(17.4, 26.3)			
9 years or more	99/1258	8.6	(6.2, 11.8)			
Muslim						
Non-muslim	149/919	14.3	(8.6, 22.8)	2.28	1	0.131
Muslim	923/4570	21.1	(17.2, 25.6)			
Any children in home <= 14						
No children/no children <=14	307/1505	18.7	(14.8, 23.3)	0.47	1	0.495
At least one child <=14	764/3987	20.3	(16.4, 24.8)			
Any (other) smokers in the home						
No (other) smokers in the home	468/2175	19.6	(15.1, 25.2)	0.02	1	0.896
At least one (other) smoker in the home	610/3347	19.9	(16.8, 23.5)			
Anyone (else) uses smokeless tobacco in the home						
No one (else) uses smokeless tobacco	344/2264	20.6	(15.2, 27.2)	0.20	1	0.652
At least one (other) person uses smokeless tobacco	734/3258	19.2	(16.0, 22.9)			

aged 25–39 (OR = 2.30, 95% CI: 1.49–3.54) or aged 40–54 (OR = 3.67; 95% CI: 1.76–7.65) or aged 55 and above (OR = 4.25; 95% CI: 2.27–7.95), being a resident of a Dhaka slum (OR = 5.86; 95% CI: 3.73–9.21) or non-tribal/non-border areas outside Dhaka (OR = 3.42; 95% CI: 1.94–6.03), being illiterate (OR = 3.37; 95% CI: 1.99–5.71), holding positive opinion towards societal approval of SLT use (OR = 5.84; 95% CI: 3.38–10.09), holding positive opinion towards SLT use by women (OR = 2.63; 95% CI: 1.53–4.54), believing that SLT is addictive (OR = 2.96; 95% CI: 1.51–5.81), and believing SLT is less harmful than bidi (OR = 2.22; 95% CI: 1.36–3.62). In addition, people who believed that SLT was less harmful had 2.12 times greater

Table 3. Smokeless tobacco use by attitudes toward smokeless tobacco among Bangladeshi residents (weighted), 2011.

				Rao-Scott ChiSq Test		
	Freq.	**%**	**(95% CI)**	**ChiSq**	**df**	**p value**
Societal attitudes toward smokeless tobacco						
Society approves	203/490	40.1	(30.3, 50.7)	41.26	2	<0.001
Society disapproves	708/4372	15.9	(12.3, 20.4)			
Neither	77/437	15.2	(11.0, 20.6)			
It is acceptable for women to use smokeless tobacco						
Agree/strongly agree	237/535	42.6	(33.2, 52.5)	46.98	1	<0.001
Otherwise	793/4858	16.0	(12.9, 19.7)			
Smokeless tobacco is Addictive						
Agree/strongly agree	1032/5179	19.8	(16.0, 24.2)	8.56	1	0.003
Otherwise	30/239	8.8	(5.0, 15.1)			
Smokeless tobacco is less harmful than cigarettes						
Less harmful	265/731	40.1	(30.2, 50.9)	48.11	2	<0.001
More harmful	128/944	15.0	(9.9, 22.2)			
No difference	549/3322	15.3	(12.1, 19.2)			
Smokeless tobacco is less harmful than bidi						
Less harmful	316/845	39.7	(30.4, 49.8)	37.69	2	<0.001
More harmful	104/801	14.1	(7.9, 24.0)			
No difference	518/3326	14.8	(11.4, 19.0)			
Opinion of smokeless tobacco use						
Otherwise	32/129	26.3	(18.8, 35.4)	3.18	1	0.074
Bad/very bad	1001/5242	18.7	(15.1, 23.0)			
Smokeless tobacco causes mouth cancer						
Otherwise	171/634	26.5	(19.3, 35.3)	3.55	1	0.060
Yes	898/4841	18.4	(14.5, 23.1)			
Smokeless tobacco causes gum disease						
Otherwise	184/804	22.2	(15.7, 30.5)	1.32	1	0.251
Yes	879/4665	18.6	(15.0, 22.8)			
Smokeless tobacco causes difficulty in opening mouth						
Otherwise	296/1397	22.2	(16.3, 29.5)	1.43	1	0.233
Yes	775/4078	18.2	(14.4, 22.8)			

odds of using smokeless compared to people who thought smokeless was more harmful than cigarettes ($p = 0.014$) (omnibus test).

Discussion

This study examined the socio-demographic and attitudinal factors associated with SLT use and found that one in every five Bangladeshi adults use SLT. Our sample is nationally representative as the distribution of respondents by division, age group and sex compares well against census estimates from Bangladesh for 2011 (Table S1) [24]. Our findings have some variations with the two earlier studies [16,19]. As there are methodological differences across studies, a direct comparison of rates needs to be interpreted cautiously.

Our findings show that the overall prevalence of SLT use (20%) is identical to the WHO 2004 study (19.7%) [19]. However, the prevalence of SLT use in our study is lower than the reported estimates (27.2%) in the GATS 2009 study [16] and another 2009 estimate (29.6%) [25]. These differences might be due to the methodological differences across the studies and the timing when the survey was conducted. Moreover, wave 3 survey was conducted in 2011; during the period when several tobacco control programs were funded by the Bloomberg Global Initiative. However, in both the GATS survey and our survey, we observed an apparent rise compared to the rate of 2004. This increasing trend might be due to the increasing taxation on cigarettes, as people from low socioeconomic status smoke more and are responsive to price [23] and the relatively low cost of SLT products. This might be also due to the lack of public awareness and inappropriate knowledge about the harmful effects of SLT use. Also, currently most anti-tobacco campaigns in Bangladesh focuses on cigarette or bidi smoking without any information about SLT use. This creates an opportunity for SLT being offered as an alternative tobacco product for smokers to use instead of cigarette or bidi. This alternative product would be appealing to many smokers who are dependent on nicotine or those who wanted to quit smoking. In this study, 9% of all smokers who had

Table 4. Odds of being a current smokeless tobacco user (weighted; n = 4702), Bangladesh 2011.

			Wald ChiSq Test		
	Odds Ratio	**(95% CI)**	**ChiSq***	**df**	**p value**
Sex					
Male	1.00	-	6.79	1	0.009
Female	1.96	(1.18, 3.24)			
Age					
15–24	1.00	-	21.95	3	<0.001
25–39	2.30	(1.49, 3.54)			
40–54	3.67	(1.76, 7.65)			
55+	4.25	(2.27, 7.95)			
Sampling area					
Dhaka non-slum sample	1.00	-	66.59	3	<0.001
Dhaka slum sample	5.86	(3.73, 9.21)			
Non-tribal, non-border areas outside Dhaka	3.42	(1.94, 6.03)			
Tribal & border areas outside Dhaka	3.11	(0.74, 13.03)			
Income					
<5,000 taka	1.00	-	3.38	3	0.337
5,000 to<10,000	0.89	(0.57, 1.38)			
10,000+ taka	1.21	(0.76, 1.95)			
Not stated	0.83	(0.42, 1.65)			
Highest level of education					
9 years or more	1.00	-	24.20	2	<0.001
1 to 8 years	2.60	(1.76, 3.84)			
Illiterate	3.37	(1.99, 5.71)			
Societal attitudes toward smokeless tobacco					
Neither	1.00	-	79.16	2	<0.001
Society disapproves	1.37	(0.90, 2.07)			
Society approves	5.84	(3.38, 10.09)			
Acceptable for women to use smokeless tobacco					
Otherwise	1.00	-	12.15	1	<0.001
Agree/strongly agree	2.63	(1.53, 4.54)			
Smokeless tobacco is addictive					
Otherwise	1.00	-	9.99	1	0.002
Agree/strongly agree	2.96	(1.51, 5.81)			
Smokeless tobacco is less harmful than Cigarettes					
No difference	1.00	-	7.45	2	0.024
More harmful	0.77	(0.33, 1.82)			
Less harmful	1.63	(0.82, 3.22)			
Smokeless tobacco is less harmful than bidi					
No difference	1.00	-	13.18	2	0.001
More harmful	1.24	(0.37, 4.13)			
Less harmful	2.22	(1.36, 3.62)			
Anyone (else) uses smokeless tobacco in the home					
No one (else) uses smokeless tobacco	1.00	-	1.39	1	0.239
At least one (other) person uses smokeless tobacco	1.63	(0.72, 3.66)			

*Omnibus test.

made a serious quit attempt reportedly used SLT to support their most recent quit attempt (data not shown). Also, the Tobacco Control Act (TCA) 2005 initially did not specify SLT in defining tobacco products. Thus most of the measures taken since 2005 to control tobacco use in Bangladesh focused on tobacco smoking. The Amendment to the TCA in 2013 has made provision for the reference to SLT specifically. The rules for the Amendment are in the process of drafting and yet to reflect the measures targeted to SLT control. The oversight of SLT control in the TCA is one of the many reasons that have contributed to the growth of SLT consumption in Bangladesh.

The increased likelihood of SLT use among the illiterate and less educated Bangladeshis may indicate that similar factors are involved in the initiation of SLT use and smoked tobacco among Bangladeshis [16,19,22]. Similar socioeconomic differences in SLT use were also reported in India [26,27]. In an earlier study, we reported that Bangladeshis with low socioeconomic status were more likely to be exposed to tobacco smoke pollution [22]. It is likely that less educated Bangladeshi adults are less aware of tobacco or SLT-related health hazards and find themselves in conditions which predispose them to use SLT. It is also possible that the limited anti-tobacco educational campaigns available in Bangladesh are not reaching this group of people. Also, the sale of SLT products is not monitored cautiously in Bangladesh making it easier for manufacturer and retail stores to promote the products openly to specific populations. Further studies should explore strategies that are used to promote SLT in Bangladesh to guide the development of policy measures.

In this study, Bangladeshis who believed SLT use was less harmful than smoked tobacco (i.e. bidi) used SLT, suggesting that low perception of risk played a key role in encouraging them to use SLT. In other studies misconceptions about the harmlessness of SLT use have led to increased social acceptability and uptake of SLT products [28,29]. Future prevention strategies should focus on increasing Bangladeshis' awareness of the relative harms of all tobacco products including SLT use.

The observation that SLT use increases with age is consistent with previous reports [16,19,26]. This increased likelihood of SLT use is related to the social acceptance of SLT use by the older people and a greater appeal of cigarette among the younger generations who may be taking up smoking instead of SLT use. Also, this may be due to increased level of nicotine addiction among the population. Following the addiction theory [30], one might have used SLT in few social occasions hooking him/her to the nicotine to develop dependency; overtime he/she will experience growing craving for nicotine and the need for SLT or other tobacco products. Some of this population might switch to tobacco or other smoked tobacco products and some would continue with SLT use. A good proportion of tobacco smokers or quitters may also supplement their tobacco dependency habit by SLT use. In this study, a small proportion of cigarette (4.4%) or bidi (9.2%) smokers who made a serious quit attempt used SLT to support their efforts. Use of SLT may provide a supplementation or substitution of nicotine intake for cigarette smokers [31] encouraging their continued use; this scenario could be particularly true in situations in which smoking is not socially acceptable, but SLT use is.

This study had several limitations. First, because of the cross-sectional design of the study only associations could be explored without any causal relationship. Second, all data on the use of SLT were based on self-reports collected by using an interviewer-administered structured questionnaire. Due to social stigma associated with tobacco and SLT use, people may under-report SLT use [27]. However, self-reported SLT use among adults is a reliable measure and has high agreement with biochemical assessment [32]. Finally, data were collected by trained interviewers who followed written interviewer guidelines. Any difference between their understanding and explanation of the questions asked could result in bias in information collected. However, such bias was minimized by the periodical observation of interviews by the senior research team members and bi-weekly meetings with the interviewers during which any unusual observation was discussed and resolved. Despite these limitations, our study provides recent information on the use of SLT among Bangladeshi adults, which would support evaluation of tobacco control policies in Bangladesh and development of appropriate intervention measures.

Conclusion

In conclusion, this study identified several important predictors of SLT use in Bangladesh, including being female, increasing age, being illiterate, residing in the Dhaka slum or non-tribal/ non-border areas outside of Dhaka, holding positive opinion towards societal approval of SLT use or SLT use by women, and believing SLT is less harmful than bidi. Findings from this study suggest that coordinated efforts of governmental and non-governmental organizations, targeting both smoked tobacco and SLT use reduction and cessation, could be modified to reach each level of population including those who are marginalized, female, less educated and elderly. As most tobacco control programs target mainly cigarette or bidi smoking, coordinated programs are needed that will also include SLT use within the tobacco control policy and prevention strategies. Future studies, possibly qualitative in nature, would be useful to understand the environmental, cultural and societal factors associated with SLT use, particularly among women and among the residents of a Dhaka slum and non-tribal/non-border areas outside Dhaka. Future research should understand the depth of beliefs about SLT use among the public and identify potential interventions that would be acceptable to them. Given the wide acceptance of SLT use by women in Bangladeshi culture, interventions to raise awareness of the harms of SLT use should target women as a key group. At the same time, national programs should focus on changing social norms by addressing inappropriate attitudes and perceptions of risk towards SLT use among the Bangladeshis. Similar to the effective policies for smoked tobacco, policies such as increasing excise tax and restricting marketing of SLT to targeted population including minors, should also be initiated. These interventions should complement the existing intervention strategies aimed at reducing SLT use among the public in Bangladesh.

Acknowledgments

The authors would like to acknowledge the team members from University of Waterloo and University of Dhaka for their contributions in the ITC Bangladesh Project.

Disclaimer: The authors alone are responsible for the views expressed in this article and they do not necessarily represent the views, decisions or policies of the institutions with which they areaffiliated. The data analyzed in this paper are from the ITC Project (itcproject.org) where the ITC data access policy can be found.

Author Contributions

Conceived and designed the experiments: ASA PD NN GTF. Performed the experiments: NN UHR ACKQ. Analyzed the data: PD ASA. Wrote the paper: ASA PD NN GTF.

References

1. Psoter WJ, Morse DE (2001) Annual per capita apparent consumption of tobacco products in the United States: 1900–1990. Prev Med 32(1), 1–9.
2. International Agency for Research on Cancer (IARC) (2007) Smokeless tobacco and some tobacco-specific N-Nirtosamines, vol 89 of IARC Monographs on the Evaluation of Carcinogenic Risks to Humans. World Health Organization International agency for Research on Cancer, Lyon, France: 89.
3. Gupta PC, Ray CS (2003) Smokeless tobacco and health in India and South Asia. Respirology 8, 419–431.
4. Department of Health and Human Services (DHHS) (1986) The Health Consequences of Using Smokeless Tobacco: A Report ofthe Advisory Committee to the Surgeon General. Washington, DC: Public Health Service. DHHS publication NIH 86-2874.
5. International Agency for Research on Cancer (IARC) (1985) Tobacco Habits Other than Smoking: Betel Quid and Areca Nut Chewing and Some Related Nitrosamines. Lyon, France: International Agency for Research on Cancer.
6. Office on Smoking and Health (OSH) (1988) The Health Consequences of Smoking: Nicotine Addiction. A Report of the Surgeon General. Atlanta, Ga: National Center for Chronic Disease. Prevention and Health Promotion. DHHS publication CDC 88-8406.
7. Pau AKH, Croucher R, Marcenes W, Rahman R, Shajahan S (2003) Tobacco cessation, oral pain, and psychological distress in Bangladeshi women. Nicotine & Tobacco. Research 5, 419–423.
8. Bolinder G, Alfredsson L, Englund A, de Faire U (1994) Smokeless tobacco use and increased cardiovascular mortality among Swedish construction workers. Am J Public Health 84, 399–404.
9. Hergens MP, Lambe M, Pershagen G, Ye W (2008) Risk of hypertension amongst Swedish male snuff users: a prospective study. J Intern Med 264(2), 187–94.
10. Persson PG, Carlsson S, Svanström L, Ostenson CG, Efendic S, et al. (2000) Cigarette smoking, oral moist snuff use and glucose intolerance. J Intern Med 248(2), 103–10.
11. Quandt SA, Spangler JG, Case LD, Bell RA, Belflower AE (2005) Smokeless tobacco use accelerates age-related loss of bone mineral density among older women in a multi-ethnic rural community. Journal of Cross-Cultural Gerontology 20(2), 109–125.
12. England LJ, Kim SY, Tomar SL, Ray CS, Gupta PC, et al. (2010) Non-cigarette tobacco use among women and adverse pregnancy outcomes. Acta Obstetricia et Gynecologica Scandinavica 89(4), 454–464.
13. World Health Organization (WHO) (2011) Who report on the global tobacco epidemic, 2011. Warning about the dangers of tobacco. Geneva, Switzerland: World Health Organization. Retrieved from http://www.who.int/tobacco/global_report/2011/en/.
14. World Health Organization (WHO) (2007) Impact of Tobacco-Related Illnesses in Bangladesh. New Delhi, India: World Health Organization, South East Asia Region.
15. Alam DS, Jha P, Ramasundarahettige C, Streatfield PK, Niessen LW, et al. (2013) Smoking-attributable mortality in Bangladesh: proportional mortality study. Bull World Health Organ 91(10), 757–64.
16. World Health Organization (WHO) (2009) Bangladesh. Global Adult Tobacco Survey: Bangladesh Report 2009, Dhaka, Bangladesh: WHO – Bangladesh.
17. John RM, Sung HY, Max W (2009) Economic cost of tobacco use in India, 2004. Tobacco control 18, 138–143.
18. Choudhury K, Haniff SMA, Mahmood SS (2007) Sociodemographic characteristics of tobacco consumers in a rural area of Bangladesh. J Health Popul Nutr 25, 456–464.
19. Zaman MM, Nargis N, Perucic AM, Rahman K (Editors) (2007) Impact of Tobacco Related Illness in Bangladesh. World Health Organization, Regional Office for South East Asia, New Delhi. (http://intranet/LinkFiles/Tobacco_Free_Initiative_Health_Cost_bangladesh.pdf).
20. Rahman MA, Mahmood MA, Spurrier N, Rahman M, Choudhury SR, et al. (2012) Why Do Bangladeshi People Use Smokeless Tobacco Products? Asia Pac J Public Health. May, 1–13.
21. Fong GT, Cummings KM, Borland R, Hastings G, Hyland A, et al. (2006) The conceptual framework of the International Tobacco Control (ITC) Policy Evaluation Project. Tobacco Control, 15, i3–11. doi:10.1136/tc.2005.015438.
22. Abdullah AS, Hitchman SC, Driezen P, Nargis N, Quah ACK, et al. (2011) Socioeconomic differences in exposure to tobacco smoke pollution (TSP) in Bangladeshi households with children: Findings from the International Tobacco Control (ITC) Bangladesh Survey. International Journal of Environmental Research and Public Health 8, 842–860.
23. Nargis N, Ruthbah UH, Hussain AK, Fong GT, Huq I, et al. (2013) The price sensitivity of cigarette consumption in Bangladesh: evidence from the International Tobacco Control (ITC) Bangladesh Wave 1 (2009) and Wave 2 (2010) surveys. Tob Control. Oct 8. doi:10.1136/tobaccocontrol-2012-050835.
24. Bangladesh Bureau of Statistics (BBS) (2014) Bangladesh Population and Housing Census 2011- a preliminary report. Available: http://www.bbs.gov.bd/Home.aspx. Accessed May 12, 2014.
25. Hussain AKM G (2012) Prevalence and patterns of tobacco use in Bangladesh from 2005–2209: Findings form a pre- and post-Tobacco Control Act analysis. Presented at the 15th Workd Conference on Tobacco or Health (WCTOH), Singapore. March 20–24, 2012.
26. Rooban T, Elizabeth J, Umadevi KR, Ranganathan K (2010) Sociodemographic correlates of male chewable smokeless tobacco users in India: a preliminary report of analysis of National Family Health Survey, 2005–2006. Indian J Cancer. Jul;47 Suppl 1: 91–100.
27. Rani M, Bonu S, Jha P, Nguyen SN, Jamjoum L (2003) Tobacco use in India: prevalence and predictors of smoking and chewing in a national cross sectional household survey. Tob Control. Dec;12(4): e4.
28. Sussman S (1989) Two social influence perspectives of tobacco use development and prevention. Health Educ Res 4(2), 213–23.
29. Gale M, Boyd IDG (1989) Smokeless tobacco use by youth in the US. Journal of School Health 59: 189–94.
30. Stolerman IP, Jarvis MJ (1995) The scientific case that nicotine is addictive Psychopharmacology (Berl) 117(1)2–10; discussion 14–20.
31. Tomar SL, Giovino GA (1988) Incidence and predictors of smokeless tobacco use among US youth. Am J Public Health 88: 20–26.
32. Agaku IT, Vardavas C, Connolly G (2013) Proposed cutoff for identifying adult smokeless tobacco users with urinary total 4-(methylnitrosamino)-1-(3-pyridyl)-1-butanonol: an aggregated analysis of NHANES 2007–2010 data. Nicotine Tob Res. 15(11): 1956–61. doi:10.1093/ntr/ntt083. Epub 2013 Aug 16.

The Effects of Chronic Cigarette Smoking on Gray Matter Volume: Influence of Sex

Teresa R. Franklin[¶1]*, **Reagan R. Wetherill**[¶1], **Kanchana Jagannathan**[1], **Barbara Johnson**[1], **Joel Mumma**[1], **Nathan Hager**[1], **Hengyi Rao**[2], **Anna Rose Childress**[1]

1 Perelman School of Medicine at the University of Pennsylvania, Department of Psychiatry, Philadelphia, Pennsylvania, United States of America, **2** Perelman School of Medicine at the University of Pennsylvania, Center for Functional Neuroimaging, Philadelphia, Pennsylvania, United States of America

Abstract

Cigarette smoke contains nicotine and toxic chemicals and may cause significant neurochemical and anatomical brain changes. Voxel-based morphometry studies have examined the effects of smoking on the brain by comparing gray matter volume (GMV) in nicotine dependent individuals (NDs) to nonsmoking individuals with inconsistent results. Although sex differences in neural and behavioral features of nicotine dependence are reported, sex differences in regional GMV remain unknown. The current study examined sex differences in GMV in a large sample of 80 NDs (41 males) and 80 healthy controls (41 males) using voxel-based morphometry. Within NDs, we explored whether GMV was correlated with measures of cigarette use and nicotine dependence. High-resolution T1 structural scans were obtained from all participants. Segmentation and registration were performed in SPM8 using the optimized DARTEL approach. Covariates included age and an estimate of total global GMV. Differences were considered significant at $p \leq 0.001$, with a whole brain FWE-corrected cluster probability of $p < 0.025$. Among NDs compared to Controls less GMV was observed in the thalamus and bilateral cerebellum and greater GMV was observed in the bilateral putamen and right parahippocampus. Lower thalamic GMV was observed in both female and male NDs compared to Controls. Female NDs also had lower GMV in the left cerebellum and in the ventral medial and orbitofrontal cortices with no areas of greater GMV. Male NDs had lower GMV in bilateral cerebellum and greater GMV in bilateral parahippocampus and left putamen. Within male NDs, GMV in the left putamen was correlated with number of pack years. This study, conducted in a large cohort, contributes to our knowledge of brain morphology in nicotine addiction and provides additional evidence of sex-specific effects on GMV in NDs. Identifying brain vulnerabilities with respect to sex provides a methodological framework for personalized therapies to improve relapse rates for both sexes.

Editor: Yu-Feng Zang, Hangzhou Normal University, China

Funding: This study was supported by grants received from National Institutes of Health (R21 DA032022 (HR), R21 DA25882 (TF), R03 DA027098 (HR), R01 HL102119 (HR), R01 DA029845 (TF), R01 DA030394-01A1 (TF)) and Pfizer Pharma (Investigator-initiated Award) (TF) and a pilot grant from the Institute for Translational Medicine and Therapeutics (ITMAT) of the University of Pennsylvania (HR). The funders had no role in study design, data collection and analysis, decision to publish, or preparation of the manuscript.

Competing Interests: Hengyi Rao is a PLOS ONE editorial board member. This does not alter the authors' adherence to PLOS ONE Editorial policies and criteria. One of the authors' sources of funding is Pfizer Pharma. This does not alter the authors' adherence to PLOS ONE policies on sharing data and materials. Further, there are no restrictions on sharing of data and/or materials.

* Email: teresafr@mail.med.upenn.edu

¶ TRF and RRW are joint first authors on this work

Introduction

Cigarette smoking is the leading cause of preventable morbidity and premature mortality worldwide [1]. Although most nicotine dependent individuals (NDs) express the desire to quit smoking, relapse rates remain high [2,3]. Preclinical studies indicate that chronic exposure to nicotine, the addictive component in cigarettes, causes significant neurochemical and pathological brain changes in fetal and adolescent rats [4,5,6]. In addition to nicotine's potential harmful effects, cigarette smoke contains numerous toxic chemicals that could contribute to the significant adverse health consequences in individuals who are chronic long-term cigarette smokers, including anatomical and chemical brain changes [7,8,9]. Understanding the vulnerabilities of the nicotine-dependent brain will aid in the development of successful treatment strategies to help us conquer this devastating and difficult to treat addiction.

Voxel-based morphometry (VBM) studies have examined the effects of chronic smoking on the brain by comparing gray matter volume (GMV) in otherwise healthy nicotine dependent individuals (NDs) to nonsmoking individuals (Controls) with inconsistent results [10,11,12,13,14,15,16]. Inconsistencies may be related to differences in methodologies and/or the populations studied. For example, although some studies identified the thalamus as a region of lower GMV in NDs [11,12], this was not observed in other studies [13,14,15,17]. Further, not all studies showed correlations with relevant smoking-related behavior. Specifically, Gallinat et al. (2006) reported that greater number of pack-years were associated with less GMV in frontal and temporal lobes; whereas, Zhang et al. (2011a) found an association between greater number of pack-years and less GMV in the left prefrontal cortex, but only in high pack-year NDs [14]. These studies, and others, suggest structural abnormalities in ND that may be related to lifetime cigarette exposure and that additional study in larger cohorts is necessary.

Although previous research highlights the adverse effects of cigarette smoking on neural structure, sex differences were not examined. Sex-specific patterns of regional GMV differences among smokers and between smokers and healthy individuals might be expected, given that numerous studies report sex differences in regional cortical and subcortical volumes in various brain disorders [18,19] including drug and alcohol dependence [20,21]. Preclinical and clinical studies indicate that females are more vulnerable to cigarette smoking initiation, nicotine dependence and have more difficulty quitting than males [22,23]. Although the exact mechanisms underlying these sex differences remain unknown, research suggests that sex differences in neural functioning and organization may influence aspects of nicotine dependence [24,25]. Knowledge of sex-specific neurophysiological anomalies in GMV associated with nicotine and cigarette smoking may provide a methodological framework for personalized therapies to improve relapse rates.

To this end, the goal of the current study was to examine differences in GMV and sex differences in GMV between NDs and matched Controls. Based on the known sex-specific differences in brain function and nicotine dependence, we hypothesized that male and female smokers would show different patterns of GMV alterations. Within ND individuals, we explored whether regional GMV was associated with cigarette use and nicotine dependence. The VBM tool in Statistical Parametric Mapping software (SPM8; Wellcome Department of Cognitive Neurology; http://www.fil.ion.ucl.ac.uk/spm) was used to accomplish this goal.

Methods

1. Subjects

Physically healthy NDs and Controls were recruited via advertisements, flyers, and referrals for fMRI studies at the University of Pennsylvania. After completing an initial telephone screen, individuals were given a description of their respective study and written informed consent was obtained. Screening procedures included a history and physical examination and a psychological assessment. The Fagerstrom Test for Nicotine Dependence (FTND) [26] assessed severity of nicotine dependence among NDs. Exclusion criteria included current DSM-IV Axis I diagnoses (other than nicotine dependence in smokers), lifetime history of head injury with loss of consciousness for more than 3 minutes, significant alcohol or drug history, contraindications for MRI, and clinically significant medical conditions. Urine drug screens verified the absence of illicit drugs in all subjects and the absence of nicotine and its major metabolite, cotinine, in Controls. Eighty NDs (41 males) and 80 Controls (41 males) matched by age, sex, and education years, met inclusion/exclusion criteria (Table 1). The study adhered to the Declaration of Helsinki and was approved by the University of Pennsylvania Institutional Review Board.

2. MR Acquisition

NDs smoked a cigarette to satiety approximately 45 minutes prior to scan acquisition. Imaging data were acquired on a Siemens 3 Tesla Trio whole-body scanner (Erlangen, Germany) at the Hospital of the University of Pennsylvania using a product eight-channel array coil. High-resolution T1-weighted anatomical

Table 1. Characteristics of nicotine-dependent cigarette smokers and non-smoking controls.

	NDs (n = 80)				Controls (n = 80)			
	Male		*Female*		*Male*		*Female*	
	n	%	n	%	n	%	n	%
	41	**51.3**	**39**	**48.7**	**41**	**51.3**	**39**	**48.7**
	Mean	*SD*	*Mean*	*SD*	*Mean*	*SD*	*Mean*	*SD*
Age (years)	35.7	11.1	31.9	10.6	33.2	7.5	30.9	7.2
Education level	14.1	2.0	14.8	2.4	13.6	2.2	14.2	2.0
Years smoking	16.0	11.3	12.0	8.4	–	–	–	–
CPD[a]	16.1	6.1	13.2	5.6	–	–	–	–
FTND	4.6	1.7	4.3	1.9	–	–	–	–
Pack years[b]	13.0	9.9	7.9	6.0	–	–	–	–

SD, standard deviation; CPD, cigarettes smoked per day; FTND, Fagerstrom Test for Nicotine Dependence; Pack-years, smoking years X CPD/20.
[a]Male NDs>female NDs, $t(79) = 2.21$, $p = 0.03$.
[b]Male NDs>female NDs, $t(79) = 2.81$, $p = 0.007$.

images were obtained using a three dimensional- magnetization prepared rapid acquisition gradient echo (3D-MPRAGE) sequence (TR = 1620 ms, TE = 3 ms, flip angle = 15°, 160 contiguous slices of 1.0 mm).

3. Data Processing

Data were preprocessed using statistical mapping software, version 8 (SPM8; Wellcome Department of Cognitive Neurology, London, UK; www.fil.ion.ucl.ac/spm) implemented in MatlabR2013 (MathWorksInc., Natick, MA, USA). Each subject's MR images were checked for structural abnormalities and reoriented to the anterior-posterior commissure line. Reorientated images were segmented into gray matter, white matter and cerebral spinal fluid in native space using the New Segmentation algorithm implemented in SPM8. This iterative procedure results in more accurate tissue classification. The resulting rigidly aligned and resliced gray and white matter tissue maps were imported into DARTEL (Diffeomorphic Anatomical Registration using Exponentiated lie Algebra), an advanced high-dimensional diffeomorphic registration algorithm within SPM8 that has been shown to improve spatial precision [27,28]. Subsequently, the study-specific gray matter templates were created from the imported maps of all subjects. The final average template was generated after six iterations by averaging all of the aligned images. During successive iterations, flow fields for each subject's images were yielded to parameterized deformations by warping to the template and then these were employed in the modulation step. The gray matter map of each subject was transformed to Montreal Neurological Institute (MNI) space by applying the deformation parameters. Next, Jacobian modulation was applied to the warped images of gray matter. The normalized modulated images were then smoothed with an 8-mm full width half maximum isotropic Gaussian kernel for statistical analyses. Data were visually inspected following each pre-processing step to ensure integrity.

4. Data analysis

Statistical parametric maps were created in SPM8 to perform between-group comparisons using the gray matter tissue segmentation output by DARTEL. A 2×2 full factorial model was used to explore differences in GMV between NDs and Controls, NDs and Controls by sex, and group X sex interactions. As it has been demonstrated that both age and total global brain measures yield significant effects on regional GMV [29,30], covariates included age and an estimate of total global GMV. Whole-brain GMV analyses were conducted using random field-based cluster-size testing, with structural differences considered significant if $p \leq 0.001$, with a whole brain FWE-corrected cluster probability of $p < 0.025$. GMV in clusters that differed between NDs and Controls were extracted using the MarsBar region of interest toolbox (http://marsbar.sourceforge.net/) and exported to IBM SPSS Statistics 19.0 (Armonk, NY) to investigate possible associations between GMV and cigarette use and dependence.

Results

Table 1 provides subject characteristics. Analysis of variance (ANOVA) was used to compare subject characteristics across groups. There were no significant differences between NDs and Controls on age, sex, or education years. Consistent with previously reported sex-specific differences in smoking behavior [31,32,33], male NDs smoked a greater number of cigarettes per day and had higher pack-years than their female counterparts. Total global GMV was not different between NDs and Controls (591.50 mm^3, SD 68.56 and 603.67 mm^3, SD 73.58, $p = 0.27$). As expected, total global GMV was greater in male NDs (629.02 mm^3, SD 60.03) compared to female NDs (553.96 mm^3, SD 55.01; $p<0.001$) and male Controls (639.11 mm^3, SD 68.62) compared to female Controls (561.87 mm^3, SD 52.64; $p<0.001$).

Table 2 provides a full summary of GMV differences. Among NDs compared to Controls, less GMV was observed in the thalamus, extending through to the medial orbitofrontal cortex, and bilateral cerebellum whereas greater GMV was observed in bilateral putamen and right parahippocampus (see Figure 1 and http://franklinbrainimaging.com: Available upon publication). There were sex-specific volume differences between NDs and Controls. Female NDs had less GMV than female Controls in the thalamus, left cerebellum, left ventrolateral prefrontal cortex, and medial orbitofrontal cortex. There were no brain regions in which female NDs had greater GMV than female Controls. ND males had significantly less GMV in the thalamus and bilateral cerebellum and significantly greater GMV in the bilateral parahippocampus (extending into the left putamen) compared to male Controls. There were no significant group X sex interactions.

Within the group of ND individuals, correlation analyses revealed that number of pack years was positively correlated with GMV in the left putamen in males ($r = .38$, $p = 0.018$). Additionally, GMV in the left cerebellum approached a significant inverse correlation with number of pack years in males ($r = -.31$, $p = 0.054$). No significant associations were found between GMV and cigarettes per day and FTND among all NDs or among male or female NDs.

Discussion

The purpose of this study was two-fold. Given the impact that chronic cigarette smoking may have on brain structure, the first goal was to conduct a systematic GMV study in a large cohort of NDs compared to Controls using an advanced registration method that provides greater sensitivity than traditional VBM. Additionally, given the importance of the influence of sex on brain structure and function in a variety of disorders, a second goal was to characterize sex differences in GMV in NDs, extending our knowledge of brain morphology in nicotine addiction. Among NDs compared to Controls, less GMV was observed in the thalamus, extending through to the medial orbitofrontal cortex (mOFC) and bilateral cerebellum whereas greater GMV was observed in bilateral putamen and right parahippocampus. Less thalamic GMV was observed in both female and male NDs. Female NDs also had lower GMV in the left cerebellum and in the ventral medial cortex and mOFC with no areas of greater GMV. Male NDs had lower GMV in bilateral cerebellum and greater GMV in bilateral parahippocampus extending into the left putamen. Positive associations were observed between pack years and GMV in the left putamen in male NDs. Additionally, GMV in the left cerebellum approached a significant inverse correlation with pack years in male NDs.

The strongest difference between NDs and Controls identified in the current report was observed in the thalamus wherein less GMV was detected in NDs as a group and in both male and female NDs. In humans, the thalamus has the highest density of nicotinic acetylcholine receptors of any brain region [34,35], and thus, constant bombardment of these receptors by chronic cigarette smoking may make it a prime target for potential morphometric anomalies. Indeed, cigarette smoking has been shown to correlate with increased nicotine binding in the human thalamus [36]. Alternatively, and not mutually exclusive, this region may be particularly susceptible to one or more of the numerous carcinogens found in cigarette smoke (e.g., acetalde-

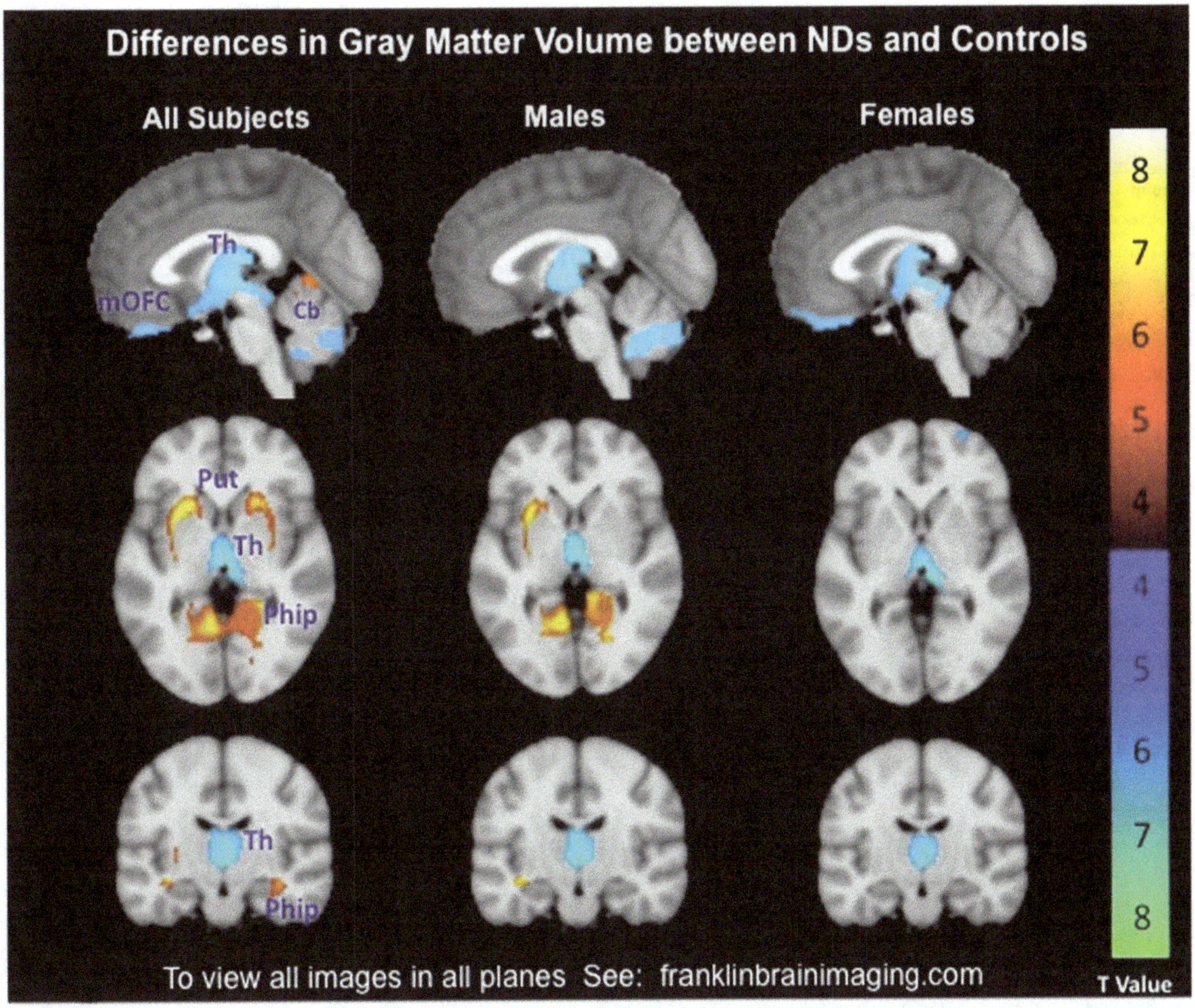

Figure 1. Differences in gray matter volume (GMV) between nicotine dependent (NDs; n = 80) and control subjects (Controls; n = 80) shown in all subjects and separately by sex (NDs, n = 41 male; Controls, n = 41 male). Representative MRI sagittal, axial, and coronal brain slices analyzed in SPM8 and overlain on the Montreal Neurological Institute brain. Slice shown is centered within the thalamus (x, y, z; 0, −16, 0). Hot colors represent regions of greater GMV, while cool colors represent regions of less GMV in NDs compared to Controls. T values range from 4.42 to 8.06, significant in whole brain analysis at $p<0.001$, and FWE cluster-corrected $p<0.025$. Images are displayed neurologically. An interactive visual display of all brain data in all three planes can be found at http://franklinbrainimaging.com (Available upon publication).

hyde, arsenic, benzene) [9]. The finding of less thalamic GMV is consistent with the findings of some studies [11,12] but not all [10,14,15]. Given that cigarette smoking behavior is multi-faceted and complex, and that various aspects of the behavior are modulated by both known [37,38,39] and unknown factors, we speculate that differences in other characteristics across studies are contributing to the variable results.

The cerebellum was also identified as a region wherein less GMV was observed in NDs compared to Controls; however, sex-specific analyses show this finding to be stronger and bilateral in male NDs. Yu and colleagues (2011) studied only males and also identified a region of the cerebellum (bilateral) as a region of lower GMV in ND [13]. Kuhn and colleagues (2012) conducted a GMV study in NDs versus Controls specifically targeting the cerebellum [17]. The study, conducted in both sexes, showed significantly less GMV in the right cerebellum compared to Controls, with peak coordinates similar to those observed in the current study. Our results provoke speculation that the cerebellar effects observed by Kuhn et al. (2012) may be sex-specific. NDs show greater density of nicotine binding in the cerebellum (from 70–200%) compared to nonsmoking individuals [40], and brain blood flow in the cerebellum is increased by cigarette smoking [41,42]. Further, plasma nicotine levels, which are elevated by smoking cigarettes, correlate with increased cerebellar blood flow [41]. Thus, potential pathophysiological effects associated with chronic smoking could at least partially account for this result. The effect may be stronger in males because of their greater exposure to cigarettes (i.e., greater number of pack-years).

The cluster of less thalamic GMV in NDs extended medially through the brain to the medial frontal gyrus, including the mOFC. GMV in prefrontal regions was unchanged in male NDs compared to male Controls but was less in female NDs compared to female Controls. Most previous studies have demonstrated reduced prefrontal GMV in NDs [10,11,12,16] while some studies

Table 2. Clusters of gray matter volume differences between NDs and Controls.

Region	Cluster size (voxels)	MNI coordinates			*T*-value	*p value FWE cor*
		x	*y*	*z*		
Group effect						
NDs<Controls						
Thalamus	1851	4	−18	2	8.06	0.001
Medial prefrontal cortex [a]		2	36	−30	4.78	
L Cerebellum	2827	−40	−70	−42	6.19	0.001
R Cerebellum	1987	30	−50	−50	4.83	0.001
NDs>Controls						
L Putamen	777	−28	8	−8	7.16	0.001
R Putamen	546	22	18	4	5.44	0.007
R Parahippocampus	2319	20	−40	−8	6.32	0.001
Sex effect						
Females: NDs<Controls						
Thalamus	891	6	−26	−2	7.07	0.001
L Cerebellum	943	−40	−72	−42	4.80	0.001
Ventral medial prefrontal cortex	540	36	60	−10	4.48	0.007
Medial orbitofrontal cortex	857	−6	24	−28	4.42	0.001
Females: NDs>Controls						
No significant clusters						
Males: NDs<Controls						
Thalamus	777	4	−14	0	5.45	0.001
R Cerebellum	1909	28	−54	−50	5.15	0.001
L Cerebellum	1627	−32	−64	−52	4.60	0.006
Males: NDs>Controls						
R Parahippocampus	660	18	−38	−8	6.30	0.001
L Parahipppocampus	472	−34	−10	−14	5.28	0.012
L Putamen[b]		−30	10	−2	5.13	

All clusters are significant in whole brain analysis at $p<0.001$, and FWE cluster-corrected $p<0.025$.
Coordinates listed are in Montreal Neurological Institute (MNI) space. L, left; R, right.
[a]extended from within the thalamic cluster.
[b]extended from within the left parahippocampal cluster.

have not [14,15]. Our results showing that this finding may be 'carried' by female NDs, may help explain these inconsistencies. Some support for this idea is provided by Yu and colleagues (2011), who studied only males, and did not find differences between NDs and Controls in prefrontal regions [13]. Given the role of the medial ventral regions of the prefrontal cortex in reward [43,44] and the development and maintenance of addiction [45,46], it is surprising that this finding was observed only in females, however resting cerebral blood flow (CBF) differs between male and female NDs in the mOFC [24], which could potentially lead to differences in regional GMV. Further, the mOFC is heavily involved in inhibition of behavior [47]. Less GMV in this region in female NDs may be related to the greater difficulty female NDs have in quitting smoking compared to male NDs [22].

In the present study, NDs had more GMV than Controls in the bilateral putamen. Striatal abnormalities are thought to underlie habitual, compulsive drug seeking and use [48,49] and other psychiatric disorders characterized by repetitive, compulsive behaviors [50,51]. Further, a meta-analysis has shown that severity of compulsivity has been associated with greater putamen GMV [52]. As such, the greater putamen GMV observed in NDs may be associated with long-term, compulsive cigarette smoking behavior. This suggestion is mildly supported by the finding of a positive association between pack years and GMV in the left putamen in male NDs.

In the present study, the parahippocampus showed greater GMV in NDs compared to Controls, but sex-specific analyses showed greater GMV in the parahippocampus only in male NDs. In direct comparisons between sexes we have shown that appetitive smoking cues (reminders to smoke) evoke greater bilateral hippocampal/amygdalar activation among males [24]. The hippocampus and amygdala are structures associated with emotional and drug memories [53,54] and as such, our previous findings may be explained by sex-specific memory-related differences to smoking cues. Specifically, females may be more efficient at retrieving autobiographical memories [55,56], while males show greater hippocampal activation to autobiographical memories [57]. Thus, males may require greater memory-related, hippocampal-amygdalar brain activity when retrieving cue-associated memories. Increased activity in brain is theoretically coupled to the delivery of life-sustaining blood and nutrients. One might tentatively speculate that chronic increased activity in this region, may lead to a relative expansion in GMV.

We hypothesized that the toxic chemicals found in tobacco smoke cause detrimental effects on brain morphology. Using pack-years as an estimate of lifetime cigarette smoke exposure, we explored whether associations existed between GMV and cigarette exposure. Associations between GMV and pack years were observed only in males; positive associations were observed in the putamen and negative associations were observed in the cerebellum. These results are inconsistent with the extant literature, which itself is inconsistent. Specifically, Gallinat et al. (2006) reported that greater pack-years were associated with less GMV in frontal and temporal lobes; whereas, Zhang et al. (2011a) found an association between greater pack-years and less GMV in the left prefrontal cortex, but only in high pack-year NDs [11,14]. In a separate report, Zhang et al. (2011b) observed a trend in dorsolateral prefrontal cortex, yet no correlations were observed in the ROI analysis conducted by Brody and colleagues [10]. Combined, the existing literature and our report do not provide conclusive evidence that exposure to cigarette smoke, as defined by pack-years, affects brain morphometry. This is not completely unexpected due to the intrinsic confounds of human neuroimaging studies where subjective measures are used to draw associations between behavior and brain. Pack-years is a measure derived by the subjective responses of individuals to only two items regarding smoking history. The measure assumes that smoking behavior has not changed since initiation and that accurate reports can be provided. Although perfecting the pack-year measure will not abolish all of its inherent flaws, a better measure could and should be developed to examine the effects of cigarette smoke exposure on GMV.

As with any study conducted in drug-dependent individuals, inferences about what differences between groups in GMV signify cannot exclude the possibility that brain volume differed prior to cigarette smoking initiation. Pre-existing differences in GMV could predispose an individual to a number of aspects of drug use including experiencing increased positive responses to the reinforcing properties of the drug, reduced negative responses to its aversive properties, and/or reduced ability to inhibit aberrant behavior.

It should be noted that GMV differences between NDs and Controls in this and other studies could at least in part be a transient difference modulated by recent smoking. The use of T1-weighted scans to identify change in brain structure *in vivo* in humans has vulnerability: the T1 relaxation time for arterial blood and gray matter are not clearly distinguishable and therefore, apparent reported GMV findings might be at least partially related to changes in CBF or other physiological signals [58,59]. For example, we observed medication-induced decreases in GMV in the cingulate and other regions that overlapped with changes in CBF following just one dose of medication [60]. If a single dose of medication can alter brain volume as indexed by VBM, it is conceivable that recent smoking could have a similar effect, especially in light of evidence that cigarette smoking induces regional alterations in CBF [41,42,61]. In the current study, NDs smoked a cigarette approximately 45 minutes prior to scan acquisition. Given that physiological responses to cigarette smoking dissipate within 20 min [plasma nicotine levels peak at 5 minutes and return to a steady concentration within 10 minutes [41] and myocardial blood flow measured after smoking returns to normal within 50 minutes [62], this should not be a confounding factor, but it cannot be ruled out.

This study is limited in that we did not obtain a full alcohol and/or illicit drug history on the subjects. However, having a significant alcohol and/or drug history was an exclusion criterion for both groups and urine drug screens verified the absence of illicit drugs in all subjects.

This study, conducted in a large cohort of NDs and matched Controls, contributes to our knowledge of brain morphology in nicotine addiction by providing in-depth analyses using an advanced registration technique and by expanding our knowledge on sex-specific effects in cigarette smokers. Identifying brain vulnerabilities with respect to sex provides a methodological framework for personalized therapies to improve relapse rates for both males and females.

Acknowledgments

The authors would like to thank the clinical and support staff, with special thanks to Melanie Maron (Study Coordinator), at the Center for the Studies of Addiction, Perelman School of Medicine at the University of Pennsylvania and the MRI technical staff at the Hospital of the University of Pennsylvania.

Author Contributions

Conceived and designed the experiments: TF RRW AC. Performed the experiments: BJ JM NH HR TF. Analyzed the data: KJ TF RRW. Contributed reagents/materials/analysis tools: HR TF AC. Contributed to the writing of the manuscript: TF RRW HR AC JM BJ KJ.

References

1. Centers for Disease Control and Prevention (2008) Smoking-Attributable Mortality, Years of Potential Life Lost, and Productivity Losses–United States, 2000–2004.
2. Baillie AJ, Mattick RP, Hall W (1995) Quitting smoking: estimation by meta-analysis of the rate of unaided smoking cessation. Australian journal of public health 19: 129–131.
3. Hughes JR, Shiffman S, Callas P, Zhang J (2003) A meta-analysis of the efficacy of over-the-counter nicotine replacement. Tobacco control 12: 21–27.
4. Dwyer JB, McQuown SC, Leslie FM (2009) The dynamic effects of nicotine on the developing brain. Pharmacology & therapeutics 122: 125–139.
5. Trauth JA, Seidler FJ, McCook EC, Slotkin TA (1999) Adolescent nicotine exposure causes persistent upregulation of nicotinic cholinergic receptors in rat brain regions. Brain research 851: 9–19.
6. Slotkin TA (2002) Nicotine and the adolescent brain: insights from an animal model. Neurotoxicology and teratology 24: 369–384.
7. Swan GE, Lessov-Schlaggar CN (2007) The effects of tobacco smoke and nicotine on cognition and the brain. Neuropsychology review 17: 259–273.
8. Longstreth WT, Jr., Bernick C, Fitzpatrick A, Cushman M, Knepper L, et al. (2001) Frequency and predictors of stroke death in 5,888 participants in the Cardiovascular Health Study. Neurology 56: 368–375.
9. The National Toxicology Program on behalf of the Secretary HaHS, Kathleen Sebelius (2011) Report on Carcinogens. Department of Health and Human Services.
10. Brody AL, Mandelkern MA, Jarvik ME, Lee GS, Smith EC, et al. (2004) Differences between smokers and nonsmokers in regional gray matter volumes and densities. Biological psychiatry 55: 77–84.
11. Gallinat J, Meisenzahl E, Jacobsen LK, Kalus P, Bierbrauer J, et al. (2006) Smoking and structural brain deficits: a volumetric MR investigation. The European journal of neuroscience 24: 1744–1750.
12. Liao Y, Tang J, Liu T, Chen X, Hao W (2012) Differences between smokers and non-smokers in regional gray matter volumes: a voxel-based morphometry study. Addiction biology 17: 977–980.
13. Yu R, Zhao L, Lu L (2011) Regional grey and white matter changes in heavy male smokers. PloS one 6: e27440.
14. Zhang X, Salmeron BJ, Ross TJ, Geng X, Yang Y, et al. (2011a) Factors underlying prefrontal and insula structural alterations in smokers. NeuroImage 54: 42–48.
15. Zhang X, Salmeron BJ, Ross TJ, Gu H, Geng X, et al. (2011b) Anatomical differences and network characteristics underlying smoking cue reactivity. NeuroImage 54: 131–141.
16. Morales AM, Lee B, Hellemann G, O'Neill J, London ED (2012) Gray-matter volume in methamphetamine dependence: cigarette smoking and changes with

abstinence from methamphetamine. Drug and alcohol dependence 125: 230–238.

17. Kuhn S, Romanowski A, Schilling C, Mobascher A, Warbrick T, et al. (2012) Brain grey matter deficits in smokers: focus on the cerebellum. Brain structure & function 217: 517–522.
18. Cahill L (2006) Why sex matters for neuroscience. Nature reviews Neuroscience 7: 477–484.
19. Cosgrove KP, Mazure CM, Staley JK (2007) Evolving knowledge of sex differences in brain structure, function, and chemistry. Biological psychiatry 62: 847–855.
20. Rando K, Tuit K, Hannestad J, Guarnaccia J, Sinha R (2013) Sex differences in decreased limbic and cortical grey matter volume in cocaine dependence: a voxel-based morphometric study. Addiction biology 18: 147–160.
21. Pfefferbaum A, Rosenbloom M, Deshmukh A, Sullivan E (2001) Sex differences in the effects of alcohol on brain structure. The American journal of psychiatry 158: 188–197.
22. Becker JB, Hu M (2008) Sex differences in drug abuse. Frontiers in neuroendocrinology 29: 36–47.
23. Lynch WJ, Sofuoglu M (2010) Role of progesterone in nicotine addiction: evidence from initiation to relapse. Experimental and clinical psychopharmacology 18: 451–461.
24. Wetherill RR, Young KA, Jagannathan K, Shin J, O'Brien CP, et al. (2013) The impact of sex on brain responses to smoking cues: a perfusion fMRI study. Biology of sex differences 4: 9.
25. Wetherill RR, Jagannathan K, Shin J, Franklin TR (2014) Sex differences in resting state neural networks of nicotine-dependent cigarette smokers. Addictive behaviors 39: 789–792.
26. Fagerstrom KO, Schneider NG (1989) Measuring nicotine dependence: a review of the Fagerstrom Tolerance Questionnaire. Journal of Behavioral Medicine 12: 159–182.
27. Ashburner J (2007) A fast diffeomorphic image registration algorithm. NeuroImage 38: 95–113.
28. Mak HK, Zhang Z, Yau KK, Zhang L, Chan Q, et al. (2011) Efficacy of voxel-based morphometry with DARTEL and standard registration as imaging biomarkers in Alzheimer's disease patients and cognitively normal older adults at 3.0 Tesla MR imaging. Journal of Alzheimer's disease : JAD 23: 655–664.
29. Good CD, Johnsrude I, Ashburner J, Henson RN, Friston KJ, et al. (2001) Cerebral asymmetry and the effects of sex and handedness on brain structure: a voxel-based morphometric analysis of 465 normal adult human brains. NeuroImage 14: 685–700.
30. Good CD, Johnsrude IS, Ashburner J, Henson RN, Friston KJ, et al. (2001b) A voxel-based morphometric study of ageing in 465 normal adult human brains. NeuroImage 14: 21–36.
31. Drum ML, Shiovitz-Ezra S, Gaumer E, Lindau ST (2009) Assessment of smoking behaviors and alcohol use in the national social life, health, and aging project. The journals of gerontology Series B, Psychological sciences and social sciences 64 Suppl 1: i119–130.
32. Kandel DB, Chen K (2000) Extent of smoking and nicotine dependence in the United States: 1991–1993. Nicotine & tobacco research : official journal of the Society for Research on Nicotine and Tobacco 2: 263–274.
33. Buist AS, Connett JE, Miller RD, Kanner RE, Owens GR, et al. (1993) Chronic Obstructive Pulmonary Disease Early Intervention Trial (Lung Health Study). Baseline characteristics of randomized participants. Chest 103: 1863–1872.
34. Picard F, Sadaghiani S, Leroy C, Courvoisier DS, Maroy R, et al. (2013) High density of nicotinic receptors in the cingulo-insular network. NeuroImage 79: 42–51.
35. Paterson D, Nordberg A (2000) Neuronal nicotinic receptors in the human brain. Progress in neurobiology 61: 75–111.
36. Breese CR, Marks MJ, Logel J, Adams CE, Sullivan B, et al. (1997) Effect of smoking history on [3H]nicotine binding in human postmortem brain. The Journal of pharmacology and experimental therapeutics 282: 7–13.
37. Bergen AW, Conti DV, Van Den Berg D, Lee W, Liu J, et al. (2009) Dopamine genes and nicotine dependence in treatment-seeking and community smokers. Neuropsychopharmacology : official publication of the American College of Neuropsychopharmacology 34: 2252–2264.
38. Franklin TR, Wang Z, Li Y, Suh JJ, Goldman M, et al. (2011) Dopamine transporter genotype modulation of neural responses to smoking cues: confirmation in a new cohort. Addiction biology 16: 308–322.
39. Wetherill RR, Jagannathan K, Lohoff FW, Ehrman R, O'Brien CP, et al. (2012) Neural correlates of attentional bias for smoking cues: modulation by variance in the dopamine transporter gene. Addiction biology.
40. Court JA, Lloyd S, Thomas N, Piggott MA, Marshall EF, et al. (1998) Dopamine and nicotinic receptor binding and the levels of dopamine and homovanillic acid in human brain related to tobacco use. Neuroscience 87: 63–78.
41. Domino EF, Ni L, Xu Y, Koeppe RA, Guthrie S, et al. (2004) Regional cerebral blood flow and plasma nicotine after smoking tobacco cigarettes. Progress in neuro-psychopharmacology & biological psychiatry 28: 319–327.
42. Zubieta JK, Heitzeg MM, Xu Y, Koeppe RA, Ni L, et al. (2005) Regional cerebral blood flow responses to smoking in tobacco smokers after overnight abstinence. The American journal of psychiatry 162: 567–577.
43. Rolls ET (2004) The functions of the orbitofrontal cortex. Brain and cognition 55: 11–29.
44. Kringelbach ML, Rolls ET (2004) The functional neuroanatomy of the human orbitofrontal cortex: evidence from neuroimaging and neuropsychology. Progress in neurobiology 72: 341–372.
45. Goldstein RZ, Tomasi D, Rajaram S, Cottone LA, Zhang L, et al. (2007) Role of the anterior cingulate and medial orbitofrontal cortex in processing drug cues in cocaine addiction. Neuroscience 144: 1153–1159.
46. Volkow ND, Fowler JS (2000) Addiction, a disease of compulsion and drive: involvement of the orbitofrontal cortex. Cerebral cortex 10: 318–325.
47. Rolls ET (2004) The functions of the orbitofrontal cortex. Brain Cogn 55: 11–29.
48. Koob GF, Volkow ND (2010) Neurocircuitry of addiction. Neuropsychopharmacology : official publication of the American College of Neuropsychopharmacology 35: 217–238.
49. Everitt BJ, Robbins TW (2005) Neural systems of reinforcement for drug addiction: from actions to habits to compulsion. Nature neuroscience 8: 1481–1489.
50. Hollander E, Anagnostou E, Chaplin W, Esposito K, Haznedar MM, et al. (2005) Striatal volume on magnetic resonance imaging and repetitive behaviors in autism. Biological psychiatry 58: 226–232.
51. Scarone S, Colombo C, Livian S, Abbruzzese M, Ronchi P, et al. (1992) Increased right caudate nucleus size in obsessive-compulsive disorder: detection with magnetic resonance imaging. Psychiatry research 45: 115–121.
52. Radua J, Mataix-Cols D (2009) Voxel-wise meta-analysis of grey matter changes in obsessive-compulsive disorder. The British journal of psychiatry : the journal of mental science 195: 393–402.
53. Mackiewicz KL, Sarinopoulos I, Cleven KL, Nitschke JB (2006) The effect of anticipation and the specificity of sex differences for amygdala and hippocampus function in emotional memory. Proceedings of the National Academy of Sciences of the United States of America 103: 14200–14205.
54. Chase HW, Eickhoff SB, Laird AR, Hogarth L (2011) The neural basis of drug stimulus processing and craving: an activation likelihood estimation meta-analysis. Biological psychiatry 70: 785–793.
55. Andreano JM, Cahill L (2009) Sex influences on the neurobiology of learning and memory. Learning & memory 16: 248–266.
56. Seidlitz L, Diener E (1998) Sex differences in the recall of affective experiences. Journal of personality and social psychology 74: 262–271.
57. Piefke M, Weiss PH, Markowitsch HJ, Fink GR (2005) Gender differences in the functional neuroanatomy of emotional episodic autobiographical memory. Human brain mapping 24: 313–324.
58. Salgado-Pineda P, Delaveau P, Falcon C, Blin O (2006) Brain T1 intensity changes after levodopa administration in healthy subjects: a voxel-based morphometry study. British journal of clinical pharmacology 62: 546–551.
59. Yamasue H, Abe O, Kasai K, Suga M, Iwanami A, et al. (2007) Human brain structural change related to acute single exposure to sarin. Annals of neurology 61: 37–46.
60. Franklin TR, Wang Z, Shin J, Jagannathan K, Suh JJ, et al. (2012) A VBM study demonstrating 'apparent' effects of a single dose of medication on T1-weighted MRIs. Brain structure & function.
61. Rose JE, Behm FM, Westman EC, Mathew RJ, London ED, et al. (2003) PET studies of the influences of nicotine on neural systems in cigarette smokers. The American journal of psychiatry 160: 323–333.
62. Czernin J, Sun K, Brunken R, Bottcher M, Phelps M, et al. (1995) Effect of acute and long-term smoking on myocardial blood flow and flow reserve. Circulation 91: 2891–2897.

Blocking TRPV1 in Nucleus Accumbens Inhibits Persistent Morphine Conditioned Place Preference Expression in Rats

Li-Jun Heng[1,2], Bo Huang[1], Heng Guo[3], Lian-Ting Ma[2], Wei-Xin Yuan[1], Jian Song[2], Peng Wang[1,2], Guo-Zheng Xu[2]*, Guo-Dong Gao[1]*

1 Department of Neurosurgery, Tangdu Hospital of Fourth Military Medical University, Xi'an, Shaanxi, China, **2** Department of Neurosurgery, Wuhan General Hospital of Guangzhou Military Command, Wuhan, Hubei, China, **3** Department of Neurosurgery, PLA Chengdu General Hospital, Chengdu, Sichuan, China

Abstract

The function of TRPV1 (transient receptor potential vanilloid subfamily, member 1) in the central nervous system is gradually elucidated. It has been recently proved to be expressed in nucleus accumbens (NAc), a region playing an essential role in mediating opioid craving and taking behaviors. Based on the general role of TRPV1 antagonist in blocking neural over-excitability by both pre- and post-synaptic mechanisms, TRPV1 antagonist capsazepine (CPZ) was tested for its ability to prohibit persistent opioid craving in rats. In the present study, we assessed the expression of TRPV1 in nucleus accumbens and investigated the effect of CPZ in bilateral nucleus accumbens on persistent morphine conditioned place preference (mCPP) in rats. We also evaluated the side-effect of CPZ on activity by comparing cross-beam times between groups. We found that morphine conditioned place preference increased the TRPV1 expression and CPZ attenuated morphine conditioned place preference in a dose-dependent and target-specific manner after both short- and long-term spontaneous withdrawal, reflected by the reduction of the increased time in morphine-paired side. CPZ (10 nM) could induce prolonged and stable inhibition of morphine conditioned place preference expression. More importantly, CPZ did not cause dysfunction of activity in the subjects tested, which indicates the inhibitory effect was not obtained at the sacrifice of regular movement. Collectively, these results indicated that injection of TRPV1 antagonist in nucleus accumbens is capable of attenuating persistent morphine conditioned place preference without affecting normal activity. Thus, TRPV1 antagonist is one of the promising therapeutic drugs for the treatment of opioid addiction.

Editor: Yael Abreu-Villaça, Universidade do Estado do Rio de Janeiro, Brazil

Funding: This work is supported by National Natural Science Foundation of China (31070940 to GDG, 31100778 to LJH), Military 12th Five-year Program of China (BWS11J006 to GZX), Scientific Research Foundation for the Returned Overseas Chinese Scholars, State Education Ministry (SRFROCS1711 to LJH), Tangdu Outstanding Talents Surporting Project (Tangdu5084 to LJH) and China Postdoctoral Science Foundation. The funders had no role in study design, data collection and analysis, decision to publish, or preparation of the manuscript.

Competing Interests: The authors have declared that no competing interests exist.

* Email: gaogd@outlook.com (GDG); xu-gz@163.com (GZX)

These authors contributed equally to this work.

Introduction

Opioid addiction is a type of complex brain disorder, which is characterized by uncontrollable opioid craving and compulsive opioid seeking and taking behavior regardless of consequences. High incidence of drug craving and relapse to drug seeking and taking behaviors is the main obstacle for treatment [1]. As traditional therapy fail to work well in preventing relapse in opioid addicts, more effective and target-specific pharmacotherapies with little side effect are in demand.

TRPV1 (transient receptor potential vanilloid subfamily, member 1) is a nonselective cation channel that could be activated by heat, proton, capsaicin and endogenous ligands endovanilloids [2–4]. TRPV1 distributed in a variety of areas in the central nervous system [5–8]. It has been gradually established that TRPV1 had important role in a series of physiological and pathological status, such as neural development, anxiety and depression. There is still limited information about the function of central TRPV1 in drug addiction, especially in opioid addiction. Previous research suggested that repeated systematic blockade of TRPV1 by capsazepine (CPZ), a TRPV1 antagonist, significantly reduced naloxone-induced withdrawal symptoms [9]. However, there was no further tests of the effect of CPZ on morphine craving or relapse, which is the core process of addiction [1]. Recently, it has been reported that TRPV1 antagonist decreased cocaine-induced cocaine-seeking behavior [10]. Both findings suggest the engagement of TRPV1 in drug addiction behaviors. However, considering the limitation of the animal model used, the difference between opioid and psychostimulant dependence [11] and the peripheral effects accompanying systematic delivery of TRPV1 blocker, further studies are needed to clarify the central action site and behavioral role for TRPV1 in opioid relapse.

Nucleus accumbens (NAc) was known as a critical region in mediating opioid relapse, and has been found to express TRPV1 [5,6]. Anatomical and electrophysiological studies suggest the possible subcellular localization of NAc TRPV1 is mainly in the presynaptic terminals and the cell bodies [5,6,12,13]. Presynaptic TRPV1 has been proved to facilitate glutamate release and accordingly potentiate glutamatergic transmission in widespread brain areas [13–21]. Importantly, the enhancement of glutamatergic synaptic strength via increased presynaptic release in NAc is an essential neuroadaptation during withdrawal associated with opioid dependence [22]. Blockade or attenuation of NAc glutamatergic transmission to reduce the excitatory drive may prevent relapse to opioid use [23–25]. In another aspect, TRPV1 present in the cell bodies are proposed to modulate neuronal activity [20]. TRPV1 agonist could increase the spike frequency of neurons in ventral tegmental area [26]. These observations strongly suggested that NAc TRPV1 antagonism might perform anti-relapse effect by limiting neuronal activity and diminishing the efficacy of excitatory inputs from presynaptic terminals, which could reduce morphine conditioned place preference (mCPP) expression [27].

Taken together, the TRPV1 receptor in nucleus accumbens could be a potential target for preventing opioid relapse. In the present study, we test the effect of blocking TRPV1 in NAc on persistent mCPP expression in rats and assess the influence of TRPV1 antagonist on motor activity in the same subjects.

Materials and Methods

Subjects and surgery

Male Sprague–Dawley rats (initial weight 200–250 g; Centre of Experimental Animals, Fourth Military Medical University, Xi'an, Shaanxi, China) were individually housed in a temperature- and humidity-controlled vivarium on a 12-hour light/dark cycle. All rats were allowed ad libitum access to food and water. Rats were acclimated to handling daily and allowed to adapt for at least 3 days before the experiment. This study was carried out in strict accordance with the Chinese Animal Welfare Act. The protocol was approved by the Committee on the Ethics of Animal Experiments of Tangdu Hospital of Fourth Military Medical University (Permit Number: TD-5084). All surgery was performed under chloral hydrate anesthesia, and all efforts were made to minimize suffering.

Rats were anesthetized with chloral hydrate (400 mg/kg, i.p.) and implanted with cannulas (0.67 mm of external diameter; Rewardsales, Shenzhen, Guangdong, China) positioned 1.5 mm above each target. The coordinates (Paxinos and Watson, 2005) were as follows respectively: NAc core: anteroposterior (AP), + 1.5 mm and mediolateral (ML), ±1.6 mm from bregma; dorsoventral (DV), −6.0 mm from the skull surface; Dorsal striatum (DS): AP, +0.9 mm; ML, ±3.4 mm; DV, −3.8 mm. The cannulas were anchored to the skull with stainless steel screws and dental cement. A stainless steel probe with a plastic cap was inserted into each cannula to keep them unblocked and prevent infection. Rats were allowed to recover from surgery for at least 5d before morphine conditioned preference training. Food intake and body weights were assessed before and after the surgery.

Morphine conditioned place preference

All experiments were performed in a dimly lit room. The CPP apparatus is composed of two equally sized wooden chambers(25.3×20.1×20.3 cm) separated by a guillotine door. The two chambers differ in their color and floor texture to provide distinct contexts that were paired with morphine or saline injections. One chamber consisted of white walls and a smooth PVC-covered floor with hollow tranverse lines. The other chamber had black walls and a coarse PVC-covered floor with hollow longitudinal lines. The procedure consisted of three different phases: preconditioning test (day 1), conditioning (day 2-day 6), and postconditioning tests, as indicated in Results. In the preconditioning test, each rat was placed in the white compartment with the door open to allow the animal to freely explore the apparatus for 15 min. Animals showing a strong unconditioned preference (>540 s in any chamber), which were 7 of the 135 rats totally used, were discarded. In the subsequent 5 days, conditioning was conducted using a counterbalanced protocol, such that one-half of the animals in each experimental group were conditioned to the spontaneously preferred side and the other half to the spontaneously nonpreferred side. In each conditioning day, the animals received an injection of either morphine (1 mg/kg, 3 mg/kg, 10 mg/kg, s.c.) or saline (1 ml/kg, s.c.) at 9:00–9:30 and were confined for 45 min in the assigned chamber before returning to their home cages. Six hours later, the animals received an injection of vehicle solution (saline, 1 ml/kg, s.c.) and were confined to the alternative chamber for 45 min. In the postconditioning phase, the expression of CPP was tested in withdrawal day 1, 7 (1 w, short-term withdrawal), 14 (2 w) and 21 (3 w, long-term withdrawal) after the last training session. The postconditioning test consisted of placing the animal into the white chamber and allowing it to freely access both chambers for 15 min. Videos of all 15 min tests were captured online and analyzed offline. The amount of time that the animals spend in the conditioned chamber was recorded as CPP score (in seconds).

Intra-NAc application of CPZ

All rats firstly received mCPP training with 10 mg/kg morphine as described earlier. CPZ was dissolved in DMSO and stored at the concentration of 100 μM, which was diluted to different concentrations for intracranial injection with at most 0.1% DMSO in final solution. Vehicle solutions were prepared accordingly. CPZ (0.1 nM, 1 nM, 10 nM) or vehicle was injected bilateral intra-NAc daily from 3 days before the mCPP expression test during short-term (1 w) or long-term (3 w) withdrawal. CPZ (1 μl) was delivered over 3 min for each side of target. The CPP test was

Table 1. The food intake and body weight of animals after surgery (Means±SEM).

Measured parameters	Control	Surgery
Food intake (g/d)	23.01±4.93	22.76±4.09
Initial body weight (g)	208.96±10.07	211.10±11.28
Body weight after recover (g)	219.92±7.16*	221.20±9.51*

*$p<0.05$, compared to the initial body weight.

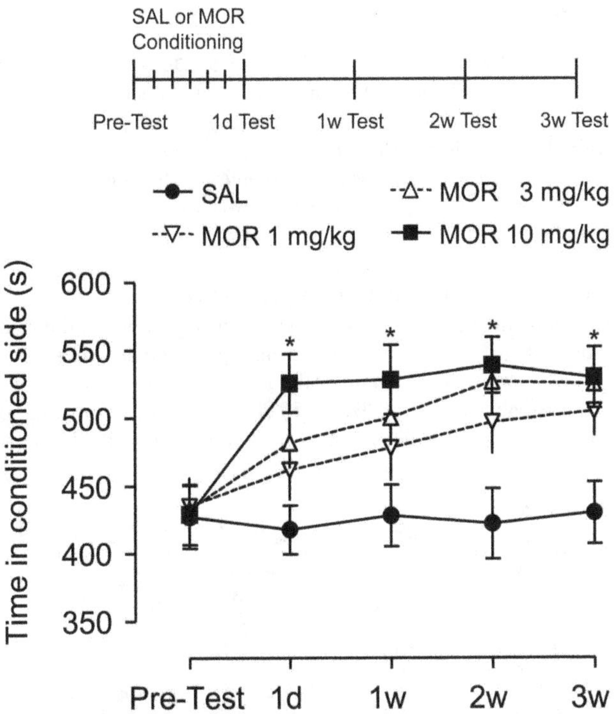

Figure 1. Repeated morphine conditioning induced persistent conditioned place preference (CPP) during withdrawal. Morphine conditioned place preference scores (time spent in drug-paired chamber) increased during morphine withdrawal. Sustained increase of mCPP score during morphine withdrawal occurred in high-dose morphine group (10 mg/kg) but not in low- (1 mg/kg) or moderate-dose (3 mg/kg) groups (n = 3). *$p<0.01$, *vs* SAL group. SAL, saline; MOR, morphine.

performed 30 min after the last CPZ injection. Furthermore, to examine the target specific effect of CPZ on mCPP, CPZ (10 nM) was injected unilateral NAc or bilateral DS before mCPP test during short-term (1 w) withdrawal.

Motor activity assessment

To assess the effects of CPZ on motor activity, crossline times were counted manually from the video of mCPP test after CPZ injection. Crossline times was defined as sum of the counts of the subject moving cross the two putative transverse lines trisecting each chamber and the counts of the subject crossing the guillotine door.

Immunoelectron microscopy

After the behavior test, rats were anesthetized with chloral hydrate (400 mg/kg, i.p.) and perfused intracardially with 100 ml of physiological saline (0.9% NaCl), followed by perfusion with a fixative containing 0.05% glutaraldehyde, 4% paraformaldehyde and 15% picric acid. The brain was removed from the skull and post-fixed in the above fixative without glutaraldehyde at room temperature for 2 hours. Vibratome sections 50 μm in thickness were cut from the blocks. Following washing in 0.01 M PBS, the sections were cryoprotected in 30% sucrose until they sunk. The sections were washed in 0.01 M PBS and incubated in blocking solution (5% NGS+5% BSA) at room temperature for 3 hours. After washing in 0.01 M PBS, the sections were incubated in rabbit anti-TRPV1 antibodies (1:150, Santa Cruz Biotechnology) and containing 1% BSA for 48 hours at 4°C. Following incubation with the primary antiserum, the sections were processed for immunogold labeling of rabbit TRPV1 antiserum. The tissue was rinsed in PBS and incubated overnight at 4°C in a 1:50 dilution of colloidal gold conjugated to goat anti-rabbit IgG (Nanoprobes) in 1% BSA. The sections were rinsed in PBS and post-fixed in 2% glutaraldehyde for 45 minutes. They were then rinsed in deionized water 10 times, and the gold particles were silver intensified by a 9-minute incubation in an HQ Silver silver enhancer (Nanoprobes). After rinsing in deionized water and 0.1 M PB 6 times, the sections were osmicated (0.5% OsO4, 1 hour, room temperature), dehydrated and embedded in Durcupan. After examination by light microscopy, the areas of interest were re-embedded and ultrathin-sectioned for electron microscopy. Ultrathin serial sections were collected on formvar-coated single slot grids, stained with lead citrate and washed in distilled water. Sections were observed under an electron microscope (JEM-1230).

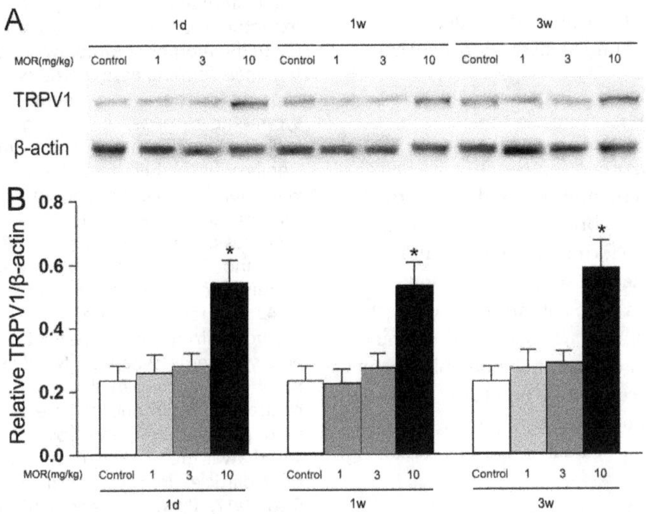

Figure 2. Analysis of western blot results of TRPV1 expression in the nucleus accumbens (NAc). (A) Representative blots of TRPV1. β-actin showed similar protein loading in each group. (B) Densitometric analyses of TRPV1 expression in NAc. The changes were expressed as the ratio to β-actin. Data represent Mean±SEM (n = 3), *$p<0.01$, *vs* control group.

The quantity of the symmetric and asymmetric synapses established by TRPV1-positive axon terminals was examined in the NAc. Serial ultrathin sections were made from a depth of ~3 μm from the surface of the vibratome sections. Every 8th section the TRPV1-stained terminals were analyzed in order, following the rules of systematic random sampling, to avoid sampling the same axon terminals. The number of TRPV1 terminals forming symmetric and asymmetric synapses was calculated for each group and normalized to 3000 μm^2 to quantify the exact changes in the number of stained terminals in each group. To assess any changes occurring in the density of TRPV1 per terminal, the number of gold particles located in the membrane of the axon terminals was counted and normalized to 1 μm of the terminal's perimeter. Image-Pro Plus 6.0 was used to make the above measurements.

Western blot

After sacrifice, the brain was dissected, chilled on a glass plate on ice and then cut into slices. The trace of the entry needle was checked to confirm the injection site. According to Atlas of The Rat Brain by George Paxinos & Charles Watson, the area of Bregma ±1.6 mm was removed from the slices and cut limited tissue of NAc, and homogenized in ice-cold homogenizing buffer (50 mM Tris-Cl, pH 7.4, 150 mM NaCl, 5 mM EDTA, 0.1% SDS, 1% NP-40, 1% deoxycholate, 1% Triton X-100, 10 mM PMSF, 50 mM sodium vanadate and 0.1% protease inhibitors cock-tail (Roche, Switzerland)). After centrifugation at 12,000×g for 15 min at 4 °C, the supernatant was collected and the protein content was subsequently assayed by using a BCA Protein Assay Kit (Pierce, Rockford, IL, USA). Equal quantities of total protein (75 μg per lane) were separated by sodium dodecyl sulfate-polyacrylamide gel electrophoresis (SDS-PAGE), followed by transfer to nitrocellulose membranes. The membranes were incubated in 5% milk at room temperature for 2 h. Blots were then incubated with rabbit polyclonal antibody against TRPV1 (1:1000, Santa Cruz Biotechnology), or β-actin (1:2000). After washing with buffer, the blots were incubated in anti-rabbit (Zhong Shan, Beijing, China, 1:1000) secondary antibody conjugated with horseradish peroxide in TBS-T with 5% milk at 4 °C overnight. The blots were visualized using a West Pico Chemiluminescent Kit (Pierce, Rockford, IL, USA), and the density of protein bands quantified by transmittance densitometry using volume integration with LumiAnalyst Image Analysis software.

Histology

At the end of the behavioral experiments, rats were anesthetized with chloral hydrate (400 mg/kg, i.p.) and perfused intracardially with 10% PBS-buffered formalin. The brains were removed, post-fixed overnight in a 30% sucrose/formalin solution, and then cryoprotected in 30% sucrose/saline. To verify the location of the cannula tips, 40 μm coronal sections were cut through the targeted area (NAc or DS), and stained with cresyl violet, and examined under a light microscope. Rats with off-target cannula placements in only one side of Nac were involved in the Uni-off Nac group for analyses. Rats with incorrect cannula placements were excluded from the study. Overall, six rats were excluded for this reason.

Data analysis

Data were expressed as Mean ±SEM. Statistical analyses were performed using repeated measures analysis of variance (ANOVA) followed by Duncan *post hoc* tests for multiple comparisons. The accepted level of statistical significance is $p<0.05$.

Results

Food intake and body weight after surgery

As shown in Table.1, the daily food intake of surgery animals was similar with control group after the surgery under anesthetized with chloral hydrate. All animals showed increasing body weight after 5-day raise. There were not significant differences of both initial and recovering body weight between control and surgery groups.

Morphine conditioned place preference

Higher mCPP scores were observed in morphine conditioned groups (Fig.1). In 1 mg/kg and 3 mg/kg morphine groups, the mCPP expression was numerically increased, but this difference was not significant ($F=0.375$, $p=0.960$). However, comparing to control group, significantly higher mCPP scores in all the 4

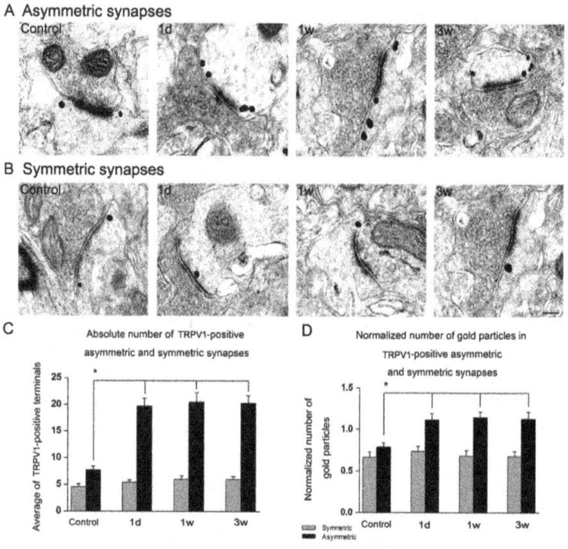

Figure 3. Quantitative changes in TRPV1 expression at the ultrastructural level in morphine withdrawal groups. High-power electron micrographs from the NAc of different groups showing TRPV1 immunogold labeling in the axon terminals forming asymmetric, excitatory-type synapses (A) and symmetric, inhibitory-type synapses (B). In the morphine withdrawal groups the number of gold particles on terminals forming asymmetric synapses increased (A). Graph (C) shows changes in the average number of TRPV1-positive asymmetric and symmetric synapses in each group. The number of TRPV1-positive asymmetric synapses in the morphine withdrawal groups was significantly higher than the control group. However, no difference was found in the normalized number of TRPV1-positive symmetric synapses among all groups. The number of TRPV1-positive symmetric synapses of control were 4.72±0.77, 4.72±0.47 and 4.74±1.00 for 1 d, 1 w and 3 w group respectively. The number of TRPV1-positive asymmetric synapses of control were 7.74±1.38, 7.75±0.77 and 7.74±1.28 for 1 d, 1 w and 3 w group respectively. Graph (D) shows the normalized number of gold particles in TRPV1-positive asymmetric and symmetric synapses. No difference appeared in the normalized number of gold particles in TRPV1-positive symmetric synapses. In contrast, a significant increase occurred in the normalized number of gold particles in TRPV1-positive asymmetric synapses of morphine withdrawal groups versus control group. The normalized number of gold particles in TRPV1-positive symmetric synapses of control were 0.68±0.17, 0.68±0.03 and 0.69±0.04 for 1 d, 1 w and 3 w group respectively. The normalized number of gold particles in TRPV1-positive asymmetric synapses of control were 0.78±0.07, 0.79±0.13 and 0.79±0.03 for 1 d, 1 w and 3 w group respectively. Scale: 200 nm. Data represent Mean±SEM (n = 3), *$p<0.05$, *vs* control group.

postconditioning tests performed at 1 d, 1 w, 2 w, 3 w after last training session were observed in high-dose (10 mg/kg) morphine conditioned group ($F = 8.144$, $p = 0.006$). There was no significant difference for mCPP score among four time point of postconditioning tests in 10 mg/kg morphine group ($p > 0.05$), which indicated that morphine with 10 mg/kg induced a persistent and relatively stable mCPP expression. We chose 10 mg/kg morphine for conditioning training in the CPZ-intervening experiments.

Morphine increased TRPV1 expression in NAc meurons

Levels of TRPV1 in the nucleus accumbens were detected by Western blot and quantitatively analyzed (Fig. 2). Control group revealed the moderate expression of TRPV1 in the nucleus accumbens. There were not significant changes of TRPV1 expression in 1 mg/kg and 3 mg/kg morphine treated groups. However, TRPV1 immunoreactivity was increased markedly in 10 mg/kg morphine withdrawal animals compared with the control group ($F = 79.288$, $p < 0.01$). There were not significant differences of TRPV1 immunoreactivity between 1 week and 3 week morphine withdrawal groups ($p > 0.05$).

Increased TRPV1 located in asymmetric synapses

Transmission electron microscopy was used to examine the expression of TRPV1 in synapse. The immunogold-positive axon terminals were found in both asymmetric synapses (excitatory-type) and symmetric synapses (inhibitory-type) (Fig. 3,Peters et al., 1991).

Two vibratome sections from each of three rats in each group were calculated for the absolute number of TRPV1 positive asymmetric and symmetric synapses, and each vibratome section was normalized to 3000 μm^2. Compared to the control group, a significant increase was found in the number of TRPV1 positive asymmetric synapses in the morphine withdrawal groups (Fig.3C, $F = 75.321$, $p < 0.05$), but no significant change was found in the number of TRPV1 positive symmetric synapses in morphine withdrawal groups (Fig.3C, $p = 0.622$).

To quantify the changes in the number of immunogold particles in certain terminals of the NAc of rats, the number of gold particles in the membranes of TRPV1 stained axon terminals forming symmetric or asymmetric synapses was counted and normalized to the unit perimeter (1 μm) of the axon terminal membrane. Significant increase was observed in the number of immunogold particles in axon terminals forming asymmetric synapses between the control group and morphine withdrawal groups (Fig.3D, $F = 36.547$, $p < 0.05$). In contrast, the number of immunogold particles showed no difference in axon terminals forming symmetric synapses between the control group and morphine withdrawal groups (Fig.3D, $p = 0.056$).

Intra-NAc CPZ decreased persistent mCPP expression in a target specific manner

To determine whether NAc endovanilloid receptor TRPV1 is involved in the expression of mCPP, rats were given bilaterally repeated intra-NAc injections of different doses of TRPV1 antagonist CPZ during morphine withdrawal. When CPZ was applied during short-term morphine withdrawal, as shown in

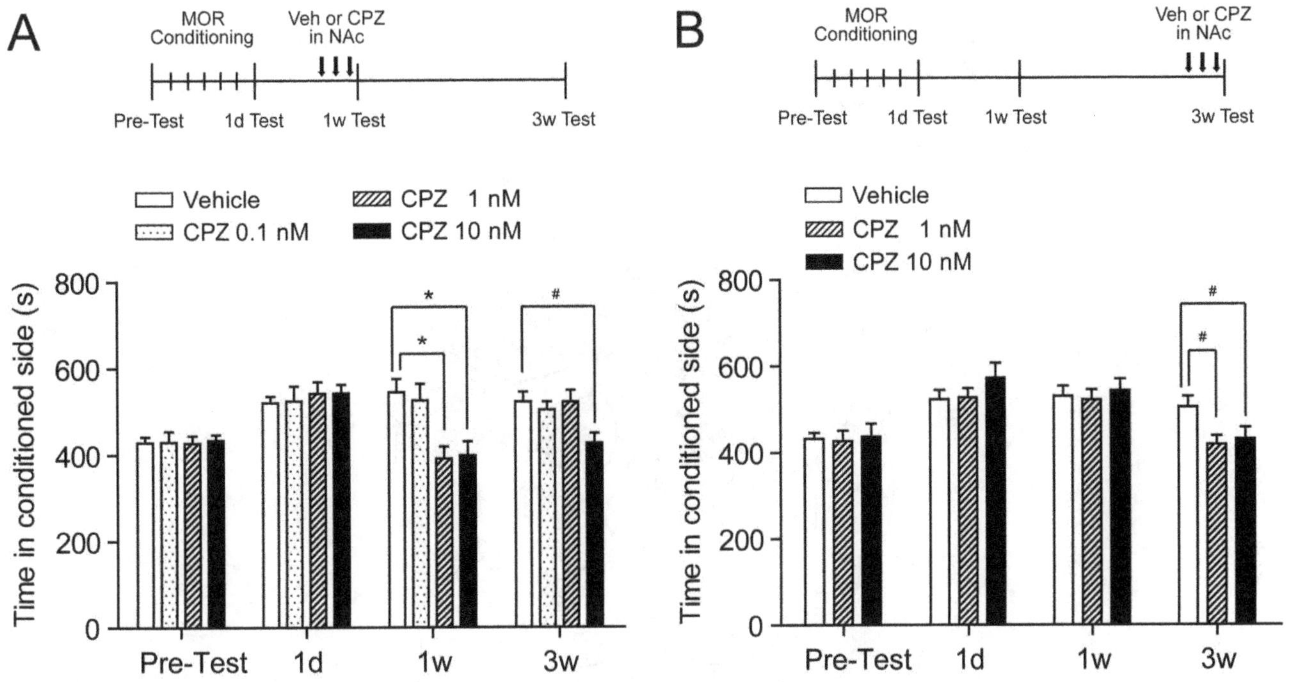

Figure 4. TRPV1 antagonist CPZ administered in bilateral NAc core decreased persistent morphine CPP after both short-(1 w) and long-term(3 w) withdrawal. (A) Dose-dependent effect of CPZ on persistent mCPP expression. Repeated high-dose CPZ (10 nM) injection during short-term morphine withdrawal could induce a complete and prolonged inhibition on mCPP expression. The moderate-dose CPZ (1 nM) has similar but temporary prohibiting effect on mCPP expression, as it could only be observed at 1 w but not 3 w of morphine withdrawal. The low-dose CPZ (0.1 nM) has no influence on mCPP. The upper schedule panel shows the rats were trained conditioned to morphine and received repeated CPZ injections in NAc core after short-term(1 w) withdrawal (n = 11 of Vehicle and CPZ 0.1 nM group, n = 10 of CPZ 1 nM group, and n = 9 of CPZ 10 nM group). (B) CPZ (1 nM and 10 nM) administration eliminated mCPP (n = 7). The upper schedule panel shows the rats were conditioned to morphine and received CPZ injections in NAc core after long-term(3 w) withdrawal. *$p < 0.01$, *vs* control group; #$p < 0.05$, *vs* control group. MOR, morphine; Veh, vehicle; CPZ, capsazepine; NAc, nucleus accumbens.

Fig. 4A, both 1 nM and 10 nM of CPZ significantly decreased mCPP expression at 1 w test (CPZ 1 nM, 370.9±20.2 s; CPZ 10 nM, 371.9±32.5 s; vehicle, 562.0±28.9 s; $F = 12.28$, $p<0.01$) (Fig. 4A). but the inhibitory effect of 1 nM CPZ was completely eliminated when tested at 3 w with the mCPP score reverted similar to control level (CPZ 1 nM, 522.6±26.4 s; vehicle, 523.3±22.5 s; $p>0.05$) (Fig. 4A). However, the inhibition of 10 nM CPZ could last to 3 w after morphine withdrawal (CPZ 10 nM, 426.8±23.2 s; vehicle, 523.3±22.5 s; $p<0.05$) (Fig. 4A). No active effect of low dose of CPZ (0.1 nM) was observed when tested at 1 w ($p>0.05$) (Fig. 4A). We used higher dose (1 nM or 10 nM) of CPZ for experiments during long-term (3 w) withdrawal. After three times injection, significant inhibition of mCPP expression was observed in both dose of CPZ (CPZ 1 nM, 418.4±19.9 s; CPZ 10 nM, 430.9±26.9 s; vehicle, 505.1±24.6 s; $F = 14.86$, $p<0.05$) (Fig. 4B). Thus, blocking TRPV1 in NAc disrupts the mCPP expression in both short- and long-term withdrawal. Figure 5 showed the Distribution of infusion sites in nucleus accumbens core.

To investigate whether CPZ inhibition on mCPP is a target-specific effect, we applied CPZ (10 nM) randomly in unilateral NAc, or bilateral DS during short-term (1 w) morphine withdrawal. Data from rats initially prepared for the bilateral CPZ administration study but with off-NAc cannula placements in only one side confirmed with staining was also analyzed here. As depicted in Figure 6A, in Uni-NAc group, no alteration of mCPP was detected after CPZ injection (CPZ, 549.1±29.7 s; vehicle, 539.0±15.9 s; $F = 0.245$, $p = 0.959$). Similarly, CPZ injection did not decrease mCPP in the Uni-off NAc group (Fig. 6A). Furthermore, when we examined the CPZ effect on mCPP in

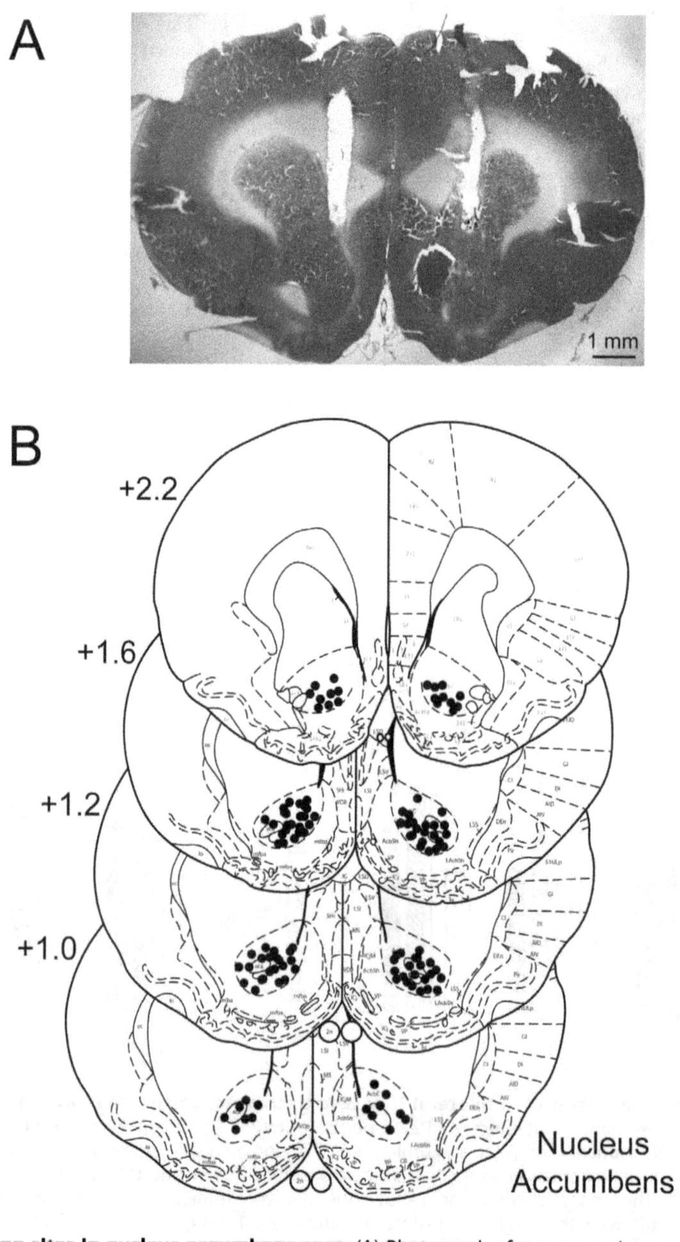

Figure 5. Distribution of infusion sites in nucleus accumbens core. (A) Photograph of representative cannula placements. The cannulas are implanted 1.5 mm above the target. (B) Schematic representations of vehicle or capsazepine injection sites in nucleus accumbens core at the labeled coronal planes. The numbers are the coordinates anterior (+) to bregma in millimeters according to Paxinos and Watson (2005).

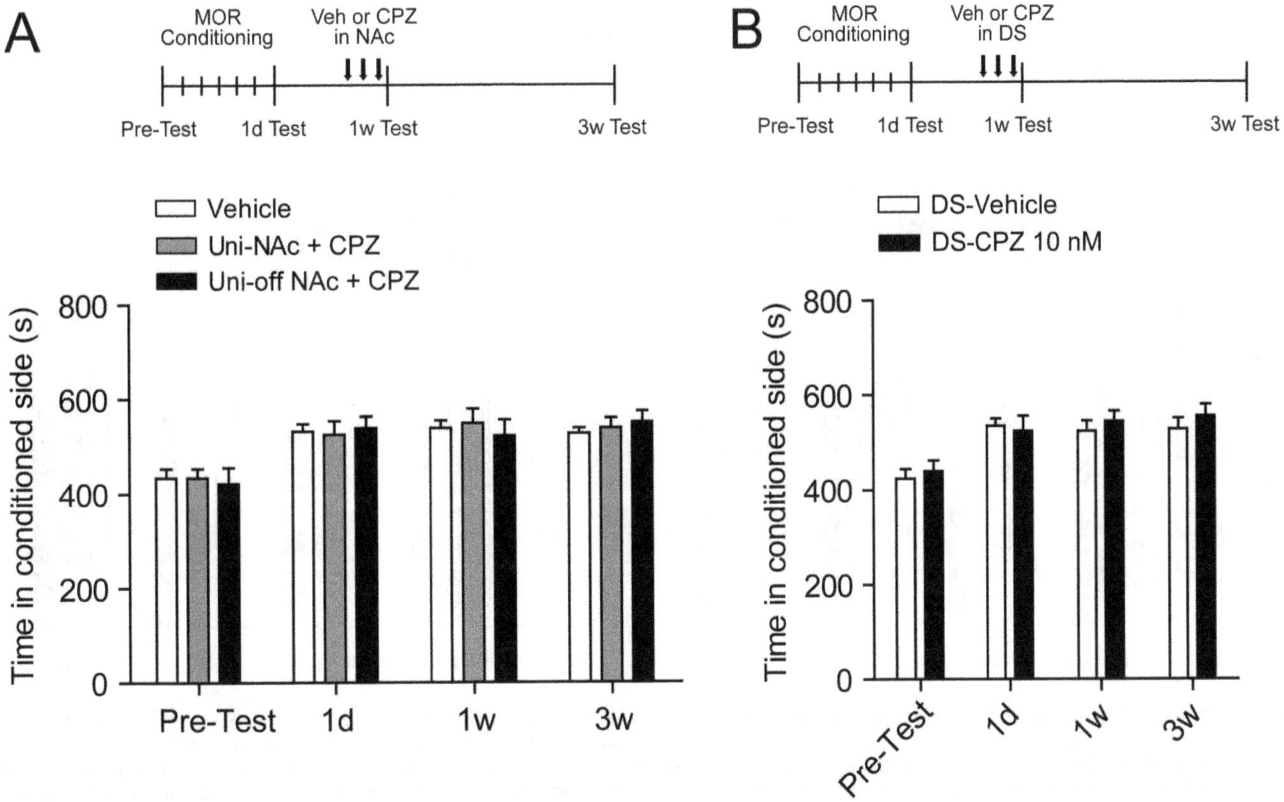

Figure 6. Injection of TRPV1 antagonist CPZ in unilateral of NAc or DS did not change persistent mCPP expression after short-term(1 w) withdrawal. (A) Unilateral NAc CPZ injection (10 nM) or one side off-target during bilateral NAc CPZ infusion (1 nM or 10 nM) failed to affect the sustained mCPP. The upper panel shows the scheme for morphine conditioning, CPZ treatment and mCPP test. Values are Mean ±SEM (n = 7 of Vehicle and Uni-NAc+CPZ group and n = 3 of Uni-off NAc+CPZ group). (B) CPZ (10 nM) injection in DS failed to influence persistent morphine CPP. The upper panel shows rats were conditioned to morphine and received CPZ injections in bilateral DS after short-term withdrawal. Values are mean ±SEM (n = 6 of DS-Vehicle group and n = 7 of DS-CPZ 10 nM group). MOR, morphine; Veh, vehicle; CPZ, capsazepine; NAc, nucleus accumbens; Uni, unilateral; DS, dorsal striatum.

the target outside NAc, we found the effective dose of CPZ (10 nM) in DS failed to influence the persistent mCPP expession ($F = 0.261$, $p = 0.853$) (Fig. 6B).

To assess the possible effect of intra-NAc CPZ on motor activity, which could indirectly influence mCPP expression, crossline times of the rats during mCPP tests were analyzed. As shown in Fig.7, there was no statistical difference ($F = 1.13$, $p > 0.05$) in crossline times among all groups after CPZ injection in both short-term (1 w) and long-term (3 w) withdrawal. The results confirmed that the alteration of all parameters in the mCPP expression test did not result from changes in motor abilities of rats.

Discussion

It is suggested that the NAc glutamatergic system is a key candidate for mediating morphine withdrawal-related addictive behaviors [28,29]. Alcantara et al. reported that morphine treatment increase the number of synapses of NAc, which was due primarily to an increase in the number of asymmetric synapses, and Asymmetric synapses in the accumbens are characteristic of glutamatergic synapses formed by inputs from other area such as prefrontal cortex, hippocampus and so on [30]. In the present study, we demonstrated that TRPV1 was increased in the nucleus accumbens of rats after morphine conditioned. Significant increase was observed in the number of immunogold particles in axon terminals forming asymmetric synapses between the control group and morphine withdrawal groups. In contrast, it showed no difference in axon terminals forming symmetric synapses, which suggested that the TRPV1 expression at asymmetric synapses might involve in morphine induced CPP. Antagonism of TRPV1 by the selective TRPV1 antagonist CPZ suppressed persistent mCPP expression in rats either during short-term or long-term morphine withdrawal. This inhibitory effect is target-specific, unique for NAc. Conversely, effective doses of CPZ in NAc did not cause significant side-effect on motor activity of the subjects, suggesting the decrease of mCPP expression is not due to motor inhibitory properties of TRPV1 antagonist. Collectively, these results not only extend our understanding on the role of central TRPV1 in drug addiction, but also indicate that TRPV1 antagonist may be a promising type of medication for inhibiting morphine conditioned behaviour.

Morphine withdrawal increased TRPV1 expression in NAc meurons

TRPV1 is a calcium-permeable cation channel [31,32]. In the central nervous system, TRPV1 is widely expressed in brain regions including postsynaptic dendrite spines, cell somata [33], and in various layers of the cortex [6,34]. Previous studies suggested that activation of postsynaptic TRPV1 channels triggered long-term depression in the NAc [12]. Activation of TRPV1 receptors is coupled to glutamate release, which in turn

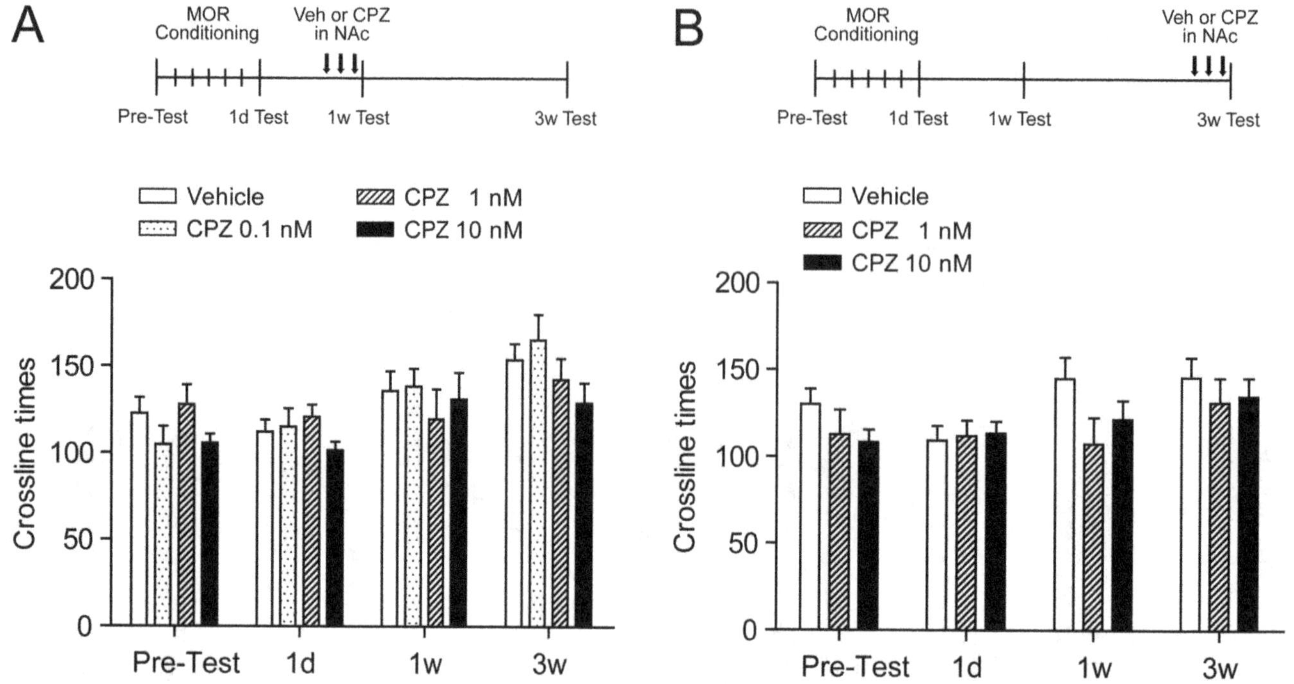

Figure 7. TRPV1 antagonist CPZ administered in bilateral NAc fail to affect normal activity after both short-(1 w) and long-term(3 w) withdrawal. (A) All doses of CPZ tested failed to influence the activity of animal measured by photobeam breaks during the 15-min mCPP test (n = 11 of Vehicle and CPZ 0.1 nM group, n = 10 of CPZ 1 nM group, and n = 9 of CPZ 10 nM group). The upper schedule panel shows the rats were trained conditioned to morphine and received repeated CPZ injections in NAc core after short-term (1 w) withdrawal. (B) Both effective doses of CPZ (1 nM and 10 nM) in eliminating sustained mCPP expression fail to affect activity (n = 7). The upper schedule panel shows the rats were conditioned to morphine and received CPZ injections in NAc core after long-term (3 w) withdrawal.Values are mean ±SEM. MOR, morphine; Veh, vehicle; CPZ, capsazepine; NAc, nucleus accumbens.

affects the release of GABA, dopamine, and other catecholamines [35,36]. Activation of TRPV1 in the ventral tegmental area caused excitation of dopaminergic neurons and increased dopamine release in NAc after a painful stimulus [26]. AMPA receptors and GABAA receptors activation are associated with facilitation of motivated behaviors [37].

In the present study, we found that morphine with 10 mg/kg induced persistent and relatively stable mCPP expression lasting from short-term (1 w) to long-term (3 w) withdrawal, which dose has been continuously confirmed to induce sustained mCPP expression in rodents [38,39]. Accordingly, the expression of TRPV1 in the NAcc was elevated in morphine conditioned animals and maintained in high levels after 1 w and 3 w withdrawal compared to the control group. The increased TRPV1 distributed on the presynaptic membrane of asymmetric synapses. The results indicated that increasing expression of TRPV1 on the presynaptic membrane of asymmetric synapses in NAcc might play an important role in morphine conditioned place preference.

Intra-NAc CPZ reduced mCPP expression

To confirm the role of TRPV1 in morphine induced conditioned place preference, we injected TRPV1 antagonist CPZ intra-NAc and found that blocking TRPV1 in NAc disrupts the mCPP expression in both short- and long-term withdrawal. Previous study has shown that repeated systematic administration of CPZ could reduce naloxone-induced acute withdrawal symptoms in mice [9]. These findings together reveal the important role of TRPV1 in both psychological and physical aspects of opioid-related behaviors.

At least two possible mechanisms may underlie the inhibitory behavioral effect of TRPV1 antagonist in NAc on mCPP. Firstly, blockade of TRPV1 in NAc may prevent it from overdrive by excitatory inputs essential for CPP. Previous studies have shown that potentiation of glutamatergic inputs on NAc medium spiny neurons is a critical type of neuroadaptation happened during prolonged opioid withdrawal and is associated with relapse [22,24,40]. Furthermore, fully or partially blockade of glutamatergic inputs has been proved to disrupt reinstatement to opioid seeking and taking behaviors [23–25,40]. It has been proved that TRPV1 activation facilitate presynaptic neurotransmitter release in variety of brain regions [3,13–17,19–21] and the existence of TRPV1 mRNA in main glutamatergic areas innervating NAc [7]. In the present study, significant increase of the number of TRPV1 positive asymmetric synapses was observed and more immunogold particles in axon terminals in the morphine conditioned rats, which suggested that the inhibitory effect of TRPV1 antagonist on synaptic efficacy should be taken into account when evaluating its inhibitory effect on CPP. Supporting this idea, our finding that the time window for the effectiveness of NAc TRPV1 antagonist on mCPP persisting from short- to long-term drug withdrawal overlapped with the period for NAc glutamate inputs potentiation reported before [22,41]. Secondly, reduction of NAc neuronal activity by TRPV1 antagonist may also contribute to its effect on mCPP expression. Wu et al [22] reported the increase of intrinsic excitability in NAc neurons during opioid withdrawal, which suggested an enhanced response capability of these neurons. In agreement with these data, increased NAc immediate early gene expression during opioid withdrawal and reinstatement supports the upregulation of NAc neural reactivity during withdrawal

[42,43]. Conversely, blocking NAc activity could reduce mCPP expression and prevent opioid relapse [27]. As is shown previously, membrane depolarization and increase of spiking are essential manifestations after central TRPV1 activation [20,26], which is mediated by its modulatory on K^+ and Ca^{2+} conductance or direct Ca^{2+} and Na^+ influx via the channel itself. Accordingly, blockade of NAc TRPV1, may contribute to limit neural activity in this region, which was confirmed to have relapse-preventing effect [27]. Further studies are necessary to elucidate the above and other mechanisms involved in the action of central, especially NAc, TRPV1 antagonism on drug addiction.

Intra-NAc CPZ administration did not affect on motor activity

Our data showed that the effective dose of NAc CPZ in preventing mCPP expression failed to influence the locomotor activity. Consistent with previous studies [44,45], we showed together that this dose range of CPZ is not sufficient to produce behavioral effect on general activity in rats when given alone. However, stimulation of TRPV1 by application of its ligand externally has been shown to suppress spontaneous activity in rodents [15,45–47]. Moreover, blockade of TRPV1 by CPZ has been proved to attenuate hypolocomotor effect of anandamide [47,48], a ligand for both cannabinoid receptor and TRPV1, which revealed that anandamide induced activity disruption is caused by a TRPV1-dependent mechanism. Collectively, these findings indicate that targeting central TRPV1 may modulate activity of the subject. Nevertheless, discrepancies between these findings and our result implicated that blocking TRPV1 by endogenous ligands in the brain, at least in NAc, may not be sufficient to affect activity, in another word, tonic TRPV1 activation in NAc isn't involved in regulating basal activity. The finding that TRPV1 gene knockout mice showed normal locomotor activity further supports this viewpoint [12]. Thus, blocking TRPV1 in NAc will result in non-effect on activity and the inhibition of CPZ on prolonged mCPP expression is not due to its influence on moving ability of the rats.

In conclusion, the present study indicated the importance of TRPV1 in the NAc in morphine addiction. The increased expression of TRPV1 in the presynaptic membranes of asymmetric synapses in NAc during morphine withdrawal may be one of the mechanisms of mCPP expression. We further demonstrated the inhibitory effect of NAc TRPV1 antagonism on prolonged mCPP expression, which confirmed the involvement of NAc TRPV1 in persistent opioid addiction. Our results support for further mechanism assessment and developing novel treatment targeting central, especially NAc, TRPV1 for mCPP prevention.

Author Contributions

Conceived and designed the experiments: LJH GZX GDG LTM. Performed the experiments: LJH BH HG. Analyzed the data: LJH WXY JS PW. Contributed to the writing of the manuscript: LJH GDG GZX.

References

1. O'Brien CP (1997) A range of research-based pharmacotherapies for addiction. Science 278: 66–70.
2. Wu LJ, Sweet TB, Clapham DE (2010) International Union of Basic and Clinical Pharmacology. LXXVI. Current progress in the mammalian TRP ion channel family. Pharmacol Rev 62: 381–404.
3. Matta JA, Ahern GP (2011) TRPV1 and synaptic transmission. Curr Pharm Biotechnol 12: 95–101.
4. Ho KW, Ward NJ, Calkins DJ (2012) TRPV1: a stress response protein in the central nervous system. Am J Neurodegener Dis 1: 1–14.
5. Micale V, Cristino L, Tamburella A, Petrosino S, Leggio GM, et al. (2009) Altered responses of dopamine D3 receptor null mice to excitotoxic or anxiogenic stimuli: Possible involvement of the endocannabinoid and endovanilloid systems. Neurobiol Dis 36: 70–80.
6. Roberts JC, Davis JB, Benham CD (2004) [3H]Resiniferatoxin autoradiography in the CNS of wild-type and TRPV1 null mice defines TRPV1 (VR-1) protein distribution. Brain Res 995: 176–183.
7. Tian YH, Lee SY, Kim HC, Jang CG (2010) Repeated methamphetamine treatment increases expression of TRPV1 mRNA in the frontal cortex but not in the striatum or hippocampus of mice. Neurosci Lett 472: 61–64.
8. Cristino L, de Petrocellis L, Pryce G, Baker D, Guglielmotti V, et al. (2006) Immunohistochemical localization of cannabinoid type 1 and vanilloid transient receptor potential vanilloid type 1 receptors in the mouse brain. Neuroscience 139: 1405–1415.
9. Nguyen TL, Nam YS, Lee SY, Kim HC, Jang CG (2010) Effects of capsazepine, a transient receptor potential vanilloid type 1 antagonist, on morphine-induced antinociception, tolerance, and dependence in mice. Br J Anaesth 105: 668–674.
10. Adamczyk P, Miszkiel J, McCreary AC, Filip M, Papp M, et al. (2012) The effects of cannabinoid CB1, CB2 and vanilloid TRPV1 receptor antagonists on cocaine addictive behavior in rats. Brain Res 1444: 45–54.
11. Badiani A, Belin D, Epstein D, Calu D, Shaham Y (2011) Opiate versus psychostimulant addiction: the differences do matter. Nat Rev Neurosci 12: 685–700.
12. Grueter BA, Brasnjo G, Malenka RC (2010) Postsynaptic TRPV1 triggers cell type-specific long-term depression in the nucleus accumbens. Nat Neurosci 13: 1519–1525.
13. Musella A, De Chiara V, Rossi S, Prosperetti C, Bernardi G, et al. (2009) TRPV1 channels facilitate glutamate transmission in the striatum. Mol Cell Neurosci 40: 89–97.
14. Benninger F, Freund TF, Hajos N (2008) Control of excitatory synaptic transmission by capsaicin is unaltered in TRPV1 vanilloid receptor knockout mice. Neurochem Int 52: 89–94.
15. de Lago E, de Miguel R, Lastres-Becker I, Ramos JA, Fernandez-Ruiz J (2004) Involvement of vanilloid-like receptors in the effects of anandamide on motor behavior and nigrostriatal dopaminergic activity: in vivo and in vitro evidence. Brain Res 1007: 152–159.
16. Marinelli S, Di Marzo V, Berretta N, Matias I, Maccarrone M, et al. (2003) Presynaptic facilitation of glutamatergic synapses to dopaminergic neurons of the rat substantia nigra by endogenous stimulation of vanilloid receptors. J Neurosci 23: 3136–3144.
17. Marinelli S, Vaughan CW, Christie MJ, Connor M (2002) Capsaicin activation of glutamatergic synaptic transmission in the rat locus coeruleus in vitro. J Physiol 543: 531–540.
18. Mori F, Ribolsi M, Kusayanagi H, Monteleone F, Mantovani V, et al. (2012) TRPV1 channels regulate cortical excitability in humans. J Neurosci 32: 873–879.
19. Sasamura T, Sasaki M, Tohda C, Kuraishi Y (1998) Existence of capsaicin-sensitive glutamatergic terminals in rat hypothalamus. Neuroreport 9: 2045–2048.
20. Xing J, Li J (2007) TRPV1 receptor mediates glutamatergic synaptic input to dorsolateral periaqueductal gray (dl-PAG) neurons. J Neurophysiol 97: 503–511.
21. Yokoyama T, Saito T, Ohbuchi T, Hashimoto H, Suzuki H, et al. (2010) TRPV1 gene deficiency attenuates miniature EPSC potentiation induced by mannitol and angiotensin II in supraoptic magnocellular neurons. J Neurosci 30: 876–884.
22. Wu X, Shi M, Wei C, Yang M, Liu Y, et al. (2012) Potentiation of synaptic strength and intrinsic excitability in the nucleus accumbens after 10 days of morphine withdrawal. J Neurosci Res 90: 1270–1283.
23. Ma YY, Chu NN, Guo CY, Han JS, Cui CL (2007) NR2B-containing NMDA receptor is required for morphine-but not stress-induced reinstatement. Exp Neurol 203: 309–319.
24. LaLumiere RT, Kalivas PW (2008) Glutamate release in the nucleus accumbens core is necessary for heroin seeking. J Neurosci 28: 3170–3177.
25. Bossert JM, Gray SM, Lu L, Shaham Y (2006) Activation of group II metabotropic glutamate receptors in the nucleus accumbens shell attenuates context-induced relapse to heroin seeking. Neuropsychopharmacology 31: 2197–2209.
26. Marinelli S, Pascucci T, Bernardi G, Puglisi-Allegra S, Mercuri NB (2005) Activation of TRPV1 in the VTA excites dopaminergic neurons and increases chemical- and noxious-induced dopamine release in the nucleus accumbens. Neuropsychopharmacology 30: 864–870.
27. Esmaeili MH, Sahraei H, Ali-Beig H, Ardehari-Ghaleh M, Mohammadian Z, et al. (2012) Transient inactivation of the nucleus accumbens reduces both the expression and acquisition of morphine-induced conditioned place preference in rats. Pharmacol Biochem Behav 102: 249–256.
28. Siggins GR, Martin G, Roberto M, Nie Z, Madamba S, et al. (2003) Glutamatergic transmission in opiate and alcohol dependence. Ann N Y Acad Sci 1003: 196–211.

29. Gass JT, Olive MF (2008) Glutamatergic substrates of drug addiction and alcoholism. Biochem Pharmacol 75: 218–265.
30. Alcantara AA, Lim HY, Floyd CE, Garces J, Mendenhall JM, et al. (2011) Cocaine- and morphine-induced synaptic plasticity in the nucleus accumbens. Synapse 65: 309–320.
31. Caterina MJ, Schumacher MA, Tominaga M, Rosen TA, Levine JD, et al. (1997) The capsaicin receptor: a heat-activated ion channel in the pain pathway. Nature 389: 816–824.
32. Szallasi A, Blumberg PM (1999) Vanilloid (Capsaicin) receptors and mechanisms. Pharmacol Rev 51: 159–212.
33. Toth A, Boczan J, Kedei N, Lizanecz E, Bagi Z, et al. (2005) Expression and distribution of vanilloid receptor 1 (TRPV1) in the adult rat brain. Brain Res Mol Brain Res 135: 162–168.
34. Mezey E, Toth ZE, Cortright DN, Arzubi MK, Krause JE, et al. (2000) Distribution of mRNA for vanilloid receptor subtype 1 (VR1), and VR1-like immunoreactivity, in the central nervous system of the rat and human. Proc Natl Acad Sci U S A 97: 3655–3660.
35. Jin YH, Bailey TW, Li BY, Schild JH, Andresen MC (2004) Purinergic and vanilloid receptor activation releases glutamate from separate cranial afferent terminals in nucleus tractus solitarius. J Neurosci 24: 4709–4717.
36. Li DP, Chen SR, Pan HL (2004) VR1 receptor activation induces glutamate release and postsynaptic firing in the paraventricular nucleus. J Neurophysiol 92: 1807–1816.
37. Yuan WX, Heng LJ, Ma J, Wang XQ, Qu LJ, et al. (2013) Increased expression of cannabinoid receptor 1 in the nucleus accumbens core in a rat model with morphine withdrawal. Brain Res 1531: 102–112.
38. Li YQ, Li FQ, Wang XY, Wu P, Zhao M, et al. (2008) Central amygdala extracellular signal-regulated kinase signaling pathway is critical to incubation of opiate craving. J Neurosci 28: 13248–13257.
39. Milekic MH, Brown SD, Castellini C, Alberini CM (2006) Persistent disruption of an established morphine conditioned place preference. J Neurosci 26: 3010–3020.
40. Shen H, Moussawi K, Zhou W, Toda S, Kalivas PW (2011) Heroin relapse requires long-term potentiation-like plasticity mediated by NMDA2b-containing receptors. Proc Natl Acad Sci U S A 108: 19407–19412.
41. Bajo M, Crawford EF, Roberto M, Madamba SG, Siggins GR (2006) Chronic morphine treatment alters expression of N-methyl-D-aspartate receptor subunits in the extended amygdala. J Neurosci Res 83: 532–537.
42. Koya E, Spijker S, Voorn P, Binnekade R, Schmidt ED, et al. (2006) Enhanced cortical and accumbal molecular reactivity associated with conditioned heroin, but not sucrose-seeking behaviour. J Neurochem 98: 905–915.
43. Kuntz KL, Patel KM, Grigson PS, Freeman WM, Vrana KE (2008) Heroin self-administration: II. CNS gene expression following withdrawal and cue-induced drug-seeking behavior. Pharmacol Biochem Behav 90: 349–356.
44. Aguiar DC, Terzian AL, Guimaraes FS, Moreira FA (2009) Anxiolytic-like effects induced by blockade of transient receptor potential vanilloid type 1 (TRPV1) channels in the medial prefrontal cortex of rats. Psychopharmacology (Berl) 205: 217–225.
45. Lee J, Di Marzo V, Brotchie JM (2006) A role for vanilloid receptor 1 (TRPV1) and endocannabinnoid signalling in the regulation of spontaneous and L-DOPA induced locomotion in normal and reserpine-treated rats. Neuropharmacology 51: 557–565.
46. Di Marzo V, Lastres-Becker I, Bisogno T, De Petrocellis L, Milone A, et al. (2001) Hypolocomotor effects in rats of capsaicin and two long chain capsaicin homologues. Eur J Pharmacol 420: 123–131.
47. Panlilio LV, Mazzola C, Medalie J, Hahn B, Justinova Z, et al. (2009) Anandamide-induced behavioral disruption through a vanilloid-dependent mechanism in rats. Psychopharmacology (Berl) 203: 529–538.
48. Tzavara ET, Li DL, Moutsimilli L, Bisogno T, Di Marzo V, et al. (2006) Endocannabinoids activate transient receptor potential vanilloid 1 receptors to reduce hyperdopaminergia-related hyperactivity: therapeutic implications. Biol Psychiatry 59: 508–515.

Social and Economic Characteristics of Street Youth by Gender and Level of Street Involvement in Eldoret, Kenya

Rebecca Sorber[1], Susanna Winston[2,3], Julius Koech[4], David Ayuku[5], Liangyuan Hu[6], Joseph Hogan[4,6], Paula Braitstein[1,4,7,8,9*]

1 School of Medicine, Indiana University, Indianapolis, Indiana, United States of America, **2** Department of Pediatrics, Warren Alpert School of Medicine, Brown University, Providence, Rhode Island, United States of America, **3** Rhode Island Hospital-Hasbro Youth's Hospital, Providence, Rhode Island, United States of America, **4** AMPATH Consortium, Eldoret, Kenya, **5** Department of Behavioral Sciences, School of Medicine, College of Health Sciences, Moi University, Eldoret, Kenya, **6** Department of Biostatistics, Brown University, Providence, Rhode Island, United States of America, **7** Department of Medicine, School of Medicine, College of Health Sciences, Moi University, Eldoret, Kenya, **8** Dalla Lana School of Public Health, University of Toronto, Toronto, Ontario, Canada, **9** Regenstrief Institute, Inc., Indianapolis, Indiana, United States of America

Abstract

Background: Street-connected youth are a neglected and vulnerable population, particularly in resource-constrained settings. The development of interventions and supports for this population requires insight into how they live. This study describes the social and economic characteristics of a convenience sample of street youth (SY) in Eldoret, Kenya.

Methods: Participants were eligible if they were aged 12–21, living in Eldoret, spending days only (part-time), or nights and days on the street (full-time) and able and willing to consent or assent. Data were collected using a standardized interview conducted in English or Kiswahili. Binary dependent variables were having been arrested and/or jailed, and first priority for spending money (food vs. other). Nominal categorical dependent variables included major source of support, and major reason for being street-involved. Multivariable analysis used logistic regression models to examine the association of gender and level of street-involvement with social and economic factors of interest adjusting for age and length of time on the street. Data were analyzed using SAS 9.3.

Results: Of the 200 SY enrolled, 41% were female, mean age of 16.3 years; 71% were on the street full-time, and 29% part-time. Compared with part-time SY, full-time SY were more likely to have been arrested (Adjusted Odds Ratio [AOR]: 2.33, 95% Confidence Interval [95%CI]:1.01–5.35), name food as their first spending priority (AOR: 2.57, 95%CI:1.03–6.45), have left home due to violence (AOR: 5.54, 95%CI: 1.67–18.34), and more likely to report friends on the street as a major source of support (AOR: 3.59, 95% CI: 1.01–12.82). Compared with females, males were more likely to have ever been arrested (AOR: 2.66, 95%CI:1.14–6.18), and to have ever been jailed (AOR: 3.22, 95%CI:1.47–7.02).

Conclusions: These results suggest a high degree of heterogeneity and vulnerability among SY in this setting. There is an urgent need for interventions taking into consideration these characteristics.

Editor: Stephen E. Gilman, Harvard School of Public Health, United States of America

Funding: This work was supported in part by Award Number R01HD060478 from the Eunice Kennedy Shriver National Institute of Child Health and Human Development. Additional funding came from a 2011 international developmental grant from the Lifespan/Tufts/Brown Center for AIDS Research. This project was specifically supported by Grant Number P30AI042853 from the National Institute of Allergy and Infectious Diseases. The content is solely the responsibility of the authors and does not necessarily represent the official views of the Eunice Kennedy Shriver National Institute of Child Health and Human Development, the National Institute of Allergy and Infectious Diseases, or the National Institute of Health. Further funding was provided by Framework in Global Health, Brown University Global Health Initiative. Dr. Winston received support from the National Institute on Drug Abuse [grant 5T32DA013911]. The funders had no role in study design, data collection and analysis, decision to publish, or preparation of the manuscript.

Competing Interests: Paula Braitstein, PhD is a PLOS ONE Editorial Board Member. The authors confirm that this does not alter the authors' adherence to all the PLOS ONE policies on sharing data and materials, as detailed online in the guide for authors.

* E-mail: pbraitst@iu.edu

Introduction

The prevalence of children and adolescents (youth) living and working on the streets of the world's cities is a widespread and escalating problem. Due to the transient nature of their lifestyle, estimating the size of street youth populations is difficult [1], but within Kenya alone, the number of street youth has been reported to be as large as 300,000 [2]. However, the label "street youth" implies a homogeneous population and does not have the same meaning and connotation in all locations [1]. Often, street youth are grouped in two major categories: 1) those who live on the streets part-time, often referred to as 'on the street', who spend their days on the street but sleep at home with family, are believed to represent approximately 60% of the street youth population in resource-constrained settings; and 2) youth who live on the streets full-time, called 'of the street', who spend their days and nights on the street and maintain few or no ties with family, and make up the remaining 40% [3].

Although the full-time versus part-time distinction has historically dominated the classification of street youth since being accepted by UNICEF in 1986 [3], very little work has been done to characterize these sub-populations with consequent debates on how to name and describe street-connected youth [4,5]. It has been suggested that street involvement may be a gradient that begins with a child first going to the street to support his or her family, eventually engaging in less and less family contact until he or she is living and working on the street full-time [6]. However, knowledge on whether and to what extent these transitions exist, the effect of experiences causing homelessness on the degree of street-connectedness, among other important questions related to this population, is limited due to a dearth of longitudinal studies on this population [7]. The financial independence that some youth are able to attain through street life has been identified as a factor contributing to a high attrition rate from rehabilitation programs [7], but few studies have attempted to characterize how street youth obtain and allocate money. Further, while factors motivating youth to adopt street life, such as poverty, domestic conflict, civil conflict, substance use in the home, and, to a lesser extent, orphanhood have been investigated, the vast majority of these studies have been done primarily on male populations with little to no attention given to females or with any gender analysis or analysis of how these reasons influence the level of involvement on the street [8–11].

The main objective of this analysis was therefore to describe the social and economic characteristics of street youth in Eldoret, Kenya, and to examine variations in these factors by gender and level of street involvement. These data may assist program implementers and policy-makers in developing tailored interventions for this vulnerable population.

Methods

Human Subjects Protection

This study received ethical approval from the Kenyan Institutional Research and Ethics Committee of Moi Teaching and Referral Hospital and Moi University College of Health Sciences (Eldoret, Kenya), the Indiana University Institutional Review Board (Indianapolis, USA), and the Miriam Hospital Institutional Review Board (Providence, USA). Approval for the study was also obtained from the District Children's Officer (DCO) in Eldoret. Recruited individuals interested in participating in the study were either accompanied or referred to the study clinic by the outreach worker for screening and consenting. If an individual was noted to be impaired as a result of substance use at the time of contact with the outreach worker, they were asked to delay going to the clinic until they were no longer 'high'. At the study clinic, all prospective participants underwent a comprehension assessment to ensure the youth understood the nature of their participation in a research study, the study procedures, and their right to withdraw at any time or withhold any answers [12]. Prospective participants failing this comprehension assessment because of substance use were invited to return at another time and informed of the reason they were not enrolled in the study. Those prospective participants passing this screening phase were enrolled. Participants over 18 provided written informed consent. Those under 18 provided written assent in the presence of a child advocate, with the District Youth's Officer providing general written consent for their participation as de facto guardian. There were two prospective participants who failed to meet the criteria for understanding and were not enrolled. None refused participation in the study.

Study Design

This is a secondary analysis of data collected for a cross-sectional study on the sexual health of street-connected youth [13].

Study Setting

Eldoret is a rapidly growing city in western Kenya with an estimated population of 289,380, making it Kenya's fifth largest city [14]. Located within Eldoret are Moi University School of Medicine (Kenya's second largest medical school), Moi Teaching and Referral Hospital (MTRH), and the Academic Model Providing Access to Healthcare (AMPATH) Program, a large HIV care and treatment program [15,16]. Eldoret is the administrative center of Uasin Gishu County, where 51.8% of the population lives under Kenya's poverty line, exceeding the national average of 47.2% [14].

Study Population

To participate in this study, street youth had to meet the following inclusion criteria: aged 12–21, living in Eldoret, Kenya, spending days only or days and nights on the street, and able and willing to consent or assent. Participants spending only their days on the street were designated part-time street youth while those on the streets day and night were designated full-time street youth.

Recruitment and Enrolment

Recruitment and enrollment was conducted from September 2011–June 2012. Youth were informed about the study through community networks, street youth support services, contacts of researchers, and by street outreach workers familiar with the population. Participants were recruited and enrolled by the street outreach workers using convenience sampling until the target sample size of 200 participants was met. Prospective participants were recruited from known 'hang-out spots' and places where children sleep (known locally as 'barracks') during the day. To address gender disparity, participants were also recruited and enrolled at Berur, an Eldoret community organization that works specifically with street girls. The study was conducted at a study clinic for high-risk youth located at Moi Teaching and Referral Hospital Berur, all of which provide healthcare or services to street youth.

Measures and Sources of Data

Study personnel interviewed each participant privately and administered a structured questionnaire. Data were manually collected. Interviews were approximately 45 minutes in length and conducted in Kiswahili or English. The clinical encounter captured data on sociodemographics: gender (male/female), age category (12–15, 16–18, 19 years and above), parental vital status (both alive, mother died, father died, both died), person(s) they were living with prior to coming to the street, educational history (ever gone to school (yes/no), desire to return to school (yes/no). Characteristics related to their street-involvement were also gathered, including whether they were on the streets part-time or full-time, cumulative time spent on the street (1–2 years, 2–5 years, >5 years), arrest history (yes/no), jail history (yes/no), and whether they have been to a rehabilitation center (yes/no). The variables pertaining to social support were what their major source of social support was (family member, street friend, non-street friend, pastor/teacher/doctor, non-governmental or community-based organization (NGO)), and belonging to a street gang or social group (yes/no). The environmental assessment section of the questionnaire collected information on amount of money earned per day (<50 KES, 50–100 KES, >100 KES), things purchased with available money (food, drugs or alcohol, send money home, other), and first priority for available money (same). For sources of income and things purchased, participants were allowed to select as many responses as applicable. Primary dependent variables of interest were: 1) history of arrest and detention (ever, yes/no); 2) first priority for spending money (food vs. all other commodities); 3) major source of support (family members, friends on the street, other); 4) primary reason for coming to the street (poverty at home, alcoholism or violence in the home, other).

Data Analysis

Data from the questionnaire were hand-entered into EpiInfo software (Version 6) following initial checks for errors and inconsistencies. Data cleaning was conducted looking for outliers, inconsistencies, and missing or wrong data. Categorical variables were summarized using proportions while continuous variables were examined using means and medians together with standard deviation and inter-quartile range (IQR), respectively. The χ^2test was used to test for associations between categorical and dichotomous variables; Fisher's exact test was used alternatively if some cells had expected value of less than 5.

Primary dependent variables were selected based on their priority in terms of potential program or policy relevance, their statistical significance in bivariate analyses, and feasibility in a logistic regression (e.g. heterogeneity in response). Non-dichotomous variables of interest were dichotomized based on relevant cut-offs (for continuous variables) or categories (for categorical ones). Multivariable analysis used both binary (for binary variables) and multinomial (for nominal variables) logistic regression models to examine the association of gender and level of street involvement with these primary dependent variables of interest, adjusting for age and length of time on the street. All analyses were conducted using SAS version 9.3.

Results

Of the 200 street youth enrolled in the study, 41% were female with a mean age of 16.3 years. Overall, 71% of the study population was on the street full-time although this varied significantly by gender: 85% of boys were on the street full-time compared to 52% of girls ($p<0.001$).

Sociodemographic characteristics

Table 1 summarizes the sociodemographics of the study population, disaggregated by gender and level of street-involvement. Males tended to be younger than females (51% of boys were aged 12–15 years compared to 32% of girls); there was no significant difference in age between those on the street full-time and part-time. A majority of both genders had a history of some school attendance (87% boys, 79% girls), with more boys than girls saying that they would like to return to school given the chance (73% boys, 58% girls). More girls than boys said that both of their parents were deceased (19% boys, 35% girls), and more youth on the street full-time reported being double orphans (28%) compared to those on the street part-time (18%). The largest proportion of both sexes said they lived with their mother only before coming to the street (30% boys, 36% girls). The largest proportion of part-time street youth reported living with their mother only prior to street involvement (44%); however full-time street youth most commonly reported having lived with family other than their parents (35%).

Characteristics of street-involvement

Table 2 details characteristics of street-involvement among the study population. Poverty was the most cited reason for leaving home by females (58%) and was the second most cited reason by males (30%). Alcoholism or violence was the most common reason for boys leaving home, and the second most common reason for girls (37% boys, 15% girls). A large fraction of both part-time and full-time street youth left home citing poverty (61% part-time, 34% full-time), but an equally large proportion of full-time street youth reported leaving home as a result of alcoholism or violence (36%, compared to 7% for part-time street youth). Few youth reported leaving home as a result of civil conflict (0% part-time, 4% full-time). The majority of both sexes reported being on the street full-time (85% of boys, 52% of girls). A majority of both genders had been on the street for more than 2 years, with a larger fraction of males compared to females in this category (82% boys v. 70% girls). In terms of street involvement, the full-time street youth had been on the streets longer, with 82% saying they had been on the streets for more than 2 years, compared with 65% of part-time street youth.

More girls than boys and more part-time than full-time street youth reported to be primarily supported by a family member (28% girls, 13% boys; 42% part-time, 10% full-time). Boys and full-time street youth said they were primarily supported by street friends (12% girls, 28% boys; 5% part-time, 28% full-time). Approximately half of the entire population, both girls and boys and full-time and part-time street youth, reported that non-governmental organizations were their major source of support, while less than 10% of any category reported that a pastor, teacher or doctor supported them.

Membership in a street social group or gang was more common amongst boys (98%) than girls (73%), and amongst. full-time (97%) than part-time street (67%) youth. By gender, 76% and 68% of boys reported having been arrested or jailed, respectively, compared to 57% and 46% of girls. By street involvement, 76% and 65% of full-time street youth said that they had been arrested or jailed, respectively. The corresponding numbers for part-time street youth were 47% and 44%.

Economic Characteristics

Table 3 summarizes the reported sources of money for the study population, and spending habits and priorities. Large fractions of both males and females reported begging (53% and 64%, respectively) and casual labor (40% and 53%) as sources of money. Other significant income generating activities for males were recycling metals (73%), carrying luggage (64%), and watching cars (45%). Overall, males had more diverse sources of income when compared with the female group. Significantly more females than males reported involvement in prostitution (15% females, 1% males). In addition to begging, both part and full-time street youth reported high involvement in a wide variety of income generating activities, but full-time street youth had a larger fraction engaged in informal employment, including recycling various materials, watching cars, and carrying luggage (15–60% full-time, 7–25% part-time).

Males also earned, on average, more than females, with 90% of males earning more than 50 KES per day (0.59 USD), while only 73% of females earned a similar amount. Full-time street youth earn more on average than their part-time counterparts, with 89% of them earning >50 KES daily, compared with 68% of part-time street youth.

Table 1. Sociodemographic characteristics of the study population by gender and level of street involvement (N = 200).

	Gender			Level of street involvement		
	Male n = 119; n (%)	Female n = 81; n (%)	P-value	Part-time n = 57; n (%)	Full-time n = 143; n (%)	P-value
Sex						
Male	-----	-----	Not applicable	18 (31.6)	101 (70.6)	**<0.001**
Female	-----	-----		39 (68.4)	42 (29.4)	
Missing	0 (0%)	0 (0%)		0 (0.0)	0 (0.0)	
Age group (years)						
12–15	61 (51.3)	26 (32.1)	**0.007**	29 (50.9)	58 (40.6)	0.184
>15	58 (48.7)	55 (67.9)		28 (49.1)	85 (59.4)	
Missing	0 (0.0)	0 (0.0)		0 (0.0)	0 (0.0)	
Has attended school						
Yes	104 (87.4)	64 (79.0)	0.112	48 (84.2)	120 (83.9)	0.959
No	15 (12.6)	17 (21.0)		9 (15.8)	23 (16.1)	
Missing	0 (0.0)	0 (0.0)		0 (0.0)	0 (0.0)	
Wants to return to school						
Yes	87 (73.1)	47 (58.0)	**0.019**	41 (71.9)	93 (65.0)	0.201
No	31 (26.1)	29 (35.8)		13 (22.8)	47 (32.9)	
Don't know	1 (0.8)	5 (6.2)		3 (5.3)	3 (2.1)	
Missing	0 (0.0)	0 (0.0)		0 (0.0)	0 (0.0)	
Parent vital status						
Single orphan	64 (53.8)	33 (40.7)	0.032	29 (50.9)	68 (47.6)	0.267
Double orphan	22 (18.5)	28 (34.6)		10 (17.5)	40 (28.0)	
Both alive	33 (27.7)	20 (24.7)		18 (31.6)	35 (24.5)	
Missing	0 (0.0)	0 (0.0)		0 (0.0)	0 (0.0)	
Persons lived with before coming to the street						
Mother only	35 (29.7)	29 (35.8)	0.367	25 (44.6)	39 (27.3)	0.093
Father only	9 (7.6)	3 (3.7)		1 (1.8)	11 (7.7)	
Both parents	29 (24.6)	17 (21.0)		14 (25.0)	32 (22.4)	
Other relatives	30 (25.4)	25 (30.9)		12 (21.4)	43 (30.1)	
Well-wishers	2 (1.7)	3 (3.7)		1 (1.8)	4 (2.8)	
Father/stepmother, mother/stepfather	13 (10.9)	4 (4.9)		3 (5.3)	14 (9.8)	
Missing	1 (0.8)	0 (0.0)		0 (0.0)	0 (0.0)	

When money was available, a majority of all groups said that they bought food (99% boys, 84% girls; 99% full-time, 77% part-time). While 63% of boys and 60% full-time street youth said they would buy drugs with their money, only 28% of girls and 23% of part-time street youth said the same. Part-time street youth were much more likely to say they took a portion of their money home (51% part-time, 11% full-time). When asked about which choice took first priority when money was available, 90% of boys and full-time street youth picked food, compared to 78% of girls and 72% of part-time street youth. Glue, alcohol, and other drugs were not cited as a priority by a majority of any group.

Multivariable Analyses

Tables 4 and 5 describe the association of gender and level of street-involvement with key social and economic characteristics using both binary (Table 4, for binary effects) and multinomial logistic regression for non-ordered categorical effects (Table 5). Compared with part-time street youth, full-time street youth were more likely to have been arrested (Adjusted Odds Ratio [AOR]: 2.33, 95% Confidence Interval [95% CI]: 1.01–5.35), name food as their first spending priority (AOR: 2.57, 95% CI: 1.03–6.45), to report that friends on the street were their major source of support (AOR: 3.59, 95% CI: 1.01–12.82), and to have left home due to alcoholism or violence (AOR: 5.54, 95% CI: 1.67–18.34). Compared with females, males were more likely to have ever been arrested (AOR: 2.66, 95% CI: 1.14–6.18), and to have ever been jailed (AOR: 3.22, 95% CI: 1.47–7.02).

Discussion

These findings suggest a heterogeneous yet highly vulnerable street youth population in this resource-constrained setting. The social and economic characteristics of each subgroup are distinct, but all of the youth profiled here appear resourceful, employing a

Table 2. Street-involvement characteristics of the study population by gender and level of street involvement (N = 200).

	Gender			Level of street involvement		
	Male n = 119; n (%)	Female n = 81; n (%)	P-value	Part-time n = 57; n (%)	Full-time n = 143; n (%)	P-value
Major reason for coming to the street						
Poverty in the home	36 (30.2)	47 (58.0)	**<0.001**	35 (61.4)	48 (33.6)	**<0.001**
Alcoholism, violence, or abuse in the home	47 (39.5)	12 (14.8)		4 (7.0)	55 (38.5)	
Boredom/abandoned	22 (18.5)	10 (12.4)		6 (10.5)	26 (18.2)	
Peer pressure/orphaned/thrown out because of stealing	14 (11.8)	12 (14.8)		12 (21.1)	14 (9.8)	
Missing	0 (0.0)	0 (0.0)		0 (0.0)	0 (0.0)	
Daily time spent on the street						
Part-time	18 (15.1)	39 (48.2	**<0.001**	—	—	Not applicable
Full-time	101 (84.9)	42 (51.8)		—	—	
Missing	0 (0.0)	0 (0.0)		—	—	
Cumulative time on the street						
1-2 yrs	22 (18.5)	24 (29.6)	0.177	20 (35.1)	26 (18.2)	**0.036**
2-5 yrs	50 (42.0)	28 (34.6)		18 (31.6)	60 (42.0)	
>5 yrs	47 (39.5)	29 (35.8)		19 (33.3)	57 (39.9)	
Missing	0 (0.0)	0 (0.0)		0 (0.0)	0 (0.0)	
Major source of support						
Family member	15 (12.6)	23 (28.4)	**0.004**	24 (42.1)	14 (9.9)	**<0.001**
Street friend	33 (28.2)	10 (12.4)		3 (5.3)	40 (28.4)	
Non-street friend	11 (9.4)	4 (4.9)		3 (5.3)	12 (8.5)	
Pastor/teacher/doctor	6 (5.0)	1 (1.2)		4 (7.0)	3 (2.1)	
NGO	52 (44.4)	43 (53.1)		23 (40.4)	72 (50.4)	
Missing responses	2 (1.7)	0 (0.0)		0. (0.0)	2 (1.4)	
Belongs to a gang or street social group						
Yes	117 (98.3)	59 (72.8)	**<0.001**	38 (66.7)	138 (96.5)	**<0.001**
No	2 (1.7)	22 (27.2)		19 (33.3)	5 (3.5)	
Missing	0 (0.0)	0 (0.0)		0 (0.0)	0 (0.0)	
Ever been arrested						
Yes	90 (75.6)	45 (56.6)	**0.003**	27 (47.4)	108 (75.5)	**<0.001**
No	29 (24.4)	36 (44.4)		30 (52.6)	35 (24.5)	
Missing	0 (0.0)	0 (0.0)		0 (0.0)	0 (0.0)	
Been to jail or juvenile detention						
Yes	81 (68.1)	37 (45.7)	**0.002**	25 (43.9)	93 (65.0)	**0.006**
No	38 (31.9)	44 (54.3)		32 (56.1)	50 (35.0)	
Missing	0 (0.0)	0 (0.0)		0 (0.0)	0 (0.0)	
Been to rehabilitation center or children's home						
Yes	75 (63.0)	53 (65.4)	0.728	32 (56.1)	96 (67.1)	0.144
No	44 (37.0)	28 (34.6)		25 (43.9)	47 (32.9)	
Missing	0 (0.0)	0 (0.0)		0 (0.0)	0 (0.0)	

wide range of strategies to meet their needs on the street. Such knowledge can assist in developing interventions targeted towards the diverse strengths and vulnerabilities of this population.

Gender

It has previously been hypothesized that, for Kenyan girls, adopting street life indicates disintegration of the family unit and societal victimization [8]. While we did not observe that girls left home primarily as a result of alcoholism or violence, the girls had fewer resources and coping skills when compared with their male counterparts. The girls in our study were more likely to be double orphans and were less likely to have schooling to fall back on or to join street social networks. Our female participants reported less daily income compared with boys, consistent with past research that found street girls had fewer economic opportunities and earned less money than boys for performing similar activities [17].

Table 3. Economic characteristics of the study population by gender and level of street involvement (N = 200).

	Gender		Level of street involvement	
	Male	Female	Part-time	Full-time
	n = 119; n (%)	n = 81; n (%)	n = 57; n (%)	n = 143; n (%)
Sources of money				
Begging	63 (52.9)	52 (64.2)	31 (54.4)	84 (58.7)
Stealing or pickpocketing	2 (1.7)	1 (1.2)	3 (5.3)	0 (0.0)
Metals recycling	87 (73.1)	9 (12.4)	10 (17.5)	86 (60.1)
Plastics recycling	32 (26.9)	10 (12.4)	6 (10.5)	36 (25.2)
Papers recycling	23 (19.3)	3 (3.7)	4 (7.0)	22 (15.4)
Selling plastic bags	2 (1.7)	2 (2.5)	0 (0.0)	4 (2.8)
Selling drugs	1 (0.8)	2 (2.5)	1 (1.7)	2 (1.4)
Watching cars	53 (44.5)	3 (3.7)	11 (19.3)	45 (31.5)
Carrying luggage and bags	76 (63.9)	6 (7.4)	14 (24.6)	68 (47.6)
Casual labor	47 (39.5)	43 (53.1)	24 (42.1)	66 (46.2)
Prostitution	1 (0.8)	12 (14.8)	5 (8.8)'	8 (5.6)
Given money by relatives/friends	2 (1.7)	10 (12.4)	7 (12.3)	5 (3.5)
Making ornaments	0 (0.0)	7 (8.6)	7 (12.3)	0 (0.0)
Collecting charcoal/cigarettes	2 (1.7)	2 (2.5)	0 (0.0)	4 (2.8)
Other	9 (7.6)	7 (8.6)	6 (10.5)	10 (17.5)
Missing	0 (0.0)	0 (0.0)	0 (0.0)	0 (0.0)
Amount earned daily (KES)				
<50	12 (10.1)	22 (27.2)	18 (31.6)	16 (11.2)
50-100	51 (42.9)	21 (25.9)	17 (29.8)	55 (38.5)
100-500	55 (46.2)	33 (40.7)	18 (31.6)	70 (49.0)
>500	1 (0.8)	0 (0.0)	0 (0.0)	1 (0.7)
Don't know	0 (0.0)	5 (6.2)	4 (7.0)	1 (0.7)
Missing	0 (0.0)	0 (0.0)	0 (0.0)	0 (0.0)
Things bought with earned money				
Food	118 (99.2)	68 (84.0)	44 (77.2)	142 (99.3)
Glue, alcohol, or other drugs	75 (63.0)	23 (28.4)	13 (22.8)	85 (59.4)
Take money home	24 (20.2)	21 (25.9)	29 (50.9)	16 (11.2)
Clothes/shoes/soap/lotion	46 (38.7)	35 (43.2)	14 (24.6)	67 (46.9)
Save for other necessities	10 (8.4)	6 (7.4)	4 (7.0)	12 (8.4)
Rent/bus fare	6 (5.0)	1 (1.2)	1 (1.8)	6 (4.2)
Other	18 (15.1)	6 (7.4)	7 (12.3)	17 (11.9)
Missing	0 (0.0)	0 (0.0)	0 (0.0)	0 (0.0)
First priority for available money				
Food	107 (89.9)	63 (77.8)	41 (71.9)	129 (90.2)
Glue, alcohol, or other drugs	8 (6.7)	2 (2.5)	1 (1.8)	9 (6.3)
Take money home	2 (1.7)	6 (7.7)	7 (12.3)	1 (0.7)
Other	2 (1.7)	6 (7.7)	4 (7.0)	4 (2.8)
Refused to answer	0 (0.0)	1 (1.2)	1 (1.8)	0 (0.0)
Missing	0 (0.0)	3 (1.3)	3 (5.3)	0 (0.0)

The frequency of girls reporting engagement in prostitution is worrisome and potentially underreported, indicating a unique vulnerability of this subpopulation, especially in the context of otherwise limited options for income generation.

Male street youth by no means have an easy lifestyle, experiencing significantly increased interaction with legal authorities and the detention system. However, the responses of the boys in our study supports the ideas set forth by previous research, portraying a group of boys who, in the face of hardship, are able to develop diverse strategies for earning money and form strong support networks of friends [8].

Table 4. Unadjusted (UOR) and Adjusted Odds Ratios (AOR) and 95% Confidence Intervals (CI) for associations of gender and level of street involvement with key social and economic indicators among street-connected youth aged 12–21 (N = 200).

	UOR	95%CI	AOR	95%CI
Ever arrested (n = 200)				
Gender (male vs. female*)	1.80	0.94–3.47	2.66	1.14–6.18
Street involvement (full vs. part-time*)	2.78	1.40–5.51	2.33	1.01–5.35
Ever been to jail (n = 200)				
Gender (male vs. female*)	2.11	1.13–3.91	3.22	1.47–7.02
Street involvement (full vs. part-time*)	1.82	0.93–3.55	1.38	0.63–3.02
First priority for money (food vs. all other responses) (n = 197)				
Gender (male vs. female*)	1.58	0.65–3.81	1.28	0.50–3.27
Street involvement (full vs. part-time*)	2.48	1.02–6.04	2.57	1.03–6.45

(Binary multivariable logistic regression analysis for the association of gender and level of street involvement with binary indicators adjusted for age and length of time on the street).
*reference category.

It should be noted that the gender-specific trends observed here are likely not entirely unique to the street youth population. For example, the general prison population in Eldoret is predominantly male; females in the general population have fewer opportunities for diversified income generation compared with males [18,19]. Regardless, these gender differences are important to understanding the needs and circumstances of this particular population, and should be considered when devising reintegration and rehabilitation strategies for street youth.

Level of street involvement

The data suggest that full-time street youth have used the streets to replace a home life and work to take care of themselves. These youth, isolated from family, generally join social groups for support (86% of boys and 82% of girls). A previous study of the Eldoret street child population found that full-time street youth maintain a large group of friends which provide functions expected from a family [20]. We see full-time street youth working more, earning more, and preferentially purchasing vital items such as food more commonly than the part-time street youth. Despite the fact that a large portion of full-time street youth do purchase drugs, it is important to note how few of them reported a preference for purchasing drugs—survival, rather than substance use, appears to be paramount to these youth, a theme consistent in the literature [21–23].

Because of their focus on survival and strong dependence on peer networks, full-time street youth are the distinctly more vulnerable population. This is particularly in evidence given the high likelihood that they came to the streets because of the need to leave a home environment of violence and/or alcoholism, and the high probability of being arrested and jailed. Compared with part-time street youth, a larger proportion of full-time street youth purchase drugs, presumably for their own use. Substance use within this population has been identified both as a coping mechanism as well as a component of a shared street culture that exists among street social groups [9,24].

Policy Implications

There are several policy implications to these findings, particularly relevant for local and national governments. First,

Table 5. Unadjusted (UOR) and Adjusted Odds Ratios (AOR) and 95% Confidence Intervals (CI) for associations of gender and level of street involvement with key social and economic indicators among street-connected youth aged 12–21 (N = 200).

Covariate	Dependent variable	UOR (95%CI)	AOR (95%CI)
	Major source of support (n = 198)		
Gender (male vs. female*)	family member	0.74 (0.32–1.68)	0.66 (0.27–1.63
Gender (male vs. female*)	friend on the street	1.79 (0.79–4.08)	2.15 (0.89–5.21)
Street status (full vs. part-time*)	family member	0.22 (0.10–0.51)	0.24 (0.10–0.55)
Street status (full vs. part-time*)	friend on the street	3.79 (1.06–13.55)	3.59 (1.01–12.82)
	Major reason for coming to the street (n = 200)		
Gender (male vs. female*)	poverty	0.51 (0.25–1.04)	0.52 (0.24–1.12)
Gender (male vs. female*)	violence	1.71 (0.72–4.08)	1.78 (0.70–4.56)
Street status (full vs. part-time*)	poverty	0.77 (0.36–1.63)	0.78 (0.36–1.68)
Street status (full vs. part-time*)	violence	5.24 (1.60–17.17)	5.54 (1.67–18.34)

(Multinomial logistic regression analysis for the association of gender and level of street-involvement with non-ordered categorical indicators adjusted for age and length of time on the street.).
*Reference category.

we found that very high proportions of the study population, both male and female, have been arrested and spent time in jail or detention facilities. The incarceration of youth in general and females in particular is known to be fraught with poor conditions, breaches of their human rights, and a distinct lack of emphasis on rehabilitation [25,26]. Researchers, national bodies, and international human rights groups have reported that police and security forces have abused children on the streets of cities all over the world [27]. Additionally, detention of youth is known to be associated with poor psychological outcomes, impaired reintegration into society, and a high rate of recidivism [28]. For youth who already come from an environment of violence and neglect, the consequences of detention on top of this may create serious obstacles to societal reintegration that are insurmountable. Without a comparison group from the general population, the increase in interaction with legal authorities experienced by street youth is difficult to quantify. However, regardless of relative frequency, the high proportion of youth arrested and incarcerated seen in this population is a major policy issue that needs to be urgently addressed. Local and national governments must find alternative strategies to handling the 'epidemic of street youth' in a way that maximizes protection and rehabilitation, and minimizes detention and abuse.

The global population of street-connected youth continues to increase with few improvements in their situation [2,29–32]. Our results challenge the commonly held assumption that many youth end up on the street as a result of ethnic violence, delinquency or boredom [6,33,34]. The fact that the majority of youth in our study cite poverty, violence and alcoholism as the primary reasons for leaving home, points to the need for policies that help to support families to care for the children they are responsible for and through more extensive child-protection initiatives. Preventing youth from having to come to the street should be the top priority for policy makers.

Presently, local governments in Kenya are endeavoring to forcibly return street youth back to where they come from, a process that can be thought of as 'universal reunification'. Universal reunification of street youth with their families (or whoever is found when they are taken there) without a risk assessment of the home environment has shown limited benefit and can be detrimental [35–37]. Whether youth leave home as a result of abusive conditions or as a result of poverty, our data suggest that the vast majority end up on the street because of seriously adverse home environments. Local governments must consider the capacity of households and communities for reintegrating these youth without additional support. A simplistic repatriation strategy is likely to fail. Moreover, the current trend by local governments to deter or prevent non-governmental (NGO) and community-based organizations from supporting street-connecting youth is likely to have a detrimental impact on youth given that half of the population in our study reported that their primary source of support was from these agencies. Local and national governments should be encouraged to work with academic and NGO stakeholders to find the best preventive and rehabilitation/reintegration strategies that are in the best interests of the youth.

Strengths & Limitations

One of the major strengths of this study is its relatively large proportion of female street youth, one of the largest in current literature. Another is the high rate of response to all portions of the interview questionnaire by the participants. Both may be attributed to the strong trust and established relationship between our study team and the street-connected youth community in Eldoret [15,38–41], including our use of street-based outreach workers and their assistance of the youth in matters unrelated to research. Our study also goes beyond traditional analyses of youth's motivations for adopting street life and their subsequent risk of abusing substances [42]. This population is understudied and there are few data to guide program implementers and policy makers; this study helps to fill that gap. This analysis does not address the sexual behaviors, substance use or mental health of this population. These are extremely important issues that we are addressing through separate analyses, studies, and publications [13,43–47].

One of the main limitations of this study is inherent to the use of a convenience sample and cross-sectional data. For example, our study has identified a much larger proportion of street-connected youth being on the street full-time compared to what has traditionally been reported [3,5]. As our data were based on a cross-sectional convenience sample, caution should be used in generalizing from this to the whole population of street youth. This study has the potential for selection bias toward those youth easiest to access and a failure to enroll those youth more difficult to reach. Additionally, due to the dynamic and transient nature of the street youth population, their characteristics and experiences are constantly in flux; a convenience sample of cross-sectional data from these individuals may not reflect the full story or may become quickly outdated. There may have been some responder bias if participants answered questions according to what they thought the interviewer wanted to hear. However, it should be noted that the interviewer, a medical officer, was well-trained in interview techniques and participants had nothing to gain or lose from the nature of their responses. The cross-sectional design has inherent limitations, including an inability to draw conclusions about the temporal nature of the exposures and outcomes examined. The cultural and geographical heterogeneity within resource-constrained settings means that it cannot be assumed that the trends observed in the Eldoret population are immediately generalizable to all street youth. The categorization of whether or not a child spends nights on the street utilizes a simple binary metric (full-time, part-time). While widely accepted, distilling the varied experiences of street children into these two categories has been criticized as an oversimplification that fails to fully address family ties and entrenchment in street life [48]. While we accept this limitation, these data nevertheless provide a more nuanced perspective into the social and economic characteristics of street-connected youth in this setting compared to most other available data on them. Finally, by enrolling youth ages 12 and above, we excluded young children, of whom there are many on the street. Caution should be used in interpreting these data.

Conclusions

These data suggest that this street youth population is heterogeneous and resourceful, yet highly vulnerable. Despite frequently reported statistics connecting Kenya's street youth population with ethnic violence or boredom, few youth actually reported these as reasons for adopting street life. The majority of youth who participated in this study left home either because of poverty or alcoholism and violence in the home. In either case, a failure of familial support, be it financial, emotional, or both appears to have driven them to search for something more on the streets. These data emphasize the urgent need for governments and other stakeholders seeking to intervene on behalf of these youth to address the various social and economic factors pulling them to the streets and obstructing their societal reintegration. A fundamental and detailed understanding of this population's heterogeneity will help to inform social reintegration policies and programs by recognizing and addressing the diverse needs of these young people.

Acknowledgments

Special thanks also go out to the staff of the OSCAR Clinic, especially Dominic Makori; Lauryn Njuguna Muthoni MBChB, Amon Chirchir, MBChB; the staff and leadership of Moi Teaching and Referral Hospital; and Philip Nzenge, former District Youth's Officer of Uasin Gishu County.

Author Contributions

Conceived and designed the experiments: RS SW. Performed the experiments: SW. Analyzed the data: RS JK PB. Contributed reagents/materials/analysis tools: DA. Wrote the paper: RS PB SW. Provided technical assistance with the analysis: LY. Provided senior biostatistical oversight: JH.

References

1. CSC (2009) Who is a "street child"? London, UK: Consortium for Street Children.
2. IRIN (2007) Youth in Crisis: Coming of Age in the 21st Century. Nairobi, Kenya: United Nations Integrated Regional Informing Network.
3. UNICEF (1986) Children in Especially Difficult Circumstances. New York.
4. Embleton L, Mwangi A, Vreeman R, Ayuku D, Braitstein P (2013) The epidemiology of substance use among street children in resource-constrained settings: a systematic review and meta-analysis. Addiction 108: 1722–1733.
5. United Nations Human Rights Office of the High Commissioner (2012) Protection and promotion of the rights of children working and/or living on the street. Geneva: Office of the United Nations High Commissioner for Human Rights.
6. Aptekar L (1994) Street Children in the Developing World: A Review of Their Condition. Cross-Cultural Research 28: 195–224.
7. Johnson H, Kisslinger T, Oneko S, Heuser A (2005) Responses to child vulnerability. Moshi, Tanzania: Mkomboze Center for Street Children.
8. Aptekar L, Ciano-Federoff LM (1999) Street Children in Nairobi: Gender Differences in Mental Health. In: M. Rafaelli RL, editor.Developmental issues among homeless and working street youth: New Directions in Childhood Development.San Francisco, CA: Jossey Bass. pp. 35–46.
9. Embleton L, Atwoli L, Ayuku D, Braitstein P (2013) The Journey of Addiction: Barriers to and Facilitators of Drug Use Cessation among Street Children and Youths in Western Kenya. PLoS ONE 8: e53435.
10. Lalani S (2009) Life on the Street: The Chokora of Eldoret. Brighton, UK: University of Sussex.
11. WERK (2002) The Story of Children Living and Working on the Streets of Nairobi. Nairobi, Kenya: Women Educational Researchers of Kenya.
12. Embleton L, Ott MA, Winston S, Kamanda A, Chirchir AK, et al. (2013) Ethical approaches to consent in conducting research in street youth in resource constrained settings. International Association for Adolescent Health (IAAH) 10th World Congress. Istanbul, Turkey.
13. Winston S, Chirchir A, Muthoni L, Ayuku D, Braitstein P (2012) Sexual risk and HIV prevalence in street-involved youth in western Kenya. IDWeek: Advancing Science, Improving Care. San Diego, CA: Infectious Disease Society of America.
14. KODP (2011a) Kenya County Fact Sheets Dec 2011. Kenya Open Data Project.
15. Ayaya S, Esamai FO (2001) Health Problems of Street Children in Eldoret, Kenya. East African Medical Journal 78: 624–629.
16. Einterz R, Kimaiyo HNKM, Khwa-Otsyula BO, Esamai F, Quigley F, et al. (2007) Responding to the HIV Pandemic: The Power of an Academic Medical Partnership. Academy of Medicine 82: 812–818.
17. EMDH (2009) Survey on Children in Street Situation in Juba. Geneva, Switzerland: Enfants du Monde—Droits de l'Homme.
18. Albee A (1994) Support to Women's Productive and Income-. New York NY: UNICEF.
19. Kinyanjui DWC, Atwoli L (2013) Substance use among inmates at the Eldoret prison in Western Kenya. BMC Psychiatry 13: 53.
20. Ayuku D (2005) Family Networks of Street Children and School Children of Eldoret, Kenya. East African Journal of Public Health 2: 6–9.
21. Ensing A, Strehl T (2010) Street-Working and Street-Living Children in Peru: Quantitative Report, Lima. International Research on Working Children (IREWOC).
22. Lugalla J, Mbwambo JK (1999) Street Children and Street Life in Urban Tanzania: The Culture of Surviving and its Implications for Children's Health. International Journal of Urban and Regional Research 23: 329–344.
23. UNICEF (2001) 2001 ZIM: A Study on Street Children in Zimbabwe. New York, NY: UNICEF.
24. Cottrell-Boyce J (2010) The Role of Solvents in the Lives of Kenyan Street Children: An Ethnographic Perspective. African Journal of Drug & Alcohol Studies 9: 93–102.
25. DCI (2008) Protecting the Rights of Children in Conflict With the Law: Research on Alternatives to the Deprivation of Liberty in Eight Countries: Defence for Children International, Institut Universitaire Kurt Bosch–University Fridbourg Master of Advanced Studies in Children's Rights Program.
26. HRW (2001) Rights at Risk: Issues of Concern for Kenyan Children. Report for the Committee on the Rights of the Child by Human Rights Watch.
27. UNICEF (2012) The State of the World's Children: Urbanization. Geneva: United Nations Children's Fund.
28. Holman B, Ziedenberg J (2006) The Dangers of Detention: The Impact of Incarcerating Youth in Detention and Other Secure Facilities. Justice Policy Institute.
29. KNYP (2002) Kenya National Youth Policy: Final Draft. Nairobi, Kenya: Ministry of Home Affairs, Heritage and Sports.
30. Ray P, Davey C, Nolan P (2011) Still on the Street, Still Short of Rights. Consortium for Street Children & Plan.
31. UN (1989) Convention on the Rights of the Child. Office of the United Nations High Commissioner for Human Rights.
32. Steffan B (2012) A Generation Out of Place: The Chronic Urban Emergency in Rift Valley, Kenya. London, UK: Save the Children, UNICEF.
33. UMP (2000) Streetchildren and Gangs in African Cities: Guidelines for Local Authorities. UN Habitat: Urban Management Programme.
34. Steffen B (2012) The Chronic Urban Emergency in Rift Valley, Kenya: Report from profiling children connected to the streets in Rift Valley Province. In: Children St, editor: UNICEF, Save the Children.
35. Jacob J, Smith T, Hite S, Cheng SY (2004) Helping Uganda's street children. Journal of Chldren and Poverty 10: 3–22.
36. Slesnick N, Dashora P, Letcher A, Erdem G, Serovich J (2009) A Review of Services and Interventions for Runaway and Homeless Youth: Moving Forward. Child Youth Service Review 31: 732–742.
37. Dekel R, Peled E, Spiro SE (2003) Shelters for houseless youth: A follow-up evaluation. Journal of Adolescence 26: 201–212.
38. Ayuku D, Odero W, Kaplan C, De Bruyn R, De Vries M (2003) Social network analysis for health and social interventions among Kenyan scavenging street children. Health Policy Plan 18: 109–118.
39. Ayuku D, Ettyang G, Odero W (2004a) Psychosocial and Nutritional Status of Street Children in Comparision to School Children: A Case of Eldoret Town. African Journal of Food, Agriculture, Nutrition, Development 4: 1–11.
40. Ayuku D, Kaplan CD, Baars HMJ, de Vries MW (2004b) Characteristics and personal social networks of the "on"the street, "of" the street, shelter and school children in Eldoret, Kenya. International Social Work 47: 293–311.
41. Ayuku D, De Vries MW, Mengech HN, Kaplan CD (2004c) Temperament characteristics of street and non-street children in Eldoret, Kenya. Afr Health Sci 4: 24–30.
42. Embleton L, Mwangi A, Vreeman R, Ayuku D, Braitstein P (2013) The epidemiology of substance use among street children in resource-constrained settings: a systematic review and meta-analysis. Addiction.
43. Aalsma MC, Carpentier MY, Azzouz F, Fortenberry JD (2012) Longitudinal effects of health-harming and health-protective behaviors within adolescent romantic dyads. Soc Sci Med 74: 1444–1451.
44. Atwoli L, Ayuku D, Koech J, Hogan J, Vreeman RC, et al. (2014) Impact of domestic care environment on trauma and post-traumatic stress among orphans in western Kenya. PLoS ONE [Electronic Resource].
45. Braitstein P, Ayaya S, Nyandiko WM, Kamanda A, Koech J, et al. (2013) Nutritional status of orphaned and separated children and adolescents living in community and institutional environments in Uasin Gishu County, Kenya. PLoS ONE 8: e70054.
46. Embleton L, Atwoli L, Ayuku D, Braitstein P (2013) The Journey of Addiction: Barriers to and Facilitators of Drug Use Cessation among Street Children and Youths in Western Kenya. PLoS ONE 8: e53435.
47. Embleton L, Ayuku D, Atwoli L, Vreeman R, Braitstein P (2012) Knowledge, attitudes, and substance use practices among street children in Western Kenya. Subst Use Misuse 47: 1234–1247.
48. Muchini B (1994) Morality and Street Children in Harare: University of Zimbabwe.

Permissions

All chapters in this book were first published in PLOS ONE, by The Public Library of Science; hereby published with permission under the Creative Commons Attribution License or equivalent. Every chapter published in this book has been scrutinized by our experts. Their significance has been extensively debated. The topics covered herein carry significant findings which will fuel the growth of the discipline. They may even be implemented as practical applications or may be referred to as a beginning point for another development.

The contributors of this book come from diverse backgrounds, making this book a truly international effort. This book will bring forth new frontiers with its revolutionizing research information and detailed analysis of the nascent developments around the world.

We would like to thank all the contributing authors for lending their expertise to make the book truly unique. They have played a crucial role in the development of this book. Without their invaluable contributions this book wouldn't have been possible. They have made vital efforts to compile up to date information on the varied aspects of this subject to make this book a valuable addition to the collection of many professionals and students.

This book was conceptualized with the vision of imparting up-to-date information and advanced data in this field. To ensure the same, a matchless editorial board was set up. Every individual on the board went through rigorous rounds of assessment to prove their worth. After which they invested a large part of their time researching and compiling the most relevant data for our readers.

The editorial board has been involved in producing this book since its inception. They have spent rigorous hours researching and exploring the diverse topics which have resulted in the successful publishing of this book. They have passed on their knowledge of decades through this book. To expedite this challenging task, the publisher supported the team at every step. A small team of assistant editors was also appointed to further simplify the editing procedure and attain best results for the readers.

Apart from the editorial board, the designing team has also invested a significant amount of their time in understanding the subject and creating the most relevant covers. They scrutinized every image to scout for the most suitable representation of the subject and create an appropriate cover for the book.

The publishing team has been an ardent support to the editorial, designing and production team. Their endless efforts to recruit the best for this project, has resulted in the accomplishment of this book. They are a veteran in the field of academics and their pool of knowledge is as vast as their experience in printing. Their expertise and guidance has proved useful at every step. Their uncompromising quality standards have made this book an exceptional effort. Their encouragement from time to time has been an inspiration for everyone.

The publisher and the editorial board hope that this book will prove to be a valuable piece of knowledge for researchers, students, practitioners and scholars across the globe.

List of Contributors

Caroline Barone
Division of Newborn Medicine, Department of Pediatrics, Floating Hospital for Children at Tufts Medical Center, Boston, Massachusetts, United States of America

Anja Vogelgesang
Division of Newborn Medicine, Department of Pediatrics, Floating Hospital for Children at Tufts Medical Center, Boston, Massachusetts, United States of America
Hanover Medical School, Hanover, Germany

Christiane E. L. Dammann
Division of Newborn Medicine, Department of Pediatrics, Floating Hospital for Children at Tufts Medical Center, Boston, Massachusetts, United States of America

Cristina Scapin
Division of Newborn Medicine, Department of Pediatrics, Floating Hospital for Children at Tufts Medical Center, Boston, Massachusetts, United States of America
Genetic and Cellular Biology Division, Dibit. Sanaffaele Scientific Institute, Milan, Italy

Anna Blumental Perry
Department of Surgery, Tufts Medical Center, Boston, Massachusetts, United States of America
Department of Biomedical Sciences, Mercer School of Medicine and Department of Laboratory Oncology Research, Anderson Cancer Institute, Memorial University Medical Center, Savannah, Georgia, United States of America

Elaine Tam
Sackler School of Graduate Biomedical Sciences, Tufts University School of Medicine, Boston, Massachusetts, United States of America

Iqra Ishtiaque
University Medical and Dental College, Faisalabad, Pakistan

Kashif Shafique
School of Public Health, Dow University of Health Sciences, Karachi, Pakistan
Institute of Health and Wellbeing, Public Health, University of Glasgow, Glasgow, United Kingdom

Zia Ul-Haq
Institute of Health and Wellbeing, Public Health, University of Glasgow, Glasgow, United Kingdom
Institute of Public Health and Social Sciences, Khyber Medical University, Peshawar, KPK, Pakistan

Abdul Rauf Shaikh
Department of Community Medicine, Dow University of Health Sciences, Karachi, Pakistan

Naveed Ali Khan
Department of Surgery, Dow University of Health Sciences, Karachi, Pakistan

Abdul Rauf Memon
Department of Medicine, Dow University of Health Sciences, Karachi, Pakistan

Saira Saeed Mirza
Department of Epidemiology, University of Rotterdam, Rotterdam, the Netherlands

Afra Ishtiaque
King Edward Medical University, Lahore, Pakistan

Yan Han, Man To Ling, Huawei Mao, Jian Zheng, Kwok Tai Lam, Yuan Liu, Wenwei Tu and Yu-Lung Lau
Department of Paediatrics and Adolescent Medicine, Li Ka Shing Faculty of Medicine, University of Hong Kong, Hong Kong Special Administrative Region, People's Republic of China

Ming Liu
State Key Laboratory of Respiratory Diseases, Guangzhou Institute of Respiratory Diseases, First Affiliated Hospital, Guangzhou Medical College, Guangzhou, People's Republic of China

Wakako Umene-Nakano, Reiji Yoshimura, Kenji Hayashi, Hikaru Hori, Atsuko Ikenouchi-Sugita, Asuka Katsuki, Kiyokazu Atake and Jun Nakamura
Department of Psychiatry, University of Occupational and Environmental Health, Kitakyushu, Japan

Shingo Kakeda, Keita Watanabe, Joji Nishimura, Junji Moriya, Satoru Ide, Issei Ueda and Yukunori Korogi
Department of Radiology, University of Occupational and Environmental Health, Kitakyushu, Japan

Hidehiko Takahashi
Department of Psychiatry, Kyoto University Graduate School of Medicine, Kyoto, Japan

Osamu Abe
Department of Radiology, School of Medicine, Nihon University, Tokyo, Japan

Yan-Min Xu
Department of Psychology, Normal College of Shenzhen University, Shenzhen, China

Hai-Chen Yang, Li-Guo Qi, Jin- Hong Guo and Tie-Bang Liu
Shenzhen Institute of Mental Health, Shenzhen Kangning Hospital, Shenzhen
Mental Health Center, Shenzhen, China

Fu Li, Fang Deng and Xiao-Bo Liu
Affiliated Mental Health Center, Tongji Medical College of Huazhong University of Science and Technology, Wuhan, China

Hong-Hui Chen
Affiliated Mental Health Center, Tongji Medical College of Huazhong University of Science and Technology, Wuhan, China
Health and Family Planning Commission of Wuhan Municipality, Wuhan, China

Cholendra Arja and Kodanda Reddy Kanala
Department of Anthropology, Division of Human Genetics, Sri Venkateswara University, Tirupati, Andhra Pradesh, India

Rajasekhara Reddy Ravuri
Department of Human Genetics, Punjabi University, Patiala, Punjab, India

Venugopal N. Pulamaghatta and Chandrasekhar Adimoolam
Anthropological Survey of India, Southern Regional Centre, Mysore, Karnataka, India

Krishna Mohan Surapaneni
Department of Biochemistry, Saveetha Medical College and Hospital, Faculty of Medicine, Saveetha University, Chennai, Tamil Nadu, India

Premanand Raya
Premananda Allergy and Chest Hospital, Tirupati, Andhra Pradesh, India

Fariborz Mobarrez, Lukasz Antoniewicz, Jeanette Kuhl and Magnus Lundbäck
Karolinska Institutet, Department of Clinical Sciences, Division of Cardiovascular Medicine, Danderyd Hospital, Stockholm, Sweden

Jenny A. Bosson
Department of Public Health and Clinical Medicine, Division of Medicine/Respiratory Medicine, Umeå University, Umeå, Sweden

David S. Pisetsky
Medical Research Service, Durham VA Hospital, Durham, North Carolina, United States of America
Department of Medicine, Duke University Medical Center, Durham, North Carolina, United States of America

Robert F. Foronjy, Abdoulaye J. Dabo and Patrick Geraghty
St. Luke's Roosevelt Hospital, Mount Sinai Health System, Division of Pulmonary and Critical Care Medicine, New York, New York, United States of America

Clifford C. Taggart and Sinead Weldon
Centre for Infection and Immunity, School of Medicine, Dentistry and Biomedical Sciences, Queen's University Belfast, Belfast, Northern Ireland, United Kingdom

Alize J. Ferrari, Amanda J. Baxter, Meredith G. Harris and Harvey A. Whiteford
University of Queensland, School of Population Health, Herston, Queensland, Australia
Queensland Centre for Mental Health Research, Wacol, Queensland, Australia

Rosana E. Norman
University of Queensland, School of Population Health, Herston, Queensland, Australia
Queensland Children's Medical Research Institute, University of Queensland, Herston, Queensland, Australia

Theo Vos
University of Queensland, School of Population Health, Herston, Queensland, Australia
Institute for Health Metrics and Evaluation, University of Washington, Seattle, Washington, United States of America

Greg Freedman and Emily Carnahan
Institute for Health Metrics and Evaluation, University of Washington, Seattle, Washington, United States of America

Jane E. Pirkis
Melbourne School of Population and Global Health, University of Melbourne, Melbourne, Australia

Louisa Degenhardt
Melbourne School of Population and Global Health, University of Melbourne, Melbourne, Australia
National Drug and Alcohol Research Centre, University of New South Wales, Sydney, Australia

Andrew Page
School of Science and Health, University of Western Sydney, Campbelltown, New South Wales, Australia

Wilson Suraweera
Centre for Global Health Research, St Michael's Hospital, Toronto, Canada

Jayadeep Patra and Prabhat Jha
Centre for Global Health Research, St Michael's Hospital,Toronto, Canada
Dalla Lana School of Public Health, University of Toronto, Toronto, Canada

Jürgen Rehm
Dalla Lana School of Public Health, University of Toronto,Toronto, Canada
Centre for Addiction and Mental Health, Toronto, Canada

Henk Koning
Pediatric Pulmonology and Pediatric Allergology, Beatrix Children's Hospital, University of Groningen, University Medical Center Groningen (UMCG), Groningen, the Netherlands
Laboratory of Allergology and Pulmonary Diseases, Department of Pathology and Medical Biology, University of Groningen, University Medical Center Groningen (UMCG), Groningen, the Netherlands

Brigitte W. M. Willemse and Gerard H. Koppelman
Pediatric Pulmonology and Pediatric Allergology, Beatrix Children's Hospital, University of Groningen, University Medical Center Groningen (UMCG), Groningen, the Netherlands
GRIAC research institute, University of Groningen, University Medical Center Groningen (UMCG), Groningen, the Netherlands

Antoon J. M. van Oosterhout, Uilke Brouwer, Lisette E. den Boef, Renée Gras, Marco van der Toorn and Martijn C. Nawijn
Laboratory of Allergology and Pulmonary Diseases, Department of Pathology and Medical Biology, University of Groningen, University Medical Center Groningen (UMCG), Groningen, the Netherlands
GRIAC research institute, University of Groningen, University Medical Center Groningen (UMCG), Groningen, the Netherlands

Marjan Reinders-Luinge, Corry-Anke Brandsma and Machteld N. Hylkema
Department of Pathology and Medical Biology, University of Groningen, University Medical Center Groningen (UMCG), Groningen, the Netherlands
GRIAC research institute, University of Groningen, University Medical Center Groningen (UMCG), Groningen, the Netherlands

Ian Sayers
GRIAC research institute, University of Groningen, University Medical Center Groningen (UMCG), Groningen, the Netherlands

Jillian C. Nissen and Kyungmin Ji
Department of Pharmacological Sciences, School of Medicine, Stony Brook University, Stony Brook, New York, United States of America

Zhen Gao and Stella E. Tsirka
Department of Pharmacological Sciences, School of Medicine, Stony Brook University, Stony Brook, New York, United States of America
Program in Neuroscience, School of Medicine, Stony Brook University, Stony Brook, New York, United States of America

Abdul Rashid
Department of Public Health Medicine, Penang Medical College, Georgetown, Penang, Malaysia

Azizah Ab Manan, Noorlia Yahya and Lailanor Ibrahim
Penang State Health Department, Georgetown, Penang, Malaysia

Jiuqing Cheng and Claudia González-Vallejo
Department of Psychology, Ohio University, Athens, Ohio, United States of America

Michelle J. Hansen, Sheau Pyng J. Chan, Shenna Y. Langenbach, Lovisa F. Dousha, Jessica E. Jones, Selcuk Yatmaz, Huei Jiunn Seow, Ross Vlahos, Gary P. Anderson and Steven Bozinovski
Lung Health Research Centre, Department of Pharmacology and Therapeutics, the University of Melbourne, Victoria, Australia

Vinay Nangia
Suraj Eye Institute, Nagpur, Maharashtra, India
Department of Ophthalmology, Medical Faculty Mannheim of the Ruprecht-Karls-University Heidelberg, Mannheim, Germany

Jost B. Jonas and Songhomitra Panda-Jonas
Suraj Eye Institute, Nagpur, Maharashtra, India
Department of Ophthalmology, Medical Faculty Mannheim of the Ruprecht-Karls-University Heidelberg, Mannheim, Germany

Prakash Behere
Suraj Eye Institute, Nagpur, Maharashtra, India
Department of Psychiatry, Datta Meghe Institute of Medical Sciences, Wardha, Maharashtra, India

Marcella Rietschel and Torsten Paul
Department of Genetic Epidemiology in Psychiatry, Central Institute of Mental Health, Medical Faculty Mannheim of the Ruprecht-Karls-University Heidelberg, Mannheim, Germany

Tsunehito Higashi, Yosuke Mai, Takahiro Horinouchi, Koji Terada, Akimasa Hoshi, Prabha Nepal, Takuya Harada, Mika Horiguchi, Chizuru Hatate and Soichi Miwa
Department of Cellular Pharmacology, Graduate School of Medicine, Hokkaido University, Sapporo, Hokkaido, Japan

Yoichi Noya and Yuji Kuge
Central Institute of Isotope Science, Hokkaido University, Sapporo, Hokkaido, Japan

Tinglin Yan, Lu Li, Baiyu Sun, Fei Liu and Peng Yang
Department of Forensic Medicine, Xi'an Jiaotong University, School of Medicine, Xi'an, Shaanxi, PR China

Teng Chen, Tao Li and Xinshe Liu
Department of Forensic Medicine, Xi'an Jiaotong University, School of Medicine, Xi'an, Shaanxi, PR China
The Key Laboratory of Health Ministry for Forensic Science, Xi'an Jiaotong University, Shaanxi, PR China

Charmion I. Cruickshank-Quinn, Michael Armstrong and Nichole Reisdorph
Integrated Department of Immunology, National Jewish Health and University of Colorado School of Medicine, Denver, Colorado, United States of America

Spencer Mahaffey
Integrated Department of Immunology, National Jewish Health and University of Colorado School of Medicine, Denver, Colorado, United States of America
Department of Pharmacology, School of Medicine, University of Colorado Denver, Aurora, Colorado, United States of America

Richard Reisdorph
Integrated Department of Immunology, National Jewish Health and University of Colorado School of Medicine, Denver, Colorado, United States of America
Department of Pediatrics, National Jewish Health, Denver, Colorado, United States of America

Matthew J. Justice
Departments of Medicine and of Biochemistry and Molecular Biology, Indiana University, Indianapolis, Indiana, United States of America

Irina Petrache
Departments of Medicine and of Biochemistry and Molecular Biology, Indiana University, Indianapolis, Indiana, United States of America
Richard L. Roudebush VA Medical Center, Indianapolis, Indiana, United States of America

Grant Hughes
Department of Biostatistics and Informatics, University of Colorado Denver, Aurora, Colorado, United States of America

Russell P. Bowler
Department of Medicine, National Jewish Health, Denver, Colorado, United States of America

Abu S. Abdullah
Boston University School of Medicine, Boston Medical Center, Boston, Massachusetts, United States of America
School of Public Health, Guangxi Medical University, Nanning, China

Pete Driezen
Propel Centre for Population Health Impact, University of Waterloo, Waterloo, Ontario, Canada

Ummul H. Ruthbah
Department of Economics, University of Dhaka, Dhaka, Bangladesh

Nigar Nargis
Department of Economics, University of Dhaka, Dhaka, Bangladesh
World Health Organization, Geneva, Switzerland

Anne C. K. Quah
Department of Psychology, University of Waterloo, Waterloo, Ontario, Canada

Geoffrey T. Fong
Department of Psychology, University of Waterloo, Waterloo, Ontario, Canada
Ontario Institute for Cancer Research, Toronto, Ontario, Canada

Teresa R. Franklin, Reagan R. Wetherill, Kanchana Jagannathan, Barbara Johnson, Joel Mumma Nathan Hager and Anna Rose Childress
Perelman School of Medicine at the University of Pennsylvania, Department of Psychiatry, Philadelphia, Pennsylvania, United States of America

Hengyi Rao
Perelman School of Medicine at the University of Pennsylvania, Center for Functional Neuroimaging, Philadelphia, Pennsylvania, United States of America

Bo Huang, Wei-Xin Yuan and Guo-Dong Gao
Department of Neurosurgery, Tangdu Hospital of Fourth Military Medical University, Xi'an, Shaanxi, China

Li-Jun Heng and Peng Wang
Department of Neurosurgery, Tangdu Hospital of Fourth Military Medical University, Xi'an, Shaanxi, China
Department of Neurosurgery, Wuhan General Hospital of Guangzhou Military Command, Wuhan, Hubei, China

Lian-Ting Ma, Jian Song and Guo-Zheng Xu
Department of Neurosurgery, Wuhan General Hospital of Guangzhou Military Command, Wuhan, Hubei, China

Heng Guo
Department of Neurosurgery, PLA Chengdu General Hospital, Chengdu, Sichuan, China

Rebecca Sorber
School of Medicine, Indiana University, Indianapolis, Indiana, United States of America

Paula Braitstein
School of Medicine, Indiana University, Indianapolis, Indiana, United States of America
AMPATH Consortium, Eldoret, Kenya
Department of Medicine, School of Medicine, College of Health Sciences, Moi University, Eldoret, Kenya
Dalla Lana School of Public Health, University of Toronto, Toronto, Ontario, Canada
Regenstrief Institute, Inc., Indianapolis, Indiana, United States of America

Susanna Winston
Department of Pediatrics, Warren Alpert School of Medicine, Brown University, Providence, Rhode Island, United States of America
Rhode Island Hospital-Hasbro Youth's Hospital, Providence, Rhode Island, United States of America

Julius Koech
AMPATH Consortium, Eldoret, Kenya

Joseph Hogan
AMPATH Consortium, Eldoret, Kenya
Department of Biostatistics, Brown University, Providence, Rhode Island, United States of America

David Ayuku
Department of Behavioral Sciences, School of Medicine, College of Health Sciences, Moi University, Eldoret, Kenya

Liangyuan Hu
Department of Biostatistics, Brown University, Providence, Rhode Island, United States of America

Index

www.ingramcontent.com/pod-product-compliance
Lightning Source LLC
LaVergne TN
LVHW060538210926
848485LV00005B/1221